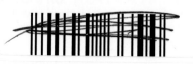

Epidemiologic Methods
for the Study of
Infectious Diseases

Epidemiologic Methods for the Study of Infectious Diseases

Edited by

James C. Thomas, M.P.H., Ph.D.
Department of Epidemiology
School of Public Health
University of North Carolina
Chapel Hill, North Carolina

David J. Weber, M.D., M.P.H., M.H.A.
Department of Medicine
School of Medicine
and
Department of Epidemiology
School of Public Health
University of North Carolina
Chapel Hill, North Carolina

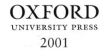

OXFORD
UNIVERSITY PRESS
2001

OXFORD

UNIVERSITY PRESS

Oxford   New York
Athens   Auckland   Bangkok   Bogotá   Buenos Aires   Calcutta
Cape Town   Chennai   Dar es Salaam   Delhi   Florence   Hong Kong   Istanbul
Karachi   Kuala Lumpur   Madrid   Melbourne   Mexico City   Mumbai
Nairobi   Paris   São Paulo   Shanghai   Singapore   Taipei   Tokyo   Toronto   Warsaw

and associated companies in
Berlin   Ibadan

Published by Oxford University Press, Inc.,
198 Madison Avenue, New York, New York, 10016
http://www.oup-usa.org

Library of Congress Cataloging-in-Publication Data
Epidemiologic methods for the study of infectious diseases /
edited by James C. Thomas, David J. Weber.
p. ; cm.   Includes bibliographical references and index.
ISBN 0-19-512112-0
1. Epidemiology—Research—Methodology.
I. Thomas, James C. (James Conley), 1954-II.
Weber, David J. (David Jay), 1951–
[DNLM: 1. Communicable Diseases—epidemiology.
2. Epidemiologic Methods.
WC   100 E635 2000]   RA652.4.E73 2001   614.4′07′2—dc21   00-056505

2 4 6 8 9 7 5 3 1

Printed in the United States of America
on acid-free paper

Preface

The period from 1977 to 1981 marked a turning point in the attitude of the public health community towards infectious diseases. The last case of smallpox was identified in 1977. A fatal infectious disease that had once been pandemic had been eradicated from the planet. There was widespread optimism that we could eliminate or control infectious diseases with the "magic bullets" of vaccines and antibiotics. Confident that infectious diseases were no longer a major threat, departments of epidemiology in schools of public health were turning their attention and reallocating their resources to chronic disease research.

The first reports of acquired immunodeficiency syndrome (AIDS) appeared in 1981. This new fatal infection quickly became pandemic. The complex nature of the organism soon dampened our collective optimism about our ability to control infectious diseases. Other newly identified infections, such as Ebola virus and Hanta virus, and reemergent infections, such as tuberculosis, reinforced the realization that infectious diseases were not so easily put into a bottle. Funding for research in infectious diseases began to increase, and faculty to study them and teach related research methods were again in demand.

Faculty in schools of public health found more applicants with an interest in infectious diseases applying to their departments. Enrollments began to grow in courses on the epidemiology of infectious diseases and additional courses were developed. Yet there was no textbook on methods for studying the epidemiology of infectious diseases. Methods developed for studying chronic diseases, such as case-control studies, and their application to cancer and cardiovascular disease were the mainstay of most curricula and textbooks. There was no infectious disease corollary, for example, to the volumes entitled *Statistical Methods in Cancer Research* (Breslow, 1980; Breslow, 1987). The available textbooks on infectious diseases addressed the life cycles of the pathogens and the distribution of infectious diseases (e.g., *Viral Infections of Humans* and *Bacterial Infections of Humans* [Evans and Kaslow, 1997; Evans, 1991]), or the quantitative methods of transmission simulation (e.g., *Infectious Diseases of Humans: Dynamics and Control* [Anderson and May, 1992]). None, however, was appropriate for teaching students in a masters program in epidemiology how to conduct epidemiologic research on infectious diseases. It is our aim that this book will help fill that gap.

The level of content in this book assumes a familiarity with basic epidemiologic concepts, such as study design types and sources of error. Thus, this is not an introductory text in epidemiology; it builds on the foundation of those texts.

The complexity of AIDS has brought new challenges to virtually every life science, and at least a few people within each of the sciences have gained an interest in infectious diseases epidemiology. Thus, the diversity of backgrounds has increased among those studying epidemiology. The first section of our book provides fundamental information to bring each epidemiology student up to a necessary starting point for studying infectious diseases. For those who are not well acquainted with the biological sciences, there are chapters on the biological concepts central to infectious diseases and the immune responses to infection. The application (and quantification) of biological concepts to disease transmission in populations is introduced in the chapter on population dynamics. This is followed by a chapter overviewing study design implications that are generic to infectious diseases. Causal concepts underlie every epidemiologic study. The chapter on causation provides a historical perspective on the evolution of ideas about the causes of infectious diseases and their epidemics.

The second section of the book covers sources of data and issues of measurement for epidemiologic studies of infectious diseases. The chapter on sources of data provides a description and an assessment of the strengths and weaknesses of various national data sets. The process of routinely collecting data to monitor trends is described in the chapter on disease surveillance. Our ability to identify the presence of, and to characterize microbes is one of the most rapidly evolving fields in epidemiology. The chapter on microbial molecular techniques provides an overview of the state of the science at the time of the printing of this book. The assessment of the reliability and validity of these and other measurement tools is discussed in the chapter on the evaluation of diagnostic criteria.

Infectious diseases can be grouped by type of organism (e.g., viruses, bacteria, parasites, etc.), symptoms (e.g., respiratory, dermatological, etc.), and mode of transmission. We have used this latter group of categories to highlight the variety of methodological concerns that pertain to different infectious organisms. The chapters in this section focus on research methods that are particular to respiratory, fecal-oral, vector-borne, and sexual transmission. Each of these chapters is designed to provide basic information for a researcher who is new to the study of a particular transmission type.

In contrast to the third section, which mainly addresses methods in observational research, the fourth section deals with studies that entail an intervention. The section begins with a description of the methods used in outbreak investigations. Intervention is implied in studies of outbreaks; they are conducted in order to identify and modify factors that have caused a cluster of infections. The chapters on clinical trials and community interventions describe the methods of evaluating interventions aimed at the level of individuals (especially as they relate to pharmaceuticals) and the level of communities. Particular attention is given to the evaluation of one type of intervention in the chapter on immunization.

In the fifth and final section, we include chapters on topics of special interest. Two of the chapters address research priorities that derive from demographic trends in the United States. With more people joining the work force, fewer young children are attended to at home during work hours. The first chapter in this section presents research methods for studies of infections in child-care settings. The American population is also getting older as "baby boomers" near retirement. The chapter on infections among the elderly describes the biological aspects of infections among the elderly and their methodological implications. Since the emergence of AIDS is behind much of the renaissance of infectious diseases epidemiology, there is much to be said about the study of this infection in addition to the material presented in the chapter on sexual transmission. The chapter on HIV and AIDS covers many of the issues. Finally, from a global perspective, infectious diseases are most common in developing countries. For people from developed countries who are interested in international research, the practical aspects of research in developing countries are described in the chapter on research collaborations in developing countries.

This book is only the beginning of all that can be said about epidemiologic research methods for infectious diseases. In many chapters, the reader is referred to other texts for more information on relevant topics. Our hope is that this book will complement other texts to better prepare a new generation of researchers.

J.C.T.
D.J.W.

Chapel Hill, N.C.

REFERENCES

Anderson RM, May RM. Infectious Diseases of Humans: Dynamics and Control. New York: Oxford University Press, 1992.

Breslow NE, Day NE. Statistical Methods in Cancer Research. Volume I—The Analysis of Case-Control Studies. Switzerland: International Agency for Research on Cancer, 1980.

Breslow NE, Day NE. Statistical Methods in Cancer Research. Volume II—The Analysis of Cohort Studies. London: International Agency for Research on Cancer, 1987.

Evans AS, Kaslow RA (eds.). Viral Infections of Humans: Epidemiology and Control, 4th Edition. New York: Plenum, 1997.

Evans AS, Brachman, PS (eds.). Bacterial Infections of Humans: Epidemiology and Control, 3rd Edition. New York: Plenum, 1998.

Acknowledgments

This book grew out of 15 years of teaching a course entitled "Introduction to Methods in Infectious Disease Epidemiology" in the Department of Epidemiology of the School of Public Health at the University of North Carolina. We thank the students who have taken that course over the years for encouraging us to develop a textbook and for giving us insights into the appropriate breadth and depth of material for such a book.

This book is the product of our second attempt to write it. We are grateful especially for those authors who agreed to write a chapter during the first attempt, who waited patiently through an interim period of reorganization and retooling on the part of the editors, and then persisted in their efforts to complete their chapter in the second and final attempt at the book.

A number of doctoral students in the UNC Department of Epidemiology reviewed and commented on chapter manuscripts, gathered information for some chapters, and constructed some of the figures and tables. They include Penny Howards, MSPH, Sonia Napravnik, MSPH, Christina Peterson, MSPH, Lynne Sampson, MSPH, and Olga Sarmiento, MD, MPH. We are indebted in particular to Dr. Sarmiento who carefully read and commented on nearly every chapter and its respective links to other chapters in the book. Any errors or oversights in the book do not reflect on her work or the work of the other students, however; all final edits were done at the hands of the editors.

For her unfailing cheerfulness, promptness, and conscientious work in formatting and attention to many other details, we thank Ms. Katherine Watson.

We thank our spouses for believing us when we said we would complete the book and for encouraging us when we feared we might not.

Contents

Contributors

O.G.W. BERLIN, PH.D.
Adjunct Associate Professor of Epidemiology
School of Public Health
University of California at Los Angeles
Los Angeles, California

MADHAV P. BHATTA, M.P.H
Doctoral Student
John J. Sparkman Center for International
    Public Health Education
University of Alabama
Birmingham, Alabama

KARIN E. BYERS, M.D., M.S.
Assistant Professor of Medicine
Allegheny General Hospital
Pittsburgh, Pennsylvania

GARY B. CALANDRA
Senior Director
Clinical Research
Merck Research Labs
Bluebell, Pennsylvania

ROBERT T. CHEN, M.D, M.A.
Chief Medical Officer
Vaccine Safety and Development Activity
Epidemiology and Surveillance Division
National Immunization Program
Centers for Disease Control and Prevention
Atlanta, Georgia

TERENCE L. CHORBA, M.D., M.P.H., M.P.A.
Director of Project RETRO-CI in Abidjan
International Activities Branch
Centers for Disease Control and Prevention
Division of HIV/AIDS Prevention-Surveillance
    and Epidemiology
Atlanta, Georgia

RALPH L. CORDELL, PH.D
Epidemiologist
Hospital Infections Program
Centers for Disease Control and Prevention
Atlanta, Georgia

D. PETER DROTMAN, M.D, M.P.H
Senior Medical Officer
National Center for Infectious Diseases
Centers for Disease Control and Prevention;
Department of Family & Preventive
    Medicine
Emory University School of Medicine;
Infectious Diseases Section, Department
    of Medicine
Veterans Affair Medical Center
Atlanta, Georgia

BARRY M. FARR, M.D., M.SC.
The William S. Jordan, Jr. Professor of Medicine
    & Epidemiology
University of Virginia Health Systems
Charlottesville, Virginia

ROBERT H. FLETCHER, M.D., M.P.H.
Professor of Ambulatory Care and Prevention,
*   and of Epidemiology*
Harvard School of Public Health
Boston, Massachusetts

JAMES D. FOLDS, PH.D.
Professor & Vice Chair
Department of Pathology and
*   Laboratory Medicine*
UNC Hospitals
University of North Carolina
Chapel Hill, North Carolina

RICHARD L. GUERRANT, M.D.
Professor of Medicine
Head, Division of Geographic Medicine
University of Virginia School of Medicine
Charlottesville, Virginia

HARRY A. GUESS, M.D., PH.D.
Vice President, Epidemiology
Merck Research Labs
Bluebell, Pennsylvania
Adjunct Professor of Epidemiology
*   & Biostatistics*
University of North Carolina
Chapel Hill, North Carolina

JACK M. GWALTNEY, JR., M.D.
Professor of Internal Medicine
Health Sciences Center
University of Virginia School of Medicine
Charlottesville, Virginia

M. ELIZABETH HALLORAN, M.D., M.P.H., SC.D.
Professor of Biostatistics
Rollins School of Public Health
Emory University
Atlanta, Georgia

SCOTT B. HALSTEAD, M.D.
Adjunct Professor of Preventive Medicine
*   & Biostatistics*
Uniformed Services
University of Health Sciences
Washington, D.C.

LAURA C. HANSON, M.D., M.P.H.
Associate Professor
Division of General Medicine
Program on Aging
University of North Carolina
Chapel Hill, North Carolina

J. OWEN HENDLEY, M.D.
Professor of Pediatrics
University of Virginia Health Systems
Charlottesville, Virginia

LOREEN A. HERWALDT, M.D.
Associate Professor
Department of Internal Medicine
University of Iowa College of Medicine
University of Iowa Hospitals and Clinics
Iowa City, Iowa

KIMBERLY L. KANE, PH.D.
Scientific and Technical Director
Department of Virology, Immunology
*   and Molecular Biology*
Northside Medical Center
Western Reserve Care Systems
Cleveland, Ohio

M. LOUISE LAWSON, PH.D.
Assistant Professor of Pediatrics
Center for Pediatric Research
Children's Hospital of The King's Daughters
Eastern Virginia Medical School
Norfolk, Virginia

DANA LOOMIS, PH.D.
Associate Professor of Epidemiology
School of Public Health
University of North Carolina
Chapel Hill, North Carolina

L. BERNARDO MENAJOVSKY, M.D., M.S.
Assistant Professor of Medicine
Associate Program Director
Internal Medicine Residency Program
Department of Medicine
Thomas Jefferson University
Philadelphia, Pennsylvania

AMY C. MORRISON, PH.D.
Post-Graduate Researcher
Department of Entomology
University of California at Davis
Davis, California

WALTER A. ORENSTEIN, M.D., M.P.H.
Director, National Immunization Program
Centers for Disease Control and Prevention
Atlanta, Georgia

AMY L. PEACE-BREWER, PH.D.
Assistant Director of Clinical Microbiology
*   & Immunology*
McLendon Clinical Laboratories
UNC Healthcare Systems
University of North Carolina
Chapel Hill, North Carolina

MICHAEL A. PFALLER, M.D.
Professor
Department of Pathology
University of Iowa College of Medicine
University of Iowa Hospitals and Clinics
Iowa City, Iowa

LARRY K. PICKERING, M.D., F.A.A.P.
Professor of Pediatrics
CHKD Chair in Pediatric Research
Director, Center for Pediatric Research
Eastern Virginia Medical School
Children's Hospital of The King's
  Daughters
Norfolk, Virginia

WILLIAM A. RUTALA, PH.D., M.P.H.
Professor
Division of Infectious Diseases
University of North Carolina (UNC)
  School of Medicine
Director
Hospital Epidemiology
Occupational Health & Safety
  Program
UNC Health Care System
Chapel Hill, North Carolina

FRANK J. SORVILLO, M.P.H., PH.D.
Associate Professor
Department of Epidemiology
School of Public Health
University of California at Los Angeles
Los Angeles, California

MARC A. STRASSBURG, PH.D.
Chief Epidemiologist
Public Health
Los Angeles County Department
  of Health Services
Los Angeles, California

SARA STRATTON, M.P.H.
Executive Director
Healthy Start Coalition of Hardee,
  Highlands, and Polk Counties, Inc.
Winter Haven, Florida

JAMES C. THOMAS, M.P.H., PH.D.
Associate Professor of Epidemiology
School of Public Health
University of North Carolina
Chapel Hill, North Carolina

STEN H. VERMUND, M.D., PH.D.
Professor of Epidemiology and International
  Health, Medicine, & Nutrition Sciences
Director, Division of Geographic Medicine
Director of the John J. Sparkman Center for
  International Public Health Education
University of Alabama
Birmingham, Alabama

MARIA J. WAWER, M.D.
Professor of Public Health
Center for Population and Family Health
Joseph L. Mailman School of Public Health
Columbia University
New York, New York

DAVID J. WEBER, M.D., M.H.A., M.P.H.
Professor of Epidemiology
School of Public Health
Professor of Medicine and Pediatrics
School of Medicine
University of North Carolina
Chapel Hill, North Carolina

STEFAN WEBER, M.D., M.S.
Associate Faculty Member
Institute of Medical Microbiology and Hygiene
Dresden Medical School
Dresden, Germany

RICHARD WENZEL, M.D., M.SC.
Professor and Chairman
Department of Internal Medicine
Medical College of Virginia
Virginia Commonwealth University
Richmond, Virginia

HOWARD WIENER, PH.D., M.P.H.
Post-Doctoral Trainee
University of Alabama
Birmingham, Alabama

STEVE WING, PH.D.
Associate Professor of Epidemiology
School of Public Health
University of North Carolina
Chapel Hill, North Carolina

Part I

FOUNDATIONS

1

Biological Basis of Infectious Disease Epidemiology

DAVID J. WEBER and WILLIAM A. RUTALA

When a physician is called to work in a place, his first problem is to study the hygienic potentialities which affect the state of health of the inhabitants. It is, in fact, these hygienic conditions which contribute towards the development and frequency of some diseases and the improbability and rarity of others, and which more or less modify the symptoms of every disease.
—Peter Ludwig Panum
Observations made during the epidemic of measles
on the Faroe Islands in the year 1846

An understanding of infectious disease epidemiology cannot be distilled to a discussion of an infectious agent inflicting disease on susceptible human hosts. Although understanding infectious pathogens is important, other factors involving the host and the environment contribute to the transmission of infectious agents, disease production, and the outcome of an infection. Infection represents a complex interplay between host factors, characteristics of the infectious agent, and environmental influences. This complex interaction has been modeled as a triangle (Jackson 1996) (Fig. 1–1), a wheel (Fig. 1–2, Jackson 1996), a tetrahedron (Fig. 1–3) (Rothenberg 1990), or a chain (Fig. 1–4) (Jackson 1996). Regardless of which model one uses to describe the interaction of humans with infectious agents and their environment, a person's state of health represents a dynamic equilibrium—a balance of forces.

This chapter reviews the important biologic factors relevant to the study of infectious disease epidemiology. Readers interested in a more detailed description of the following topics are referred to several excellent volumes on basic microbiology (Murray 1999), clinical infectious diseases (Reese 1996, Evans 1997, Evans 1998, Feigin 1998, Mandell 2000), and immunology (Paul 1999). *The Control of Communicable Diseases Manual*, published by the American Public Health Association, provides a brief description of the major infectious diseases with an emphasis on prevention and control measures (Chin 2000).

CHAIN OF INFECTION

In order for infection to occur, a chain of events must take place (Tables 1–1 and 1–2). First, there must be a susceptible host. Although people live in a sea of microorganisms, they generally stay healthy because of nonspecific (intrinsic) and specific host defenses (see Chapter 2). Second, an infectious agent capable of causing infection must be present. Third, the pathogenic microorganism must have a reservoir where it can propagate (i.e., live, reproduce, and die in the natural state). Potential reservoirs

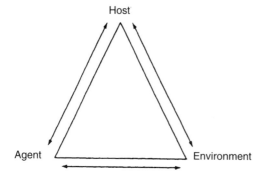

Figure 1–1. Triangle model of infectious diseases.
Source: Adapted from Jackson 1996.

include humans, animals, and the environment. Fourth, there must be portal of exit from the reservoir and portal of entry into a susceptible host. The portals of exit from a human or animal reservoir are the respiratory tract, the genitourinary tract, the gastrointestinal tract, skin and mucous membranes, transplacental (i.e., mother to fetus), and blood. Microbes gain entrance via these same portals, although blood-borne transmission requires percutaneous injury or mucous membrane contamination. As illustrated in Table 1–1, the route of agent shedding often predicts the portal of entry to the subsequent host. Some agents only cause disease when presented to the host by specific means. *Shigella dysentery*, which causes severe diarrhea, must be ingested; other agents such as *Staphylococcus aureus* can cause disease via multiple portals of entry, including respiratory tract (pneumonia), skin (furuncle), gastrointestinal tract (food poisoning), and blood (bacteremia). Fifth, an organism must be transmitted, directly or indirectly, from one place to another.

TRANSMISSION

Infections may result from either exogenous flora (i.e., microorganisms having an animal, human, or environmental reservoir) or endogenous flora. Endogenous flora may be either normal commensals of skin, respiratory tract, gastrointestinal tract, or genitourinary tract or present in relatively inactive forms within the body (i.e., latent infections). Endogenous microflora represent a frequent source of infection when the delicate balance between agent and host is disturbed (e.g., by chemotherapy for cancer). Relatively few pathogens are able to evade host defenses and cause latent infection. The most common of these are the herpes viruses (*Herpes simplex*, *Varicella zoster*, cytomegalovirus, Epstein-Barr virus), human immunodeficiency viruses (HIV-1 and HIV-2), *Mycobacterium tuberculosis*, and some fungi (*Cryptococcus neoformans*, *Histoplasma capsulatum*, *Blastomyces dermatitidis*).

Transmission generally refers to the mechanism by which exogenous pathogens reach

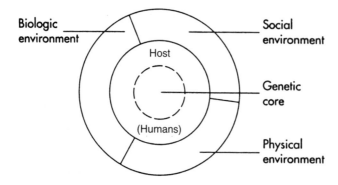

Figure 1–2. Wheel model of infectious diseases.
Source: Adapted from Jackson 1996.

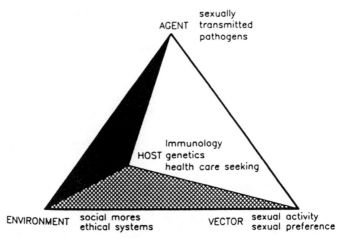

Figure 1–3. Tetrahedron model of infectious diseases. *Source*: Adapted from Rothenberg 1990.

and infect a susceptible host. Transmission may occur by one or more of four routes: contact, common vehicle, airborne, or vector-borne (Tables 1–1 and 1–3). In contact spread, the host has contact with the source that is either direct, indirect, or droplet. Direct contact includes such activities as touching, kissing, and sexual activity. Indirect contact requires an intermediate object, which is usually inanimate, in the transmission of the pathogen from the source to the patient. Droplet spread refers to transmission by respiratory droplets and requires relative proximity (<3 feet). Vertical transmission or transmission from an infected mother to fetus (i.e., in utero transmission) is considered either a category of contact transmission or a separate mode of transmission (see later). Common vehicles may include the following: ingested water or food, medical instruments, or infused products such as blood. Airborne transmission refers to passage of a pathogen through the air for long distances. Such pathogens may have a human

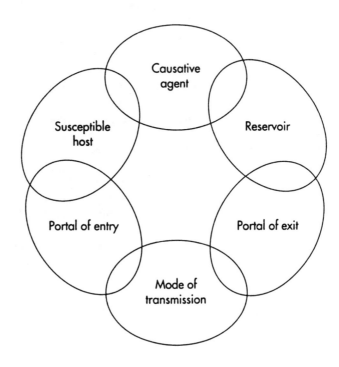

Figure 1–4. Chain model of infectious diseases. *Source*: Adapted from Jackson 1996.

Table 1–1 Key Terms in Understanding the Cycle of Infection

Infectious Agent	Viruses, Bacteria, Fungi, Protozoa, Helminths
Portals of exit	Skin/blood, respiratory secretions, urine, feces, semen/cervical secretions
Means of transmission	Contact (direct, indirect, droplet, vertical), common vehicle, airborne, vector-borne
Portals of entry	Skin, respiratory tract, gastrointestinal tract, genitourinary tract, in utero (transplacental)
Source	Human, animal, environment
Susceptible host	Specific (B- or T-cell mediated) immunity not present, immune compromised host, defects in specific and/or nonspecific host defense mechanisms

or environmental reservoir. Vector-borne spread refers to the transmission of an infectious agent by an arthropod. This transmission may simply be mechanical transfer of microorganisms on the external appendages of the vector. Alternatively, the vector may internalize the agent requiring subsequent regurgitation, defecation (e.g., riduviid bug, which is the vector for *Trypanosoma cruzi*, the causative agent of Chagas' disease), or penetration of the skin or mucosal surface (e.g., mosquito, which is the vector for *Plasmodium vivax*, a causative agent of malaria). Vector-borne infectious agents, in general, are highly adapted to their vector host. The infectious agent may be harbored by the vector without biologic interaction between the vector and the agent (e.g., yellow fever virus) or there may be biologic transmission in which the pathogen undergoes biologic changes within the vector (e.g., malaria).

Direct contact between humans may lead to transmission of an infectious agent via several mechanisms. Close contact may result in transmission of external parasites such as scabies or mites. Exchange of saliva via kissing may transmit such diseases as mononucleosis and oral Herpes simplex. Sexual activity is an efficient means for transmitting several diseases such as gonorrhea, syphilis, and chancroid. Vertical transmission (i.e., from an infected mother to her fetus or child) may occur via in utero transmission, at the time of birth via passage through a contaminated birth canal, or postnatally via breast milk. In utero transmission of infectious agents is fortunately uncommon. However, several infectious agents may be transmitted from an infected mother

to her fetus transplacentally. These include syphilis, toxoplasmosis, rubella, cytomegalovirus, and human immunodeficiency virus. Other agents may be transmitted to the fetus by its passage through a contaminated birth canal, including group B streptococcus, *Listeria*, *Neisseria gonorrhoeae*, *Chlamydia*, and various gram-negative bacilli. Finally, some infectious agents may be transmitted to neonates via breast milk (e.g., HIV).

While some infectious agents are transmitted by only a single route, others may be transmitted by multiple routes. In general, the most common diseases transmitted by sexual activity such as gonorrhea and syphilis have no other significant routes of transmission. Tularemia provides an example of a disease transmitted by multiple routes. The causative agent, *Francisella tularensis*, may be transmitted from its animal reservoirs to human by cutaneous contact with infected animal products (e.g., rabbit skins), ingestion of contaminated food or water, ocular contact with infected animal products, inhalation of dust from contaminated soil, bites from infected animals such as the cat or squirrel, and by biting arthopods such as the wood tick, dog tick, deerfly, or mosquito.

In describing the transmission of an infectious agent, vague terms such as person-to-person, household, horizontal, and intimate contact should be avoided, as they may include both physical contact such as handshaking and embracing as well as droplet spread and contact with recently contaminated surfaces.

For some infectious diseases, the route(s) of transmission remain largely unknown, such as *Helicobacter pylori*. Identification

Table 1–2 Importance of Understanding the Cycle of Infection for Control of Infectious Diseases

Pathogen	Disease	Portal of Exit	Transmission	Portal of Entry	Control
Influenza virus	Pneumonia	Respiratory secretions	Airborne	Respiratory tract (inhalation)	Vaccine, tissue to decrease airborne particles
Polio virus	Polio	Stool	Contact: Fecal-oral Common vehicle: Water	Gastrointestinal tract (ingestion)	Vaccine
Rabies virus	Rabies	NR	Contact: Animal bite	Skin (animal bite)	Immunize cats, dogs; immunize at risk humans; postexposure prophylaxis for humans after an animal bite or other exposure
Bordetella pertussis	Whooping cough	Respiratory secretions	Droplet	Respiratory tract (inhalation)	Vaccine; postexposure prophylaxis
Clostridium tetani	Neonatal tetanus	NR	Contact	Skin: umbilical cord (toxin)	Maternal immunization; sterile transection of umbilical cord
Neisseria gonorrhoeae	Gonorrhea	Genital secretions	Sexual	Genital tract	Screening of high-risk and symptomatic persons, followed by treatment
Mycobacterium tuberculosis	Tuberculosis	Respiratory secretions	Airborne	Respiratory tract (inhalation)	Contact tracing with treatment; screening with treatment of latent infection
Rickettsia rickettsii	Rocky Mountain spotted fever	Skin (via tick bite)	Tick-borne	Skin (via tick bite)	Prevention and early removal of ticks
Salmonella typhi	Enteric fever	Stool	Contact: Fecal-oral Common vehicle: Food	Gastrointestinal tract (ingestion)	Vaccine; separation of fecal waste from water supply; good hygiene
Treponema pallidum	Syphilis	Genital secretions	Sexual	Genital tract	Screening of high-risk and symptomatic persons, followed by treatment
Cryptosporidium sp.	Diarrhea	Stool	Contact: Fecal-oral Common vehicle: Water; food	Gastrointestinal tract (ingestion)	Separation of fecal waste from water supply; filter water supply; pasteurize juice
Plasmodium falciparum	Malaria	Skin (mosquito bite)	Vector (mosquito)	Skin (mosquito bite)	Mosquito spraying; reduce mosquito bites (netting, insect repellant); antimalarial prophylaxis

NR, not relevant for humans.

Table 1–3 Mechanisms of Disease Transmission, Examples

Airborne	Direct	Indirect	Droplet	Vertical	Vector-Borne	Common Vehicle
Influenza	HIV (sexual)	Papilloma virus (warts via contaminated surfaces)	Rhinovirus	HIV	Eastern equine encephalitis (mosquito)	Hepatitis A (food)
Measles	Rabies (via bite)	Hepatitis B (via needle sharing)	Pertussis	Rubella	Rocky Mountain spotted fever (tick)	Salmonellosis (food, water)
Tuberculosis	Gonorrhea (sexual)	*Clostridium difficile*	Meningococcal infection	Syphilis	Lyme disease (tick)	Cryptosporidiosis (food, water)
Cryptococcosis	Syphilis (sexual)			Toxoplasmosis	Malaria (mosquito)	

of the route of transmission from the source to the host may provide crucial information for designing control measures.

UNDERSTANDING A PATHOGEN'S LIFE CYCLE

Understanding the life cycle of pathogens is crucial to developing an appropriate study or intervention strategy. Prior to describing the various possible life cycles several key terms must be defined. The *reservoir* is the niche which the pathogen normally inhabits (i.e., where it lives, reproduces). Reservoirs of human infection may be humans, animals, insects, or the environment. The *source* is the means by which the pathogen is directly transmitted to humans. Sources may be animate or inanimate and may include other humans, animals, insects, food or water, medications, or medical devices. The reservoir and the source may be identical (e.g., as with most sexually transmitted agents) or different. For example, the reservoir of *Salmonella typhi* is always humans, but sources of infection are usually contaminated food or water. The reservoir of *Salmonella enteritidis* is animals, but like *S. typhi* they usually pass to humans via contaminated food or water. However, *S. enteritidis* may be trans-

mitted by direct contact with infected animals such as turtles. Within the life cycle of a pathogen, humans may serve as an essential link (e.g., most sexually transmitted agents, *Mycobacterium tuberculosis*, or *Plasmodium vivax* [malaria]) or may represent a dead end host, in which case human infection is accidental (e.g., rabies, Eastern equine encephalitis, tetanus).

Interrupting the life cycle of a pathogen is often an effective means to control the disease (Table 1–4). In general, one may interrupt the life cycle at multiple points. How best to intervene depends on many factors including the effectiveness of the planned intervention strategies, immediate benefits to infected humans, cost, rapidity with which the intervention will reduce infection and/or disease incidence, and environmental concerns. One can use schistosomiasis as an example of the importance of understanding the life cycle for guiding intervention strategies. The life cycle of *Schistosoma* spp. is complex. Humans pass eggs via the stool or urine. These eggs hatch into miracidia when exposed to fresh water and seek out a snail intermediate host. Following a developmental stage in the snail, cercaria are released into the water where they seek out a human host and initiate infection by penetrating

Table 1–4 Possible Life Cycles of Pathogens

Life Cycle	Examples
Human → Human	*Treponema pallidum* (syphilis), *Neisseria gonorrhoeae* (gonorrhea), *Mycobacterium tuberculosis* (tuberculosis)
Human → Environment → Human	*Ascaris lumbricoides* (roundworm), (whipworm)
Human → Arthropod → Human	*Plasmodium vivax* {intermediate host, mosquitoes} (malaria), Dengue virus (breakbone fever)
Human → Animal → Human	*Schistosoma* spp. {intermediate host, snails} (schistosomiasis)
Human → Animal → Animal → Human	*Paragonimus westermani* {intermediate hosts, snails and then crabs or crayfish}
Environment ↳Human (accidental)	*Sporothrix schenckii* (sporotrichosis, rose pruner's disease), *Coccidioides immitis* (coccidioidomycosis, valley fever)
Animal → Animal ↳Human (accidental)	Rabies virus (rabies), *Pasteurella multocida* (pasteurellosis)
Animal → Environment → Animal ↳Human (accidental)	*Cryptosporidium* sp., *Toxoplasma gondii* (toxoplasmosis)
Animal → Arthropod → Animal ↳Human (accidental)	*Rickettsia rickettsii* {intermediate host, ticks} (Rocky Mountain spotted fever), Eastern equine encephalitis {intermediate hosts, mosquitoes} (arboviral encephalitis)

the skin. The life cycle of this pathogen can be interrupted by treating infected humans thereby eliminating the pathogen, by providing safe sewage disposal thereby preventing the eggs from hatching and/or the miracidia from reaching their snail host, by eliminating the host snails (e.g., via the use of molluscacides, introduction of predators, elimination of snail habitat), or by providing safe water for drinking and bathing thereby preventing the cercaria from finding a human host and initiating infection.

Several epidemiologic tools may be useful in guiding the decision on where to intervene to interrupt the life cycle of a pathogen including modeling disease transmission, decision analysis, and cost-effectiveness analysis. In general, interventions that do not rely on volitional changes in human behavior (e.g., mosquito control) are likely to be more successful than interventions requiring behavior modification (e.g., condom use for sexually transmitted disease prevention).

THE KEY TRIANGLE

As stated earlier, infection results from a complex interaction of the host, the agent, and the environment. Infectious disease epidemiologists must understand these factors and assess their individual importance in the transmission of specific infectious diseases (Table 1–5).

THE HOST

Humans are simultaneously dependent on and threatened by the microorganisms that surround them. Host factors often dictate which individuals exposed to an infectious agent will become infected, develop disease, resolve the infection, or die as a result of infection.

Characterization of Host Defenses

Host resistance may be divided into specific and nonspecific immunity. Specific immune mechanisms include humoral (antibodies) and cell-mediated immunity (see Chapter 2). Nonspecific host defense mechanisms include the skin and mucous membranes, which provide

barrier protection; the mucous membranes, which secrete destructive enzymes such as lysozyme, immunoglobulins, and other compounds with antimicrobial properties; the complement system, a protein cascade, which leads to initiation of the inflammatory response, clearance of immune complexes, opsonization of microorganisms, and killing of certain gram-negative bacilli; leukocytes, which are granulocytic white blood cells capable of phagocytosis and killing of microorganisms; cytokines (e.g., interleukins 1 and 2, tumor necrosis factor, interferons), which are able to induce fever, T- and B-cell proliferation, immunoglobulin synthesis, and to interfere with viral synthesis.

Defects of host defenses are a major predisposing factor for infection. Specific defects are often associated with specific infectious agents (Table 1–6). Host defense abnormalities may be congenital (e.g., sickle cell anemia), acquired (e.g., Hodgkin's disease, malnutrition), or due to an infectious agent (e.g., human immunodeficiency virus). Iatrogenic breaches of morphologic integrity, such as the placement of an intravenous catheter for medications, are a major cause of hospital-acquired infections.

Immunosuppression due to medication is increasingly common owing to the increase of solid organ transplantation (e.g., heart, lung, kidney) that requires the administration of immunosuppressive medications to prevent rejection of the "foreign" organ, and more aggressive chemotherapy for malignant tumors. The risk of infection developing in an immunocompromised patient is a result of an interaction between two major factors: the patient's exposure to pathogens and the patient's net state of immunosuppression. Factors influencing the exposure to pathogens include other persons (especially important are children), pets, occupational exposures, travel exposure, and habits (e.g., swimming, hiking, fishing, hunting, camping). Factors influencing the net state of immunosuppression include the underlying disease; the effects of therapy; the presence or absence of granulocytopenia (i.e., <1000 granulocytic white blood cells); presence or absence of injury to the primary host defense

Table 1-5 Understanding the Key Triangle: Host, Pathogen, and Environment

Host Factors			Pathogen Factor	Environmental Factors	
Intrinsic Factors	Behavior Factors/Extrinsic Factors			Physical Environment	Social Environment
Age	Habits (smoking, alcohol consumption, drug use)		Pathogenicity	Urban vs. rural	Sexual network
Gender	Diet		Infectivity	Tropical vs. temperate	Crowding
Race	Sexual activities		Infective dose	Climate	Medical availability
Genetic makeup	Occupation		Immunogenicity	Remoteness	Education
Physiology	Recreational activities		Evasiveness	Vector presence	Public health resources
Immune responsiveness	Animal exposure		Environmental stability		
	Chemotherapy				
	Immunosuppressive medications				
	Immunizations				

Table 1-6 Impact of Specific Host Defense Abnormalities

Host Defense	Defect	Pathogens with Increased Incidence	Disease(s)
Skin	Disruption (e.g., wound)	*Streptococcus pyogenes*	Cellulitis
Skin	Disruption (e.g., wound)	*Staphylococcus aureus*	Cellulitis, furuncle, abscess
Skin	Disruption (e.g., wound)	*Clostridium tetani*	Tetanus
Gastric acid	Achlorhydria	*Salmonella* sp.	Enteric fever
Genital mucosa	Disruption (e.g., from sexually transmitted disease)	HIV	AIDS
Neutrophils	Neutropenia	*Staphylococcus aureus*	Sepsis
		Gram-negative bacilli	Sepsis
Complement	Deficient levels (late components)	*Neisseria* sp. infections	Sepsis
Spleen	Splenectomy	*Streptococcus pneumoniae*	Sepsis
Immunoglobulin (IgG)	Deficient levels	*Streptococcus pneumoniae*	Sepsis
Cell-mediated immunity	Underlying disease (HIV), immunosuppressive medications	*Mycobacterium tuberculosis*	Tuberculosis
Cell-mediated immunity	Underlying disease (HIV), immunosuppressive medications	*Pneumocystis carinii*	Pneumonia
Cell-mediated immunity	Underlying disease (HIV), immunosuppressive medications	*Listeria monocytogenes*	Listeriosis

barrier to infection, the intact mucocutaneous surfaces; metabolic factors such as state of nutrition; and the immunomodulating effects of certain microbial invaders, particularly viruses (Kontoyiannis 1995). The latter includes cytomegalovirus, Epstein-Barr virus, hepatitis viruses, HIV, *Capnocytophaga*, *Plasmodium* spp., and *Histoplasma capsulatum*. The chronic administration of immunosuppressive medications not only increases the incidence and severity of acute infection, but also results in chronic, progressive disease of a form essentially unknown in normal hosts even though the invading microorganisms are common in all populations.

Age

Age is an important predictor of disease incidence for two major reasons: First, exposure is often highly related to age. Figure 1-5 displays the age distribution by gender of the human immunodeficiecy virus (HIV) infection. As with other sexually transmitted diseases, the age-specific incidence peaks between 20 and 40 years of age. A small peak is apparent in childhood corresponding to vertically (mother-to-child) transmitted cases. Although this disease is more prevalent in males in some countries due to the initial association with unsafe sexual practices by gay men, the incidence in male and female children who acquire infection from their infected mothers is equal. Second, immunity to disease is highly correlated with age (see Chapter 2). In general, both extremes of age have a higher incidence of infectious diseases. Young children are partially protected against acquiring many infectious agents by maternally derived antibody transferred via the placenta. However, this immunity wanes over 6 to 15 months. The relationship between young age and in-

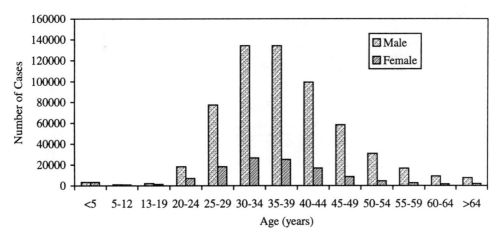

Figure 1–5. HIV infection cases by sex and age at diagnosis. *Source*: Adapted from CDC 1999.

fection is clearly illustrated by the classic childhood exanthems; measles, rubella, and varicella (chickenpox). These viral infections occur predominantly in young children who lack immunity and are exposed to infected peers. Older individuals are more likely immune and less likely to become exposed. Older individuals have a higher frequency of infectious diseases due to comorbid states (e.g., diabetes), waning immunity, longer exposure time for latent infections (e.g., tuberculosis), and altered immune state. Tuberculosis is an example of a disease dramatically more frequent among older persons (Fig. 1–6). In describing the relationship between age and disease incidence it is important that age-specific incidence rates be calculated.

The relationship between age and infection is not always simple. For example, age enters into both the incidence of bacterial meningitis and the relative contribution of different organisms at different ages (Schuchat 1997, Wenger 1990). Young children have both a higher incidence of bacterial meningitis and a different set of pathogens. Neonatal meningitis is most commonly due to group B streptococcus, *E. coli*, and *Listeria*. Meningitis among older children and adults is most commonly due to *Streptococcus pneumoniae* and *Neisseria meningitidis*.

This evolution of relative risk represents poorly understood interactions between immunity, exposure, and associated medical conditions.

Age also affects the outcome of infection, as exemplified by the common childhood viral illnesses of the past. Measles, varicella (Wharton 1996), mumps, and hepatitis A are more likely to cause significant morbidity with increased age of acquisition. The age-specific incidence of Rocky Mountain spotted fever and case-fatality rate illustrate the important point that age-specific incidence and age-specific mortality may not be colinear (Bernard 1982). The highest incidence of Rocky Mountain spotted fever is among older children and younger adults but the highest mortality is among older adults. Again, in general, individuals at the extremes of life tend to have a higher case fatality rate (i.e., proportion of persons dying as a function of all persons infected).

The use of vaccines and other interventions may significantly alter the age-specific incidence of disease. The introduction of pertussis vaccine has resulted in less disease in younger individuals but a relatively increased frequency of disease in young adults. Immunization may substitute a generally benign childhood illness for disease with sig-

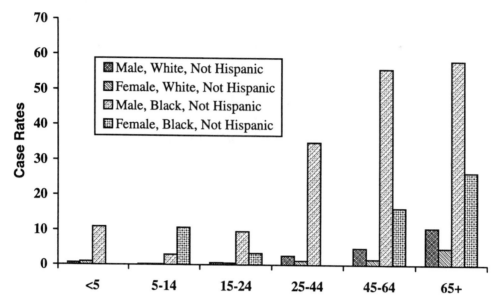

Figure 1–6. Tuberculosis case rates per 100,000 population by race/ethnicity, sex, and age: United States, 1997.
Source: Adapted from Centers for Disease Control and Prevention. Reported Tuberculosis in the United States 1997.

nificant sequelae among a susceptible older population with waning vaccine associated immunity. This issue needs to be considered as newer vaccines such as varicella and hepatitis A are introduced.

Although age is commonly considered a risk factor for infectious disease acquisition and/or morbidity, age may merely serve as a marker for the presence of physiologic factors causally related to disease acquisition. For example, Saviteer and colleagues (1988) showed that the incidence of hospital acquired pneumonia increased with age. However, careful investigations of some infectious diseases has revealed that age per se was not associated with an increased incidence of infection but rather older individuals were more likely to have risk factors associated with disease acquisition. For example, Hanson and colleagues (1992) demonstrated that when all the important risk factors for nosocomial pneumonia were assessed, age was not an independent risk factor; rather the higher incidence in the elderly was due to a greater frequency of risk factors (e.g., smoking, chronic lung disease, decreased mental status). Increasingly, we are coming to realize that physiologic age, not chronologic age, is the important predictor of infection risk.

Gender
Almost all infectious diseases occur more frequently among individuals of one sex versus the other. Sex-specific differences in disease frequency may represent differences in exposure, anatomy and physiology, or as yet unknown factors. Diseases related to out-of-doors exposures such as the tick-transmitted diseases Rocky Mountain spotted fever and tularemia are more common in males than females. While anatomy obviously dictates the risk of pelvic inflammatory disease and epididymitis caused by *Neisseria gonorrhoeae*, disseminated gonorrhea is more common in women, perhaps because of prolonged asymptomatic infection or because local defenses in the female genital tract are not as effective in containing infection to local tissues.

Acquisition of schistosomiasis, a parasitic infection harbored by snails, is related to exposure to contaminated water. Cultural dicta may govern exposure, since such tasks as gathering water for cooking and drinking, laundering of clothing, harvesting rice, and fishing may be gender-specific.

In some cases the reason for sex differences is unclear. Thus the incidence of tuberculous diseases is similar in men and women up to age 24, but thereafter men are increasingly likely to develop tuberculosis mainly as a result of reactivation (Fig. 1–6). Whether this represents a cohort effect with differential exposure in the distant past or a more significant waning of immune surveillance (i.e., ability of host defenses to contain viable tubercule bacilli within local granuloma) among men is unclear. Patterns of tuberculosis in populations also demonstrate that various host factors can act independently as risk factors. Independent risk factors for tuberculosis include older age, male sex, and nonwhite race (Fig. 1–6).

Ethnicity

Although the incidence of many infectious diseases is greater among certain races or ethnic groups, these differences are often explained by differences in socioeconomic status that dictate differences in exposure, immunity, and access to medical care, including vaccines. Selective pressures brought on by centuries of exposure may explain the relative resistance of Caucasians to tuberculosis and Africans to malaria. Certain genetic traits that may enhance or retard the acquisition of infectious agents may be more prevalent in certain ethnic groups (see below). Different immune response gene haplotypes may be present in different ethnic groups and affect the susceptibility to infectious agents.

Genetics

The relationship between heredity and infectious disease susceptibility and pathophysiology is also complex. Genetic traits may result in reduced or enhanced suscepti-

bility to infection or disease if infected. Terminal complement deficiencies (C5, C6, C7, or C8), for instance, may predispose to recurrent infection with *Neisseria gonorrhoeae* and *N. meningitidis* (Lokki 1995). Individuals who lack both Duffy blood group antigens (a and b) are resistant to *Plasmodium vivax* malaria, since these antigens are required for attachment of the agent (Hadley 1997). Other genetically acquired disorders may present with seemingly unrelated manifestations yet have an altered risk of developing disease. Individuals with sickle cell trait (heterozygotes) have less severe infections with *Plasmodium falciparum* (Gendrel 1991) malaria, but persons with sickle cell disease (homozygotes) are at higher risk of serious infections due to *Streptococcus pneumoniae* and *Haemophilus influenzae* (Onwubalili 1983). Growing evidence suggests an association between certain histocompatibility antigen classes and increased risk for tuberculosis, paralytic poliomyelitis, leprosy, and chronic hepatitis B antigenemia. The gene, HLA B27, has been strongly linked to reactive arthropathy following certain gastrointestinal infections (Gonzalez 1999).

Physiology

Besides age, gender, and ethnicity, the dynamic equilibrium represented by health status may be tipped by both subtle and not so subtle influences. Diabetics are at increased risk for respiratory, urinary tract, and skin infections (Joshi 1999). They have a higher frequency of infections with group B streptococcus, *Salmonella enteritidis* (gastroenteritis), *Mycobacterium tuberculosis* (pneumonia), *Candida* sp. (infections of the vagina and mouth), *Pseudomonas aeruginosa* (aggressive infections of the outer ear canal with invasion of adjacent bone), and Mucor (invasive fungal infection of the paranasal sinuses) when ketoacidosis is present. Subtle body temperature differences may ordain the site of agent replication and disease manifestations. Heat sensitivity limits leprosy caused by *Mycobacterium leprae* to the skin and nasal mucosal membrane. Indeed, inducement of fever by infecting the host with malaria has been used with variable success in the therapy of tertiary syphilis and Lyme disease.

Diet and Nutrition

Specific dietary habits may influence the host's risk of infection. *Diphyllobothrium latum* or fish tapeworm, for instance, occurs only in individuals who ingest raw or undercooked fish (Ruttenber 1984). Other infections are endemic but may be more common in persons eating certain foods. For example, ingestion of raw shellfish is associated with several infections including hepatitis A and viral gastroenteritis (Wanke 1987); *Mycobacterium bovis* infection is associated with ingestion of unpasteurized cow's milk in lesser developed countries (Cosivi 1998); and brucellosis is associated with ingestion of unpasteurized cheese made from goat's milk (Young 1983).

Good nutritional status is critical to the maintenance of good health. Malnutrition contributes significantly to infectious disease–related morbidity in developing countries. Only recently has malnourishment been recognized as a contributing cause of postoperative sepsis and death. Vitamin A deficiency may impair maturation of T lymphocytes, diminish secretory immune responses to polysaccharide antigens, diminish complement activity, and impair the antimicrobial action of phagocytic cells leading to increased morbidity due to measles (Semba 1994). Zinc deficiency has been linked to an increased risk of diarrhea, pneumonia, and malaria (Black 1998).

Intercurrent or Preexisting Infections

Certain infections occur more frequently or even exclusively in hosts who are recovering from or currently infected with another infectious agent. Viral infections of the upper respiratory tract may damage the mucous membranes with destruction of the cilia-bearing epithelial cells resulting in an increased risk of pneumonia caused by two common respiratory pathogens, *Streptococcus pneumoniae* or *Staphylococcus aureus*.

Schistosoma haematobium, a fluke that causes urinary bladder wall abnormalities, predisposes the host to other urinary tract infections including those with *Salmonella*, an unusual urinary tract pathogen (Lambertucci 1998). Hepatitis delta agent replication is dependent on a simultaneous infection with hepatitis B virus that provides the delta agent with its surface antigen coat (Taylor 1999). Without concomitant hepatitis B replication, the delta agent cannot replicate or cause disease.

Human Behavior

The host's actions are not always in his or her best interest. Neonatal tetanus may result from cord contamination of the umbilical stump due to use of nonsterile instruments to cut the cord (Gurkan 1999) or placing materials such as "ghee" (clarified butter) on an umbilical wound (Bennett 1999). Customs including circumcision, scarification, ear piercing, and tattooing may lead to tetanus unless appropriate sterile techniques are used (Sow 1993). Smoking induces airway inflammation and significantly predisposes to both upper and lower respiratory tract disease. Smoking is one of the major risk factors for chronic bronchitis (Niroumand 1998), and environmental smoke (passive smoking) is an important risk factor for upper respiratory tract infections in children (Gryczynska 1999, Hajnal 1999). A wide spectrum of viral (e.g., HIV, hepatitis B, C, D), bacterial (e.g., endocarditis due to *Staphylococcus aureus* or cellulitis due to group A streptococci), and fungal (e.g., endocarditis due to *Candida* sp.) infections complicate injecting drug use (Contoreggi 1998). Even mundane activities such as maintaining proper hygiene, careful trimming of toe nails, and appropriate care of contact lenses are important in reducing the host's risk of infection.

Human activities are the only significant risk factors for sexually transmitted diseases. Factors associated with an increased risk of sexually transmitted diseases (including HIV infection) include such activities as multiple partners, failure to use condoms, exchange of sex for money, and receptive anal intercourse. Behavioral interventions are therefore crucial to the control of these infections.

AGENT

Classification

Infectious agents range from self-replicating proteinaceous materials (prions), to sub-viral particles (the viroid/virusoid-like delta hepatitis agent), viruses, bacteria (including *Chlamydia, Rickettsia,* and *Mycoplasma*), fungi (yeast and molds), protozoans, helminths (flukes, worms), and ectoparasites (lice, fleas, mites, bedbugs, and ticks). Detailed classification is based on morphology, growth requirements, antigenic character, and, increasingly, nucleic acid organization and sequence. When new syndromes or new agents are recognized, hypothesis generation is based on the characteristics of well-recognized disease processes or agents. Important clues regarding route of transmission, pathophysiology, treatment, laboratory diagnosis (antigenicity, immune response, culture techniques, nucleic acid sequence), potential role of vectors and/or reservoirs, and control measures may be surmised. For example, initial investigation and public health recommendations for the illness in the Southwest United States caused by a Hantaan virus-like agent were based on knowledge about other similar viral infections.

Intrinsic characteristics of the agent

Each infectious agent has intrinsic characteristics that may dictate host range, mode of transmission, and ability to produce disease that are independent of any host interaction. Such basic considerations include size, requirements for replication (intracellular versus extracellular, nutrients), as well as temperature, humidity, and pH tolerance. Susceptibility to temperature, detergents, and desiccants varies widely and obviously influences potential modes of transmission. While *N. gonorrhoeae* and HIV do not survive for prolonged periods outside the host, the spores of *Bacillus anthracis*, the agent

causing anthrax, can survive in soil for years and *Clostridium botulinum* spores can endure boiling for hours.

Agents produce substances that either help avert host defenses mechanisms or directly cause disease manifestations. Toxins are responsible for the symptoms experienced with diphtheria, tetanus, scarlet fever, and some types of food poisoning including *Clostridia botulinum, Clostridia perfringes,* and *Staphylococcus aureus*. Diphtheria toxin production requires the agent to possess a lysogenic phage that encodes the toxin. Vaccines directed at toxin-produced diseases generally comprise inactivated toxin stimulating a protective immune response. Serious host injury may result from the circulating toxins produced by *Staphylococcus aureus* (Staphylococcal toxic shock syndrome) or group A *Streptococcus pyogenes* (streptococcal toxic shock syndrome) that function as super-antigens (Stevens 1996, Manders 1998), and the effects of local toxins on the colonic mucosa produced by *Clostridium difficile* (necrotizing enterocolitis) (Taege 1999).

Other agents synthesize and secrete one or more substances that aid in the survival of the agent or combine to produce pathologic changes. Enzymes may be produced that destroy red and white blood cells (hemolysins and leukocidins, respectively), disrupt connective tissue (hyaluronidase, collagenase), cleave nucleic acids (nuclease), avert killing of the agent by leukocytes (catalase), or stimulate either clot formation or lysis (coagulase and streptokinase, respectively). Nonenzymatic products such as siderophores, which scavenge for iron, allow the agent to compete in the host environment.

Other structural components of the agent also contribute to pathogenicity. Motility, for instance, may be an important factor in infection and disease production. The presence of a polysaccharide capsule may help the agent avoid phagocytosis. Fingerlike projections on bacterial surfaces called fimbriae may enhance the adherence of the bacteria to host membranes (e.g., *E. coli* strains causing urinary tract infections). Endotoxins refer to the integral lipopolysaccharide component of certain bacterial cell walls that can trigger a complex series of cascades including complement activation, alteration in vascular tone and permeability, as well as coagulation and fibrinolysis producing fever, inflammation, and sometimes shock.

Susceptibility to available antibiotics may be genetically determined. Unfortunately, selection pressures, mutations, genetic recombination, and plasmid exchange between bacteria have lead to resistance to antibiotics. Antibiotic resistance may result from production of enzymes that degrade the antibiotics, altered cell surface permeability, enhanced efflux pumps, or alteration in the antibiotic target sites, which reduces or prevents binding (Hawkey 1998, Gold 1996). The growing tide of antibiotic resistance among the most common community- and hospital-acquired microorganisms is alarming and carries potentially grave public health consequences (Hawkey 1998, Gerberding 1999, Virk 2000).

Thus mere identification of an agent by genus and species may inadequately define the pathogen without additional description of serotype, genotype, phenotype, phage type, toxin production, or antibiotic resistance pattern. *Staphylococcus aureus* may produce an array of distinct clinical presentations, from local skin infections to food poisoning, endocarditis, toxic shock syndrome, depending on the location of infection and production of specific virulence factors.

Extrinsic characteristics of the agent
The host agent relationship may be *symbiotic*, *commensal*, or *parasitic* depending on the agent, the host, the environment, and the circumstances. *Escherichia coli*, for instance, may be commensal in the vaginal tract, may establish a symbiotic relationship in the gastrointestinal tract synthesizing vitamin K, but may be parasitic in the urinary and respiratory tracts.

Certain characteristics of the agent are best described in relationship to a specific host. The identical strain of *Streptococcus pneumoniae*, for instance, may pose vastly different consequences in mice and humans,

for instance. Host specificity refers to limited host range of some agents. *Salmonella typhi* has a predilection for humans, while *S. dublin* infects predominantly cattle. *Clostridia botulinum* types A, B, E, and F may cause human disease, whereas types C and D infect other animals. Smallpox, hepatitis B, polio, and measles are examples of diseases whose causative agents exclusively infect humans.

Several terms define the interaction between agent and host. *Infection and infectivity* refers to the ability of the agent to invade and multiply in a host. The *infective dose* refers to the theoretical number of organisms required to establish an infection in a group of hosts of the same species. Even such a seemingly simplistic concept is complicated by the multitude of host and agent factors discussed previously as well as mode of transmission. The infective dose of *Staphylococcus aureus*, for example, is dependent on the virulence factors produced. Even a virulent organism presents variable risks when presented to intact skin, a clean wound, a clean wound with a foreign body (suture), a necrotic wound, the respiratory tract, or the bloodstream. In the laboratory, infective dose is described by the minimum number of agents required to cause infection in 50% of hosts (ID_{50}). Stomach acidity adversely affects the survival of some bacteria (*Salmonella*) more than others (*Shigella*). Thus neutralization of gastric acid by disease, medication, or diet may affect on the host's susceptibility to *Salmonella* more than *Shigella*. From a practical standpoint, a gauge of infectivity is estimated by the *secondary attack rate*—the proportion of exposed susceptible hosts who develop disease. Infectivity represents a continuous spectrum from measles and chickenpox, which are highly infectious, to rubella and the common cold, which are of intermediate infectivity, and tuberculosis, leprosy, and Creutzfeldt-Jakob disease, which are of low infectivity.

Clinical presentation may (tuberculosis, syphilis, Herpes simplex) or may not (hepatitis A, *Salmonella*, polio) influence infectivity. The number, size, and degree of inflammation and healing of syphilis and *H. simplex* genital ulcers presumably influence the level of infectivity. Severity of illness, however, does not alter the risk of transmission of such infectious agents as hepatitis C or polio.

Colonization is the persistence, often with multiplication, of an agent on a mucosal surface without an apparent host reaction. *Contamination*, on the other hand, generally refers to the presence of an agent on the surface of the body or an inanimate object (i.e., fomite) such as an eating utensil, toy, or handkerchief that may serve as a source of infection. While the distinction between infection and colonization or contamination is important, it is not always simple. Intubated patients on a respirator often develop colonization of their upper respiratory tract with gram-negative organisms that are also the most common cause of lower respiratory tract disease. Identification of these organisms in respiratory secretions is not synonymous with infection and disease.

Pathogenicity represents the proportion of infections that result in clinically apparent infection or *disease*. Again, host factors, infecting dose, route of transmission contribute to this continuous spectrum. Highly pathogenic agents include rabies, measles, chickenpox, and the common cold while polio and tuberculosis are of low pathogenicity.

Virulence can be conceptualized as the proportion of clinically apparent cases resulting in significant clinical manifestations. Measurement might include days absent from work/school, specific sequelae, or mortality referred to as *case fatality rate*. When death is used as the measurement of virulence, the difference between pathogenicity and virulence becomes apparent. Rabies is both highly pathogenic and virulent; the common cold is highly pathogenic but rarely virulent, and poliovirus might be classified as moderately virulent despite having a low pathogenicity.

The pathogenesis or mechanism by which an agent causes disease is often multifactorial but may include: (1) direct tissue invasion, (2) induction of an inflammatory response, (3) direct cellular destruction, (4) toxin production, (5) immune perturbation, hypersensitivity, or allergic reaction (post Strepococcal glomerulonephritis, dengue hemorrhagic fever), (6) immune suppression, and (7) obstruction or mass effect.

The characteristics of the agent, the host, and the environment interact in a complex manner to determine the natural history of an infectious disease. This interaction determines the latent period, incubation time, and period of infectivity.

ENVIRONMENTAL FACTORS

The "environment" encompasses all areas in which the host and agent interact. This milieu has been categorized into three areas: physical, describing the geography and the climate; biologic, made up of plants, animals, and other life forms; and socioeconomic, which describes the interactions of host species. Such classification oversimplifies the identification and the characterization of the complex interplay of environmental factors.

As discussed previously, the environment modifies or dictates host, agent, reservoir and vector ranges, and behaviors. In this current age of jet travel, bodies of water, mountain ranges, and deserts no longer represent barriers to the dissemination of plants, animals, microbes, or disease. Influenza has caused pandemics spreading around the globe during a single season. Plants and animals may be transported either inadvertently (rodents, insects) or purposefully (kudzu, tropical fish) from indigenous areas to locations without natural predators, disease, or competition for food, allowing for unrestricted spread. Humans may also change their environment through travel or directly such as deforestation, building water reservoirs, or introducing new fauna or flora to their surroundings. Many of the recently recognized human pathogens have been associated with changes to our environment.

Temperature (average and range), humidity, precipitation, as well as altitude and latitude, which affect solar radiation and ultraviolet exposure, directly and indirectly affect the risk of infection. Agents, reservoirs, and vectors generally tolerate a limited range of conditions. Hookworm ova deposited in the soil require both warmth and humid conditions for maturation and hatching. The temperature tolerance of malarial parasites and their mosquito vectors may not be identical with the parasites requiring relatively warmer temperatures for maturation. Thus some areas may be infested with the mosquito yet not be plagued by malaria. Global warming poses the theoretical spread of both the vector and the parasite to higher latitudes and altitudes.

The incidence of respiratory infections tends to be higher during the colder months in temperate areas and during the rainy season in the tropics. Even within the colder months, the relative incidence of many viral pathogens fluctuates. Rhinoviruses tend to cause outbreaks in the early fall and spring, while coronaviruses and influenza are more prominent in the winter. Increased crowding indoors during colder months presumably contributes to this seasonality, but changes in relative humidity may also be important. Viruses surrounded by a lipid bilayer (envelope) survive better under lower relative humidity conditions found in the coldest months.

Climate and geography and human manipulation also dictate the distribution of plant and animal life, which in turn, influences recreation, agriculture, occupational pursuits, diet, behavior, and economy. Plague, caused by the bacterium *Yersinia pestis*, has caused multiple pandemics devastating the human population and altering the course of history. Crowding and poor sanitation provided a suitable environment when in 1346 the black death rode into Europe from Central Asia in the guise of *Y. pestis*–infected rodents and their fleas transported by the returning Mongols. A more recent example is the emergence of Lyme disease caused by a spirochetal organism, *Borrelia burgdorferi*. Reclamation of farmland in the northeast United States for forest and housing communities has led to a juxtaposition of humans and deer, mice, and ticks, creating ideal conditions for disease transmission.

Socioeconomic factors are strongly linked with the risk of infectious agents transmitted by fecal-oral, respiratory, vertical, and sexual routes, but dissecting the etiology of this association are problematic. Housing, sanitation, population density, diet, level of education, occupation, availability of health services, and cultural attributes are just a few of the variables that contribute to these "socioeconomic" differences.

GEOGRAPHIC DISTRIBUTION OF DISEASE

The host, agent, vector, reservoir, and route of transmission all affect the geographic distribution of an infectious disease. Host behaviors (e.g., communal bathing), rituals (e.g., scarification), occupation (e.g., hunting, fishing), water supply, diet (e.g., raw fish), as well as pet and domestic animal exposure influence the geographic distribution of disease. Even population density and size influence disease persistence. A small, closed population of individuals previously infected by measles, which induces lifelong immunity, will not support further infection.

Geologic differences can also be attributed to temperature, humidity, and rainfall, as discussed earlier. The distribution of West African and East African trypanosomiasis is related to the breeding habits of the tsetse fly vectors. Most dramatically, the distribution of bartonellosis is limited by the range of the vector sandflies confined to the river valleys of the Andes Mountains at altitudes between 2000 and 8000 feet.

THE NATURAL HISTORY OF INFECTIOUS DISEASES

A variety of host responses may occur when a susceptible host is exposed to an infectious agent (Friis 1999) (Fig. 1–7). These are often depicted as an iceberg, with the largest number of responses occurring subclinically. Host responses are very variable, ranging from exposure without multiplication of the pathogen (e.g., response in a person who has received live polio vaccine to a challenge with wild polio) to colonization without infection

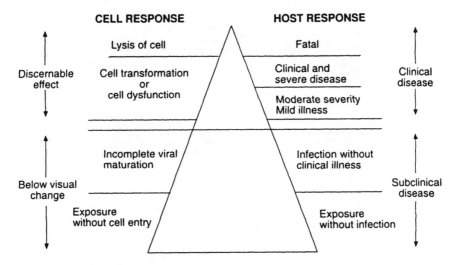

Figure 1–7. Iceberg concept of infection.
Source: Adapted from Friis and Sellers 1999.

(i.e., replication of the pathogen without invasion or host response) to illness (ranging from mild to severe). The severity of disease varies tremendously among infectious disease pathogens, being very low for some agents such as rhinoviruses (i.e., common cold) and very high for others such as smallpox (Fig. 1–8).

Clinical Infection

The factors that affect whether a person exposed to a pathogen will develop clinical illness include nonspecific and specific (i.e., antibody and cell-mediated) immunity, route of exposure, inoculum (i.e., dose of pathogen), and pathogenicity of the microbe. Once the microbe successfully invades the host, a period of replication occurs before clinical symptoms develop. The latent period is defined as the time from infection until the infectious period starts (Fig. 1–9).

The period of time from exposure to a source of infection to the first signs of symptoms of clinical illness is called the incubation

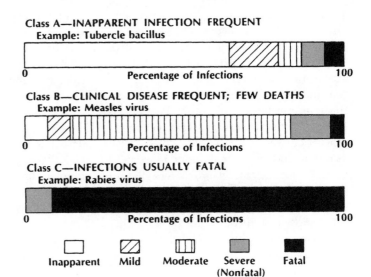

Figure 1–8. Distribution of clinical severity for different infectious diseases. *Source*: Adapted from Mausner and Kramer 1985.

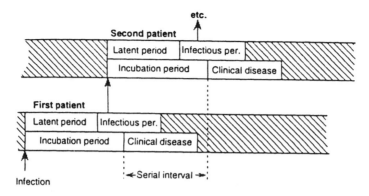

Figure 1–9. The relationship of some important time periods.
Source: Adapted from Giesecke 1994.

period. The factors influencing the incubation period include the specific pathogen, inoculum dose, portal of entry, mechanism of tissue injury, and immune response. The incubation period may be calculated if the source of exposure is known (e.g., contaminated food source) or if multiple generations of infection occur via person-to-person transmission (Fig. 1–9). The incubation period is useful in infectious disease epidemiology because it helps define the agent causing an outbreak, aids in differentiating common-source from person-to-person transmission, impacts on the window of time during which postexposure prophylaxis (if available) may be effective, determines the time during which an exposed person is at risk for developing infection, and assists in determining the time during which the person is infectious.

The incubation period must be differentiated from the communicable period (i.e., the time during which the infected person may transmit infection) (Table 1–7). Persons infected with many viral agents become infectious prior to development of symptoms such as rash including such childhood illnesses as varicella, measles, and parvovirus B-19 (fifth disease). The communicable period may last only a few days or may persist for years (e.g., tuberculosis) or through the person's lifetime (e.g., human immunodeficiency virus, cytomegalovirus). It is important to note that not all infectious diseases are communicable (i.e., can be transmitted via person-to-person spread). This includes vector-borne diseases (e.g., malaria, Rocky Mountain spotted fever, Lyme disease) and some diseases acquired from the environment (e.g., tetanus, cryptococcal infection).

The infectiousness of an infected person refers to how likely that person is to transmit infection and is best measured by the secondary attack rate. Diseases such as measles and varicella have secondary attack rates above 80% among susceptible exposed persons. A disease such as leprosy is only rarely ($\ll 1\%$) communicable. The virulence of the pathogen refers to how likely the agent is to cause severe disease. Examples of diseases with low virulence include rhinoviruses (i.e., common cold) and parvoviruses (i.e., warts). Examples of diseases with mortality greater than 50% include smallpox, Ebola virus infection, and rabies. Infectiousness and virulence are not linked and infectious agents may be of low infectivity and low virulence (e.g., parvovirus), low infectivity and high virulence (e.g., leprosy), high infectivity and low virulence (e.g., rhinoviruses), and high infectivity and high virulence (e.g., smallpox).

PREVENTING INFECTIOUS DISEASES

The ultimate goal of studying infectious diseases is to implement interventions that prevent infection or ameliorate infection. In

Table 1–7 Incubation Periods and Period of Communicability for Selected Infectious Diseases

Disease	Average Incubation Period (range)	Period of Communicability
Diphtheria	2–5 d (occasionally longer)	Variable, <2 weeks to >4 weeks
Hepatitis A	28–30 d (15–50 d)	Latter half of incubation period till a few days after onset of jaundice
Hepatitis B	60–90 d (45–180 d)	Weeks prior to symptoms till clearance of HbsAg (days to lifelong)
Influenza	1–3 d	3–5 days from clinical onset in adults
Lyme disease	7–10 d (3–32 d)	No person-to-person transmission
Measles	~10 d (7–18 d)	1 day prior to prodromal period to 4 days after rash
Pertussis	7–20 d	Onset of cough till ~3 weeks
Rocky Mountain spotted fever	7–10 d (3–14 d)	No person-to-person transmission
Rubella	14–17 d (14–21 d)	1 week prior to rash till 4 days after onset of rash
Syphilis	~3 weeks (10 d–3 months)	During time when skin lesions of primary and secondary syphilis present
Typhoid fever	8–14 d (3 d–1 month)	As long as viable bacteria in excreta (usually from first week through convalescence, 2%–5% become chronic carriers)
Varicella	14–16 d (8–21 d)	1–2 days before rash till all lesions dried and crusted

Source: Adapted from Chin J., 2000.

this regard, it is important to remember that although many infections are successfully treated with antimicrobials, prevention is superior to therapy. Mausner and Kramer (1985) define several levels of prevention (Fig. 1–10). Primary prevention (appropriate in the stage of susceptibility) is prevention of disease by altering susceptibility or reducing exposure for susceptible individuals. Secondary prevention (applied in early disease, i.e., preclinical and clinical stages) is the early detection and treatment of disease. Tertiary prevention (appropriate in the stage of advanced disease or disability) is the alleviation of disability resulting from disease and attempts to restore effective functioning.

Primary Prevention

Prevention of the occurrence of disease consists of measures that fall into two major categories: general health promotion and specific protective measures (Mausner and Kramer 1985). General health promotion includes provision of conditions at home, work, and school that favor healthy living (e.g., good nutrition, adequate clothing, shelter, rest, and recreation). It also includes health education such as safe sex, preventive medicine, and personal hygiene. Specific health measures include immunizations, environmental sanitation (e.g., purification of water supplies), and protection against accidents and occupational hazards.

Immunizations are the best example of a successful primary intervention technique. Immunizations have been listed as the greatest public health achievement of the twentieth century (CDC 1999b). Vaccines currently recommended for universal use in the United States include mumps, measles, rubella, varicella, polio, *Haemophilus influenzae* type b, hepatitis B, diphtheria, pertussis, tetanus, and conjugate pneumococcal vaccine (CDC 2000). The universal use of vaccines in the United States has resulted in a dramatic decrease in vaccine preventable diseases (CDC 1999c) (Table 1–8). Smallpox has been eradicated from the world. Polio is likely to be eradicated in the next decade.

Prophylactic therapy of persons exposed

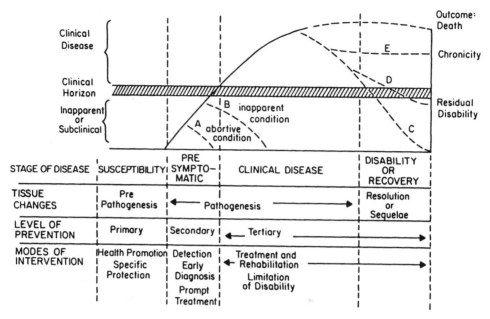

Figure 1–10. Schematic representation of the natural history of infection. *Source*: Adapted from Mausner and Kramer 1985.

to infections who are in the incubating stage of illness has been highly successful in reducing the risks of disease transmission. Examples of infections for which postexposure prophylaxis is available and has been highly successful include hepatitis A, rabies, invasive meningococcal infection, and pertussis.

Secondary Prevention

Secondary prevention refers to the early detection and prompt treatment of disease. Infectious diseases represent the best example of the successful therapy of disease preventing morbidity and mortality. In addition to benefiting the sick infected person, treatment with antibiotics reduces the risk of contacts. For example, detection of chronic infections such as syphilis and tuberculosis and appropriate therapy may dramatically decrease the overall incidence of these diseases.

Tertiary Prevention

Tertiary prevention consists of limitation of disability and rehabilitation where disease has already occurred and left residual damage. For example, the use of artificial respirators saved many persons with paralytic polio in the era before polio vaccine. Rehabilitative services have improved the lives of persons with congenital infections such as rubella and syphilis.

SUMMARY

The examples provided are not intended to suggest that host, agent, and environmental factors contribute only to the epidemiology of unusual agents, transmitted by curious vectors in some isolated environmental niche. For example, the epidemiology of urinary tract infections, a common infection in adult women, exemplifies the complex interplay between host, agent, and environment.

The environment (community-acquired versus nosocomial or hospital-acquired) is a critical determinant in the incidence and relative contribution of various urinary pathogens. While *E. coli* and *Staphylococcus saprophyticus* are the predominant pathogens in an outpatient population, *Klebsiella, Enterobacter, Enterococcus,* and *Pseudomonas* are

Table 1–8 Impact of Vaccines Recommended Before 1990 for Universal Use in Children—United States

Disease	Baseline 20th Century Annual Morbidity	1998 Morbidity	% Decrease
Smallpox	48,164	0	100
Diphtheria	175,885	1	100
Pertussis	147,271	7405	95.0
Tetanus	1314	41	96.9
Poliomyelitis (paralytic)	16,316	0	100
Measles	503,282	100	100
Mumps	152,209	666	99.6
Rubella	47,745	364	99.2
Rubella (congenital)	823	7	99.1
Haemophilus influenzae type b	20,000	1194	94.0

Source: Adapted from the Centers for Disease Control and Prevention, 1999c.

more often isolated from hospitalized patients. Cross-infection, especially between patients with indwelling Foley catheters on broad spectrum antibiotics, contributes to this phenomenon.

Many host related factors affect the risk of urinary tract infections. The incidence of infection is greater in women than in men, who are more often affected as children and in old age. Women who inherit the P blood group have a receptor allowing for the adherence of certain fimbriated *E. coli*. Physiologic considerations include pregnancy, diabetes mellitus, and menopause, which increase the risk of infection. Compromised immune status and possibly altered inflammatory responses contribute to risk. For example, damage to the bladder epithelium by schistosomiasis may predispose to infection as may conditions that impair urinary flow such as catheters, prostatic enlargement, stones, and strictures from previous gonococcal infections. Sexual activity and instrumentation (i.e., use of indwelling catheters) of the urinary tract increase the risk of infection.

The most common urinary pathogens have virulence factors that contribute to their pathogenicity. Specific fimbriae, adhesions, motility, and urease production are factors that may confer virulence. Alteration in the normal flora may predispose to

yeast infection, and broad spectrum antibiotic exposure may lead to infection with an antibiotic resistant organism.

In conclusion, the goal of public health is to alter the natural history of disease in order to prevent or ameliorate the disease. Infectious disease epidemiologists use an understanding of the biology of infectious diseases and the principles of epidemiology to design and conduct studies that ultimately will aid in the control of infections.

REFERENCES

Bennett J, Ma C, Traverso H, et al. Neonatal tetanus associated with topical umbilical ghee: covert role of cow dung. International Journal of Epidemiology. 28(6):1172–1175, 1999.

Bernard KW, Helmick CG, Kaplan JE, et al. Surveillance of Rocky Mountain spotted fever in the United States, 1978–1980. Journal of Infectious Diseases 146(2):297–299, 1982.

Black RE. Therapeutic and preventive effects of zinc on serious childhood infectious diseases in developing countries. American Journal of Clinical Nutrition, 68(2 Suppl):476S–479S, 1998.

Centers for Disease Control and Prevention. *HIV/AIDS Surveillance Report.* 11 (1): 1-42, 1999a.

Centers for Disease Control and Prevention. Ten Great Public Health Achievements-United States, 1900–1999 *MMWR.* 48 (12): 242–243, 1999b.

Centers for Disease Control and Prevention. Impact of Vaccines Universally Recommended for Children-United States, 1990–1998 *MMWR.* 48 (12): 243–248, 1999c.

Centers for Disease Control and Prevention. Reported Tuberculosis in the United States, 1998.

Centers for Disease Control and Prevention. Reported Tuberculosis in the United States, 1998. August 1999d.

Centers for Disease Control and Prevention. Update: Raccoon Rabies Epizootic—United States and Canada, 1999.

Chin J. Control of Communicable Diseases Manual. 17th ed. American Public Health Association, 2000.

Contoreggi C, Rexroad VE, and Lange WR. Current management of infectious complications in the injecting drug user. J. Subst. Abuse Treat. 15 (2): 95–106, 1998.

Cosivi O, Grange JM, Daborn CJ, et al. Zoonotic tuberculosis due to *Mycobacterium bovis* in developing countries. Emerg. Infect. Dis. 4 (1): 59–70, 1998.

Evans AS, and Brachman PS, eds. Bacterial Infections of Humans. Epidemiology and Control. 3rd ed. New York and London: Plenum Medical Book Company, 1998.

Evans AS, and Kaslow RA, eds. Viral Infections of Humans. Epidemiology and Control. 4th ed. New York and London: Plenum Medical Book Company, 1997.

Feigin RD, and Cherry JD. Textbook of Pediatric Infectious Diseases. 4th ed. 1 vol. Philadelphia: W. B. Saunders Company, 1998.

Friis RH, Sellers TA. Epidemiology for Public Health Practice, 2nd ed. Rockville, Maryland: Aspen Publishers, 1999.

Gendrel D, Kombila M, Nardou M, et al. Protection against *Plasmodium falciparum* infection in children with hemoglobin S. Pediatr. Infect. Dis. J. 10 (8): 620–621, 1991.

Gerberding JL, McGowan JE, and Tenover FC. Emerging nosocomial infections and anitmicrobial resistance. Curr. Clin. Top. Infect. Dis. 19: 83–98, 1999.

Giesecke, J. Modern Infectious Disease Epidemiology. London: Edward Arnold, 1994.

Gold HS, and Moellering RC. Drug therapy: antimicrobial-drug resistance. N. Engl. J. Med. 335 (19): 1445–1453, 1996.

Gonzalez S, Martinez-Borra J, and Lopez-Larrea C. Immunogenetics, HLA-B27 and spondyloarthropathies. Curr. Opin. Rheumatol. 11 (4): 257–264, 1999.

Gryczynska D, Kobos J, and Zakrzewska A. Relationship between passive smoking, recurrent respiratory tract infections and otitis media in children. Int. J. Pediatr. Otorhinolaryngol. 49 Suppl 1: S275–278, 1999.

Gurkan F, Bosnak M, Dikici B, et al. Neonatal tetanus: a continuing challenge in the southeast of Turkey: risk factors, clinical features and prognostic factors. Eur. J. Epidemiol. 15 (2): 171–174, 1999.

Hadley TJ, and Peiper SC. From malaria to chemokine receptor: the emerging physiologic role of the Duffy blood group antigen. J. Am. Soc. Hematol. 89 (9): 3077–3091, 1997.

Hajnal BL, Braun-Fahrlander C, Grize L, et al. Effect of environmental tobacco smoke exposure on respiratory symptoms in children. SCARPOL Team. Swiss Study on Childhood Allergy and Respiratory Symptoms with Respect to Air Pollution, Climate and Pollen. Schweiz. Med. Wochenschr. 129 (19): 723–730, 1999.

Hanson LC, Weber DJ, and Rutala WA. Risk factors for nosocomial pneumonia in the elderly. Am. J. Med. 92 (2): 161–166, 1992.

Hawkey PM. The origins and molecular basis of antibiotic resistance. Br. Med. J. 317 (7159): 657–660, 1998.

Jackson, M. General Principles of Epidemiology. In: Bowlus B, ed. Infection Control and Applied Epidemiology. St. Louis: Mosby-Year Book, 1996.

Joshi, N, Caputo GM, Weitekamp MR, and Karchmer AW. Primary care: infections in patients with diabetes mellitus. N. Engl. J. Med. 341 (25): 1906–1912, 1999.

Kontoyiannis DP, Rubin RH. Infection in the organ transplant recipient. Infectious Disease Clinics of North America 1995; 9(4): 811–822.

Lambertucci JR, Raves AA, Serufo JC, et al. Schistosomiasis and associated infections. Memorias do Instituto Oswaldo Cruz 1998; 93 Suppl 1:135–139.

Lokki ML, and Colten HR. Genetic deficiencies of complement. Ann. Med. 27 (4): 451–459, 1995.

Mandell G, Bennett J, and Dolin R, eds. Principles and Practice of Infectious Diseases. 5th ed. Vol. 2. Philadelphia: Churchill Livingstone, 2000.

Manders SM. Toxin-mediated streptococcal and staphylococcal disease. J. Am. Acad. Dermatol. 39 (3): 383–398, 1998.

Mausner J, Kramer S. Epidemiology—An Introductory Text, 2nd ed. Philadelphia: W.B. Saunders Co., 1985.

Murray P, Baron EJ, Pfaller MA, Tenover F, and Yolken R, eds. Manual of Clinical Microbiology. 7th ed. Washington: American Society for Microbiology, 1999.

Niroumand M, and Grossman RF. Airway infection. Infect. Dis. Clin. North Am. 12 (3): 671–688, 1998.

Onwubalili JK. Sickle cell disease and infection. J. Infec. 7 (1): 2–20, 1983.

Paul WE. Fundamental Immunology. 4th ed. Philadelphia: Lippincott Raven, 1999.

Reese R, and Betts R, eds. A Practical Approach to Infectious Diseases. 4th ed. Little, Brown and Company, 1996.

Rothenberg R. Analytic approaches to the epidemiology of sexually transmitted diseases. Sexually Transmitted Diseases. 2nd ed. McGraw-Hill, Inc., 1990.

Ruttenber AJ, Weniger BG, Sorvillo F, Murray RA, and Ford SL. Diphyllobothriasis associated with salmon consumption in Pacific Coast states. Am. J. Trop. Med. Hyg. 33 (3): 455–459, 1984.

Saviteer SM, Samsa GP, and Rutala WA. Nosocomial infections in the elderly. Increased risk per hospital day. Am. J. Med. 84 (4): 661–666, 1988.

Schuchat A, Robinson K, Wenger J, et al. Bacterial meningitis in the United States in 1995. N. Engl. J. Med. 337 (14): 970–976, 1997.

Semba RD. Vitamin A, immunity, and infection. Clin. Infect. Dis. 19 (3): 489–499, 1994.

Sow PS, Diop BM, Barry HL, Badiane S, and Coll/Seck AM. Tetanus and traditional practices in Dakar (report of 141 cases). Dakar Med. 38 (1): 55–59, 1993.

Stevens DL. The toxic shock syndromes. Infect. Dis. Clin. North Am. 10 (4): 727–746, 1996.

Taege AJ, and Adal KA. *Clostridium difficile* diarrhea and colitis: a clinical overview. Cleve. Clin. J. Med. 66 (8): 503–507, 1999.

Taylor JM. Hepatitis delta virus. Intervirology. 42 (2-3): 173–178, 1999.

Virk A, and Steckelberg JM. Clinical aspects of antimicrobial resistance. Mayo Clin. Proc. 75 (2): 200–214, 2000.

Wanke CA, and Guerrant RL. Viral hepatitis and gastroenteritis transmitted by shellfish and water. Infect. Dis. Clin. North Am. 1 (3): 649–664, 1987.

Wenger JD, Hightower AW, Facklam RR, Gaventa S, and Broome CV. Bacterial meningitis in the United States, 1986: report of a multistate surveillance study. The Bacterial Meningitis Study Group. J. Infec. Dis. 162 (6): 1316–1323, 1990.

Wharton M. The epidemiology of varicella-zoster virus infections. Infect. Dis. Clin. North Am. 10 (3): 571–578, 1996.

Young EJ. Human brucellosis. Rev. Infect. Dis. 5 (5): 821–842, 1983.

2

Immune Response and Methods for Detection of Infectious Diseases

AMY L. PEACE-BREWER, KIMBERLY L. KANE,
and JAMES D. FOLDS

An individual's ability to survive in a world of pathogens depends on an intact immune system. The immune system is a network of cells and proteins that are capable of identifying, as well as removing, a foreign invader. As the system is challenged by various pathogens, such as microorganisms, viruses etc., different sections of the immune system are activated to facilitate the removal of the pathogen. Each section of the immune system is adept at eliminating or clearing different types of organisms. Therefore understanding how the various sections of the immune system respond to different organisms can be useful for identifying stages of infection.

This chapter is divided into three major sections: an overview of the branches of the immune system; examples of different immune responses; and laboratory testing methodologies illustrating how one can distinguish between infection and exposure to a particular pathogen. The primary goal of the chapter is to illustrate the complexity and interdependence of the immune response to a pathogen and to address the need for careful consideration of immunologic assays that may be appropriate for determining the disease status of patients. In this brief chapter, we cannot provide an indepth description of the immune response to infections. We have cited within the text several good references for more complete information. Several of the cited texts include illustrations that further clarify the many complex mechanisms and interactions.

OVERVIEW OF THE IMMUNE SYSTEM

Innate Immunity

Innate immunity is the part of the immune system present at birth. It is simple but effective. The innate immune response is nonspecific and does not possess a memory or the ability to improve or alter itself. As a result, each exposure to an antigen results in the same response. Innate immunity includes physical barriers to infection, like the skin and its secretions, mucous membranes, and intestinal flora. There are also innate defenses provided by phagocytic cells such as polymorphonuclear cells and macrophages. The mission of these cells is to engulf and break down foreign substances. The result of this is the secretion of proteins such as cytokines and enzymes, which play an important role in protecting the host. Cytokines, like the interferons, which are secreted by phagocytic cells and chemotactic factors, like complement components, activate lymphocytes and other mononuclear cells to mount a vigorous attack against the pathogen. As a result of these coordinating defense mechanisms an individual's innate immunity is sufficient to prevent the majority of potential infections (Paul 1999).

Acquired Immunity

Acquired immunity is the part of the immune system that develops over the lifetime of an individual and represents the second line of defense. It has the ability to remember as well as the capacity to alter its response to a pathogen. As a result the host can respond more rapidly and more vigorously to a pathogen that has been encountered previously.

Acquired immunity is effective against most pathogens, including bacterial, viral, parasitic, and fungal sources. There are two major types of acquired immune responses: cellular and humoral. The cellular response is carried out by primarily T lymphocytes (or T cells) derived from the thymus. The humoral response is mediated primarily by bone marrow–derived B lymphocytes (or B cells) and the proteins they secrete called antibodies (or immunoglobulins). Other cells such as natural killer cells, and macrophages also play a role in the defense against invading pathogens. Table 2–1 describes briefly the cells that play a role in the immune response and some of their characteristics (Paul 1999; Stites 1997).

Cellular immunity

Cellular immunity is the part of the acquired response primarily mediated by T lymphocytes with the assistance of antigen presenting cells (APCs). APCs include tissue macrophages, polymorphonuclear cells (PMNs),

monocytes, and B cells. APCs are cells whose main function is to display or present portions of a pathogen (peptides) on their surface. This display of peptides alerts circulating T cells to the presence of a pathogen. This is possible with the assistance of the self major histocompatibility complex (MHC) or human leukocyte antigens (HLA). There are two types of MHC molecules: class I and class II. In general, class I molecules are responsible for the presentation of peptides originating from pathogens residing inside a cell (Paul 1999). These pathogens are typically viruses, like influenza A, or intracellular bacteria such as *Mycobacterium tuberculosis* or *Listeria monocytogenes* (Stites 1997). In contrast, peptides presented by MHC class II molecules generally originate from pathogens that were outside of the cell such as *Staphylococcus aureus* and *Escherichia coli*. These peptides are a result of the phagocytosis of bacteria or of other pathogens, which are then degraded into peptides in the phagolysosome. Formation of a peptide/MHC complex takes place inside the cell. It is formed by the binding of a peptide within the groove that is created when the MHC protein folds. This "filled" MHC molecule moves to the cell surface where it displays the pathogen-derived peptide to a T cell. Once the T cell interacts with the APC presenting the pathogen peptide, the T cell is activated and a series of events takes place that leads to the elimination of the pathogen (Paul 1999).

A T cell is able to recognize the peptide/ MHC complex using a T cell–specific surface protein known as the T cell receptor (TCR). The TCR is actually a complex of proteins. Two of the protein chains interact directly with the peptide/MHC complex while the other proteins are involved in the delivery information, resulting from the interaction, to the nucleus of the T cell. In addition to the interaction between the TCR and the peptide/MHC complex there are other proteins, known as accessory molecules, on each of the cells whose interaction results in the generation of additional signals that instruct the T cell further.

There are two types of peptides presented

Table 2-1   Selected Characteristics of the Cells of the Immune System

Cell Type	Function	Lineage Associated Immunophenotypic Markers	Cytokines Recognized	Cytokines Secreted
Macrophage/monocyte	Phagocytosis; antigen presentation	CD14, CD33	IL-2, IFN-γ, TNF-β,	IL-1, IL-6, IL-8, IL-10, IL-12, TNF-α, TGF-β
B lymphocytes	Antibody secretion; antigen presentation	CD19	IL-2, IL-4, IL-5, IL-6, IL-10	IL-1, TNF-α, TNF-β, GM-CSF
T lymphocytes				
Cytotoxic T lymphocytes	Cytotoxicity	CD3, CD8	IL-2	IFN-γ, TNF-β, TNF-α
Helper T lymphocytes				
T helper 1 (Th$_1$)	Activators of macrophages	CD3, CD4	IFN-γ, IL-12	IL-2, IFN-γ, TNF-β,
T helper 2 (Th$_2$)	Activators of B cells	CD3, CD4	IL-4	TGF-β, IL-10, IL-4, IL-5, IL-6, IL-13
Natural killer cells	Antibody-dependent cell-mediated cytotoxicity	CD16, CD56	IFN-α, IFN-β, TNF-α, IL-12	TNF-α, IFN-γ, GM-CSF

by MHC molecules. Peptides derived from pathogens and peptides derived from normal cellular proteins (self proteins). Peptides generated from self proteins result from the normal continuous cellular degradation process which occurs once a particular protein or enzyme has served its purpose. Normally all nucleated cells display peptides from normal cellular proteins with the aid of the MHC class I proteins. This provides a signal to patrolling T cells that there are no pathogens present and all is well. Hence, for the recognition process to be productive, the T cell must be able to distinguish foreign (pathogenic) substances from those that are generated from normal "self" proteins. T cells "learn" to be self-tolerant during development. T cell precursors originate in the bone marrow and travel to the thymus where they alter expression of some of their cell surface proteins and undergo positive and negative selection processes. During positive selection, T cells that are expressing functional TCRs are tested for their ability to recognize self-MHC proteins. Only those cells that recognize and bind to self-MHC molecules

continue to develop, and those cells that fail the test follow a default pathway and undergo a process known as apoptosis and die. The second test, negative selection, requires that T cells not be strongly "autoreactive"; that is, the cells must not have a strong affinity for self-peptides or self-MHC that might lead to autoimmune disease. Cells that are autoreactive are given a signal to undergo apoptosis and die, as well. Only those cells that recognize self but do not bind too strongly to it are able to exit the thymus and enter the circulation. Once the T cells enter the circulation, they are able to participate in a cellular response or help to develop an antibody-mediated response (Paul 1999).

When a T cell identifies a pathogen-derived peptide within the MHC complex, it initiates a series of protective measures. This includes the secretion of various cytokines, like IL-2, IL-4, IL-5, IL-6, IL-10, and γ interferon that activate other T cells, B cells, and antigen presenting cells (Curfs 1997). These cytokines can activate the antigen presenting cells to undergo a respiratory burst that causes an increase in their phagocytic activity. B cells receive a signal to activate, proliferate, and differentiate into either antibody secreting cells, called plasma cells, or cells with the ability to recognize the pathogen during future encounters, called memory cells. Other T cells, in the vicinity, can also be activated by the secretion of cytokines. This may lead to an increase in the expression of several surface proteins, especially the IL-2 receptor complex.

Mature T lymphocytes can be divided into subsets by function and expression of specific cell surface proteins (Table 2–1) (Paul 1999). The nomenclature for cell surface proteins consists of the letters CD, which stand for clusters of differentiation, and a number, such as 4, which denotes a specific protein. Helper T cells generally express CD4, rather than CD8, on their surface, and recognize peptide/MHC class II complexes at the cell surface. Cytotoxic T cells generally express CD8 and recognize peptide MHC class I complexes on the cell surface. Additionally, helper cells can be further subdivided into Th_1 and Th_2 subsets based on cytokine secretion (Table 2–1) (Curfs 1997).

T lymphocytes participate in multiple stages of the immune response; as a result, these cells must be highly regulated. Many theories have been proposed to explain how T cells are regulated but the simplest theory states that T cells regulate each other. For example, the secretion of a cytokine by one T cell alters the state of a neighboring T cell (Curfs 1997). The cytokine IL-4 is secreted primarily by the subset of helper T cells known as Th_2 cells. Th_2 cells tend to drive the immune response toward a more humoral (involves antibodies) response by emphasizing B cell differentiation and proliferation. In contrast gamma-interferon, secreted by a subset of T lymphocytes called Th_1 cells, drives the immune response toward a more cellular approach by activating other T cells. IL-4 and γ interferon are competitive inhibitors of each other. As a result, the focus of the immune response shifts with the balance between the cytokines. Table 2–1 lists some of the similarities and differences between the different subsets of immune

cells and may help to clarify the differences between the two T helper cell subsets (Curfs 1997; Paul 1999).

Similar to the cytokines described above, each T cell subset plays a unique role in the defense against invading pathogens. Each part is critical to the whole for the body to defend itself against pathogens. T helper cells are possibly the most crucial from the standpoint that T helper cells start the cascade of other specific immune responses. T helper cells play a crucial role in the development of antibody as well as in the activation of other T cells through initiation of the cytokine cascade. Further APCs, which function in the initial phase of the immune response, are signaled to increase their activity (or upregulate) by the γ interferon secreted by the helper T cells. This upregulation causes an increase in phagocytic activity as well as an increase in the expression of peptide/MHC complexes displayed on the surface of these cells (Paul 1999).

Cytotoxic T cells are T cells that generally express the CD8 molecule on their surface, and their TCR complexes recognize peptides bound by Class I MHC molecules that are expressed on all cell types. Cytotoxic T cells are most important in clearing viruses and killing tumor cells. They lyse virally infected cells by secreting a pore forming protein called perforin, which kills the target cell and prevents continued viral replication within that cell. Cytotoxic cells also respond to a number of cytokines that are secreted by helper cells and can be activated as an important part of the cellular immune response against these and other pathogens. Antibodies to viruses are generally of limited usefulness in clearing the virus and so the absence of cytotoxic cells, in inherited immunodeficiencies such as adenosine deaminase deficiency, for example, leads to an increase in susceptibility to viral infection (Paul 1999).

Humoral immunity
Humoral immunity is the portion of the immune response that is mediated by B lymphocytes and their secreted antibodies (Paul 1999; Stites 1997). B cells develop from stem

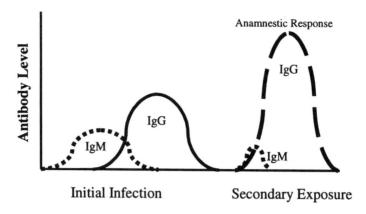

Figure 2-1. Antibody response to infection.

cells primarily in the bone marrow and, to a small degree, in the spleen and fetal liver. B cells are characterized by the expression of specific cell surface proteins. They express surface immunoglobulin, CD19, CD20, and CD22, which are lineage markers, and occasionally, CD21 and CD23, which are receptors, and CD38, CD40, and CD69, which are involved in activation. The combination of the markers expressed helps identify different subsets of B cells as well as the stage of development the cell has reached.

Within the bone marrow, the B cell precursor rearranges its immunoglobulin genes and produces two proteins, one heavy and one light, which form the immunoglobulin complex expressed on the cell surface. The B cell then moves into the circulation where it is able through use of the immunoglobulin complex to bind pathogens that are present within the circulatory or lymphatic systems. Unlike the T cell antigen receptor, the B cell immunoglobulin molecule does not need to recognize antigens in the context of self proteins, nor does the antigen need to be endocytosed and processed. For a B cell to be activated two signals must be received: one from the T helper cell and one from the interaction of the immunoglobulin with antigen. As a result of activation, the B cell can differentiate into either of two different types of B cells: a memory cell that will continue to circulate and recognize antigen in the periphery; or a plasma cell

that will dramatically increase specific antibody secretion into the blood to fight the infection. Plasma cells have a short half-life and are effective for fighting the current infection, but memory cells have a very long half-life and are able to provide an anamnestic response (i.e., a characteristic antibody response as a result of a second encounter with a pathogen) upon reexposure (Fig. 2-1).

There are five different major types (isotypes) of immunoglobulin: IgM, IgD, IgA, IgE, and IgG. Each isotype has different functions in the immune system, which adds to the versatility of the humoral response (Table 2-2) (Paul 1999; Rose 1997). Isotypes IgG1, IgG2, and IgG3 fix complement, leading to a cascade of events that results in the clearance of pathogens (described in the section on the complement cascade). IgA, IgG1, and IgG3 clear pathogens through opsonization, a process in which bacteria or other pathogens are marked for clearance by phagocytes. In contrast IgE is associated with allergy and causes histamine release. Also of note is the special ability of IgG to cross the placenta and enter the circulation of the fetus. In the primary immune response the principal immunoglobulin isotype is IgM, while IgG is the predominant isotype of the secondary (anamnestic) response (Paul 1999; Rose 1997).

Antibodies are ultimately important for the actual clearing of the organisms from the host

Table 2–2 Characteristics of Immunoglobulins

Immunoglobulin	Function and Characteristics	Serum Concentration
IgM	Primary component of initial antibody response; potent activator of complement; does not cross the placenta	120 mg/dL
IgD	Functions as membrane bound receptor for antigen	3 mg/dL
IgA	Found in secreted form in variety of body fluids; crucial role in mucosal immunity	200 mg/dL
IgE	Associated with allergic inflammatory response mediated by antigen crosslinking of IgE bound to Fc receptor on mast cells and basophils	0.05 mg/dL
IgG	Primary component of developing or anamnestic antibody response; involved in opsonization of antigens mediating clearance; crosses placenta	1000 mg/dL

through opsonization, antibody dependent cellular cytotoxicity, and complement-mediated lysis. Humoral responses are crucial for bacterial infections and for neutralizing toxins. In spite of the importance of T lymphocytes in all host defense, antibody responses are indispensable in immune responses as part of the interconnected network of immunologic cells (Paul 1999).

Complement cascade

The third component of acquired immune responses is the complement cascade. The complement cascade is a series of proteins that stimulate each other in a chain reaction leading to clearance of pathogens. Two pathways can activate this series of proteins: the classical pathway, which is activated by antibody-antigen complexes; and the alternative pathway, which does not require participation of specific immune responses. As the complement cascade is activated and enzymatic cleavage of the complement proteins occurs, some of the resulting complement protein fragments have activities that are important for adaptive antigen-specific responses. For example, some of the complement fragments have chemotactic activity, serving to call additional lymphocytes and phagocytic cells to the site of the infection. Some of the components activate a strong inflammatory response that increases transcription, translation, secretion of Il-1, and the activation of T cells. Some complement fragments stimulate the respiratory burst of phagocytic cells, thus increasing antigen

presentation. Additionally, the activity of secreted antibody is dependent on the complement cascade for lysis of invading bacteria or virally infected cells. All of these examples illustrate the crucial role complement plays in the immune response (Paul 1999).

IMMUNE RESPONSES TO INFECTIOUS DISEASES

This section describes different kinds of immune responses to specific infectious diseases: cellular, humoral, and the combination of the two.

Cellular Responses to Infection

Certain pathogens have been historically connected with cellular responses, like tuberculosis, leprosy, syphilis, viruses, helminthic parasites, and fungal infections (Stites 1997). The primary reason for linking these infections with the cellular response is that T cells seem to be more crucial for clearing the organisms than are antibodies. Methods for detecting cellular responses are limited but may still be useful in certain circumstances. Skin tests for delayed type hypersensitivity (DTH) may identify whether the patient is developing an antigen-specific DTH response, but there are few antigens that can be tested in this way (Stites 1997). Proliferation assays have been used as an indication that the T cells are functional. These tests use compounds known as mitogens that are capable of stimulating the majority of T cells nonspecifically (Rose 1997). Further, mitogen responses do not always parallel antigen-specific responses because the signaling pathways are different, and mitogens rely very little on functional TCR protein components. Additionally, mitogen assays are very susceptible to complications, because they are technically demanding and difficult to standardize. However, proliferation assays, which can also be directed against a few selected antigens, like PPD (purified protein derivative or *tuberculin*), and *Candida* sp. are still the most common laboratory method for determining an effective cellular response (Rose 1997).

There are also assays to measure products of a cellular response. For example, there are enzyme linked immunosorbent assays, ELISAs (or EIAs), for measuring cytokine secretion by the patient's cells (Cook 1998; Curfs 1997; Hermann 1995; Rose 1997). There are also methods for determining whether the patient's cells will respond to different cytokines, as a measure of the $Th_1:Th_2$ ratio or the activation state of the T cells. These tests, while fundamental for identifying patients with cellular immunity defects, are not always as useful for measuring a specific cellular response during an infection, because they are very indirect.

Viruses, primary targets of cytotoxic T cells, are among the pathogens that elicit strong cellular responses. Cytotoxic T cells recognize foreign peptides in the context of class I MHC, rather than class II MHC, like helper T cells. This difference allows cytotoxic T cells to more efficiently attack virally infected cells because all cells in the human body express class I molecules. Class II molecules are expressed only on certain subsets of cells that are most often involved in antigen presentation to T helper cells. If cytotoxic T cells were dependent upon class II, they would only be able to attack a small subset of virally infected cells. When cytotoxic T cells identify a virally infected cell they secrete perforin into the local environment. Perforin is a protein that inserts itself into the membrane of the infected cell and disrupts the membrane integrity, much like the complement components do. By lysing the infected cell,

the cytotoxic T cell is able to prevent viral replication in that cell and decrease the chance of infection of the surrounding cells. This is more efficient than antibody-dependent cytotoxicity, which would eliminate one organism at a time, and would not be effective against cells that are infected with the virus unless they are expressing intact viral proteins on their surface. Antigens inside cells are not accessible to antibody-mediated responses, and several organisms, such as *Mycobacterium tuberculosis*, have adapted to the intracellular environment to avoid the humoral response. Most viruses, such as influenza A, initiate a cell-mediated response that eventually leads to eradication of the internalized virus. Additionally, phagocytosis, which is upregulated by T cell responses, can clear dead or dying cells that are infected with a virus. The intracellular environment of the phagocytic cell is harsher and more lethal than the inside of other cells. However, these phagocytic cells are dependent upon the T cell response for their increase in function following activation. As a result, any organisms that are eliminated primarily by phagocytosis, such as *S. aureus* or *E. coli*, require a functional cellular response. That means that other pathogens, in addition to viruses, may also be cleared by cell-mediated cytotoxicity.

The notable exception to the concept of virally induced cytotoxicity is the human immunodeficiency virus (HIV). This virus is the root of many exceptions, mainly because of how severely it disrupts the function of the immune system. It is able to avoid the attack of cytotoxic T cells primarily because of its ability to prevent helper T cells from activating the cytotoxic T cells. Another symptom of the HIV disruption of the immune response is manifest early in the course of disease when HIV causes a nonspecific hyperstimulation of helper T cells before driving them into anergy (a nonresponsive state). Early in HIV infection, helper T cells proliferate expansively and randomly without antigen stimulation. This random disregulated activation and proliferation cause an imbalance in the regulation of all the other cell subsets, as might be expected. For example, cytotoxic T cells may receive inappropriate signals and cytokines from the activated helper cells that lead to their activation in the absence of a known antigen. Additionally, B cells may be instructed to proliferate and produce antibody nonspecifically. In effect, HIV infection causes an initial upregulation of the immune system, which ultimately results in a complete disregulation of the system. This extreme upregulation works eventually to "wear out" the cells involved. Essentially, the cells are exhausted, owing to inappropriate stimulation and, as a result, simply stop functioning (Paul 1999).

Other pathogens that elicit strong cellular responses include fungi and helminths. Both of these infections cause very strong inflammatory responses that are ultimately responsible for eliminating the pathogen. The T cells involved play a key role in sustaining the inflammatory response until the pathogen is completely eliminated. This response is dependent upon T helper activity and cytokine secretion (Curfs 1997; Paul 1999).

One other group of organisms that elicit strong cellular responses must be included because of the lesson in immunology they provide. Leprosy, syphilis, leishmaniasis, and tuberculosis are important diseases because the balance between the cellular and humoral responses is crucial to the development of severe disease (Stites 1997). When these pathogens elicit cellular responses, the illness is contained and may be driven into a latent or remission state. However, as the balance between cellular and humoral responses shifts toward the humoral response, these pathogens become more lethal and cause more severe disease. It is thought that the antibodies formed may actually protect the organism from attack by T cells that directly kill the invading pathogen. Antibodies are not effective, because these pathogens have developed mechanisms for evading the antibody response. Therefore in people with depressed cell-mediated immunity, these diseases can become significantly worse in spite of a functional humoral response, because the antibody response is useless for clearing the causative agent.

Thus these diseases may also see an upward trend in severity or number because of acquired immune deficiency syndrome (AIDS) which eliminates the cell-mediated response. Clearly the increase in HIV infection will lead to an increase in those illnesses that are normally prevented by functional cell-mediated responses, including illnesses that are normally stopped by innate nonspecific responses.

Humoral Responses to Infection

Some pathogens are much better at eliciting humoral responses by the host. For example, bacteria possess a number of highly antigenic surface proteins that can be recognized by antibodies. Recognition leads to the formation of antibody-antigen complexes that are cleared by the kidneys, antibody dependent cytotoxicity, or phagocytosis mediated by receptors expressed on phagocytic cells (Paul 1999).

Antibodies are not immediately detectable after infection. In a primary response antibody will not be detectable for approximately 7–14 days post infection. There are many methods for detecting strong antibody-mediated responses, but they all involve measuring the level of total antibody or specific antibody present in the serum of an infected individual. By using various ELISA techniques, it is possible to differentiate the isotypes of the responding antibodies, as well, which allows the clinician to identify the time course of the illness. IgM rises first to a moderate degree during a primary response to an antigen, followed by elevated levels of IgG that persist longer than the IgM titers. During a secondary, or anamnestic, response, the IgM again rises, but the rise in IgG is much more dramatic and rapid and quickly overshadows the IgM response (Cook 1998; Hermann 1995; Paul 1999; Rose 1997).

One caveat of the ELISA detection method is that, because this method is indirect and measures antibody produced against the pathogen rather than the pathogen itself, the ELISA requires a functional immune system to be an effective diagnostic tool. If a patient is not making antibody responses, regardless of the reason, then measuring immunoglobulin levels will not be representative of that patient's disease state (Hermann 1995; Rose 1997).

Other factors that influence the humoral response include characteristics of the invading organism or antigen (Cook 1998; Forbes 1998; Hermann 1995; Rose 1997). Some bacteria avoid the host response by adapting to the intracellular environment of phagocytic cells. By living intracellularly, bacteria are not exposed to the antibodies and complement that could lead to their lysis. Proteins are much more antigenic than are polysaccharides, which are much better than lipid moieties. Therefore encapsulated bactgeria, such as *S. pneumoniae*, and *Haemophilus* sp., are better protected from the humoral immune response because the protein antigens are covered with polysaccharides. Additionally, some polysaccharide capsules on bacteria have immunosuppressive activity, like the mucoid capsule on *Pseudomonas aeruginosa*. Capsules, in general, are effective at blocking the humoral response. Antigens with repetitive units are especially susceptible to humoral attack because repeating antigens can cross-link IgM or other surface immunoglobulin on B cells without the help of T cells. Few antigens are really T cell independent B cell antigens. Lipopolysaccharide (LPS), or bacterial endotoxin, is one of the most important T cell independent antigens, but LPS may also cause disregulation of the immune system because of its potential mitogenic activity. LPS may be able to avoid specific stimulation of the immune system by inducing a relatively nonspecific stimulation and providing a distraction. This "confuse the enemy" theme is not uncommonly used by bacteria to avoid host defense. By providing a number of antigens that may or may not be able to lead to clearance of the organism, the bacteria are able to divide the immune response into different directions, making each direction less effective.

In spite of the number of possible complications, antibody production is still a very successful method for identifying infectious diseases. A good example of a disease where antibody production is very important is Lyme disease, caused by *Borrelia burgdorferi*. In this disease IgM and IgG appear about three to six weeks following exposure and can clear the spirochetal organism from the host. Some patients who are treated with antibiotics prior to the development of a full humoral response fail to seroconvert and produce significant levels of anti-borrelial antibodies. Additionally, borreliacidal antibodies are felt to be necessary for preventing long-term illness or sequelae developing as a result of *Borrelia*. The cellular response appears to be useful for activating phagocytic cells that can contain the infection while the antibodies are being formed and lyse the *Borrelia* organisms. The absence of a humoral response to specific borrelial antigens has been linked to persistent and severe symptoms of arthritis and autoimmune phenomena following Lyme disease. Clearly, the presence of a functional humoral response is necessary for appropriate resolution of Lyme disease, and the lack of an appropriate humoral response may lead to disregulation of the antibody response and cross-reactivity leading to autoimmunity (Cook 1998; Forbes 1998; Hermann 1995; Rose 1997).

Combined Responses to Infection

Some pathogens induce strong mixed immune responses where both the cellular and humoral responses are necessary for the elimination of the organism. Almost all organisms elicit some mixed responses, but both responses are not always useful for clearing the pathogen. It is true, though, that the combination of cellular and humoral response will be different for different pathogens and routes of infection. It is also true that the clearance of the organism may be more dependent on one arm of the immune response than the other. Each individual response is unique for the organism, setting, time, and localization of the infection. Usually, a combination of the humoral and cellular responses will result in the best destruction of the organism, but some organisms will only be eliminated by a combination of both responses. Neither arm alone will eliminate the organism (Paul 1999; Stites 1997). An example of an illness where both arms of the immune response are crucial is hepatitis B virus (HBV) infection. Because this pathogen is a virus, T cell responses are important. It is also known that this pathogen stimulates a robust antibody response that aids in clearance and staging of the disease by the clinician. During HBV infection, early diagnosis can be made by detection of HBV antigens, both the surface antigen and the hepatitis B "e" antigen. At least two to three weeks are required for the development of detectable levels if IgM antibodies to the core antigen. Therefore helper and cytotoxic T cells must be able to contain the spread of the virus for the first few weeks of infection. Cytotoxic T cells kill virally infected cells, and helper T cells provide help to cytotoxic cells and B cells while also maintaining the inflammatory response at the site of infection. This can be especially difficult because HBV is subject to sanguinal transmission, and it requires constant monitoring of the blood stream for infectious and antigenic particles. After the antibody response has been initiated, there is a long recovery time during which antibody-mediated cellular cytotoxicity and phagocytosis can eliminate infected cells, and antibody-bound viral particles are unable to attach to and enter a new cell. Symptoms of inflammation remain, however, and are indicative of the continual T cell activation to clear the virus. It may take months or years for all of the virus particles to be removed, and they may never be completely eliminated. It appears to be very difficult for people with depressed cellular or humoral responses to control this infection. Thus HBV exemplifies those infections that require both arms of the immune system (Rose 1997; Stites 1997).

One other interesting disease where both cellular and humoral responses are important is trypanosomiasis. This illness is persistent because of the pathogen's ability to genetically alter its antigens and their expression. As a result, although antibody formation is essential for clearing this organism, no effective antibody memory response can be formed. The pathogen sheds its old antigen and expresses a new one that appears unrelated to the first antigen. There-fore the humoral response is continually challenged to begin again to build an effective antibody pool. Clearly, under these conditions, it would be important for the cellular response to remain viable and continue to supply cytokines to other immunologic cells. Additionally, T cells are necessary to maintain the inflammatory response that not only limits the growth of the organism but also induces the antigenic changes that occur. In this case, not only are both arms of the immune response necessary, but they must cooperate and assist each other in the clearance of the trypanosomes (Stites 1997).

These two examples are characteristic of most immune responses under normal circumstances where both cellular and humoral responses are functional and efficient. However, there are certain other characteristics of the immune response that still must be mentioned. First, there is a difference between how localized and systemic infections alter the propensity of the immune system to be slanted toward the humoral or cellular response. Certainly, secreted substances with reasonable half-lives, like antibodies, will be more effective systemically than will cells that have a limited capacity to circulate freely throughout the body and into the tissues (Paul 1999). However, cells do have the ability to return to particular locations within the secondary immune system tissues and may be able to recruit additional help from other cells in lymphoid tissues near the site of infection. It is also true that cells generally have a longer half-life than the products they secrete. Certainly, cytokines are not able to circulate in an active form, and so helper cells are necessary within the local environment of the infection to provide the growth factors needed by the other cells. Draining lymph nodes are a good example of "regional headquarters" where cells can interact and then return to the site of the localized infection. This eliminates the need to have T cells of all antigenic specificities within the tissues, even for localized infections (Curfs 1997; Paul 1999).

Another factor that plays a role in the ability of the immune system to ward off infection is the blood-brain barrier and immune-privileged sites. An immune-privileged site is one in which no immune response will be mounted under nomral conditions. The anterior chamber of the eye is one example. Theoretically, no infection will penetrate, and no immunologic cells have access to this part of the eye. Therefore if trauma results in infection, a functional immune response may not be mounted because the foreign body is not exposed to immunologic cells. In the central nervous system, the blood-brain barrier functions in a similar manner to keep immunologic cells from gaining access, and therefore pathogens localizing behind the blood-brain barrier may be protected from immunologic attack (Paul 1999).

In summarizing the immune responses to infectious pathogens, when the immune system as a whole works together in the intended manner, the host is protected against an onslaught of an almost infinite number of different pathogens and foreign substances. Through the cooperation of each and every cell within the immune system pathogens are eliminated and the severity of an infectious process either fails to be induced or is reduced.

LABORATORY DIAGNOSTIC METHODS FOR INFECTIOUS DISEASES

Laboratory methods for diagnosis of infections concentrate on either the detection of antibodies to a particular pathogen or the detection of the pathogen itself (Cook 1998; Forbes 1998; Hermann 1995; Rose 1997). Assays that detect antibody yield information about the immune status of the individual. For example, detection of IgM antibodies specific for hepatitis A in the absence of IgG antibodies may indicate an acute infeciton, whereas detection of IgG antibodies specific for hepatitis A indicates past exposure or perhaps vaccination (Cook 1998; Hermann 1995).

Methods for detecting a specific pathogen focus on either the ability to culture the organism or the ability to detect an antigenic component of the organism (Forbes 1998). While culture of a particular pathogen is diagnostic, it is limited by the quality of the specimen from which the pathogen is to be cultured as well as the identity of the pathogen itself. Not all pathogens are cultivable.

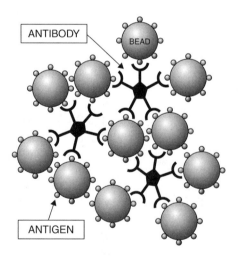

Figure 2–2. Latex agglutination. IgM antibody interacts with antigen on latex bead, resulting in lattice formation and agglutination.

As an alternative to culture direct detection of the pathogen is possible in some cases.

In either case, antibody or antigen, detection is dependent upon assays that use antibody. Assays such as latex agglutination (LA), complement fixation (CF), enzyme linked immunoassay (EIA), and fluorescent antibody (FA) tests make up the majority of the test methodologies that are used to diagnose infectious disease. These methods all aim to make the evidence of microscopic entities discernible to the unaided human eye.

The latex agglutination assay relies on the ability of antigen and antibody to agglutinate (Fig. 2–2). For example, pathogen-specific antigens are attached to an inert particle, such as latex beads. These beads are then mixed with the patient's serum. When antibodies in the patient's serum, specific for the pathogen, bind to the antigen affixed to the latex bead a lattice is formed, resulting in agglutination, which is visibly detectable as clumping (Cook 1998; Forbes 1998; Hermann 1995; Rose 1997).

Enzyme linked immunoassay is analogous to latex agglutination in its utilization of an inert surface to which antigen or antibody is attached. This assay is dependent upon the attachment of enzyme molecules that are conjugated to specific antibodies (Fig. 2–3). These antibodies then bind to their specific target, which may be antigen or antibody depending upon whether the EIA is designed to detect antigen or antibody. After binding, these enzymes in the presence of substrate will generate a colorimetric product that is proportional to the number of antigen-antibody complexes formed.

Another widely used methodology is fluorescent antibody detection. This assay detects the interaction of antigen and antibody by using antibodies that are conjugated with a fluorochrome. These interactions can be visualized using fluorescent microscopy. These assays are useful in direct visualization of antibody or antigen within specimens, culture, body fluids, or tissue (Cook 1998; Forbes 1998; Hermann 1995; Rose 1997).

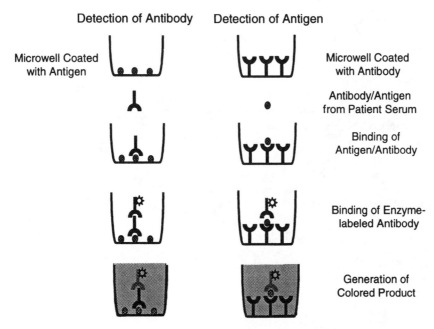

Figure 2–3. Enzyme linked assay. Diagram of the detection of antigen or antibody using an enzyme labeled antibody.

Table 2–3 Laboratory Methods to Detect Infection with Various Pathogens

Pathogen	Disease	Methods to Detect Antibody to Pathogen*	Methods to Detect Pathogen-Specific Antigen*
Viral			
Adenovirus	Respiratory infections	CF, EIA	FA, EIA
Cytomegalovirus	Associated with persistent, latent, and recurrent infections	LA, EIA	FA
Epstein-Barr virus	Infectious mononucleosis	LA, EIA	
Hepatitis A	Hepatitis	EIA	
Hepatitis B	Hepatitis	EIA	
Hepatitis C	Hepatitis	EIA	
Herpes-simplex virus-1	Lesions on skin, lips, genitalia	EIA, CF	FA, EIA
Herpes-simplex virus-2	Genital lesions	EIA, CF	FA, EIA
HIV-1	AIDS	EIA	EIA
HIV-2	AIDS	EIA	
Influenza viruses A and B	"Flu"		FA, EIA
Mumps	Viral parotitis	EIA	
Parainfluenza 1, 2, and 3	Respiratory infections		FA, EIA
Respiratory syncytial virus	Respiratory infections		FA, EIA
Rotavirus	Gastroenteritis		LA, EIA
Rubella	German measles; congenital abnormalities	LA, EIA, HI	
Rubeola	Measles	EIA	
Varicella zoster virus	Chickenpox and shingles	LA, EIA, CF	
Bacterial			
Bacterial meningitis (*Haemophilus influenzae*, *Neisseria meningitidis*, *Streptococcus agalactiae*, *Escherichia coli*, and *Streptococcus pneumoniae*)	Meningitis		LA
Bordetella pertussis	Whooping cough		FA
Borrelia burgdorferi	Lyme disease	EIA	
Campylobacter sp.	Gastroenteritis		LA, EIA
Chlamydia trachomatis	Sexually transmitted; urethritis		EIA, FA
Clostridium difficile	Colitis		LA, EIA
Group A streptococcus	Pharyngitis	LA, EIA	LA, EIA, OIA
Legionella sp.	Legionnaires' disease		EIA, FA
Neisseria gonorrhoeae	Gonorrhea		EIA
Rickettsia rickettsii	Rocky Mountain spotted fever	LA, FA	
Treponema pallidum	Syphilis	EIA	HA
Fungal			
Cryptococcus	Septicemia, meningitis		EIA, LA
Dimorphic fungi (*Blastomyces dermatiditis*, *Coccidioides immitis*, *Histoplasma capsulatum*)	Initial pulmonary infection; may be followed by multiorgan dissemination		Ouchterlony gel diffusion
Parasitic			
Cryptosporidium sp.	Gastroenteritis		EIA, FA
Giardia sp.	Diarrhea		EIA, FA
Pneumocystis carinii	Pneumonia		FA

*EIA = enzyme-linked immunoassay; CF = complement fixation; FA = fluorescent antibody; HA = hemagglutination; HI = hemagglutination inhibition; LA = latex agglutination; OIA = optical immunoassay.

Currently, for almost any pathogen that has been identified and is associated with infectious disease, methodologies exist for the determination of an individual's immune response to the pathogen or identification of the pathogen itself. Table 2–3 lists some of the most common diagnostic methodologies for infectious disease diagnosis (Cook 1998; Forbes 1998; Hermann 1995; Rose 1997). For the vast majority of these pathogens nucleic acid testing is also available.

At the center of laboratory testing for infectious disease is the antigen-antibody interaction. An understanding of the immune response and the role of both pathogen and immune system in infectious disease is crucial to understanding and interpreting laboratory tests. Laboratory tests, when interpreted using this knowledge, yield valuable information concerning the status of the individual with respect to disease. These tests can be used as tools to determine whether an

Table 2–4 Advantages and Disadvantages of General Methods for Detecting Infection

Diagnostic Test	Advantages	Disadvantages
Culture	"Gold standard"	May have low sensitivity
	Specific	Potential laboratory hazard
	Allows determination of antimicrobial susceptibility	Culture technique may not exist
	Provides material for molecular analysis	Difficult to perform in field
	Allows quantitative assessment of infection	May not be available in lesser developed cultures
		Can not detect past infection
		May not be able to distinguish colonization from infection (nonsterile site)
		May not be useful in subject on antibiotics
Antibody measurement	Routine methods often exist for measurement	Not all pathogens elicit an antibody response (e.g., prion agents)
	May allow detection of acute infection (IgM)	Usually not detectable for 1–3 weeks following infection
	May allow detection of past infection (IgG)	May lack specificity for detection of exact pathogen due to cross-reactivity
	May correlate with immunity (E.g., anti-HBsAg)	May not be able to distinguish between acute and past infection
	Safe, does not require culture of pathogen	May not reflect extent of disease (i.e., for latent infections such as herpes simplex and HIV)
Antigen detection	Indicates current infection (if from sterile site)	Not available for many pathogens
	May be adapted to detection in the field	Does not detect past infection
	Often useful despite subject being on antibiotics	May not be able to distinguish colonization from infection (nonsterile site)
	May allow quantitative assessment of infection	

individual is currently infected or has been exposed at some previous time. Further, they can provide information on the current immune status of an individual with respect to a particular pathogen. This would be important in determining whether an individual is susceptible to infection or is protected as a result of perhaps vaccination or previous infection. In summary, an understanding of the immune system and laboratory testing methodologies when used in combination provides a powerful tool for monitoring or detecting infectious disease in either a single individual or a large population.

SELECTED REFERENCES

Cook L. New assays for infectious agents replacing traditional serologic methods. Advance for Medical Laboratory Professionals. December 7: 12–15, 1998.

Curfs JHA, Meis JFGM, and Hoogkamp-Korstanje JAA. A primer on cytokines: sources, receptors, effects, and inducers. Clin. Microbiol. Rev. October: 742–780, 1997.

Forbes BA, Sahm DF, Weissfeld AS. Immunochemical methods used for organism detection. In: Forbes BA, Sahm DF, Weissfeld AS, eds. Bailey and Scott's Diagnostic Microbiology. 10th ed. St. Louis, MO: Mosby, 1998: 208–219.

Hermann JE. Immunoassays for the diagnosis of infectious diseases. In: Murray PR, Baron EJ, Pfaller MA, et al. Eds. Manual of Clinical Microbiology, 6th ed. Washington, DC: American Society for Microbiology, 1995:110–122.

Paul WE. Fundamental Immunology. 4th ed. Philadelphia: Lippincott-Raven, 1999.

Rose NR, Conway de MaGario E, Folds JD, Lane HC, and Nakamura RM, eds. Manual of Clinical Laboratory Immunology. 5th ed. Washington, DC: American Society for Microbiology, 1997.

Stites DP, Terr AI, and Parslow TG. Medical Immunology. 9th ed. Stamford, CT: Appleton and Lange, 1997.

3

Theories of Causation

DANA LOOMIS and STEVE WING

How does scientific work, including epidemiology, relate to knowing the causes of events, why things happen? How do we decide on the cause of a person's disease—was it the germ, unboiled water, inadequate knowledge about health behaviors, poor nutrition, lack of water purification, poverty, economic inequality, or a legacy of racist colonial development? And how do we make judgments not only about a particular case of disease but about the cause of disease in general? These questions are critically important because the scientific answers play a role in public health action and policy, both in justifying continuation of accepted practices and in promoting different approaches.

This chapter reviews the topic of causal thinking in epidemiology, with a focus on infectious diseases. We take a historical approach to the topic because of the important differences between explanations of the causes of disease in different places and times, and because it is widely believed that scientific knowledge is progressive, that is, it accumulates in a linear fashion toward the truth. A historical perspective allows us to evaluate not only the progressive aspects of beliefs about causation of disease but also the world views and social values upon which models of causation and prescriptions for public health practice rest.

The chapter is organized into five sections. First we discuss causal ideas before microbiology, at a time when causal theories emphasizing contagion and environment were on relatively equal footing. Next we discuss the impact of the germ theory on causal thinking in epidemiology, its monocausal implications and its later expansion into multicausal and ecological views. Because of the importance of rapid changes in health and disease states in influencing causal thinking, the third section addresses causal implications of evidence about trends in infectious disease. The fourth section summarizes the basis of current causal thinking in epidemiology, which is dominated in the English language literature by studies of risk factors for noninfectious disease. In the final section we suggest an alternative perspective that is not focused on risk factors.

CAUSAL IDEAS BEFORE MICROBIOLOGY

Modern ideas about the causes of disease emerged near the end of the nineteenth century, when developments in microbiology and medicine first coalesced to permit the identification of bacterial pathogens and the classification of the clinical manifestations they produce in humans. As the relative recency of these ideas suggests, however, there were many well-developed theories about the causes of disease before the advent of microbiology. Because epidemic disease is a visible feature of human life, cultures must have theories of disease, or epidemiologies, to explain how and why it occurs. Folk traditions were historically—and, for many people, continue to be—important sources of epidemiological explanation. Despite the importance and legitimacy of other traditions, our concern here is to understand the roots of causal thinking in contemporary public health and medicine. Thus we focus on ideas prevalent among formally trained practitioners of those disciplines in the tradition that began to develop in Europe in the nineteenth century.

Environment or Contagion?

Among physicians in early nineteenth century Europe, there were two predominant classes of explanations for the origins of mass disease: environmental theories and contagion theories. The environmental theories were rooted in the Hippocratic tradition (Greenwood 1993). Their adherents postulated that the cycles of the seasons or the quality of the air and water or general living conditions directly determined the occurrence of epidemics. The competing idea that epidemics result from person-to-person transmission of contagious matter is also ancient, but its modern expression is often traced to the fifteenth century writings of Girolamo Fracastoro, a Veronese physician. The specific nature of the contagious material was not known until the late nineteenth century, but it was postulated centuries earlier to be an autonomous agent, possibly living, that was specific to each disease, capable of being transmitted among people, and which might exist sometimes in a human host and sometimes in the environment (Fracastoro 1930).

Both environmental and contagion theories of disease were used in developing preventive measures and formulating public health policy well before the nineteenth century. During the Renaissance, environmental causes were invoked in reports issued by the Florentine government, which associated epidemic conditions with filth and noxious odors (Cipolla 1992). Some Italian cities employed environmental sanitation to control both tuberculosis and bubonic plague. On the other hand, fear of contagion simultaneously led to the practice of quarantining ships and their crews, which many ports had adopted by the eighteenth century (Rosen 1958, Dubos, 1952).

By the 1840s, an environmental theory of disease began to gain the upper hand as a motivating force for public health policy. This idea, that epidemics resulted from contaminated air, or miasma, emanating from putrefying organic matter, rose to prominence in the context of the unprecedented urbanization brought about by the industrial revolution. In early Victorian England, Edwin Chadwick and other liberal reformists depicted the vile living conditions industrialization had inflicted on the new urban working class and championed the provision of clean water, adequate housing, and effective sewerage to improve health and social welfare (Cullen 1975; Mackenzie 1981). Reforms based on environmental theories of disease were also instituted elsewhere in Europe and in the United States (Rosen 1958).

The reformist orientation associated with the miasma theory played an integral part in the development of another field that has become integral to modern epidemiology. In England and France, statistical methods provided much of the information that was used to make the case for sanitary reform. Reformers saw the new discipline of statistics, named for the study of states, as an essential part of the new, rational approach to governance that would sweep away the arbitrariness of monarchy (Hacking 1990). Interest in health and social questions motivated much of the development of statistics in the early nineteenth century, and prominent statisticians of the era, like William Farr in England and René Villerme, in France, championed reform causes (Coleman 1982; Cullen 1975).

Moral and Social Causation

Despite the dominance of the miasmatist school of thought, other theories of disease were able to coexist with it. Religious and moral explanations were especially prominent in the nineteenth century. While these ideas were not taught in professional medical curricula, they remained important in the beliefs of the public and health professionals alike. The consummate public health professional of nineteenth century England, physician, epidemiologist, and reformer William Farr, argued that, while sanitary reform was imperative, moral failure in the form of sloth and drunkenness was partly to blame for the poor state of the working class (Eyler 1979). Writing from a popular perspective, Charles Dickens was fond of portraying the triumph of individual virtue over adversity. Whereas Farr accepted the fundamental arrangements of Victorian society, however, Dickens seemed to call for a return to a traditional morality free from the corrupting influences of the industrial age.

Different moral arguments were a key aspect of another, far more radical, thread of nineteenth century causal ideas. This intellectual current, exemplified by the work of Friedrich Engels and Rudolf Virchow, consisted of environmental theories of disease rooted in political economy. When Virchow, then a young professor of medicine, was deputized in 1848 to investigate an outbreak of typhus in eastern Germany he cited poverty and economic underdevelopment as its root causes (Taylor and Rieger 1985). Virchow's statement that "medicine is a social science, and politics is nothing but medicine on a grand scale" eloquently summarized his views concerning the causes and prevention of disease (Taylor and Rieger 1985). Engels, writing in England, charac-

terized the ill health of British workers as "nothing short of murder callously committed through the instrument of industrial capitalism" (Engels 1993). Like Virchow, Engels saw the manner in which people organize themselves into societies as the fundamental determinant of health.

Despite their outward differences, the main nineteenth century ideas of disease causation had several elements in common. Both the miasmatic theory and the contagion theory visualized disease as resulting from the action of autonomous agents, extrinsic to the human organism. The kind of intervention needed to prevent disease would of course differ depending on how the agent was believed to act. But whether sick people's belongings were burned to stop contagion or privies were constructed to eliminate miasmas, disease was to be controlled through specific, often narrowly conceived, environmental changes directed toward the suspected agent. The miasmatic and political-economic views also shared an underlying faith in scientific methods and their potential to rationalize government (Engels 1993; Cullen 1975).

Despite these commonalities, the political-economic thread of Virchow and Engels was distinctly different from other scientifically oriented disease theories of its day in one critical way. It was the only theory to consider the production of health and disease in an ecological context, in that it saw illness as part of a complex social and cultural system and the control of disease as requiring consideration of that system in its entirety.

THE GERM THEORY EMERGES

For a time, the miasma theory of disease dominated the formation of public health policy. Mainstream scientists viewed contagionism as an antiquated, scientifically discredited theory (Ackerknecht 1948). Quarantine and other disease control measures derived from it were discarded in response to political liberals' arguments that they were inefficient and failed to address the true causes of disease.

Nevertheless, the idea that diseases are produced by living organisms was not abandoned. John Snow conducted a series of elegantly designed epidemiological studies of cholera epidemics in London in the 1850s, based on the hypothesis that the disease was produced by an infective agent transmitted through water contaminated with human feces (Snow 1936). The fact that this work and similarly oriented mid–nineteenth century studies, like those of Panum on measles (Panum 1940) and Budd on fevers (Budd 1984), were carried out at the height of the miasma theory's ascendancy indicates the persistence of contagion theories of disease.

A Revolution in the Laboratory

The dominance of the miasma theory was finally broken by developments in the laboratory, rather than by epidemiological research. By the 1860s, decades of careful work by numerous researchers had yielded incremental progress in the science and technology of microbiology. With this background in place, Louis Pasteur's elucidation of the mechanisms of infection and Robert Koch's developments in culture technique and descriptions of bacterial life cycles were seen as signal breakthroughs, capable of finally filling the gaps in existing knowledge about the mechanisms by which disease is produced.

Still more dramatic changes came with Koch's identification of the tubercle bacillus as the unique and specific cause of tuberculosis. With this development there was born a new disease defined on etiologic grounds, which grouped together older disease entities, including phthisis, scrofula, and Pott's disease. Tuberculosis was of overwhelming public health importance in the late nineteenth century. It was the leading cause of death in most industrialized countries, yet it was not regarded at the time as a single disease and there was no unified theory about its etiology. In an influential 1882 paper, Koch elucidated three pieces of evidence that convincingly identified the tubercle bacillus as the agent of the disease.

These observations, which came to be known as Koch's postulates, provided a previously lacking conceptual framework for identifying pathogenic agents, as follows:

1 the agent is found in every case of the disease in association with its characteristic lesions;
2 the disease can be produced by artificially introducing the agent into a symptom-free host, after isolating the agent from a diseased host and growing it in pure culture, and
3 the agent can be recovered from the new host after symptoms appear.

Koch's conceptualization of pathogenic agents as necessary and sufficient causes of disease, combined with the ideas that pathogens are living organisms capable of being passed from one person to another, and possibly from other species to humans, constituted the classical germ theory of disease.

The Focus Shifts Inward

The application of the methodology developed by Koch brought about immediate and profound changes in infectious disease research, as well as in medical and public health practice. One important change was that the focus of activity shifted from the community and the clinic to the laboratory. Microbiologic research to identify pathogens proceeded at a dizzying pace in the decades around the turn of the century, with the agents of most infectious diseases of contemporary public health importance being identified by 1910 (Rosen, 1958).

Along with this change in the emphasis of research came changes in the training of public health professionals. University departments of hygiene were transformed into centers for training and research in bacteriology, especially in Germany, where the old sanitary emphasis was virtually swept away (Winslow 1943). When new schools of public health were founded in the twentieth century, bacteriology was an essential part of the curriculum; the community aspects of health initially received little attention (Fee 1987).

The formalization of epidemiology as a discipline was largely a result of the establishment of public health curricula based on the paradigm of the germ theory. However, the epidemiology of 1920 bore little resemblance to the modern discipline. The first academic textbooks on the subject described epidemiology as concerned exclusively with infectious diseases, and curricula emphasized the investigation of outbreaks and the tracing of contacts (Frost 1941; Stallybrass 1931; Fee 1987).

In remarkable contrast to the situation during the sanitary revolution of the 1840s, statistics had little place in the new epidemiology emerging from advances in bacteriology. Charles Chapin, Rhode Island's influential health director, in 1909 exhorted epidemiologists to make more use of quantitative methods, but he was referring to calculations ranging from disinfection rates to the cost of treatment; population statistics were scarcely mentioned (Chapin 1934a).

With Koch's methodology for identifying the agents responsible for infectious diseases, there was, of course, no need for statistical methods. By definition the agent was present in every case of the disease, so the observation of only a single case could provide definitive evidence of causation. Diseases could now be redefined based on their etiologic agents, rather than their clinical manifestations (MacMahon 1970). There was also a rational basis for distinguishing infectious from noninfectious diseases based on etiology, rather than using labels like epidemic or chronic that described their time course in populations or individuals.

Redefinition of diseases by etiology brought microbiologic methods into medical practice, since isolation of the agent in culture was now required for definitive diagnosis of many diseases.

Perhaps most important of all, the microbiologic revolution dramatically changed the spectrum of disease control strategies that seemed appropriate. Although medical therapies capable of directly combating infection in the human host were slower to evolve, public health measures were quickly reoriented toward preventing transmission of pathogens. General environmental hygiene was replaced by more specific measures—such as disinfection of drinking water; quarantine was reintroduced; and sick people and their contacts were put under surveillance (Rosen 1958).

This change in direction was so profound that Charles Chapin, speaking before the American Public Health Association in 1902 (Chapin 1934b), ridiculed the public health movement's past focus on community sanitation and urged public health workers to adopt an up-to-date approach to disease prevention based on the germ theory:

The English, who carried the notion of the danger of filth to the extreme, were assumed to be the leaders in public health work, and we blindly followed the leaders. It was believed that the municipality was chiefly responsible for infectious diseases. Pure air, pure water, and a pure soil was the cry. We have learned the true nature of infection and we have learned that the parasites which are its essence rarely propagate in filth and are rarely air-borne. Instead of an indiscriminate attack on dirt, we must learn the mode of transmission of each infection, and must discover its most vulnerable point of attack.

A New Paradigm and Its Critics

Despite the tremendous advances in scientific understanding that the classical germ theory brought about, problems with it were quick to emerge. Some technical difficulties were eventually overcome. The identification of viruses was delayed until improved laboratory techniques were developed, the role of host resistance was not immediately appreciated, and modes of transmission proved difficult to untangle for some agents (Evans 1978). Yellow fever was a particularly vexing problem because it involved both viral etiology and insect vectors, but it ultimately came to be understood through a combination of field, clinical, and laboratory investigations.

Other deficiencies of the germ theory were more fundamental, but not as readily apparent. The germ theory's tendency to yield oversimplified accounts of the occurrence of disease in populations was central to some of the most penetrating critiques. People who had been schooled in the older, sanitary approach, notably William Farr and, in Germany, Max von Pettenkoffer, accepted that microbiologic agents had a role in producing epidemic disease but were unwilling to concede that they were the sole cause (Eyler 1979; Winslow 1943). Pettenkoffer was a particularly vocal critic of the germ theory, remembered today for drinking a glass of water containing *Vibrio cholerae* to prove the organism was not the cause of cholera. Although Pettenkoffer has been derided for this protest against "progress," some of his arguments about the causation of infectious diseases were later revived to illustrate the supposedly more complex causation of noninfectious diseases, as we will see later.

The potential loss of the public health movement's former emphasis on community improvement and social well-being was one important consequence of the germ theory. Modernists like Chapin championed the efficiency of public health practice based on the germ theory, which could be carried out by an elite corps of highly trained experts, rather than requiring a broad social movement.

Some patrons of the new public health clearly stood to benefit from the limited approach it engendered. The Rockefeller Foundation initiated public health programs worldwide that directed interventions specifically toward control of infectious agents. The foundation's health workers and their supporters believed that this strategy would benefit capitalist interests by producing a healthier work force without causing social disruption (Kunitz 1988; Brown 1979). The Rockefeller Foundation was also instrumental in founding schools of public health in the United States and Latin America. In the selection of Johns Hopkins University as the site of the first such school, the foundation again expressed a clear preference for a science-based public health practiced by experts in the clinic and the laboratory (Fee 1987).

The emergence of the germ theory transformed infectious disease research, public health, and medical practice, sweeping away institutions and approaches based on older paradigms. Tremendous advances in the understanding of transmission, infection, patho-

genesis, immunity and—ultimately—therapy were direct results of the germ theory. Nevertheless, the germ theory and its derivative public health programs did not succeed in all respects. Evidence suggests that they played a relatively minor role in the subsequent decline of infectious diseases in the industrialized countries.

CAUSAL THEORIES AND CHANGING PATTERNS OF MORBIDITY

Epidemiologic Transition

It is well known that mortality has declined dramatically in the twentieth century, and that this decline has been facilitated largely by a shift in the leading causes of death from infectious to noninfectious diseases. That historic change in the structure of mortality has been termed the Epidemiologic Transition.

Interventions based on causal models derived from the germ theory are often credited with the twentieth century decline in infectious disease mortality. Fueled by declining morbidity and mortality, the development of antibiotic drugs, and the successful international campaign against smallpox, optimism that all infectious disease might soon be eliminated surged following the second world war. Techniques of mass immunization had been honed during the war, and campaigns against vaccine-preventable diseases were carried out worldwide. The logic of the germ theory was also turned on insect disease vectors, using newly developed chemical pesticides as antibiotic drugs on an environmental scale. Some of the most important and intractable infectious diseases, including measles, poliomyelitis, malaria, and yellow fever, seemed to yield to this aggressive approach. In the climate of the times, it did not seem like outrageous bravado for the American epidemiologist Charles-Edward Amory Winslow to title a 1943 book on the history of public health *The Conquest of Epidemic Disease* (Winslow 1943).

The wholesale elimination of infectious diseases would constitute the strongest possible validation of the germ theory, demonstrating that it not only predicted the behavior of organisms in the laboratory but allowed people to intervene with measurable success in the real world. In fact, however, history does not support this interpretation of the germ theory's application.

The Role of Medicine

In much of North America and Europe, mortality had already begun to decline in the early or middle nineteenth century, decades before the bacteriologic revolution, and continued steadily downward for the next 100 years despite the absence of specific medical measures that were effective against the leading infectious diseases. Thanks to this prolonged decline, mortality from the major infections had already been reduced manyfold by the time sulfa drugs, antiobiotics, and vaccination came into widespread use in the middle of the twentieth century. McKeown's historical analysis of the contribution of medicine to the improvement of health in England provides a number of striking examples (McKeown 1976). Mortality from tuberculosis, which was the leading cause of death in the nineteenth century, probably began to decline before 1800 and dropped from an annual rate of 400 deaths per 100,000 population by 1840 to 50 per 100,000 in 1940; the decline accelerated in the 1940s and 1950s when streptomycin, isoniazid, and other drug therapies became available, but the overall change attributable to modern curative treatment (from 50 to around 1 per 100,000 in 1980) was much smaller in absolute terms than the reduction that had already taken place (McKeown 1976; Comstock 1982). Similar patterns, with most of the reduction in mortality taking place before the introduction of specific medical treatments, occurred for other major infections, including typhoid, measles, scarlet fever, and whooping cough (McKeown 1976; McKinlay & McKinlay 1977).

This sequence of events is not compatible with the claim that medical interventions *caused* the modern decline in infectious diseases. Antibiotics and other drug therapies clearly have had a substantial effect in the last 50 years, especially in developing countries, where the previous reduction in mortality had been smaller. However, it is necessary to look to earlier historical periods for explanations of the most significant advances in health. McKeown (1976) attributed most of the reduction in infectious disease mortality in the nineteenth and early twentieth centuries to improvements in nutrition, environmental hygiene, and slower population growth, none of which required either knowledge of the specific agents of infection or the ability to intervene directly against them.

To argue that medical therapies were less important to the 100-year decline in mortality than environmental, technological, and social changes is not to deny that pathogenic organisms have a critical role in the production of infectious diseases. However, the profound importance of these changes, which were not specifically intended to control pathogens, demonstrates the inadequacy of a simple, unicausal theory that assumes pathogenic agents are necessary and sufficient causes of disease, and argues for the need to consider epidemic disease in a larger ecologic context.

Old Problems Persist, New Ones Emerge

If the importance of the ecology of infections was not apparent 20 years ago, it should be starkly obvious today. In the optimistic days of the 1970s, it was widely assumed that less affluent countries would, through industrialization, increasing affluence, and modern medical technology, experience steadily improving health to pass through the epidemiologic transition from infectious to chronic diseases as Western Europe and North America had. In reality, many countries are suspended between the two poles of the model transition, experiencing rising rates of mortality from lung cancer, heart disease, and injuries simultaneously with lingering infectious diseases, especially among children and the poor (Frenk 1989).

At the same time, infectious diseases have reemerged as important problems in countries that were thought to have completed the epidemiologic transition. Public health workers and physicians worldwide have been taken by surprise by the resurgence of diseases thought to be under control, like tuberculosis, and the appearance of previously unknown infections involving agents like HIV and Ebola virus. Some critics, from both within and outside public health, have attributed the failure to foresee these developments to decades of narrow thinking that focused on fighting infections with drugs, but ignored the ecologic interactions among microbes, vectors, humans and other hosts, and the environment within which all of them exist. The rapid pace and large scale of environmental change are among the overlooked factors suggested as catalysts for recent environmental changes, and possibly for more to come. Popular books have helped to rekindle interest in the ecology of disease (Garrett 1994; Preston 1994). Writers have described emergent infections as the earth's "revenge" for humans' destruction of natural ecosystems, and described the paving of a highway across Central Africa as "one of the most important events of the century," which "affected every person on earth" by initiating changes in microbial ecology (Preston 1994).

The public health establishment's unpreparedness for recent epidemiologic developments underscores the deficiency of traditional models of the causes of infections in populations and the approaches they engender. More effective causal models would allow change to be anticipated and facilitate appropriate responses to it. Infectious disease researchers have recently begun to give more serious consideration to the development of more appropriate paradigms.

MULTICAUSALITY IN EPIDEMIOLOGY

Emphasis on multiple causal factors, or "multicausality," arose in response to the simplified idea that an infectious agent is the unique and sufficient cause of an infectious disease. Methods of modern risk factor epidemiology and concepts about causality of disease have developed largely in application to noninfectious diseases in which a specific necessary disease agent is not recognized. In this approach, the causes of disease are considered to be agents, exposures, or risk factors. These factors may include microbes, chemicals, nutrients; anthropometric, physiologic and genetic characteristics as well as behaviors, mental states, race, or socioeconomic status.

The method of the discipline is to observe whether disease occurs more or less commonly among individuals who have the exposure or factor than among those who do not. The broader goal of explanation of the occurrence of disease in populations is pursued by attempting to enumerate risk and protective factors (the "independent variables") and their dose-response relations with a list of disease outcomes derived primarily from clinical practice (the "dependent variables"). This research has resulted in lists of carcinogens, cardiovascular risk factors, and health risk behaviors that are targeted for modification by hygienic, behavioral, or pharmacologic intervention.

Association and Causation

When disease is observed to occur at a different rate among exposed and nonexposed populations, it is said that exposure and disease are associated. Issues of causality in modern epidemiology primarily relate to sorting exposure-disease associations into two categories, causal and noncausal. This is clearly stated in the 1964 surgeon general's report on smoking and health, an early and prominent example of this causal reasoning. The surgeon general wrote, the "elements of causation in chronic disease" are: the consistency of the association, the strength of the association, the specificity of the association, the temporal relationship of the association, and the coherence of the association.

Consistency refers to variation of the association between subgroups or across studies. Evidence of a similar relationship between a factor and disease in various groups is considered to be more suggestive of a causal role for the factor than evidence of variation in the association. Lack of substantial effect modification is important to the consistency of the association.

Strength refers to the magnitude of the difference in disease between exposed and unexposed groups. The difference in disease rates is often expressed as a rate ratio, odds ratio, degree of elevation above background rates, or the ratio of cases observed to expected based on some average experience. Closely related to strength of association and noted as a separate quality in many presentations of criteria for making judgments about causality is the concept of dose response, or the gradient of the increase in disease as exposure increases. Perhaps because of a confusion in the medical literature between the strength of an association, which is assessed by measures such as relative risk, attributable risk, or regression coefficients, and the statistical significance of the association, significance level has sometimes been considered to be relevant to consideration of causality. However, the ambiguity of such statistical tests outside certain randomized settings means that this is not an appropriate general criterion.

Specificity means that the exposure is associated with a particular disease and not with disease in general. This criterion has its origins in infectious disease epidemiology in which the organism is expected to produce particular symptoms, and therefore would not be associated with disease in general. This criterion may be quite inappropriate for exposures such as cigarette smoke or undernutrition that are involved in the pathogenesis of a wide range of outcomes.

Temporal relationship means that the exposure leads to the disease rather than vice versa. The ability to establish the temporal relationship between exposure and disease is an often cited advantage of follow-up studies over cross sectional or case-control studies.

Coherence refers to the plausibility of the association in terms of biologic, physical, and social mechanisms, including the extent to which the observed association fits in with animal studies and other epidemiologic studies of the same or related factors. Of these criteria, coherence is the least specific, the least related to the collection of epidemiological data per se, and the most crucial.

Coherence has been called biologic plausibility (Hill 1965). Even stronger than biologic plausibility is demonstration of the mechanism by which an outcome is a consequence of a determinant; this has been called directionality (Susser 1991). It is evidence of a necessary cause that most clearly distinguishes the demonstration of the roles of infectious versus noninfectious agents in production of disease. In the case of infectious disease, Koch's postulates summarize the evidence that can be marshaled to demonstrate the role of a microbial agent in a specific case of disease in an individual. The organism is necessary for production of a disease that is defined as the pathologic consequences of infection with a particular organism. The problem of causality, from the perspective of risk factor epidemiology, derives from its engagement with diseases for which a necessary cause is not recognized. These tend to be noninfectious diseases. There are exceptions to this generalization, such as asbestosis, but most noninfectious diseases are medically defined in relation to diagnosis and treatment rather than to an etiologic agent. Thus, the primary issue in distinguishing a causal from a noncausal association has to do with showing that an agent and disease are associated because the agent acts pathologically to produce disease. In the case of noninfectious conditions that have been the primary focus of risk factor epidemiology, disease production can occur in the absence of the risk factor, that is, the factor is neither necessary nor sufficient to produce disease in a particular individual (although it may be necessary to produce mass disease).

Models of Causation

Multicausal thinking about factors that are neither necessary nor sufficient to produce disease has taken various forms. Factors that influence susceptibility to infection following exposure to an infectious agent, or disease following infection, may be considered as risk factors as in the case of noninfectious diseases. Thus, the consistency, strength, temporality, and specificity of the association between a susceptibility-related factor and disease rates might be considered along with evidence of mechanisms through which increased susceptibility would be produced. The agent and susceptibility factors may be pictured as a web of causation in which many physiologic, behavioral, and environmental factors are connected by arrows to indicate the direction of relationships. Another depiction of multicausality is the component cause model, which presents disease causality in terms of specific groups of separate factors that combine to result in disease. There may be many such combinations of factors. In the case of diseases with one necessary agent, including infectious diseases, all of these groups of causal factors, typically represented by pie diagrams, include the necessary agent.

Another heuristic device that has been used to describe the causal production of disease is the ecologic triad of host, agent, and environment. This model derives from Max von Pettenkoffer's argument that infectious diseases did not have a single cause, but could instead be likened to fermentation, which requires a host (carbohydrate), agent (yeast), and environment (temperature) in the proper combination (Rosenau 1927). Infectious diseases depend on the agent, host characteristics including behaviors and susceptibility states, and environmental factors that facilitate the viability of the agent and its transmission to the host.

The host-agent-environment model of causation is one way of explicitly recognizing that the agent produces disease in a context that involves characteristics of the host and of the social, physical, and biologic environment (including other species) that influence and are influenced by the agent and the host. Causal thinking in this tradition has been less influenced by a focus on independent exposure-disease associations and the attendant criteria for distinguishing causal from noncausal associations that characterize risk factor epidemiology, and more influenced by ecologic perspectives on complex interactions of various species.

Causal Criteria and Study Design

The perspective of risk factor epidemiology, that exposures are the causes of disease in populations, is mirrored in the model for modern epidemiologic study designs, the randomized experiment. In this approach, subjects with specific characteristics, including absence of a disease or outcome of interest, can be chosen for study. Next, they can be allocated to be exposed or unexposed to a factor according to rules that, as in the well-shuffled decks of repeated card games, tend toward an even distribution of the heterogeneous study subjects between exposure groups over the course of many trials. During the period of application of controlled amounts of exposure (or nonexposure), all other conditions affecting the subjects can be held constant. Finally, the subjects are available to the researcher for determination of the outcome characteristics in members of each group, using a standardized protocol. The analysis of such a study amounts to a comparison of the frequency of the outcomes of interest in the groups. Differences in frequency that persist over many trials, or that are obtained in a small number of large trials, are attributed to the action of the experimental agent.

According to this logic, study designs that more closely approximate a randomized experiment can provide more compelling evidence of causation than less controlled designs. This hierarchy of methods for producing evidence is represented in Table 3–1. The left columns shows the traditional ranking in value of a list of typical epidemiologic study designs. The other columns indicate some of their key characteristics and the strength of the causal implication typically accorded to their evidence. Historical studies of particular cases or of populations that lack controls are considered to provide the weakest evidence. Slightly more compelling are aggregate studies that lack individual-level information on exposure and disease, such as time trend studies or international comparisons. Cross-sectional surveys collect individual data on exposures and outcomes but are unable to confirm that the exposure preceded the outcome. All these types of studies are considered to be primarily descriptive in nature and suited to generating hypotheses about specific exposure-disease associations, not to testing hypotheses, which, in this assessment, is considered to be a more rigorous

Table 3–1 Hierarchy of Modern Epidemiologic Study Designs According to the Perspective of Risk Factor Epidemiology

| Design | Comment | Traditional Evaluation | | | Potential Context Sensitivity |
		Hypothesis Generating	Hypothesis Testing	Causal Implications	
Case history	No controls	✔		Speculative	High
Aggregate	Group unit	✔		Possibly suggestive	↑
Cross-sectional	No temporal information	✔		Somewhat suggestive	
Case-control	Retrospective information	✔	✔	Moderately suggestive	
Cohort follow up	Prospective information	✔	✔	Strongly suggestive	↓
Randomized clinical trial	Experimental		✔	Firm	Absent

Source: Adapted from Ibrahim, 1985.

scientific activity with stronger causal implications. The hypothesis testing designs are defined as analytical in contrast to the less powerful descriptive designs. These are sometimes called quasi-experimental designs and attempt to collect data on exposure and outcome in more controlled settings, often involving more selected groups of study subjects.

In this approach to establishing causality of disease, factors that can be manipulated experimentally, such as therapeutic and preventive interventions, are the only factors that can receive the strongest level of support. To more closely approximate experimental conditions, observational studies often restrict samples to produce greater comparability between exposed and unexposed groups. Other variables are statistically controlled in the analysis so that differences in disease rates may be more clearly attributed to exposure and less confounded by other differences between exposure groups. Because control over measurement and monitoring of study subjects is central to the experimental model, and because of the importance of knowing that exposure precedes disease, individual follow up is important.

The focus on isolating independent exposure-disease associations, and on characteristics that are considered to be solely properties of individual humans rather than reflections of the physical and social developmental environment, mitigates against attention to the complex ecologic context in which disease and exposure emerge. Such considerations may be more evident in aggregate or case series designs that are at the low end of the hierarchy of study designs according to the risk factor perspective. This situation is depicted in the right-most column of Table 3–1, which indicates that designs which are more experimental most effectively exclude the context. The experiment, in which the exposure is determined by the experimenter, excludes the importance of where the exposure comes from, what changes occurred during its production, and why certain population groups continue to be exposed over time.

In contrast, aggregate studies of time trends in diseases and exposures, or case studies of epidemiologic transition, such as the shift from infectious to noninfectious diseases as the major public health problems, may focus attention on the ecologic context including such features as agriculture and transportation systems, occupational and environmental regulations, levels of poverty, and access to medical care in the general population. More experimental study designs achieve their control and specificity by excluding complex contexts for the purpose of assessing a particular exposure-disease relationship while holding everything else constant.

By considering the causes of disease to be agents or exposures, by establishing a hierarchy of decision making about causality that places greatest weight on experimental and quasi-experimental evidence, and by excluding ecologic relationships from primary consideration as causes of disease, risk factor epidemiology effectively excludes human social and economic organization from a central place in disease causality. The epidemiologic triad, a model largely abandoned in modern epidemiology texts that discuss criteria for determining whether or not associations are causal, had a more explicit place for social and economic forces. Such concerns continue to be represented in infectious disease studies that are focused less on risk factors and more on human ecology.

CONCLUSION

We have presented the topic of causal thinking in epidemiology from a historical perspective in order to emphasize the choices that today's researchers make in justifying the logic of their hypotheses, study designs, and approaches to data analysis. Although both laboratory and statistical technologies used by epidemiologists have become more powerful during the last century, the causal thinking that provides the philosophical basis for epidemiologic inquiry in public health has not shown similar growth and sophistication. Rather, the competing causal ideas that informed debates among contagion, miasma, moral, and political explanations of disease remain in much the same form that existed in the mid-1800s. For example, a virus, personal moral failure, and discrimination on the basis of sexual orientation and race, have all been cited as the cause of the HIV epidemic.

We strongly recommend adoption of a nuanced historical and ecologic approach to evaluating disease causality. Such an approach, while utilizing quantitative and methodological insights offered in evaluation of risk factors, should explicitly consider physical, biological, and social aspects of the context in which risk factors are considered. Placing risk factors in context may be viewed as contrary to principles of experimental design and analysis that demand that a complex myriad of factors be held constant while one or a few factors are isolated. However, this apparent contradiction can be dissolved by taking a more dialectical approach to causality, one that utilizes the strength of the experimental approach as a heuristic model, useful in a limited domain, but not a basis for an ontological model of the occurrence of disease in populations. In this way, evidence collected through experimental and quasi-experimental designs, the approach of most population-based epidemiologic studies, must be interpreted in light of the co-evolution of host, agent, and environment, human population dynamics, and ecologic and political systems.

The idea of causality is strongly connected to public health practice. Once something is identified as a cause, it becomes a potential target for intervention and disease control. Decisions about what causes disease may lead us to vaccinate against specific organisms, issue directions to boil water, disinfect the water supply, control sources of contamination, improve the food supply, or reduce poverty. In this way, scientific decisions about cause are deeply political and ethical. Rather than disguise these more complex and moral dimensions of the assessment of causality, epidemiologists are responsible to make them as clear as possible so that scientists, policymakers, and the public can engage in more open debate about the best ways to improve public health.

REFERENCES

Ackerknecht EH. Anticontagionism between 1821 and 1867. Bull. Hist. Med. 562–593, 1948.

Brown, ER. Rockefeller Medicine Men: Medicine and Capitalism in America. Berkeley: University of California Press, 1979.

Budd, William. On the Causes of Fevers (1839). Baltimore: Johns Hopkins University Press, 1984.

Chapin, CV. The need of quantitative methods in epidemiological work. In: Chapin CV, Papers of Charles V. Chapin, MD: A Review of Public Health Realities. New York: Commonwealth Fund, 1934.

Chapin, CV. Dirt, disease and health officer. In: Chapin CV, Papers of Charles V. Chapin, MD: A Review of Public Health Realities. New York: Commonwealth Fund, 1934.

Cipolla, CM, Miasmas and Disease: Public Health and the Environment in the Pre-Industrial Age. New Haven: Yale, 1992.

Coleman, W. Death is a Social Disease: Public Health and Political Economy in Early Industrial France. Madison, WI: Univ. of Wisconsin Press, 1982.

Comstock, GW. Epidemiology of tuberculosis. Am. Rev. Respir. Dis. 125: 8–15, 1982.

Cullen MJ. The Statistical Movement in Early Victorian Britain: The Foundations of Empirical Social Research. New York: Harvester Press, 1975.

Dubos R, and Dubos J. The White Plague: Tuberculosis, Man and Society. Boston: Little, Brown, 1952.

Engels F. The Condition of the Working Class in England in 1844. Oxford/New York: Oxford University Press, 1993 (originally published in 1845).

Evans AS. Causation and disease: a chronological journey. Am. J. Epidemiol. 108: 249–258, 1978.

Eyler, JM. Victorian Social Medicine: The Ideas and Methods of William Farr. Baltimore: Johns Hopkins University Press, 1979.

Fee, E. Disease and Discovery: A History of the Johns Hopkins School of Hygiene and Public Health, 1916–1939. Baltimore: Johns Hopkins University Press, 1987.

Fracastoro G. De contagione et contagiosis morbis et eorum curatione, libri III, with translation and notes by Wilmer Cave Wright. New York, London: G. P. Putnam's Sons, 1930.

Frenk J, Bobadilla JL, Sepulveda J, Lopez Cervantez M. Health transition in the middle-income countries: new challenges for health care. Health Policy and Planning 4:29–39, 1989.

Frost WH. Epidemiology. In: Maxcy KF, Ed., The Papers of Wade Hampton Frost: A Contribution to the Epidemiological Method. New York: Commonwealth Fund, 1941.

Garrett, L. The Coming Plague: Newly Emerging Diseases in a World out of Balance. New York: Farrar, Straus and Giroux, 1994.

Greenwood M. Epidemics and Crowd Diseases: An Inroduction to the Study of Epidemiology. New York: Macmillan, 1933.

Hacking I. The Taming of Chance. Cambridge: Cambridge University Press, 1990.

Hill AB. The environment and disease: association or causation? Proc. R. Soc. Med. 58: 295–300, 1965.

Ibrahim M. Epidemiology and Health Policy. Rockville, MD: Aspen Systems Corp., 1985.

Kunitz SJ. Hookworm and pellagra: exemplary diseases in the New South. J Health Soc. Behav. 29:139–148, 1988.

MacKenzie DA. Statistics in Britain 1865–1930: The Social Construction of Scientific Knowledge. Edinburgh: Edinburgh University Press, 1981.

MacMahon B, and Pugh TF. Epidemiology: Principles and Methods. Boston: Little, Brown, 1970.

McKeown T. The Role of Medicine: Dream, Mirage or Nemesis? London: Nuffield Provincial Hospitals Trust, 1976.

McKinlay JB, McKinlay SM. The questionable contribution of medical measures to the decline of mortality in the United States in the twentieth century. Milbank Mem. Fund Q. Health Soc. 55:405–428, 1977.

Panum, PL. Observations made during the epidemic of measles on the Faroe Islands in the year 1846. New York: Delta Omega Society; distributed by the American Public Health Association, 1940.

Preston, R. The Hot Zone. New York: Random House, 1994.

Rosen GA. History of Public Health. The Johns Hopkins University Press, 1993 (originally published 1958).

Rosenau MJ. Preventive Medicine and Hygiene. 5th ed. New York: Appleton-Century, 1927.

Snow J. Snow on Cholera. New York: Commonwealth Fund, 1936.

Stallybrass, CO. The Principles of Epidemiology and the Process of Infection. London: G. Routledge & Son, ltd. 1931.

Susser M. What is a cause and how do we know one? A grammar for pragmatic epidemiology. Am. J. Epidemiol. 133: 635–648, 1991.

Taylor, R, Rieger A. Medicine as social science: Rudolf Virchow on the typhus epidemic in Upper Silesia. Int. J. Health Serv. 15:547–559, 1985.

Winslow C-EA. The Conquest of Epidemic Disease: A Chapter in the History of Ideas. Madison WI: University of Wisconsin Press, 1980 (originally published 1943).

4

Concepts of Transmission and Dynamics

M. ELIZABETH HALLORAN

Transmission from one host to another is fundamental to the survival strategy of most infectious agents. Each microbe has its own life cycle, modes of transmission, population dynamics, evolutionary pressures, and molecular and immunologic interaction with its host. The transmission cycle may involve a particular insect or other vector, and consequently its ecology. Studies and interventions need to take the particular transmission, dynamics, and biology of each infectious agent into account.

Some underlying principles of transmission and dynamics, however, are common to many infectious diseases. These principles are captured in a wide variety of mathematical and statistical models. Since the human host population is the ecological niche for the infectious agent, some of the principles come from general theories of populations, evolution, and ecology (see Burnet and White 1972, McNeill 1976). Other principles have their origins in infectious disease epidemiology.

Many different questions motivate quantitative transmission models. A few examples follow.

- What is the probability that transmission will occur after a susceptible host is exposed to infection? How do transmission dynamics and interventions influence the evolution of a microbe? How do different models of transmission influence our thinking? How do different assumptions about human contact patterns influence the design and analysis of field studies?
- Under what conditions will an epidemic occur? Will an infectious agent become established in a population and either persist or die out? Will a microbe establish itself within a host and avoid immune surveillance and clearance?
- What interventions can prevent an epidemic or eliminate endemic transmission? What interventions will reduce transmission and by how much? What will the long-term effects of an intervention be in a population? What is the best intervention type and resource allocation strategy? What is the optimal timing? How do different subpopulations influence transmission of an infectious agent and choice of intervention strategies?

When the appropriate data are available, the models can be used to estimate quantities of interest to answer the above questions.

How we think about the transmission dynamics of an infectious agent within a host population influences how we design and interpret epidemiologic studies. It can influence our choice of interventions. Mixing structures, contact patterns, and subpopulations can affect both transmission dynamics and the results of studies. In this chapter, we consider some basic principles and simple models of transmission and population dynamics of infectious diseases. We focus on aspects of transmission and dynamics that have consequences for the design of studies and interpretation of results.

STATES OF INFECTION WITHIN A HOST

The natural history of infection within a host can be described with reference to either infectiousness or disease (Fig. 4–1). Both time lines begin with the successful infection of the susceptible host by the microbe. The natural history of infectiousness includes the *latent period*, the time interval from infection to becoming infectious, and the *infectious period*, during which time the host could infect another host or vector. Eventually the host becomes noninfectious, either by clearing the infection, possibly developing immunity, or by death. The host can also become noninfectious while still harboring the microbe. The host may become an infectious *carrier* if he or she recovers from disease but remains infectious (i.e., asymptomatically infected).

The natural history of disease in the infected host includes the *incubation period*, the time from infection to symptomatic disease, and the *symptomatic period*. The probability of developing symptomatic disease after becoming infected is the *pathogenicity* of the interaction of the microbe with the host. Eventually the host leaves the symptomatic state, either by recovering from the symptoms or by death. If the microbe has provoked an autoimmune response in the host, symptoms can continue even after the microbe is cleared. An *inapparent case* or *silent infection* is a successful infection that does not produce symptoms in the host. Inapparent cases can be infectious.

While the disease process and its associated time line are important to the infected person and to a physician, the dynamics of

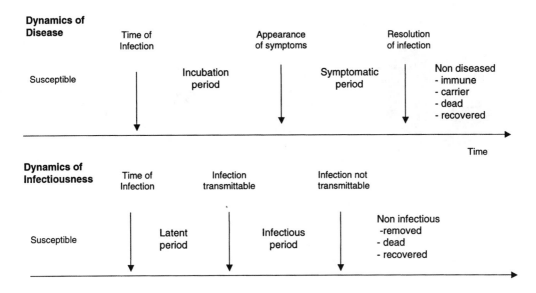

Figure 4–1. Natural history time lines for infection and disease.

infectiousness are important for propagation of the microbe and for public health. The relation of the two time lines to one another is specific to each microbe and can have important implications for study design, modeling, and public health.

For example, Elveback and colleagues (1976) developed an influenza model that distinguished between illness and infection attack rates. The infected people become infectious, but only a fraction of them develop overt disease. In many studies of infectious agents, it is easier to use overt disease as the outcome, rather than infection, since infection may be difficult to ascertain. If many infections are inapparent, however, using overt disease would result in an underestimate of the level of exposure to infection in the population. Estimation of the incubation and latent periods can be difficult because the time of infection as well as the onset of infectiousness are often difficult to observe.

Human immunodeficiency virus (HIV) poses a particular problem for public health because the virus has a short latent period and a long incubation period. A person infected with HIV can infect many people before symptoms develop. *Plasmodium falciparum*, one of the organisms that causes human malaria, has an incubation period of about 14 days, but the infective stages do not appear until about 10 days after the first symptoms. Thus early treatment of symptoms with a drug that also kills or prevents infective stages could have an important effect on transmission. In chickenpox, the latent period is about two days shorter than the incubation period. Thus by the time symptoms appear, a child can infect many other children. Keeping children with symptomatic chickenpox out of school might not have a large effect on transmission. Gonorrhea infection in women is often asymptomatic, so women often go untreated. In men, the infection is often quite painful, leading them to seek treatment. Thus the duration of infectiousness tends to be shorter in men than in women for reasons related to the different time lines of disease in men and women.

TRANSMISSION MODELS

One measure of the success of an infectious agent is how effectively it is transmitted. The *transmission probability p* is the probability that, given a contact between an infective source and a susceptible host, successful transfer of the microbe will occur so that the susceptible host becomes infected (Fig. 4–2). The transmission probability is a key quantity both in epidemiology and in infectious disease models. There are many different ways of modeling the probability of becoming infected upon repeated exposure to infection. We consider the simple binomial model

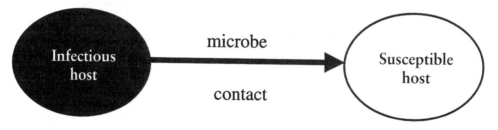

Transmission probability depends on:
- Type and definition of contact
- Microbe
- Infectious host
- Susceptible host

Figure 4–2. Transmission from an infective to a susceptible host during contact.

of transmission for discrete contacts and, briefly, a simple model in continuous time.

Binomial Models of Probability of Infection

The binomial model of transmission can help answer several questions. What is the effect of an intervention in a population? How do we interpret our assumptions about how a risk factor or intervention affects the transmission probability? How well is one infectious agent transmitted compared to another? When the appropriate data are available from field studies, the binomial model is often used to estimate the transmission probability.

The basic idea of the binomial model is that exposure to infection occurs in discrete contacts and that each contact is independent of another. We define p as the transmission probability during a contact between a susceptible person and an infectious person or other source of infection, such as an infectious mosquito. Then the probability that the susceptible person will not be infected during the contact is $q = 1 - p$. The quantity q is called the *escape probability*. For example, if the transmission probability for herpes simplex is $p = 0.30$, then the escape probability for one contact is $q = 1 - p = 0.70$. If a susceptible person makes n contacts with infectious people, then, assuming all contacts are equally infectious, the probability of escaping infection from all the n contacts is $q^n = (1 - p)^n$. The probability of being infected after n contacts with infectives is $1 - q^n = 1 - (1 - p)^n$.

Suppose a person has six successive sexual contacts with someone who has genital herpes (Fig. 4–3A). What is ithe probability that the person will have become infected after six contacts? In this example, $n = 6$. The calculation proceeds by first calculating the probability that the susceptible person will escape infection from all six contacts. Then this number is subtracted from one to get the probability that the person is infected at least once. If the probability of escaping infection from the first exposure is $q = 0.7$, then the probability of escaping infection from the second exposure is the probability of escaping the first one times the probability of escaping the second: $q \times q = 0.7 \times 0.7 = 0.49$. The probability of escaping infection from the third contact is similarly the probability of escaping infection from the first two contacts times the probability of escaping infection from the third: $q^2 \times q = 0.49 \times 0.7 = 0.34$. The probability of escaping infection from six successive contacts is $0.7^6 = 0.12$. The probability of becoming infected at least once is $1 - (1 - p)^n = 1 - (0.7)^6 = 0.88$.

We have made an important assumption here. We assumed that each successive contact was not affected by any of the previous contacts. That is, the person did not develop immunity or become more susceptible as time went on. We also assumed that all of the contacts had the same risk of transmission. These assumptions may not be fulfilled. If so, the assumptions can easily be changed and a more complicated form of the binomial model developed.

In a different problem, suppose a susceptible child attends school one day where six of the children simultaneously have influenza. What is the probability of becoming infected (Fig. 4–3B)? Assume that the probability of becoming infected from one contact with one child with influenza is $p = 0.3$. Proceeding as before, the probability of escaping infection from one child is $q = 0.7$. Now we can calculate the probability of being infected from all six children, with a $0.7^6 = 0.12$, so the probability of being infected on that day at school is $1 - q^6 = 0.88$.

Although the answers for the two examples are numerically the same, in the second example we made a different biological assumption than in the first. In the example of influenza at school, we assumed that each of the six *simultaneous* exposures to infection is the same, and that each additional child with influenza increases the probability of being infected independent of how many other infective children are present. The contacts and exposures to infection are assumed to operate the same as if they were successive and independent. The assumption of independence is commonly used in the binomial model, whether contacts are si-

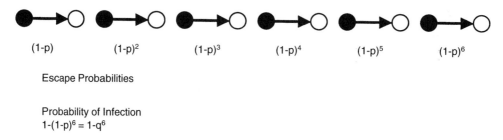

Escape Probabilities

Probability of Infection
$1-(1-p)^6 = 1-q^6$

Figure 4–3A. The probability of infection with six consecutive contacts.

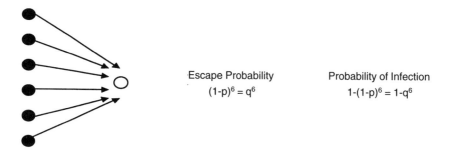

Escape Probability
$(1-p)^6 = q^6$

Probability of Infection
$1-(1-p)^6 = 1-q^6$

Figure 4–3B. The probability of infection with six simultaneous contacts.

multaneous or successive. For instance, this assumption is at the heart of the Reed-Frost model discussed later.

What if, however, biologically we think that once there is one infectious child in a classroom, then the room is saturated with infectious particles? Then adding more infectious children to the school will not increase the probability of becoming infected. We need to change our expression for the probability of becoming infected. If p is the probability of becoming infected from one infected person at school, then $q = 1 - p$ is again the escape probability from exposure to one infected. In contrast to the previous model, however, the probability of becoming infected from exposure to two or more infectives at the same time is still p and the escape probability is still $q = 1 - p$. Under these biologic assumptions, the probability of becoming infected from one child with influenza on one day is $p = 0.3$, and the probability of becoming infected from simultaneous exposure to six children with influenza

on one day is also $p = 0.3$. The Greenwood model (Greenwood 1931) makes the assumption that the probability of infection on a given day does not change with increased number of infectives. The assumption is seldom used in practice, however. We could make assumptions between the two extremes, but there are generally not enough data to support using more complex models.

As discussed in Chapter 5, Overview of Study Design, the binomial model is useful in estimating the transmission probability if data are available on the number of potentially infectious contacts that susceptibles in a study population make as well as the number of susceptibles who become infected.

Other Transmission Models

Another way to model the probability of becoming infected is simply to multiply the number of contacts with infectives (n) times the transmission probability (p), np. In the previous example of herpes, however, $np = 6 \times 0.3 = 1.8$. Since probabilities have to lie between 0 and 1, this approach obviously has limits. In particular, either n or p, or both need to be small. Another commonly used expression for the probability of not becoming infected is e^{-np}. So, the probability of becoming infected is $1 - e^{-np}$. In the herpes example above, then, the probability of not becoming infected is $e^{-6 \times 0.3} = e^{-1.8} = 0.17$ and for becoming infected is $1 - e^{-1.8} = 0.83$. Comparing this with the probability of being infected calculated from the binomial model, 0.88, we note that they are similar but not identical.

In the herpes example, the transmission probability is high, and the product of np is large. If the transmission probability is much smaller or the contact rate is much smaller, or both, then the three methods for calculating the probability of becoming infected give similar answers. Suppose again that there are six infectious contacts in one day, but that the transmission probability of the infection in question is just $p = 0.001$. Then using the binomial model, the probability of becoming infected is $1 - (1 - p)^n = 1 - (.999)^6 = 0.00599$. Using the exponential expression, the probability of becoming infected is $1 - \exp(-6 \times 0.001) = 0.00598$, and based on the simple expression, $np = 6 \times 0.001 = 0.006$. There is a little difference in the answers. In this example, the calculated np makes sense as the probability of becoming infected. The two simpler approaches are sometimes used as approximations for the binomial model. They are generally less time consuming to compute than the binomial model, which can be an issue in complex models. However, as we have just demonstrated, the approximation will not always be good. If used for estimation, all three models require the same data. In general, it is good to use the binomial model if feasible.

Continuous Models for Probabilitiy of Infection

The binomial model assumes discrete contacts or discrete units of time. Another approach to modeling the probability of becoming infected assumes that contacts occur in continuous time. This approach is usually based on the contact rate per unit time, which we denote by c. Thus cp is the probability of being infected per unit time if all the contacts are with infectious persons. Analogous to the discrete model, the expressions $\exp(-cp)$ and $1 - \exp(-cp)$ are the probabilities of escaping infection or becoming infected per unit time, respectively. If the exposure occurs over some time period Δt, then the probabilities of escape or of infection are $\exp(-cp\Delta t)$ and $1 - \exp(-cp\Delta t)$, respectively. The data needed for using this approach to estimate the transmission probability are the contact rate with infectives per unit time, the time interval, and the infection status of each person in the study.

Contacts with Persons of Unknown Infection Status

Sometimes contacts are made with persons or sources of unknown infection status. We denote the probability that an individual with whom a contact is made is infectious by P. Then the probability of being infected from a contact of unknown infection status is $\rho = pP$. The quantity ρ is not a transmission probability in the strict sense, but an infection probability. The probability of escaping infection from contact with someone of unknown infection status is $1 - \rho = 1 - pP$. Under the binomial model, the probability of becoming infected after n such contacts is $1 - (1 - pP)^n = 1 - (1 - \rho)^n$.

Suppose as in the genital herpes example above that $p = 0.3$ but that the contacts are with six individuals of unknown infection status. If the individuals are randomly chosen from a population where the prevalence of genital herpes is $P = 0.4$, then the probability of being infected after six contacts is $1 - (1 - 0.3 \times 0.4)^6 = 0.54$.

An analogous expression for the infection probability can be developed for the continuous time model. The probability of being infected per unit time is the incidence rate or hazard rate of infection. An expression for the incidence rate, I, as a function of the contact rate, the transmission probability, and the prevalence is $I = cpP$. This expression for the incidence rate as a function of prevalence is a fundamental relation of dependent happenings (Ross 1916) in infectious diseases, discussed in more detail in Chapter 5, Overview of Study Design. The probability of escaping infection within some period of time Δt is $\exp(-cpP\Delta t)$, and of being infected is $1 - \exp(-cpP\Delta t)$. At the population level, the probability of becoming infected in some period of time is closely related to the incidence proportion.

These examples show some of the options and subtleties inherent in different approaches to modeling the transmission process.

Modeling Risk Factors for the Transmission Probability

How do risk factors or interventions play a role in the probability of becoming infected during a contact between an infectious person and a susceptible person? How does the choice of models affect our answer? Suppose we are doing a study of a vaginal foam to prevent genital herpes transmission. We believe that the vaginal foam reduces the probability of transmission per sex act by 80%. We might formulate our binomial model so that foam reduces the transmission probability, p, by 80% in everyone who uses it and at every sex act with an infective. Then the transmission probability in people using foam, p_{foam}, would be 20% of that in people not using it, so that $p_{foam} = 0.20p$. Since the factor 0.20 multiplies the baseline p, we are assuming that the foam has a *multiplicative effect* on the transmission probability. The protection is not complete, since the people using foam still have a transmission probability of $0.20p$. Thus, a multiplicative effect is sometimes called *leaky*, because it denotes only partial protection, allowing microbes to get through the defense. Note that we have also assumed that the effect is the same in everyone and for every contact.

Suppose we want to evaluate the effect of using vaginal foam in a study population of 2000 sexual partnerships, where one partner is infected in each partnership. Half of the partnerships use foam, the other half do

not. We decide to use the incidence proportion ratio at the end of the study to estimate the relative risk of infection with and without foam. The first study we conduct is one month long and each partnership has exactly five contacts during that time. If $p = 0.25$, then $p_{foam} = 0.20 \times 0.25 = 0.05$. What is the expected incidence proportion at the end of one month?

In the group not using vaginal foam, the probability of becoming infected is $1 - (1 - p)^5 = 1 - 0.75^5 = 0.76$, so the expected number of infections in that group is 1000 people $\times 0.76 = 760$. In the group using foam, the probability of becoming infected is $1 - (1 - 0.05)^5 = 1 - 0.95^5 = 0.23$, so the expected number of infections in that group is 1000 people $\times 0.23 = 230$. The incidence proportion ratio we would expect to see at the end of one month is $(230/1000)/(760/1000) = 0.30$. The incidence proportion ratio, 0.30, is not equal to the multiplicative effect of the foam on the transmission probability, 0.20. The efficacy of the vaginal foam based on the incidence proportion ratio would be estimated to be $1 - 0.30 = 0.70$, not $1 - 0.20 = 0.80$, the efficacy per single contact.

What happens to the incidence proportion ratio if we continue the study for two months? Suppose that after two months, each partnership has had exactly ten sexual contacts. Now the expected number of infections in the control group is $(1 - .75^{10}) \times 1000 = 943$, while in the group using vaginal foam, it is $(1 - 0.95^{10}) \times 1000 = 401$. We expect to see an incidence proportion ratio after two months of $(401/1000)/(943/1000) = 0.43$. The incidence proportion ratio has increased from 0.30 to 0.43. The efficacy appears to be 0.57, not 0.70, as it would after one month, or 0.80, for a single contact. The intervention seems less efficacious after two months even though the effect of the vaginal foam on the transmission probability has not waned.

As the number of exposures in the two groups increase, the incidence proportion ratio will continue to increase toward one as it did from one month (five contacts) to two months (ten contacts total), and efficacy will appear to decrease. Eventually everyone in both groups will become infected under the multiplicative assumption if they are exposed often enough. This illustrates the meaning of a multiplicative or leaky model at the transmission probability level. In principle, people can still become infected if exposed often enough. A different model might assume that vaginal foam protected 80% of the users completely, while 20% not at all. In this situation, at least 80% of the 1000 people using foam in the study would never become infected. This illustrates the difference between assuming a multiplicative model where the effect is the same for everyone and assuming a heterogeneous distribution of protection. Smith and colleagues (1984) and Halloran and associates (1991, 1992) provide further discussion of this point.

Suppose we use the model in continuous time developed earlier, and we assume that the protective effect has the same multiplicative effect on the transmission probability. In this partner study the contacts are all potentially infectious, $P = 1$, thus $I(t)_{\text{foam}} = 0.20cp$. Using this expression, the incidence rate ratio will be 0.20, giving the same answer as the multiplicative effect on the transmission probability. The expected incidence proportions in the two groups are not the same as those obtained using the binomial model. For the nonfoam group, the probability of being infected after one month is $1 - \exp(-5 \times 0.25) = 0.713$ and for the foam group it is $1 - \exp(-5 \times 0.05) = 0.221$, so the expected number of infections is 221 in the group using vaginal foam and 713 in the nonfoam group. The number of expected infections is different than calculated above from the discrete binomial model. The incidence proportion ratio is $(221/1000)/(713/1000) = 0.31$ after one month, which is similar though not identical to that calculated above.

In summary, there are three important points: (1) The binomial model of infection is widely used in practice. (2) There are differences between assuming that a contact process occurs discretely or that it occurs in continuous time. It is not possible to say that one approach is better than the other. They are simply different, and sometimes produce different answers. (3) The effect of a risk factor at the level of the transmission probability might be different from the apparent effect that will be estimated if using the incidence rate ratio or the incidence proportion ratio. Care should be taken to be precise in interpreting estimated relative risks.

BASIC REPRODUCTIVE NUMBER

Another key quantity in infectious diseases is the basic reproductive number, R_0, pronounced "are-zero" or "are-naught." The concept comes from general population theory. Understanding R_0 is important for public health applications and for describing the population biology of a parasite in a population of hosts. For small microbes such as viruses and bacteria, also called *microparasitic diseases* in the population biology literature, R_0 is defined as the expected number of new infectious hosts that one infectious host will produce during his or her infectious period in a large population that is completely susceptible. R_0 does not include the new cases produced by the secondary cases, or cases further down the chain. It also does not include secondary cases who do not become infectious.

For example, if $R_0 = 6$ for mumps in a human population, then one infectious person in that population would be expected to produce six new secondary infectious cases if the population were completely susceptible. If the infectious person produced three additional cases who were not infectious, R_0 would still be 6.

For microparasitic infections, R_0 is the product of the contact rate c, the duration of infectiousness d, and the transmission probability per contact with the infectious person, p. The average number of contacts made by an infectious person is the product of the contact rate and the duration of infectiousness—cd. The number of new infections produced by one infective during his or her infectious period is the product of the number of contacts in that time interval and the transmission probability per contact:

$$R_0 = \begin{array}{c}\text{number} \\ \text{of} \\ \text{contacts} \\ \text{per unit} \\ \text{time}\end{array} \times \begin{array}{c}\text{transmission} \\ \text{probability} \\ \text{per contact}\end{array} \times \begin{array}{c}\text{duration of} \\ \text{infectiousness}\end{array} = cpd.$$

As presented here, the expression assumes that everyone who gets infected becomes infectious. A term could be included for the probability of becoming infectious after infection. The simplest assumption is that the recovery rate, r, is constant. Then the duration of infectiousness equals the reciprocal of the rate of recovery from the infectiousness, that is $d = 1/r$. Another expression for R_0 is then $R_0 = cp/r$.

R_0 summarizes many important aspects of an infectious agent in a host population in one quantity. It allows comparison of seemingly disparate diseases from the viewpoint of population biology. A value of R_0 is not specific to a microbe, but to a microbe population within a particular host population at a particular time. Contact rates relevant for respiratory transmission will be lower in rural areas than in more densely populated urban areas. So, for example, we expect the R_0 of mumps to be lower in rural than in urban areas. The R_0 of malaria may be low during the season of low mosquito density but high during the season in which mosquitoes are plentiful. The R_0 of HIV in a sexually active population of single people might be much higher than it is in a population of fairly monogamous married couples.

R_0 is dimensionless. It represents the number of new infectious cases per index infectious case (i.e., referent or original case). Without further information about the magnitude of the quantities composing R_0 we cannot conclude much about the time frame of an epidemic, the transmissibility of the microbe, or the contact rate. R_0 is about 2 to 3 for influenza in some populations and also about 2 to 3 for HIV in some populations. Influenza has a relatively high transmission probability and short duration of infectiousness. The influenza virus spreads on a different time scale than HIV, which has a low transmission probability and longer duration of infectiousness. If we were to know only that $R_0 = 3$ for both, then we

would know that they both could easiliy produce epidemics, but we would not be able to draw conclusions about the relative time frames of the two. For that, we require further information.

The R_0 for indirectly transmitted diseases depends on the product of the two components of transmission. Indirectly transmitted diseases are those in which an infectious agent is transmitted between two different host populations. An example is the vector-borne disease malaria, which is transmitted from humans to mosquitoes and back to humans.

The definition of R_0 assumes that all contacts are with susceptibles. In real populations, however, people are often immune to a parasite. Under these circumstances, the expected number of new cases produced by an infectious person is less than R_0 and is called the *effective reproductive number*, denoted by R. If x is the proportion of a randomly mixing, homogeneous population that is susceptible, R is the product of R_0 times the proportion x of the contacts made with susceptibles:

$$R = R_0 x. \tag{1}$$

Suppose that $R_0 = 3$ for influenza in a population and that one-half of the population is immune. Then the effective reproductive number for influenza is $R = 3 \times 0.5 = 1.5$. A case of influenza would produce on average only 1.5 new secondary cases rather than 3 in this population.

R_0 and Public Health

Under what conditions will an epidemic occur? In general, for an epidemic to occur in a susceptible population, R_0 must be greater than one. If R_0 is less than one, an average case will not reproduce itself, so a microbe will not spread. Since R_0 is an average, a particular infectious person could produce more than one infective case, even when R_0 is less than 1, so there may be a small cluster of cases. We would not, however, expect a self-sustaining outbreak.

When a microbe has established itself and is endemic so that, over time, the average incidence does not change, then each infectious case must be producing on average one infectious case, that is, replacing itself. Otherwise the average incidence would either be increasing or decreasing. Thus at equilibrium, on average, $R = 1$.

How might we reduce or eliminate an infectious agent from a host population? If we want to reduce transmission so that the microbe will die out, then we must keep the average number of secondary cases produced by one infectious case below 1, R is less than 1. Suppose that $R_0 = 3$ for genital herpes in a population. To prevent an epidemic, we would need to decrease the contact rate by more than a factor of three. Alternatively, if vaginal foam reduced the transmission probability by 80%, then R_0 would be reduced to $0.2 \times 3 = 0.6$ if everybody used it. Thus, an epidemic might effectively be prevented either by reducing the contact rate or by use of an effective vaginal foam. Suppose that without treatment, an average case of tuberculosis is infectious for one year. If an average case produces five other cases, then $R_0 = 5$. By using active case detection, it might be possible to find cases in the first month of being infectious and treat with antibiotics. If the treated cases become noninfectious within two weeks after beginning treatment, then they would be infectious on average for only six weeks rather than 52 weeks. The R_0 would be reduced to about $(6/52) \times 5 = 0.6$.

What fraction, f, of the population do we need to vaccinate to produce enough immune people so that the infective people will not each be able to infect on average one other person? If the fraction of susceptibles is low enough, the probability that an infective host has contact with a susceptible host before recovering will be very low. The microbe will not be able to persist. Suppose that a vaccine confers complete and lifelong immunity in everyone who is immunized. If f is the fraction vaccinated before the age of first infection, then $1 - f$ would be the maximum fraction of the population that is susceptible, not taking into account additional immune people who have already had the disease. Substituting $1 - f$ for x in expression (1) for R, in principle, we need to vaccinate a fraction f such that

$$R = R_0(1 - f) < 1,$$

to eliminate transmission. The fraction that needs to be immunized to eliminate transmission is

$$f > 1 - (1/R_0).$$

Assume that $R_0 = 3$ for influenza in a population. Under the assumption of random mixing, the fraction that needs to be immunized before the age of first infection is $f = 1 - (1/R_0) = 1 - (1/3) = 0.67$. A higher R_0 requires immunization of a higher fraction to eliminate transmission (Fig. 4–4).

In the preceding example, we assumed that vaccination conferred complete protection. However, an intervention might provide only partial protection, such as the example of using vaginal foam that we presented. In that example, protection was just 80%. A vaccine might provide only partial protection and be just 90% or even 50% efficacious. If in the influenza example the transmission probability per contact in the vaccinated people is reduced by 90%, then the probability of infection in the vaccinated is just the factor $\theta = 0.10$ of that in the unvaccinated. If $R_0 = 3.0$ and everyone is vaccinated, then $R = 0.10 \times R_0 = 0.30$. The vaccine might be successful in preventing the spread of influenza. If the protective efficacy is just 0.50, however, then $\theta = 0.50$. Even if everyone is vaccinated, $R = 0.50 \times 3.0 = 1.50$. Since R is greater than 1, we would not expect to eliminate transmission with this vaccine.

In the preceding example, we assumed that the intervention had the same effect on everyone. An intervention might reduce the transmissin probability, the contact rate, or the duration of infection the same in everyone. As mentioned earlier, though, a risk factor or intervention may have different effects in different people. A vaccine might completely protect some people but fail completely in others. Then the expression for R takes into account the heterogeneities.

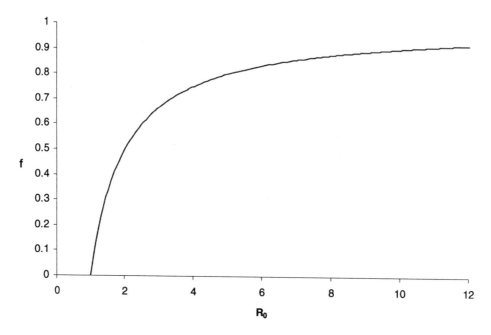

Figure 4-4. The fraction, f, of a population needed to be vaccinated with a completely protective vaccine to eliminate transmission as a function of R_0, the basic reproductive number.

In a simple example, suppose that a vaccine completely protects a proportion, h, of those who are vaccinated, while it fails in the remainder, $1 - h$, of the individuals who receive it. Suppose that, again, a fraction, f, of the population is vaccinated. Then the fraction of the population protected by immunization is hf, and $R = R_0(1 - hf)$. Then the fraction of the population that needs to be immunized to eliminate transmission is

$$f > \frac{1 - (1/R_0)}{h}.$$

Assume as in the preceding influenza example that $R_0 = 3$. Assume that the vaccination fails completely in the fraction $1 - h = 0.15$ while conferring complete and long-lasting protection in the other fraction $h = 0.85$. The fraction, f, that must be vaccinated to eliminate transmission increases to

$$f = \frac{1 - (1/R_0)}{h} = \frac{0.67}{0.85} = 0.79.$$

If the vaccine fails in 40% of the vaccinated people, then the fraction that must be vaccinated is $0.67/0.60 > 1.0$. With such a vaccine at the high failure rate, elimination of transmission would not be possible even if everyone were vaccinated.

HERD IMMUNITY

Herd immunity describes the collective immunological status of a population of hosts, as opposed to an individual organism, with respect to a given microbe (Anderson and May 1982). Herd immunity of a population can be high if many people have been immunized or have recovered from infection with immunity, or be low if most people are susceptible. If x is the proportion susceptible in expression (1), then $(1 - x)$, the proportion immune, gives some measure of the herd immunity. For any given microbe and host population, as herd immunity increases, R will decrease.

Seroprevalence of protective antibodies against an infectious agent is a measure of herd immunity. In Figure 4–5, the age-specific seroprevalences, that is, proportions of people with anti-hepatitis A virus (HAV) IgG and anti-hepatitis E virus (HEV) IgG in a collection of communities in Vietnam (Hau et al. 1999) are plotted. Seroprevalence of anti-HAV IgG rises very quickly with age, essentially reaching 1.00. The seroprevalence of anti-HEV IgG, on the other hand, is very low. The area under the histograms, adjusted for the varying sizes of the age groups, can be regarded as the level of herd immunity. The herd immunity for HAV is high and that for HEV is low. On average, 97% versus 16% of the people have antibodies against the two diseases. There is concern that the population is susceptible to an outbreak of HEV. Fine (1993) reviews herd immunity.

COMPARING INTERVENTIONS

We can also use the basic reproductive number to help choose among intervention strategies. Which intervention strategy has the largest effect on R_0? Given how much each intervention costs, which has the greatest effect for the amount of money spent? How does our choice of model for R_0 affect our conclusions?

Historically, the concept of R_0 played an important role in the choice of malaria intervention campaigns. In malaria, several interventions can be used against the vector, anopheline mosquitoes. Mosquitoes lay their eggs in water, and the hatched larvae need to breathe at the water surface. Thus either draining breeding pools or putting oil on the water surface will reduce the number of larvae that grow to adult mosquitoes. Some vector mosquitoes will bite nonhuman animals as well as humans. By increasing the number of nonhuman animals available for mosquitoes to bite, the biting rate (i.e., contact rate) on humans will be decreased. Often malaria mosquito vectors tend to bite people indoors, then rest on the walls while they excrete some of the blood fluid. This behavior makes spraying walls with insecticides a useful intervention. How can we derive an expression for R_0 for malaria, then use it to compare intervention strategies? What different aspects of the transmission cycle go into the expression?

Malaria is an indirectly transmitted dis-

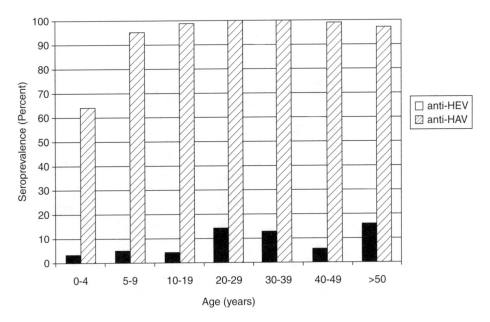

Figure 4–5. Age-specific prevalences of anti-HEV and anti-HAV immunoglobulin G in Vietnam. Source: Hau et al. 1999

ease in that it is transmitted from human to human via female anopheline mosquitoes. We can also say it is transmitted from mosquito to mosquito via the human. Thus, the R_0 expression is composed of two parts, the part from mosquito to human and the part from human to mosquito. We need the contact rates from mosquitoes to humans and from humans to mosquitoes, the two transmission probabilities, and the duration of infectiousness in mosquitoes and humans (Fig. 4–6; Table 4–1).

The expression for R_0 depends on the model we choose for a disease, that is, what components of the life cycle that we include. We consider here two simple models based on the early Ross (1911) and Ross-Macdonald (Macdonald 1957) models (see Aron and May 1982). We assume the humans become infected and infectious at some rate depending on the mosquito biting rate and transmission probability, then recover at some rate, r, without developing immunity. We do not include birth or death of humans in our expression. The duration of infectiousness of humans is $1/r$.

Mosquitoes become infected by biting infective humans. The mortality rate, μ, of mosquitoes is assumed to be independent of

whether they are infected. Mosquitoes do not recover from malaria, so the duration of infectiousness is the reciprocal of the death rate, $1/\mu$. The factor, b, is the transmission probability to humans per bite by an infectious mosquito, and c is the transmission probability to mosquito from an infective human.

To get expressions for the two contact rates, we define the quantity, a, as the number of bites per unit time on humans by a single female mosquito, or the contact rate for female mosquitoes with humans per unit time. The quantity a is a composite of the rate at which mosquitoes take blood meals and the proportion of those blood meals that are taken on humans. We assume that there is some constant number, M, of female mosquitoes and a constant number, N, of humans, so that the number of female mosquitoes per human host is $m = M/N$. The factor, $ma = aM/N$, is the rate of bites received by one human per unit time.

The component ac/r represents the part of R_0 of mosquitoes being infected by humans. The component mab/μ represents the part of R_0 of humans becoming infected by mosquitoes. Both components have the form of contact rate times transmission probability

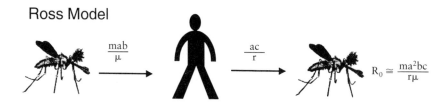

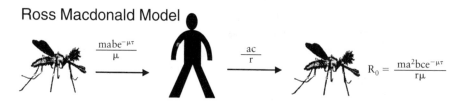

Figure 4–6. R_0 expression for two different malaria models.
Source: Mosquito image used with permission from the American Museum of Natural History.

Table 4-1 Quantities for the R_0 for Malaria

Term	Meaning
N	the size of the human population
M	the size of the female mosquito population
m	= M/N, the number of female mosquitoes per human host
a	the rate of biting on humans by a single mosquito (number of bites per unit time)
b	the transmission probability from an infective mosquito to a human
c	the transmission probability from an infective human to a mosquito
r	the recovery rate for humans
μ	the mortality rate for mosquitoes
τ	the latent period of the malaria parasite in the mosquito

times duration of infection. The basic reproductive number for the simple Ross model is

$$R_0 = \frac{ac}{r} \times \frac{mab}{\mu} = \frac{ma^2bc}{r\mu}.$$

As an example, suppose that the transmission probabilities $b = c = 0.1$, $M = 1,000,000$ mosquitoes, $N = 1000$ humans, $a = 0.1$ bites on human per day, $\mu = 0.1$ per day, and $r = 0.004$ per day. Then $R_0 = 250$, very high indeed.

This original simple model by Ross does not include the latent period (or external incubation period) in the mosquito. The latent period of the malaria parasite in mosquitoes is an important component, because it is on the order of the life expectancy of the mosquito. Thus a large proportion of the mosquitoes who become infected never become infective before they die. In the late 1940s, George Macdonald (1957) added the latent period of malaria in the mosquito to the model. If τ (pronounced "tau") is the latent period of the malaria parasite in the mosquito, the probability of a mosquito surviving the latent period to become infectious without dying is $e^{-\mu\tau}$. The expression for R_0 for the expanded Ross-Macdonald model is

$$R_0 = \frac{ac}{r} \times \frac{mabe^{-\mu\tau}}{\mu} = \frac{ma^2 bce^{-\mu\tau}}{r\mu}.$$

Suppose that the latent period $\tau = 10$ days and that the other quantities have the same values as above. Then using the Ross-Macdonald model, $R_0 = 92.0$, considerably lower than the R_0 calculated above. Thus the expression for R_0 and the underlying model can influence the value obtained for R_0.

The Ross-Macdonald R_0 played an important role in the decision of the World Health Organization to launch the malaria eradication campaign in the 1950s. This eradication campaign was based on spraying the insecticide DDT on the insides of houses to kill the mosquitoes resting after taking a blood meal, drastically increasing the mortality rate of mosquitoes, μ. Interventions up until that time had been aimed at decreasing the number of female mosquitoes, M, thus m, the number of female mosquitoes per human, by draining breeding pools or spraying water with oil. Another intervention was to add animals to the environment, so that the mosquitoes might bite the animals instead of the humans. This would reduce a, the rate of biting on humans by a single mosquito.

By seeing how these three quantities, μ, M, and a, enter into R_0, it is possible to get an idea which type of intervention would have the strongest effect. By inspection, M in ma, enters linearly into R_0. Because the biting rate of the mosquito is included twice, the squared power of a enters R_0. The life expectancy of the mosquito also enters twice into R_0, once linearly, and then exponentially. If the number of mosquitoes is reduced by one-half, R_0 will just decrease by a factor of two. If a is reduced by one-half, R_0 will decrease by a factor of four. If μ is increased by a factor of two, the decrease in R_0 will be by a factor greater than four.

Continuing the preceding example, suppose interventions change the parameters M, a, or μ by factors of 2. If the abundance of mosquitoes is reduced to M = 500,000, then R_0 = 46.3. If the biting rate is reduced to a = 0.05, then R_0 = 23.2. If the mortality rate of the mosquitoes increases by a factor of 2 to μ = 0.2, then R_0 = 16.9. Thus increasing the mortality rate, thereby reducing the life expectancy of the mosquito, has the strongest effect on R_0. The goal of the eradication program was to decrease $R_0 < 1$. In this example, to reduce R_0 so that it is less than 1, then μ must be increased to somewhat more than 0.4, for a life expectancy of about 2.5 days. Thus mortality of the mosquito needs to be increased by a factor of 4. The abundance of mosquitoes would have to be reduced by a factor of at least 92, however, to reduce R_0 below 1. We leave it as an exercise for the reader to calculate the changes in R_0 if the same interventions were used under the simple Ross model rather than the Ross-Macdonald model.

The prior calculations show how the Ross-Macdonald model could have a strong influence in embarking on the eradication campaign. Other factors, such as the beginning of the appearance of insecticide resistance, also put pressure on the campaign. The eradication campaign was abandoned in the late 1960s. After that time the goal was to achieve a new host-parasite balance. More complex models of malaria were developed that included immunity and superinfection (Dietz et al. 1974, Struchiner et al. 1989, Halloran et al. 1989). These models allow modeling of the effect of vaccination.

Factors contributing to malaria epidemics can also be understood using the Ross-Macdonald expression. The mortality rate of mosquitoes depends heavily on the weather. In particular, mosquitoes live longer in higher humidity. Also, the latent period, or extrinsic cycle, of the malaria parasite within the mosquito depends on the temperature. Thus increased humidity would reduce μ, increasing R_0. Similarly, high temperatures would reduce τ, also increasing R_0.

In this section we have shown that the computed value of R_0 depends on what is included in the model. Also, the effect of interventions can be compared using R_0, but conclusions will also depend on what is included in the model.

EVOLUTIONARY USES OF R_0

R_0 can be used to quantify evolutionary concepts. *Virulence* is a measure of the speed with which an organism kills an infected host. We denote the disease-dependent death rate, or virulence, by α. If r is the recovery rate from infectiousness, and α the virulence, then the duration of infectiousness is $d = 1/(r + \alpha)$ and $R_0 = cp/(r + \alpha)$. Since R_0 is a function of the time spent in the infective state, R_0 could decrease as virulence increases. If the microbe is highly virulent so that it kills its host quickly, then R_0 could be less than 1, and the microbe will die out. For example, suppose that the microbe does not kill the host and that the host usually recovers from infectiousness in about d = 10 days. Then r = 0.1 per day. If R_0 = 3.0 for this disease, then $cp = rR_0$ = 0.1 × 3.0 = 0.3. If instead the microbe kills the host on average in a little over three days when the host does not recover first, then α = 0.3 per day, and R_0 = 0.3/(0.1 + 0.3) = 0.75. In this case $R_0 < 1$, so the microbe will not be successful. If, on the other hand, the microbe kills the host only after about 10 days on average when the host does not recover first, then R_0 = 0.3/(0.1 + 0.1) = 1.5. In this case, $R_0 > 1$. Viewed in this way, there is evolutionary pressure on microbes to become less virulent and to develop a more benign relation to the host.

In some diseases, hosts become more infectious when they become sicker, so the transmission probability increases at the same time that virulence increases. Thus, R_0 could increase as virulence increases, putting evolutionary pressure on the agent to increase virulence. The balance depends on the particular microbe. In the above example, suppose that even though the microbe kills the host on average after about three days, the transmission probability, p, also increases by a factor of two. Then $R_0 = (c \times 2p)/(r + \alpha) = (2 \times 0.3)/(0.1 + 0.3) = 1.5$. In this case, R_0 is greater than 1, so we would expect the microbe to be successful. The increased virulence was offset by the increased transmission probability to keep $R_0 > 1$.

The *case fatality rate* is the probability of dying from a disease before recovering or dying of something else. In the notation used here, the case fatality rate is $\alpha/(r + \alpha)$ (ignores other death causes). If virulence is $\alpha = 0.3$ per day, and the recovery rate is $r = 0.1$ per day, then the expected case fatality rate is $0.3/(0.1 + 0.3) = 0.75$. This means that 75% of the people die before recovering. As virulence increases, the case fatality rate increases.

R_0 IN MACROPARASITIC DISEASES

The concept of R_0 comes from general population theory and refers to the expected number of reproducing offspring that one reproducing member of the population will produce in the absence of overcrowding. With larger parasites such as worms, called *macroparasites*, we define R_0 to be the expected number of mature female offspring that one female will produce in her lifetime. This contrasts with the definition of R_0 for microparasites, or microbes, which refers to the number of new infectious *hosts* produced by one infectious host.

For example, the disease schistosomiasis is caused by large, sexually reproducing worms called schistosomas that can live for over two decades within a human host. If a female schistosoma worm has an $R_0 = 2$ in a population of human hosts and an intermediate host population of snails, then the average female schistosoma produces two mature female worms. Most of the thousands of eggs produced by the adult female do not survive passage through the environment and the intermediate snail hosts to establish themselves in another human host. The two new successful worms could be in one new human host, or in two different hosts. The $R_0 = 2$ refers to the number of worms, not to the number of hosts. There are some further complexities in calculating thresholds,

because there must be at least one male worm in the human host for the female to reproduce.

What is important in designing interventions against macroparasitic diseases? The total number of parasites in a host is often more important than whether a host is infected, because the level of morbidity of a host can be associated with the number of parasites the host carries, or *parasite burden*. Some hosts can have very heavy infection, that is many worms, while others have very light infection. Chemotherapy that targets people with heavy parasite loads could have a greater effect on transmission and morbidity than untargeted therapy.

CAVEATS

The previous sections demonstrate that R_0 is a conceptually useful measure that provides a summary of several aspects of an infectious disease. However, the simple relations described earlier usually do not hold. Heterogeneities in the contact rates, transmission probabilities, and infectious periods produce different R_0s in different subgroups. If members of a group who live near each other are not immunized, then it is possible for transmission to occur in that group, even when transmission has been eliminated in other segments of the population. The contact rate can increase locally if people move into crowded conditions, such as into college dormitories, military barracks, or refugee camps. Especially when transmission is tenuous or near elimination, heterogeneities can play an important role in determining whether a microbe can persist in a population. Anderson and May (1991) present an extensive overview of R_0. R_0 is a relatively static concept. Further understanding of infectious diseases in populations requires study of transmission dynamics.

DYNAMICS OF INFECTION IN A POPULATION

Under some circumstances an infectious agent will invade and establish itself in a susceptible host population, with an ensuing epidemic, then die out again. Some infectious agents will invade, however, and after an initial epidemic, *persist*. They become *endemic*, with either fairly stable, possibly seasonal transmission, or other epidemic patterns. In addition to the consderations of R_0 described above, under what conditions might persistence or dying out happen?

CONTACT PROCESS AND RANDOM MIXING

To describe the spread of an infectious agent in a human population, we need to describe how the human hosts and any vectors contact each other in some way that the infectious agent can be spread. There are different ways to think about how individuals in populations make contact. One is that people behave like gas molecules with the rate of contact being determined by density. If people were pressed more closely together, as in an urban environment, they would contact each other more often than if they were less densely distributed, as in a rural environment. Hence, for diseases such as measles, influenza, or mumps that spread by airborne or droplet transmission, popula-

tion density plays a role in determining the value of R_0. Alternatively, contacts can be selected, such as in sexual contacts or injection of intravenous drugs. In this case, R_0 is determined more by social behavior. In many cases, both density and social choice will play a role in determining contact rates and mixing patterns.

Regardless of how contacts arise, the simplest assumption about the contact pattern in a population is that of *random mixing*. Figure 4-7 schematically represents random mixing, with the figures being evenly distributed in the space. Under the assumption of random mixing, every person has an equal chance of making contact with each other person. Consequently, every person also has an equal chance of being exposed to infection because every person is equally likely to make contact with an infectious person. The assumption of equal exposure to infection of people in the comparison groups, and whether it is valid, is important in many studies of interventions and risk factors affecting susceptibility. As in the prior discussion, we denote by c the constant contact rate that does not change over time in a randomly mixing population.

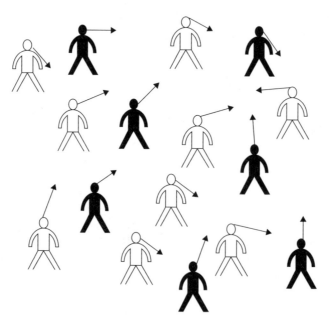

Figure 4-7. Random mixing. Solid figures denote infective people. Open figures denote susceptible people.

STATES OF THE HOST POPULATION

Suppose we choose to model an infectious disease by allowing people in the human population to pass through three different states (Fig. 4–8A,B). They start out susceptible, denoted by X, then become infected and infectious, denoted by Y, after which they recover with immunity, denoted by Z. Models of this type of infection process are called SIR models for susceptible, infected, recovered or removed. Other examples include SIS models, in which people recover without immunity to become susceptible again, and SIRS models, in which people acquire immunity, but lose it again to become susceptible. We use the notation XYZ here, rather than SIR, because we use I for incidence rate and R for incidence proportion. If these are the only three states possible, then each person in a population of N individuals is in one of these three states, where $X(t)$ is the number of susceptible people at time t, $Y(t)$ is the number of infectives, and $Z(t)$ is the number of immunes. This simple model ignores the latent and incubation periods, and assumes that infection, disease, and infectiousness occur simultaneously. This model could be a simplified representation of influenza, measles, or chickenpox.

There are two ways to enter and two ways to leave a population. Individuals can enter a population by being born into it or immigrating. Individuals can leave a population by dying or emigrating. In a closed population, there are no births, immigration, deaths, or emigration. We first consider a closed population of N initially susceptible people who are assumed to be mixing randomly with contact rate c (Fig. 4–8A). The population is analogous to a closed cohort. Initially, at time $t = 0$, everyone in the population is in the susceptible state X.

DYNAMICS OF AN EPIDEMIC

Suppose that a microbe such as an influenza virus is introduced into a closed population, so that one person enters the infectious state, Y (Fig. 4–9). Alternatively, an infectious person or several infectious persons besides the N initially susceptible might enter the population. Here we consider a simple deterministic, mass mixing model of the spread of infection. A deterministic, non-chaotic, model always gives the same answer and usually solves equations for populations rather than for discrete individuals.

The infection spreads from the first infective to the average number R_0 of susceptibles. If people recover at the rate r, then they are infectious on average for the time

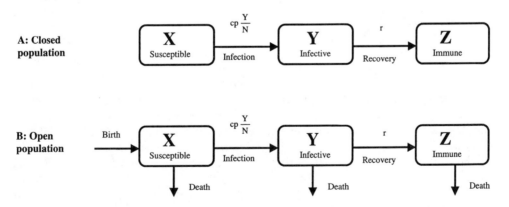

Figure 4–8A,B. Transmission model for an infectious disease in a host population. The three compartments represent susceptible (X), infective (Y), and immune (Z) hosts at time t. The total host population is of size $N = X + Y + Z$. Susceptible hosts become infected at an incidence rate (force of infection) of cpY/N, where c is the contact rate, p is the transmission probability, and Y/N is the prevalence of infective hosts at time t. The rate of recovery is r. Arrows represent transitions in and out of compartments.

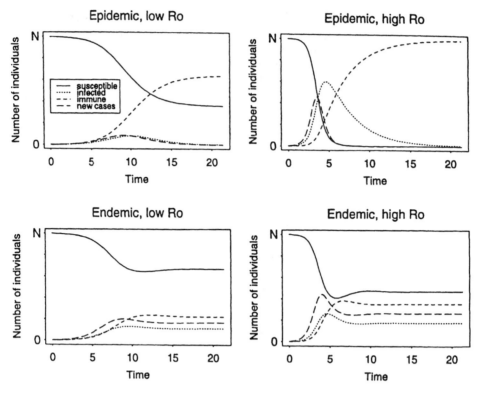

Figure 4–9. Comparison of the spread of an infectious disease in a closed or open population. The infectious agent is introduced into a population of N susceptibles. Susceptible people become infected and infectious, then develop immunity. **Top left:** Epidemic in a closed population, low R_0. The epidemic dies out before all susceptibles become infected. **Top right:** Epidemic in a closed population, higher R_0. Everyone becomes infected during the epidemic. There are no infectives left as the epidemic dies out. **Bottom left:** Epidemic followed by endemic persistence in an open population, low R_0. The infectious agent does not die out due to the supply of new susceptibles. Prevalence of susceptibles, infectives, and immune people is in dynamic equilibrium. The number of new incident cases is steady. **Bottom right:** Epidemic followed by endemic persistence in an open population, high R_0.
Source: Halloran, 1998.

period $d = 1/r$. If $R_0 > 1$, the epidemic is expected to spread. The first infective eventually recovers with immunity into state Z, while the infection spreads from those he or she infected to more susceptibles. In Figure 4–9, the number of infectives, $Y(t)$, initially increases. As the epidemic spreads, the number of susceptibles, $X(t)$, decreases, while the number of people with immunity, $Z(t)$, begins to increase. Incidence and prevalence of infection will increase until the number of susceptibles available becomes a limiting factor. Then the number of new cases and the prevalence begin to decrease until the mi-

crobe dies out and no people are left in the infective compartment, $Y(t)$. A microbe in a closed population where people recover with long-lasting immunity will inevitably die out, because the key to *persistence* in a host population is a continuous supply of susceptibles. The susceptibles can be produced either by births or immigration into the population, or by recovery without immunity or by waning of immunity after it is acquired. In this example of a closed population, however, no new susceptibles are produced.

The dynamics of the epidemic are described by three differential or difference equations that express the rate of change of the number of people in each of the three states. The rate at time t at which people leave the susceptible compartment X and become infected is simply the incidence rate, $I(t)$, or similarly the hazard rate or force of infection. The prevalence of infectives at time t, $P(t)$, is the number of infectious people, $Y(t)$, divided by the size of the population N, or $Y(t)/N$. The expression for the incidence rate as a function of prevalence in the epidemic is

$$I(t) = cpP(t) = cp\,\frac{Y(t)}{N}.$$

This is the dependent happening expression discussed in Chapter 5. The change in the number of susceptibles, the population-at-risk to become infected, $\Delta X(t)$, per small interval of time, Δt, at time t equals the incidence rate, $I(t)$, times the size of the population-at-risk, $X(t)$. The change in the number of infectives, $\Delta Y(t)$, is the difference between the number of new infections and the number of infectives developing immunity. The number of infectives developing immunity in the time interval Δt is the change in the number of immunes, $\Delta Z(t)$. The three difference equations for the epidemic model are then

change in susceptibles:

$$\frac{\Delta X(t)}{\Delta t} = -I(t)X(t) = -cp\,\frac{Y(t)}{N}X(t),$$

change in infectives:

$$\frac{\Delta Y(t)}{\Delta t} = cp\,\frac{Y(t)}{N}X(t) - rY(t),$$

change in immunes:

$$\frac{\Delta Z(t)}{\Delta t} = rY(t).$$

More commonly, differential equations are used, but we avoid the notation here.

We can associate aspects of the epidemic process with common epidemiologic measures. An estimate of the incidence rate, $I(t)$,

estimates $cpY(t)/N$. A cross-sectional study to estimate prevalence, $P(t)$, of current infection would yield an estimate of $Y(t)/N$. The number of new infections in an interval of time estimates $[cpY(t)/N]X(t)\,\Delta t$, the incidence rate times the number at risk for the event times the time interval. The epidemic process of a disease producing long-lasting immunity in a closed population is always either increasing or decreasing. An important consequence for conducting studies in epidemics in closed populations is that there is no stationary state of the disease process. Thus epidemiologic methods, study designs, or analytic methods that assume stationarity of the disease process are not applicable under epidemic conditions.

The epidemic process also depends on the population biology. Since R_0 is the product of the contact rate, the transmission probability, and the infectious period, in this model, $R_0 = cp/r$. The expected number of new cases per infective host decreases from R_0 to $R = R_0x$, where $x = X(t)/N$, the proportion still susceptible at time t. The epidemic peaks and begins to decrease when R is less than 1, so that $X(t)/N$ is less than $1/R_0$, that is, when the proportion of the population still susceptible becomes less than the reciprocal of the basic reproductive number. Not all the susceptibles need to become infected before the microbe dies out. The greater R_0, the fewer susceptibles will be left when the epidemic peaks and the fewer susceptibles will be left at the end of the epidemic (Fig. 4–10). Thus the incidence proportion, or attack rate, after an epidemic provides information on R_0. If an intervention reduced some aspect of R_0, then the intervention would result in the epidemic peaking when a greater proportion of the population was still susceptible, and fewer people would become infected before the epidemic died out.

TRANSMISSION IN AN OPEN POPULATION

An open population can have people entering, leaving, or both. In an open population, the susceptibles form a dynamic cohort with

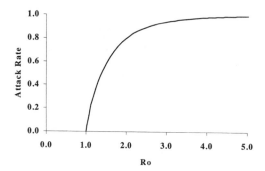

Figure 4–10. The attack rate as a function of the basic reproductive number, R_0.

the population-at-risk changing over time (see Fig. 4–8B). In an open population, if the replenishment of susceptibles is fast enough compared with the dynamics of the microbe, then the microbe will not necessarily die out. The microbe can invade the population, establish itself, persist, and become endemic. It is possible, however, that the microbe will die out if the replenishment of susceptibles is not fast enough in comparison to the spread of immunity to the microbe. Microbes can persist by hopping from one population to another, then returning to one where the susceptibles have had time to replenish themselves.

When a disease is first introduced into a population, there will be a period when the dynamics are not stationary. As stated in the section, Dynamics of an Epidemic, epidemiologic methods that assume stationarity of the disease process cannot be used during the epidemic phase. If the infectious agent has achieved a dynamic equilibrium, however, then some relations might be applicable. An open population with a dynamic cohort at risk for infection is amenable to many of the study designs regularly used in dynamic cohorts. In choosing study designs and methods of analysis, we need to consider whether the dynamics of transmission are at equilibrium or changing over time.

WITHIN HOST DYNAMICS

The dynamics of the infectious agent *within* a host also can be described by dynamic

models (Antia et al. 1996, 1998, Pilyugin et al. 1997). These models describe the interaction of the microbe with the immune cells or antibodies that might attack it, and its target cells within the host. Similar concepts from population theory are used to model the within-host dynamics of the infectious agent and to model the infectious agent circulating in the human population. For example, R_0 for a virus within a host describes the number of new viral particles successfully produced by one virus particle. The various immune compartments such as T cells, B cells, and memory cells can be included in the dynamic models.

Chain Binomial Models

The deterministic, mass action, dynamic models described above are useful for exploring scientific and biologic questions. However, they have not been used much for estimating quantities of interest. *Chain binomial* models are dynamic models developed from the simple binomial model by assuming that infection spreads from individual to individual in populations in discrete units (i.e., individual "links" of the chain) of time, producing infection chains governed by the binomial (i.e., dichotomous outcomes such as yes/no or newly infected/not newly infected) probability distribution. The expected distribution of infections in a collection of populations after several units of time can be calculated from the chained, that is, sequential, application of the binomial model. The Reed-Frost and Greenwood models are examples of chain binomial models. As mentioned before, the Reed-Frost model assumes that exposure to two or more infectious people at the same time are independent exposures. The Greenwood model assumes that exposure to two or more infectious people at the same time is equivalent to exposure to one infectious person.

As a simple example of the Reed-Frost chain binomial model, consider spread of infection in a group of three individuals, where one person is initially infected and the other two are initially susceptible (Table 4–2). We assume that the initial infective is no longer infective after the first time unit. In the first

Table 4-2 Chain Binomial Reed-Frost Model in Groups of Size 3 with 1 Initial Infective and 2 Susceptibles

Chain	Chain Probability	at p = 0.4	at p = 0.7	Total Infected
$1 \to 0$	q^2	0.360	0.090	1
$1 \to 1 \to 0$	$2pq^2$	0.288	0.126	2
$1 \to 1 \to 1$	$2p^2q$	0.192	0.294	3
$1 \to 2$	p^2	0.160	0.490	3
Total	1	1.00	1.00	

time unit, one of three things can happen: neither of the susceptibles will become infected; both of them will become infected; or just one of them will become infected. The probability that neither becomes infected is the probability that both escape infection, or q^2. In this case, the chain ends, so the probability of this chain is q^2. If both susceptibles become infected in the first time unit, the chain also ends. The probability of both becoming infected from the first exposure is p^2.

The probability that one person becomes infected while the other does not is pq. Since this can happen two ways, then the probability of just one being infected in the first time unit is $2pq$. If one of the susceptibles becomes infected in the first time unit, then this person is the new infective who can expose the last remaining susceptible. Exposure of the last remaining susceptible can result in two possible outcomes. Either the susceptible becomes infected or does not, with probabilities p and q, respectively. The *chained probabilities* then are $2pq \times p = 2p^2q$ and $2pq \times q = 2pq^2$, respectively.

In Table 4-2 the chain probabilities are calculated for two different values of p, $p = 0.4$ and $p = 0.7$. If we were to have 1000 groups of size three with one initial infective, at $p = 0.4$ we would expect 360 groups to have just one infected, 288 to have two infected, and $192 + 160 = 352$ to have three infected at the end. Similarly, at $p = 0.7$, we would expect 90, 126, and 784, respectively. Note that there are two different chains by which all three people become infected. If we were not able to observe the actual chains, we would not know which path the chain had taken. In this case, we would have only

final value data, that is, data on how many were infected in each household at the end. This is also called the final size distribution.

The R_0 in this model, assuming that the duration of infectiousness is one time unit, or d = 1, is $R_0 = pN$, or sometimes $R_0 = p(N - 1)$, if there is one initial infective. In this example, if $p = 0.4$, then $R_0 = 0.4 \times 2 = 0.8$. If $p = 0.7$, then $R_0 = 0.7 \times 2 = 1.4$. In deterministic models, if $R_0 > 1$, the epidemic will always take off. If $R_0 < 1$, the epidemic will never take off. An index that makes more sense in the probabilistic world is the probability that the epidemic will not take off.

The probability that an epidemic will not spread from the initially infected people is called the *probability of no spread*, denoted by P_{ns}. It can be calculated from the transmission probability p, or escape probability, $q = 1 - p$, the number of initially infected people in the population Y_0, and the number of initially susceptible people X_0.

The probability that a susceptible person escapes infection from all Y_0 initial infectives is q^{Y_0}. The probability that all X_0 of the susceptible people escape infection from all of the infectives is $P_{ns} = (q^{Y_0})^{X_0}$. In the above example, with $p = 0.4$, the probability of no spread is $P_{ns} = (0.6^1)^2 = 0.36$. With $p = 0.7$, $P_{ns} = (0.3^1)^2 = 0.09$. The terms *minor* and *major* epidemics distinguish situations in which there is little spread from the initial infectives from situations in which an epidemic gains momentum and is self-sustaining.

Chain binomial models can be used to estimate the transmission probability from data gathered on each generation of infection or from the final distribution of infectives within a collection of households or other small transmission units after an epidemic has occurred. Abbey (1952), Bailey (1957), and Becker (1989) discuss chain binomial models. An important assumption of the simple version of the Reed-Frost model is that the households or mixing groups are each independent of one another. Below we present an extension of the model that allows for interaction outside of the households within the community.

Stochastic Models

Stochastic models, which incorporate elements of chance, are commonly used in infectious disease modeling (Chiang 1980). For example, the Reed-Frost model can be simulated using a random number generator at each step for each person to decide whether an exposed person becomes infected. In contrast, in deterministic (i.e., nonstochastic), mass action models, fractions of a population are assigned to a particular state at any given time. In general, stochastic simulation models are useful for generating simulated data with variability so that methods of analysis can be used and compared. Stochastic computer simulations are especially useful in helping to design studies and to develop new methods of analysis (see, for example, Golm et al. 1999 or Longini et al. 1999). Deterministic models do not generate variability but can be used to understand properties of the transmission system.

In a staged Markov model, individuals rather than populations move through states. Whether a person moves to the next state in a given time unit has a certain probability and is random. The Markov property means that the probability of moving to the next state is independent of the time already spent in the current state. The relation between the stochastic formulation of epidemic models and the deterministic formulation has been studied in detail. In many situations, the deterministic model gives an average of the behavior of the stochastic model. However, more situations lead to extinction of infection in stochastic models than in deterministic models.

Complex Dynamic Models and Simulation

Many questions of interest require more complex models than we can present here. What are the age-related changes in infection and disease? What is the advantage of using a targeted versus an untargeted strategy? Will natural immunity wane if transmission is too low? If many people are vaccinated, the incidence of infection will decrease, so that the average age of infection in the susceptibles will increase. Some diseases, such as mumps, chickenpox, and rubella, are more serious if acquired at older ages. Thus the number of total cases could decrease owing to a vaccination program at the same time that the number of serious cases would increase. For example, rubella is a mild disease in children, but it can result in congenital defects if a pregnant woman becomes infected. If many, but not all, young people are vaccinated, then transmission will be reduced. The people who were not vaccinated will acquire rubella at a later age than if no one was vaccinated (Knox 1980, Ukkonen and von Bonsdorff 1988). Thus it is possible that the number of babies born with congenital defects could increase, even though fewer people contract rubella.

A similar concern about introducing varicella vaccination in the United States was raised. The question was whether vaccination, especially if the fraction vaccinated was not high, could increase the number of primary chickenpox cases in older age groups who have more severe morbidity. Halloran and colleagues (1994) studied several different scenarios and found that likely vaccination would not result in more severe cases. Models including age (Schenzle 1984) and mixing structures are required to study complex questions such as this one. The general rule is that a model has to contain the characteristics related to the question you are asking or you cannot get an answer. Anderson and May (1991) provide an extensive overview of deterministic models to study dynamics of infectious disease and interventions.

Several caveats should be kept in mind in considering the results of complex models and computer simulations. Regardless of how complex the model is, it is always a simplification of reality. Someone made choices in choosing what would be included in the model. These choices affect the results produced by the model. Models are excellent at forcing us to make both our assumptions and our ignorance explicit. Often, too few data are available to estimate the parameters, and the results usually underestimate the uncertainty of the knowledge. Regardless of these caveats, models are very useful in sharpening our thinking and especially in gaining qualitative understanding of complex processes.

USING DYNAMIC CONCEPTS TO INTERPRET STUDIES

We now illustrate how understanding the transmission dynamics of an infection can help interpret the results of a study. Two hypothetical investigators who conducted separate studies of gonorrhea in a heterosexual population of men and women come to different conclusions. The subscript m and f denote men and women, respectively. The first investigator conducted a study in clinics using a sound sampling scheme with good ascertainment. The results showed that the incidence rate and number of new clinical cases of gonorrhea are higher in men than women, $I_m > I_f$. The investigator concluded that gonorrhea is a greater problem in men than women. The second investigator conducted a population-based study that was also well designed, and found that the prevalence of gonorrhea infection is higher in women than in men, $P_f > P_m$. She concluded that the problem is greater in women. How can transmission concepts help us think about this paradox (Fig. 4–11)?

Assume that gonorrhea transmission has been fairly constant over a period of time in this population. Women can be infected with gonorrhea for a long time before they develop symptoms, whereas men develop symptoms quickly and go for treatment. Thus the infectious period in men is shorter than in women, d_m is less than d_f. Generally the transmission probability from females to males is lower than that from males to females. However, to make this point as simply as possible, we assume here that they are equal, so that $p_{fm} = p_{mf} = p$. Assume that the population has an equal number of men and women, $N_m = N_f = N$, that the rate of new partners (contact rate) is the same in both, $c_m = c_f = c$, and that men and women mix randomly with the opposite sex.

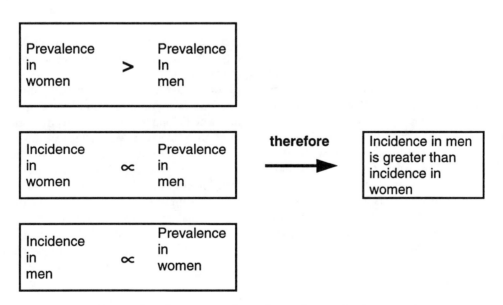

Figure 4–11. Relation of incidence rate and prevalence of gonorrhea in men and women.

Prevalence of infection in women is higher than in men, largely because the duration is longer, so there is a greater number of susceptible men than women who are at risk to become new cases $(1 - P_m) > (1 - P_f)$. Susceptible men make the same number of contacts per unit time and have the same transmission probability as the women, but their contact pool, the women, has a higher prevalence of infection, so the incidence rate is higher in the men, $I_m = cpP_f > cpP_m = I_f$. The combined effect in the men of a higher incidence rate and a greater proportion of susceptibles results in a higher number of new cases in men than in women. If we were to conduct a study in a clinic based on incidence rate or number of new cases, we would conclude that the problem is more serious in men. If we were to conduct a prevalence study in the population, we might think the problem is more pronounced in women. The males and females are related through the dynamic transmission process, and the paradox is resolved.

If we can reduce the population prevalence in women, for example, by shortening the duration of infection by early detection and treatment (Thomas et al. 1998, 1999), it would reduce the incidence rate in men, and consequently the prevalence in men. This, in turn, will reduce the incidence rate in women, and consequently contribute further to decreasing the prevalence in women. The dependence of events in infectious diseases results in interventions having greater overall effects than would be expected from just the direct effects in the individuals receiving the intervention. We leave it as an exercise for the reader to develop an expression for the basic reproductive number for this situation. What would happen to the rate of new partnerships (contact rate) c_f and c_m if there were twice as many men as women? Consider what would happen if the transmission probability from men to women, p_{mf}, were twice as high as that from women to men, p_{fm}.

NONRANDOM MIXING

We conclude this chapter by considering some more ideas on contact processes and patterns within populations. Contact patterns play a central role in determining transmission and exposure to infection. Most populations do not mix randomly but are composed of different types of small transmission units or subpopulations that mix with their own members differently than with other subpopulations. The groups could be sexual behavior groups, different age groups within a school, or households in a community. Individuals may belong to several different mixing groups, including families, schools, and neighborhoods. Our scientific questions and the purpose of our investigation will determine in large part how we choose to think about the structure of the population and how the individuals and groups within it mix. Are we modeling the long-term effects of intervention? Do we want a model of transmission that allows us to estimate meaningful parameters from the data we collect? Are we interested in understanding social networks?

Transmission Units within Populations

So far we have considered two possible mixing patterns. One was random mixing in a large population. The other, in the context of the chain binomial model, was a collection of small populations that mixed randomly within themselves but did not interact with one another (Fig. 4–12A). Now we consider a combination of the two with a larger population being composed of smaller transmission units. Individuals mix with the others in their own transmission units in one way and with members of the community who belong to other small transmission units in a different way. The transmission units could be households, sexual partnerships, schools, workplaces, or day care centers, for example (Fig. 4–12B,C,D).

In the simplest case, an individual belongs to one small transmission unit and interacts randomly with the others in the population. For example, a person may be in a steady but nonmonogamous sexual partnership and so have contact with the partner but also sexual contact with other individuals in the community at large. As another example, a person may have contact in a family

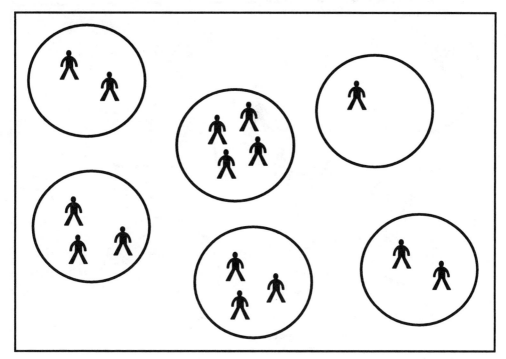

A

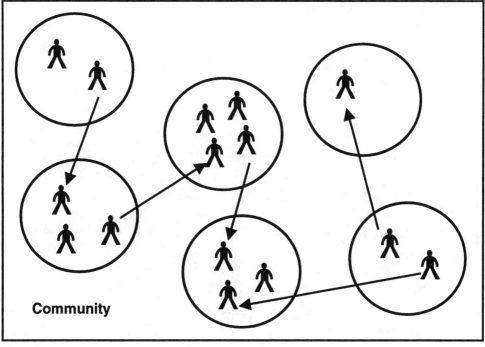

B

Figure 4–12A and B. A: Independent transmission units. B: Transmission units within a community.

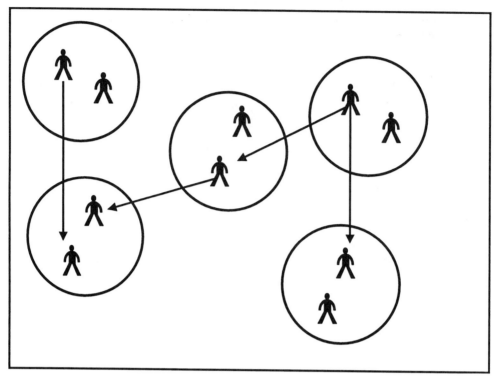

C

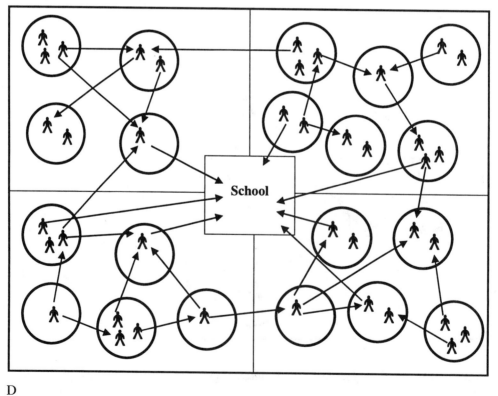

D

Figure 4–12C and D. C: Nonmonogamous sexual partnerships with contacts in the community.
D: Contact patterns in a community of households in four neighborhoods with one school.

household, but also within the community at large. When we define the community structure in this way, it allows that a susceptible individual can become infected if exposed to an infected person within the household as well as the possibility of being infected in the community at large during the course of an epidemic or over the duration of a study. Longini and Koopman (1982) formulated a model that contains both the probability of being infected within a household and within the community at large. This model can be used for studying transmission in sexual partnerships by assuming that the households are all of size two. We can allow for the fact that some people do not have steady sexual partners by allowing for singles (households of size one) as well as partnerships. This is the basis of the model for the augmented study design discussed in Chapter 5.

Subpopulations

Rather than small transmission units, we may think of a population as divided into large subgroups that mix more with their own members than with other groups. For example, we may observe two large communities that have little interchange between them. Alternatively, we may divide a population into two differently sexually active subgroups that have some contact with each other.

In a population composed of two mixing groups, group 1 and group 2 (Fig. 4–13), the contact pattern is described by a *mixing matrix* that has the same number of rows and columns as the number of mixing groups. The entries in the matrix represent the contact rates of individuals within and between the groups. The contact rate of individuals of group j with individuals of group i ($i,j = 1,2$) is denoted by c_{ij}. The mixing pattern of two groups is represented by the matrix,

$$C = \begin{pmatrix} c_{11} & c_{12} \\ c_{21} & c_{22} \end{pmatrix}.$$

On the diagonals are the contact rates within groups, c_{11} and c_{22}. The entries c_{12} and c_{21} off the diagonals represent the contact rates between the groups corresponding to that row and column.

R_0 will be higher in the group with the higher contact rate, assuming that the transmission probability and infectious period are the same in both groups. If an epidemic occurs and there is contact between the two groups, the epidemic in the group with the higher contact rates will help drive the epidemic in the group with the lower rates. The group with the higher R_0 would serve as a *core population* for transmission. Thomas and Tucker (1995) have reviewed this and other concepts of core groups for sexually transmitted diseases. The existence of a core group has consequences for intervention programs. It may be easy to reduce the average R_0 for the whole population below 1, while R_0 in the core population remains above 1, so that transmission will persist. In infectious diseases, the chain is only as weak as its strongest link.

Hethcote and York (1984) examined different strategies for reducing gonorrhea, taking into account sex workers who acted as a core group and their contacts within the general population. They found that an intervention program generally needs to be targeted at the subpopulation with the higher R_0, in this case, the core population of sex

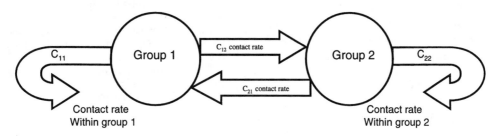

Figure 4–13. Mixing pattern of two groups in a population.

workers, to have most effect. In general, when planning interventions in situations with heterogeneous transmission or levels of infection, targeting therapy or prevention to the groups with the highest transmission or levels of infection is often most effective in reducing infection in the population at large. In the section, R_0 in Macroparasitic Diseases, we mentioned that often a small proportion of the population has a very heavy parasite burden. This is another example in which targeting the therapy enhances the effectiveness of the intervention.

Another approach to describing contact patterns is *social networks* of people (Morris and Kretzschmar 1997, Koopman et al. 2000). In this approach contacts are made through pair-formation and dissociation processes. The approach also allows that several people can be in contact with each other during an interval of time, and then dissociate. The transmission patterns produced by this *concurrency* of contacts and the resulting networks can be compared to transmission in which all contacts are sequential. In general, epidemic spread is more rapid if several people can make contact simultaneously.

Like much else in infectious diseases, contact patterns are often difficult to determine and usually are not measured. When conducting studies in infectious diseases where transmission plays a role, it is important to formulate explicitly the underlying assumptions that are being made with respect to contact patterns and exposure to infection. Since groups with different contact rates and mixing patterns could have different exposure to infection, consideration of the contact patterns could be important for interpreting measures of effect. Failure to take into account unequal exposure to infection in the groups being compared can produce biased estimates of effect. In Chapter 5, we demonstrate how differential contact rates can affect estimates of effect.

SUMMARY

Several principles of transmission and dynamics are common to many infectious diseases. These include the transmission probability, the basic reproductive number, conditions for an epidemic, and the role of contact and mixing patterns. The transmission probability is a measure of the ability of a microbe to spread from an infected to a susceptible host during a contact. The binomial model of transmission is widely used to quantify transmission concepts and to estimate the transmission probability. The basic reproductive number, R_0, describes the potential of a microbe to spread in a population. Dynamic models are used to understand the spread of infection and the role of interventions over time. Assumptions about mixing and contact patterns influence the interpretation of epidemiologic studies in infectious diseases.

Dr. Halloran was partially supported in writing this chapter by NIH grants R01-AI32042 and R01-AI40846. The mosquito image was used with permission from the American Museum of Natural History.

REFERENCES

Abbey H. An examination of the Reed-Frost theory of epidemics. Hum. Biol. 24: 201–233, 1952.

Anderson RM, and May RM, eds. Population Biology of Infectious Diseases. Berlin: Springer-Verlag, 1982.

Anderson RM, and May RM. Infectious Diseases of Humans: Dynamics and Control. Oxford: Oxford University Press, 1991.

Antia R, Koella JC, and Perrot V. Models of the within-host dynamics of persistent mycobacterial infections. Proc. R. Soc. Lond. B. 263: 257–263, 1996.

Antia R, Pilyugin SS, and Ahmed R. Models of immune memory: on the role of cross-reactive stimulation, competition, and homeostasis in maintaining immune memory. Proc. Natl. Acad. Sci. USA. 95: 14926–31, 1998.

Aron JL, and May RM. The population dynamics of malaria. In: Anderson RM, ed. Population Dynamics of Infectious Diseases: Theory and Application. London: Chapman and Hall, 1982: 139–179.

Bailey NTJ. The Mathematical Theory of Epidemics. London: Griffin, 1957.

Becker, NG. Analysis of Infectious Disease Data. London: Chapman and Hall, 1989.

Burnet M, and White DO. Natural History of Infectious Disease. 4th ed. Cambridge: Cambridge University Press, 1972.

Chiang CL. An Introduction to Stochastic Processes and Their Applications. Huntington, NY: Robert E. Krieger, 1980.

Dietz K, Molineaux L, and Thomas A. A malaria model tested in the African savannah. Bull. WHO. 50: 347–357, 1974.

Elveback LR, Fox JP, Ackerman E, et al. An influenza simulation model for immunization studies. Am. J. Epidemiol. 103: 152–165, 1976.

Fine P. Herd immunity. Epidemiol. Rev. 15: 265–302, 1993.

Golm GT, Halloran ME, and Longini IM. Semiparametric methods for multiple exposure mismeasurement and a bivariate outcome in HIV vaccine trials. Biometrics. 55: 94–101, 1999.

Greenwood M. On the statistical measure of infectiousness. J. Hyg. Camb. 31: 336–351, 1931.

Halloran ME, Struchiner CJ, and Spielman A. Modeling malaria vaccines II: population effects of stage-specific malaria vaccines dependent on natural boosting. Math. Biosci. 94: 115–149, 1989.

Halloran ME, Haber MJ, Longini IM, and Struchiner CJ. Direct and indirect effects in vaccine field efficacy and effectiveness. Am. J. Epidemiol. 133: 323–331, 1991.

Halloran ME, Haber MJ, and Longini IM. Interpretation and estimation of vaccine efficacy under heterogeneity. Am. J. Epidemiol. 136: 328–343, 1992.

Halloran ME, Cochi S, Lieu T, Wharton M, and Fehrs LJ. Theoretical epidemiologic and morbidity effects of routine immunization of preschool children with live-virus varicella vaccine in the U.S. Am. J. Epidemiol. 140: 81–104, 1994.

Hau CH, Hien TT, Tien NTK, et al. Prevalence of enteric hepatitis A and E viruses in the Mekong River Delta region of Vietnam. Am. J. Trop. Med. Hyg. 60: 277–280, 1999.

Hethcote HW, and Yorke JA. Gonorrhea transmission dynamics and control. Lecture Notes in Mathematics 56. Berlin: Springer-Verlag, 1984.

Knox EG. Strategy for rubella vaccination. Int. J. Epidemiol. 9: 13–23, 1980.

Koopman JS, Chick SE, Riolo CS, et al. Modeling infection transmission through networks in geographic and social space using the GERMS framework. J. STD. (in press) 2000.

Longini IM, and Koopman JS. Household and community transmission parameters from final distributions of infections in households. Biometrics. 38(1): 115–126, 1982.

Longini IM, Hudgens MG, Halloran ME, and Sagatelian K. A Markov model for measuring vaccine efficacy for both susceptibility to infection and reduction in infectiousness for prophylactic HIV-1 vaccines. Stat. Med. 18: 53–68, 1999.

Macdonald G. The Epidemiology and Control of Malaria. London: Oxford University Press, 1957.

McNeill WH. Plagues and Peoples. New York: Doubleday, 1976.

Morris M, and Kretzschmar M. Concurrent partnerships and the spread of HIV. AIDS. 11: 641–648, 1997.

Pilyugin S, Mittler J, and Antia R. Modeling T-cell proliferation: an investiation of the consequences of the Hayflick Limit. J. Theor. Biol. 186: 117–129, 1997.

Ross R. The Prevention of Malaria. 2nd ed. London: John Murray, 1911.

Ross R. An application of the theory of probabilities to the study of a priori pathometry, Part 1. Proc. R. Soc. Series A. 92: 204–230, 1916.

Schenzle D. An aged-structured model of pre- and post-vaccination measles transmission. IMA J. Math. Appl. Med. Biol. 1: 169–191, 1984.

Smith PG, Rodrigues LC, and Fine PEM. Assessment of the protective efficacy of vaccines against common diseases using case-control and cohort studies. Int. J. Epidemiol. 13(1): 87–93, 1984.

Struchiner CJ, Halloran ME, and Spielman A. Modeling malaria vaccines I: new uses for old ideas. Math. Biosci. 94: 87–113, 1989.

Thomas JC, and Tucker M. The development and use of the concept of a sexually transmitted disease core. J. Infect. Dis. 174 (Suppl): S134–43, 1995.

Thomas JC, Eng E, Clark M, Robinson J, and Blumenthal C. Lay health advisors: sexually transmitted disease prevention through community involvement. Am. J. Public Health. 88: 1252–1253, 1998.

Thomas JC, Lansky A, Weiner DH, Earp JA, and Schoenbach VJ. Behaviors facilitating sexual transmission of HIV and STDs in a rural community. AIDS and Behavior. 3: 257–268, 1999.

Ukkonen P, and von Bonsdorff C-H. Rubella immunity and morbidity: effects of vaccination in Finland. Scand. J. Infect. Dis. 20: 255–259, 1988.

5

Overview of Study Design

M. ELIZABETH HALLORAN

Concepts of study design in infectious disease epidemiology have much in common with those in noninfectious disease epidemiology. However, the presence of the infectious agent, separate from but interacting with the human host population, introduces further complexities. Whether a person becomes infected depends on who else in the population is already infected and infectious. Alternatively it may depend on environmental sources of infection. Sir Ronald Ross (Ross 1916) coined the term "dependent happenings" to describe the characteristic of contagious diseases that the number of people becoming newly infected depends on how many are already infected. The transmission of the infectious agent and dependent happenings produce the special aspects of study designs in infectious diseases.

Infectious disease epidemiology encompasses the study of diverse scientific questions:

- Is a disease *communicable*? What infectious organism is causing a disease? What is the mode of transmission? How effec-

tively is the infectious agent transmitted? What are the contact patterns and patterns of spread within the host population? What is the source or reservoir of a point source epidemic?

- What is the *natural history* of infection in individuals? What is the latent period, and the duration and degree of infectiousness? What is the probability of becoming symptomatic? What is the incubation period from acquisition of infection to symptoms? What is the duration of symptoms? What is the probability of dying?

- What are the *population biology*, epidemiology, and dynamics of the infectious agent and any vector? Is the microbe endemic or epidemic? Is an epidemic occurring? Is a disease reemerging? What is the age distribution of infection and disease in the host population? Are there important temporal and spatial aspects of the agent and any vectors? How diverse are genetic variants of the microbe? Is the microbe developing drug resistance or evolving owing to some other pressure? Does transmission intensity influence microbial diversity?

- What are the effects of *covariates or interventions* on infection, disease, and infectiousness? What facilitates infection (risk factors for exposure and susceptibility)? What facilitates disease progression (risk factors)? How can infection and disease be prevented? What is the effect of intervention at the individual level and at the population or community level?

The choice of study design needs to be tailored to the question being asked. Several of the questions listed above are concerned with the etiology and natural history of the infectious agent. The Henle-Koch postulates for evidence that an organism causes a disease are useful (Evans 1976). New techniques in molecular epidemiology permit more accurate tracking of transmission (Glynn et al. 1999, Small et al. 1994), studies of the natural history of the disease, and study of the evolution of microbes (Lipsitch 1997) than before. Several of the questions concern the study of the dynamics and interaction of the host population with the infectious agent population (see Chapter 4).

In this chapter, we focus on the dependent happening relation and its consequences for design and interpretation of studies in infectious disease epidemiology. For coherence of presentation, we also present some definitions and concepts from general epidemiology. In the next section, we present measures of disease frequency, with a focus on the transmission probability. We give a formal expression for the dependent happening expression and show its usefulness. In the third section, we present measures of causal effects and association, with a focus on the transmission probability ratio, and the indirect, total, and overall effects of interventions in populations. We demonstrate the difference between causal effects and association using a formal model for causal inference. We also show how the formal dependent happening relation can aid in interpreting risk ratios. In the fourth section, we present cohort study designs, focusing on those appropriate for estimating the transmission probability and the secondary attack rate. The context is developed as an expanded approach to cohort studies. We also discuss case-control studies. In the fifth section, we consider cross-sectional and community-level studies. In the last section, we touch on aspects of estimation and inference.

MEASURES OF DISEASE FREQUENCY

In this section we define several common measures of disease frequency. Specific to infectious disease epidemiology are the transmission probability, the secondary attack rate, and the basic reproductive number. Common to all fields of epidemiology are the incidence rate, hazard rate, incidence proportion, and prevalence. Because of the phenomenon of dependent happenings in infectious diseases, the common measures of disease frequency have additional intrinsic relations to one another through the underlying transmission process. We give a formal definition of the dependent happening relation as a function of the measures of disease frequency. We discuss how this relation contributes to the design and interpretation of infectious disease studies.

Transmission Probability and Secondary Attack Rate

In Chapter 4, we defined the *transmission probability, p*, as the probability that, given a contact between an infective source and a susceptible host, successful transfer of the microbe will occur so that the susceptible host becomes infected. The transmission probability in a population is

$$p = \frac{A}{n},$$

where n is the total number of contacts made between susceptibles and infectives in a population, and A is the number of infections that occur during those contacts. The transmission probability depends on characteristics of the infective source, the microbe, the susceptible host, and the type of contact.

The *secondary attack rate (SAR)* is a special case of the transmission probability. The secondary attack rate is the expected proportion of susceptibles who become infected when exposed to an infectious person. In the secondary attack rate, the contact between the infectious susceptible persons may be defined as occurring over some time period, such as the duration of infectiousness or over the period of the study. For example, the *household SAR* is the probability that a susceptible individual living in the same household with an infectious person during his or her period of infectiousness will become infected (Fine et al. 1988, Orenstein et al. 1988). The secondary attack rate is defined

$$SAR = \frac{A}{M},$$

where M is the total number of susceptible exposed persons and A is the number of persons exposed who develop disease. The *SAR* is a proportion, not a true rate.

Both the transmission probability and secondary attack rate are defined conditionally on the susceptibles being exposed to infection. Being conditional on exposure to infection distinguishes the transmission probability and secondary attack rate from the general measures of disease frequency such as incidence rate, hazard rate, and incidence proportion presented below.

The probability, ρ, of becoming infected given a contact with a source of unknown infection status is related to the transmission probability p, but it is not strictly a transmission probability. It is an infection probability. Under random mixing, the probability of becoming infected from a contact with a source of unknown infection status is $\rho = pP$, where P is the prevalence of infectious people in the population of contacts.

Incidence rate and hazard rate

The incidence rate, I, of an event in a population is the rate at which the event occurs per unit of person-time at risk. The incidence rate is

$$I = \frac{A}{T},$$

where A is the number of cases observed during a total of T units of person-time at risk. Incidence that varies over time we denote at time t by $I(t)$. If the incidence rate changes in a time interval but is estimated as an average over that interval, the estimate will not reflect the fluctuations that occur within the interval. The hazard rate is the instantaneous probability of an event occurring in a small interval of time. The hazard rate at time t is denoted by $\lambda(t)$. The hazard rate and incidence rate are defined somewhat differently, but both are measures of the probability of an event in an individual in a small unit of time at risk. The term *force of infection* is used in infectious disease epidemiology to denote either the hazard rate or the incidence rate of infection. The incidence rate in infectious diseases can vary rapidly, such as during an epidemic or due to seasonality of the vector population. The rapid changes in incidence rates are a source of some of the challenges of infectious disease epidemiology.

Incidence proportion

The *incidence proportion, R,* is the number of people who experience an event in a closed group of susceptible people over the course of study. The incidence proportion is expressed

$$R = \frac{A}{N},$$

where N is the number of people in the population and A is the number of people who experience the event. We can be explicit that the incidence proportion is measured over a time interval $(0, T)$ by writing $R(T)$. In infectious disease epidemiology, the incidence proportion is often called the attack rate (AR). The *infection* attack rate or incidence proportion is the proportion of the population who become infected. The *disease* attack rate or incidence proportion is the proportion who develop disease.

The mirror image of the incidence proportion is the survival probability, the probability of not experiencing an event in a time interval $(0, T)$. Use of the incidence proportion in the form given here requires that the population be a closed group from the beginning to the end of the study. That is, no one can leave the population. However, analytic methods in survival analysis allow estimation of the probability of experiencing an event in the time interval $(0, T)$ even when some people leave the study.

Prevalence

The *prevalence*, P, is the proportion of a population that has the disease or outcome of interest at a given time. *Seroprevalence*, also denoted P, is the proportion of a population that has a serological marker at a given time. An example is the seroprevalence of immunoglobulin G (IgG) against a specific microbe. Current seroprevalence can reflect either past or current infection, depending on which immune markers are measured. We denote prevalence at time t by $P(t)$. Prevalence of a disease or of infectious people can change rapidly with time, especially during epidemics or due to seasonality of the microbe.

Basic Reproductive Number, R_0

The *basic reproductive number*, R_0, of a microbe in a population is the expected number of new infectives produced by one infective in a large, completely susceptible population during his or her period of infectiousness. For microparasitic diseases, the basic reproductive number is expressed as

$$R_0 = cpd,$$

where c is the number of contacts per unit time, p is the transmission probability, and d is the duration of infectiousness. The basic reproductive number is a measure of the reproductive capacity of a microbe in a particular host population. It is discussed in more detail in Chapter 4.

The Dependent Happening Relation

The key relation in infectious diseases is the dependence of infection events among individuals in a population, called dependent happenings. Under random mixing, the dependent happening relation can be expressed as

$$I(t) = cpP(t), \qquad (1)$$

where $I(t)$ is the incidence rate, c is the constant contact rate, p is the transmission probability, and $P(t)$ is the prevalence of infectious persons at time t. The dependent happening relation means that the incidence rate of infection is dependent on the prevalence of infectious persons. The incidence rate also depends on the contact process and contact patterns, as well as the transmission probability.

The formal expression (1) of the dependent happening relation helps clarify our thinking about several issues. First, in designing and interpreting studies in infectious diseases, it is crucial to distinguish risk factors or interventions related to exposure to infection from those related to susceptibility. The dependent happening expression (1) makes explicit the different components related to the risk of becoming infected. All three factors on the right in relation (1) contribute to exposure to infection. If individuals increase their rate of contact, c, it could increase their exposure to infection. The transmission probability, p, depends on the degree of infectiousness of the contact as well as the type of contact, and so plays a role in determining the level of exposure to infection. The prevalence of infectious people in the population $P(t)$ also helps determine the level of exposure to infection. Behavioral changes aimed at lowering exposure to infection could be aimed at reducing the contact rate, c, altering the transmission probability, p, or reducing the probability that a person makes contact with someone who is infectious. The latter would mean being more selective about with whom one makes contact, with the effect of reducing the prevalence of infectives $P(t)$ in one's contact groups.

Susceptibility of the person at risk to become infected enters into the dependent happening relation primarily through the transmission probability, p. That is, conditional on actually being exposed to a certain level of infection, the susceptibility of the exposed person determines whether the person becomes infected. Although in any given study, the separate components of the dependent happening relation (1) may not be measured, assumptions about the relation of the incidence rate to the contact process, transmission probability, and prevalence are fundamental in designing and interpreting studies.

Second, the dependent happening relation (1) applies in epidemic and rapidly changing situations as well as in stationary situations. It does not rely on the assumption of equilibrium to be valid. Contrast this with another well-known relation from epidemiology that does rely on the assumption of equilibrium incidence rate and prevalence. If D is the average duration of disease, and I is the equilibrium incidence rate of disease, then prevalence approximately equals the product of the incidence rate and average duration (Freeman 1980):

$$P \doteq ID \qquad (2)$$

Relation (2) holds approximately for prevalence less than 0.10. At higher prevalences, the left side would be better represented by the prevalence odds. In Chapter 4 on transmission dynamics, we presented a hypothetical example of gonorrhea in men and women. The dependent happening relation (1) in that example is that incidence of infection in each gender depends on the prevalence of infectious people in the other gender. This does not require that gonorrhea is at equilibrium in the population. In contrast, at equilibrium, expression (2) says that prevalence of infection in each gender depends on the incidence and duration in the same gender. The capital D for duration of disease distinguishes it from the lower case d for duration of infectiousness. The word disease emphasizes that relation (2) is more closely related to the natural history of disease, whereas the dependent happening relation (1) is more closely related to the course of infectiousness, as discussed in Chapter 4.

Third, expression (1) not only demonstrates the relation between the transmission probability and incidence rate as measures of disease frequency but also clarifies their difference. While the transmission probability is defined conditional on exposure to infection, the incidence rate is defined as events per person time. The incidence rate as well as the incidence proportion rely on the notion that the people being studied are potentially exposed to infection, but do not require that any particular individual is actually exposed. Halloran and Struchiner (1995) call the transmission probability a *conditional* measure of disease frequency, while the incidence proportion, incidence rate, and hazard rate are *unconditional* measures. The parameters transmission probability, incidence rate, and incidence proportion form a hierarchy requiring decreasing amounts of information about the transmission and contact processes (Rhodes et al. 1996).

Fourth, the dependent happening relation for the incidence rate $I(t) = cpP(t)$ can be contrasted with the expression for the basic reproductive number, $R_0 = cpd$. Both contain the product of the contact rate and the transmission probability, cp, a fundamental expression of the transmission process. However, the incidence rate reflects the point of view of the susceptible and the probability of becoming infected per time unit. The basic reproductive number, R_0, reflects the point of view of the infectious host as the number of people he or she will infect.

Finally, the dependent happening relation (1) can be used to estimate different quantities, depending on which components have been measured. The product of the contact rate and the transmission probability equals the more easily estimable ratio of the incidence rate to the prevalence of infectives, $cp = I(t)/P(t)$. Thus we do not need to observe the underlying contact process and transmission probabilities to obtain some information about their product cp. The transmission probability can be estimated if the other three components are measured, $p = I(t)/cP(t)$. To estimate c separately from p, however, generally information is needed about the contact process. That is, c and p are not separately identifiable from cp without information on contacts.

MEASURES OF EFFECT AND ASSOCIATION

Evaluating interventions and determining risk factors for infection and disease are important goals of infectious disease epidemiology. Risk differences and risk ratios are formed from the measures of disease frequency discussed earlier. Measures of effect and association based on the transmission probability are specific to infectious diseases epidemiology, while those based on the incidence rates or incidence proportion are common to all fields. Because of the dependent happening relation, interventions in infectious diseases can also have important indirect effects on individuals not receiving the intervention directly. In this section, we focus on the measures of effect and association that are particularly important for infectious disease epidemiology. We begin with a discussion of the difference between causal effects and association.

Causal Effects Versus Association

Suppose we do a study of condom use and its relation to the risk of sexually transmitted infection. We observe that the difference between the proportion of people who contract a sexually transmitted disease in the group using condoms and the group not using condoms is 0.4. We can definitely say we have observed an association between condom use and risk of infection, and quantify the association using the observed risk difference. Can we claim, however, that condom use has a causal effect on reducing risk of infection compared to no condom use? No, we cannot say that condom use is the cause of the reduction in risk without further restrictions. To clarify the difference between association and causal effects, we turn to a formal structure for defining effects of causes.

The approach for defining the effects of causes requires that the effect of a cause be defined relative to another cause. The causes could be different treatments, preventive interventions, or risk factors. In our example, the comparison is between condom use and no condom use. The causal effect of condom

use compared to no condom use by an individual is defined as the difference between what the infection outcome would be if the person used condoms and what it would be if the person did not use condoms. This approach to defining causal effects assumes that an individual has some potential outcome for each of the various interventions or treatments under study. The causal effect in an individual is the difference between his or her potential outcomes under the two treatments (Rubin 1978, Holland 1986).

Consider four individuals who are at risk for a sexually transmitted disease. The potential outcomes of the four individuals are listed in Table 5–1. For individual i, let Y_{i0} and Y_{i1} denote the potential infection outcomes under no condom use and condom use, respectively. Then, for any individual i, the individual causal effect of condom use versus no condom use is $Y_{i1} - Y_{i0}$. For subject one in Table 5–1, it is $0 - 1 = -1$, that is, condom use prevents infection in subject 1. For subject 2, the difference in the potential outcomes is $1 - 1 = 0$. That is, there is no causal effect of condom use in subject 2. The person becomes infected in either case.

The fundamental problem of causal inference is that only one of these potential outcomes is observable in any individual, since we can observe the individual only either using condoms or not using condoms. A statistical approach to solving the fundamental problem of causal inference is to define the average causal effect in a population. The average causal effect, C, in the population is the average of the individual causal effects. This, in turn, equals the difference between

Table 5–1 Potential Outcomes under Condom Use or No Condom Use *

	Potential Outcome*	
Subject	Condom Use $(X=1)$ (Y_{i1})	No Condom Use $(X=0)$ (Y_{i0})
1	0	1
2	1	1
3	0	0
4	0	1

*0,1 denote uninfected and infected, respectively.

the average value of the potential outcomes if everyone received one intervention and the average if everyone received the other intervention. Thus

$$C = E[Y_1 - Y_0] = E[Y_1] - E[Y_0],$$

where E means the average or expected value. In Table 5–1, the average causal effect of condom use compared to no condom use as measured by sexually transmitted infection is $(1 - 3)/4 = -0.50$.

Of course we still cannot observe the potential outcomes of each individual under each intervention. What we can observe is each person's potential outcome under the intervention that he or she actually used. The potential outcomes that we do not observe are called *counterfactual*. We can observe the difference in the average potential outcomes in the people who actually used a particular intervention ($X = 1$) and the average of the potential outcomes in people who did not use the intervention ($X = 0$). We denote this actual observable difference as A, and write

$$A = E[Y_1|X = 1] - E[Y_0|X = 0],$$

where $E[Y_1|X = 1]$ is the average of the potential outcomes in people who actually received $X = 1$, and similarly for $E[Y_0|X = 0]$. In the example above, we observed a difference of 0.4 between risk of infection in the two groups, so $A = 0.4$ in the example. The value of A expresses an association between the intervention and the outcome, but does this association equal the average causal effect in the population C? The answer is, not in general. That is, in general

$$C = E[Y_1] - E[Y_0] \neq E[Y_1|X = 1] - E[Y_0|X = 0] = A,$$

except under certain conditions.

Under two important assumptions, the observable association, A, will equal the average causal effect in the population C. The first assumption is that the potential outcomes in one person are independent of the treatment assignments in the other people.

This allows Table 5–1 to have only two columns of potential outcomes for each person, one for each treatment. For instance, the assumption is that subject 1's condom use does not affect the potential outcomes of subject 2. This is sometimes called the *noninterference of units* assumption (Cox 1958). The assumption is obviously violated in many studies in infectious diseases.

The second assumption is that the intervention assignment for each individual is independent of his or her potential outcomes. An example of an independent assignment mechanism is randomization. That is, under randomization, we do not assign people whose potential outcome is infection to use condoms, while assigning people whose potential outcome is no infection not to use condoms. This would obviously bias our measure of effect. Formally, under randomization and the noninterference of units, the causal risk difference equals the observed risk difference,

$$C = E[Y_1] - E[Y_0] = E[Y_1|X = 1] - E[Y_0|X = 0] = A.$$

This statement can be interpreted that in a large population, if half of the people are randomly assigned to each of the two treatments, the difference in the observed average outcome of the two groups would be the same as if it had been possible to observe the entire population under each of the treatments. Assignment mechanisms are usually not random. That is, people decide for their own reasons whether they want to use condoms, and it could very well be associated with their probability of becoming infected. This is a simple formal argument for using randomization to estimate causal effects. It also clarifies the difference between association and causal effects.

Most studies are not randomized. Many studies are *observational*, with the investigator having little influence over the events under study. In many *experimental* or intervention studies, the investigator may have some control over allocation or the interventions or covariates of interest, but does not randomize them. The goal of observational and nonrandomized studies may be to elucidate causal effects, but since they are not randomized, the objective is difficult to achieve. Under these circumstances, the difference in the average outcomes of two groups could be due to something other than the measured risk factor or intervention. An estimated association between the outcomes of interest and the intervention or risk factors of interest could be due to unmeasured confounders.

For instance, people who use condoms may also be very careful about whom they choose for sex partners. Thus people who use condoms may also have a lower exposure to infection. Although we may observe a fourfold decrease in sexually transmitted diseases among people who use condoms compared to those who do not, the reduction may have nothing to do with condom use itself. Thus it would be incorrect to conclude that use of condoms has a causal effect on reducing sexually transmitted diseases. It would be correct to say that there is an observed association. Causal inference will generally rely on some untestable assumptions.

There are many sources of bias in observational studies. Ascertainment or selection biases result in the actual study population not being representative of the population that was targeted to be studied. Ascertainment bias can be important in infectious disease studies that ascertain transmission units through an infectious person, such as an index case. The types of infected persons so ascertained might not represent the infected population. Also, larger transmission units in a population would tend to be ascertained more often than smaller transmission units because they have more people in them. Other sources of biases and potential confounders are covered in detail in Rothman and Greenland (1998) as well as many other texts.

It is important to measure possible confounders in nonrandomized studies to take them into account in the analysis. However, it is difficult to measure all confounders. *Sensitivity analyses* can be used to quantify potential *hidden biases* due to unobserved covariates (Rosenbaum 1995, Robins et al.

1999). The point of departure for sensitivity analyses is quite often the paradigm of the randomized study and causal inference described previously. When the goal is to make causal statements based on observational studies, sensitivity analyses can provide some measure of uncertainty about the bias and how large the bias would need to be to swamp out the observed association. Although randomization helps in interpreting study results as causal effects, it does not control for all confounding of estimates. The interested reader can find more on this topic in Greenland and Robins (1986), Greenland (1987), Greenland et al. (1999), Gail (1986, 1988), and Gail et al. (1984, 1988).

Despite its general usefulness, the potential outcome approach to causal effects encounters difficulty when applied to dependent happenings, such as in infectious diseases. The assumption commonly made when using the potential outcome paradigm is that the potential outcomes in any individual are independent of the treatment assignments in other individuals. This is not true for many of the situations in infectious diseases.

Suppose a person is vaccinated and does not become infected, but if he had not been vaccinated, he would have become infected and infected another person. This second person's infection outcome is dependent on the intervention assignment of the first person. Although the assumption that the potential outcome in one person does not depend on the treatment assignment in another person is not conceptually necessary for this approach to causal inference (Rubin 1978, Rubin 1990), the problems arising when the assumption is violated have not been solved.

For example, in Table 5–1, related to potential outcomes for two treatments, the two columns need to be expanded for each individual to include all the treatment and outcome possibilities of people with whom he or she may make potentially infectious contact. However, this is not generally feasible. Quite simply put, because of the indirect effects in infectious diseases, the population causal rate ratio of receiving an intervention compared to not receiving the intervention does not necessarily equal the observed rate ratio. Another option is to condition on exposure to infection, as in the transmission probability. This solution runs into other problems. Studies that challenge humans with inoculation by the microbe are unethical if they pose more than a minimal risk, so exposure to infection can, in general, not be randomized. Halloran and Struchiner (1995) discuss in detail the problem of using the potential outcome approach to causal inference in infectious diseases. Although solutions are still being sought for applying the approach to dependent happenings, the paradigm is increasingly being used to study causal effects, association, nonadherence, and confounding. Infectious disease epidemiologists need to be familiar with its strengths and its shortcomings.

Measures of Effect and Association

Commonly, the same ratio and difference measures are used for estimating both causal effects and associations. Their interpretation is simply different. For simplicity of presentation, we generally use the term *effect* in the following discussion. In this section we present an overview of many of the commonly used risk ratios. Table 5–2 contains a summary of some important relative risk measures in infectious disease epidemiology by choice of comparison group and level of information required. In the top row are relative risk measures based on the transmission probability. These measures are specific to infectious disease epidemiology. They estimate the relative susceptibility and infectiousness associated with risk factors or covariates conditional on exposure to infection. In the bottom part of the first column are the unconditional relative risk measures based on the incidence rate, hazard rate, and incidence proportion. These relative risk measures are not specific to infectious disease epidemiology. The unconditional relative risk measures estimate either relative exposure to infection or susceptibility depending on the design of the study and assumptions regarding exposure to infection. In the bottom right portion of the table are measures of community level relative risk in which the comparison groups are transmission dynam-

ically separate populations. They include the indirect, total, and overall effects of intervention. The indirect effects of intervention are important in the dependent happening situation.

Transmission Probability Ratio

The transmission probability ratio, TPR, is a measure of the relative risk of transmission to susceptibles between different pairs of risk factors in infectives during a contact. For any given type of contact and infectious agent, we can estimate the effect of a covariate on susceptibility, infectiousness, or their combination by our choice of comparison pairs in the transmission probability ratio. We may want to compare the male-to-male, male-to-female, female-to-male, and female-to-female transmission probabilities of gonorrhea. We may want to know how transmission of influenza between children compares to that between adults, or also between children and adults. We may want to compare the ability of two types of mosquitoes to transmit malaria to humans. The goal of a study might be to estimate the effect of vaccination on reducing susceptibility and infectiousness as measured by the secondary attack rate. We can also estimate the transmission probability of differing types of contacts, infectious agents, routes of infection, or strains of an infectious agent. For instance, one clade (i.e., strain) of HIV may be more transmissible than another.

Suppose that there are two types of infectives and susceptibles making a specified type of contact for a given type or strain of microbe. We denote the two risk levels as 0 and 1. The risk factors might be vaccinated and unvaccinated, for example. Then there are four different possible combinations of the risk factors in the transmission probability. If the first subscript denotes the infectious person and the second denotes the susceptible in the contact, then the four transmission probabilities are p_{00}, p_{01}, p_{10}, p_{11}. For instance, p_{10} denotes the transmission probability of an infective with risk factor level 1 to a susceptible with risk factor level 0. The relative susceptibility as measured by the transmission probability ratio, TPR_S, is

Table 5–2 Various Measures of Relative Risk.

		Comparison Groups and Effect		
Level	Parameter Choice	Susceptibility	Infectiousness	Combined Change in Susceptibility and Infectiousness
A. Parameter conditional on exposure to infection				
I	Transmission probability, p Secondary attack rate (SAR)	$TPR_S = \dfrac{p_{01}}{p_{00}}$	$TPR_I = \dfrac{p_{10}}{p_{00}}$	$TPR_T = \dfrac{p_{11}}{p_{00}}$

B. Parameter not conditional on exposure to infection

		Study Design			
		I Direct	IIA Indirect	IIB Total	III Overall
II	Incidence rate (I)	$IR_I = \dfrac{I_{A1}}{I_{A0}}$	$IR_{IIA} = \dfrac{I_{A0}}{I_{B0}}$	$IR_{IIB} = \dfrac{I_{A1}}{I_{B0}}$	$IR_{III} = \dfrac{I_A}{I_B}$
	Hazard (λ)	$HR_I = \dfrac{\lambda_{A1}}{\lambda_{A0}}$	$HR_{IIA} = \dfrac{\lambda_{A0}}{\lambda_{B0}}$	$HR_{IIB} = \dfrac{\lambda_{A1}}{\lambda_{B0}}$	$HR_{III} = \dfrac{\lambda_A}{\lambda_B}$
III	Proportional hazards (PH)	$HR_{PH} = e^{\beta_1}$	NA	NA	NA
IV	Incidence proportion (R) Attack rates (AR)	$RR_I = \dfrac{R_{A1}}{R_{A0}}$	$RR_{IIA} = \dfrac{R_{A0}}{R_{B0}}$	$RR_{IIB} = \dfrac{R_{A1}}{R_{B0}}$	$RR_{III} = \dfrac{R_A}{R_B}$

Adapted from Halloran et al., Am J Epidemiol 146:789–803, 1997.

The subscripts 0 and 1 describe two levels of risk. The subscripts S, I and T denote susceptibility, infectiousness, and combined effects, respectively. The Cox proportional hazards estimator is denoted by e^{β_1}. Time has been omitted from the table for notational clarity.

measured by comparing the transmission probabilities to susceptibles with different covariates from infectives. The relative infectiousness, TPR_I, of infected people with the two covariate levels is measured by comparing the transmission probabilities from infectives with different covariate levels to susceptibles. To measure the combined effect of the covariates, TPR_T, the transmission probability between people who are both covariate level 1 is compared to that between people in which both are covariate level 0. The transmission probability ratios are:

relative susceptibility: $TPR_S = \dfrac{p_{i1}}{p_{i0}}$;

relative infectiousness: $TPR_I = \dfrac{p_{1j}}{p_{0j}}$;   (3)

and combined effect: $TPR_T = \dfrac{p_{11}}{p_{00}}$.

The transmission probability ratios are in the top row of Table 5–2. In general, there could be several levels of covariates, with p_{ij} denoting the transmission probability from an infective with covariate status i to a susceptible with covariate status j.

One of the covariates might be considered a control or baseline value. Table 5–3 presents an example from a measles vaccine study of the secondary attack rates from vaccinated or unvaccinated index cases to vaccinated or unvaccinated susceptibles. Recall that the secondary attack rate is a special case of a transmission probability, so we can use the SAR_{ij} in place of the p_{ij} in the expressions for the transmission probability ratios. We use the subscripts 0 and 1 to denote unvaccinated and vaccinated, respectively. As an example, consider the data in Table 5–3. The secondary attack rate if both the index case and the exposed children are unvaccinated is $SAR_{00} = 0.38$. If both are vaccinated,

Table 5–3 Secondary Attack Rates by Vaccination Status of the Index Child and the Vaccination Status of the Exposed Children in a Measles Epidemic in Senegal, 1994–1995

Index Case	Secondary Attack Rate		
	Vaccinated, Exposed Children	Unvaccinated, Exposed Children	All Children
Vaccinated	6/83 (0.07)	3/17 (0.18)	9/100 (0.09)
Unvaccinated	41/374 (0.11)	47/124 (0.38)	88/498 (0.18)
Total	47/457 (0.10)	50/141 (0.35)	97/598 (0.16)

From Cisse et al. 1999.

$SAR_{11} = 0.07$. If we calculate TPR_S separately for children exposed to unvaccinated or vaccinated index cases, the estimates are $TPR_S = SAR_{01}/SAR_{00} = 0.11/0.38 = 0.29$ and $TPR_S = SAR_{11}/SAR_{10} = 0.07/0.18 = 0.39$, respectively. Without stratifying on infective vaccination status, the effect of vaccination on susceptibility is estimated as $TPR_S = SAR_{\cdot 1}/SAR_{\cdot 0} = 0.10/0.35 = 0.29$. The dot in the subscript indicates summation over both the 0 and the 1 strata. The interpretation is that the average transmission probability to vaccinated children is 0.29 that of the transmission probability to unvaccinated children. The analogous calculations for the effect of vaccination on infectiousness are $TPR_I = SAR_{10}/SAR_{00} = 0.07/0.11 = 0.64$, $TPR_I = SAR_{11} = SAR_{01} = 0.18/0.38 = 0.47$, and $TPR_I = SAR_{1 \cdot} = SAR_{0 \cdot} = 0.09/0.18 = 0.50$, respectively. The vaccine seems to have a stronger effect on susceptibility than on infectiousness. The ratio of the transmission probability if both the index case and the exposed children are vaccinated compared to if both are unvaccinated is $TPR_T = SAR_{11}/SAR_{00} = 0.07/0.38 = 0.18$.

The corresponding vaccine efficacies based on the transmission probability ratios can be calculated from $VE_S = 1 - TPR_S$, $VE_I = 1 - TPR_I$, and $VE_T = 1 - TPR_T$ (Halloran et al. 1997). In this case, the average vaccine efficacy for susceptibility is $VE_S = 1 - 0.29 = 0.71$, the average vaccine efficacy for infectiousness is $VE_I = 1 - 0.50 = 0.50$, and the efficacy if both are vaccinated compared to if neither are vaccinated is $VE_T = 1 - 0.18 = 0.82$.

A slightly different approach to the TPR_S can be used in the binomial models described in Chapter 4. Assume that the effect of the covariates on infectiousness and susceptibility are multiplicative on the transmission probability, and that the two effects are independent. Denote the relative susceptibility of risk factor level 1 to 0 by θ, so that $TPR_S = \theta$, and the relative infectiousness of level 1 to 0 by ϕ, so that $TPR_I = \phi$. By the assumption that the two effects are independent, then $TPR_T = \theta\phi$. Assume that p_{00} is the baseline transmission probability, denoted simply by p. The transmission probability between an infective of covariate status μ and a susceptible of covariate status ν is written $\theta^\nu \phi^\mu p$. For example, if both people in the contact are of covariate status 0, this reduces simply to $p = p_{00}$. If the infectious person has covariate status $\mu = 1$ and the susceptible person has covariate status $\nu = 0$, then the expression reduces to $\phi p = p_{10}$. A simple extension of the binomial model to include covariates is to insert the appropriate expression for the transmission probability for each contact observed. The expression can be solved using numerical methods for the estimates of p, θ, and ϕ to obtain the desired TPR_S. Other more complex models for estimating transmission probability ratios are mentioned in the Study Designs section.

Incidence and Hazard Rate Ratios

Consider the situation that there is just one covariate with two levels, denoted by 0 and 1. The incidence rate ratio at time t is

$$IR(t) = \frac{I_1(t)}{I_0(t)},$$

where $I_0(t)$ and $I_1(t)$ are the incidence rates in the two covariate groups. The hazard rate ratio is $\lambda_1(t)/\lambda_0(t)$. If the hazard rate ratio in the two groups is constant over time, the proportional hazards model is said to hold (Cox 1972). The proportional hazard ratio is often denoted e^β, where β is the estimated parameter. In the proportional hazards model, the baseline hazard rate in the two groups cancels out and does not need to be estimated. The incidence rate ratio and hazard rate ratio do not condition on exposure to infection. They are not specific to infectious diseases. In Table 5–2 the incidence rate ratio and hazard rate ratio are the second and third row of parameters. The fourth row contains the proportional hazard parameter, but only under the column for direct effects. Vaccine efficacy estimated by the incidence rate ratio is $VE_{IR}(t) = 1 - IR(t)$. Vaccine efficacy can also be estimated from the hazard rate ratio.

Relative Incidence Proportion

Assume again that there is just one covariate with two levels, denoted by 0 and 1. The incidence proportion ratio at time T in a study that goes from time $(0, T)$ is

$$RR(T) = \frac{R_1(T)}{R_0(T)},$$

where $R_0(T)$ and $R_1(T)$ are the incidence proportions up to time T in the two covariate groups. The bottom row in Table 5–2 contains the incidence proportion ratio. The incidence proportion ratio does not require information on exposure to infection and is not specific to infectious disease epidemiology. It is sometimes called the attack rate ratio. Vaccine efficacy can be estimated from $VE_{RR}(T) = 1 - RR(T)$.

Conditional Versus Unconditional Relative Risks Measures

The relative risk measures require differing levels of information for their estimation. The greatest difference is between the conditional parameters, such as the transmission probability ratio, and the unconditional parameters, such as the incidence rate ratio and the incidence proportion ratio. To estimate the TPR, information on contacts between susceptibles and infectives and knowledge of infection events is generally required. The transmission probability ratios are specific to infectious diseases. For estimation of the incidence rate ratio, the time at which each event occurs and the time at potential risk are required. Similar time-to-event data are needed to estimate the relative hazard rates. For the incidence proportion ratio, only information on whether an event occurs by the end of the study is required. Thus the ordering of the rows in Table 5–2 corresponds to a hierarchy of information needed for estimating the relative risks (Rhodes et al. 1996).

In designing a study, a choice needs to be made about which relative risk measure will be used in the analysis to help determine what data to collect. The primary choice is between using the transmission probability ratio or one of the unconditional measures, such as the incidence rate ratio. We can use the dependent happening relation (1) to clarify some of the implications of using the incidence rate ratio. Analogous arguments would apply to the hazard rate ratio and the incidence proportion ratio. We expand the dependent happening relation (1) to include two covariate groups. We let $I_1(t)$ in covariate group 1 be the product of the contact rate c_1, the transmission probability from an average infectious person with whom they make contact, $p_{\cdot 1}$, and the prevalence of infection in those people with whom they make contact, $P^1(t)$. The index is in the superscript to indicate it is the prevalence in those people with whom people in covariate group 1 make contact. This might not be covariate group 1 itself. Similarly, the incidence rate $I_0(t)$ in covariate group 0 is the product of the contact rate c_0, the transmission probability $p_{\cdot 0}$, and the prevalence in their contacts, $P^0(t)$. The incidence rate ratio can then be expressed

$$IR(t) = \frac{I_1(t)}{I_0(t)} = \frac{c_1\, p_{\cdot 1}\, P^1(t)}{c_0\, p_{\cdot 0}\, P^0(t)}. \quad (4)$$

Although the incidence rate ratio compares the incidence rates in two groups of susceptibles, its interpretation is not limited to being a measure of the relative susceptibility of the two groups. In expression (4), the incidence rate ratio could differ from 1 for a variety of reasons. The contact rates, c_0 and c_1, of the comparison groups could differ. The transmission probabilities, $p_{\cdot 0}$ and $p_{\cdot 1}$, could differ either because the susceptibility of the comparison groups differs, the groups make different types of contacts, or they make contacts with infective people of differing infectiousness. The proportion of contacts the groups make with infective people $P_0(t)$ and $P_1(t)$ could differ because they circulate in differing subpopulations. For example, we might observe that the incidence rate of yellow fever is three times higher in men than in women. The higher incidence rate in men could result from: a higher contact rate with the mosquito vector for yellow fever; men may be more susceptible to developing yellow fever when exposed; or men may spend time in areas where a higher proportion of the yellow fever vector mosquitoes are infected.

Consider again a study of the effect of condoms on sexually transmitted infection. Assume that condom use reduces infectiousness, so that the transmission probability to people whose partners use condoms is $p_1 = 0.25 p_0$. Assume we conduct a study in which we do measure contacts of the study subjects with infectives. Assume that there are 100 contacts between infectives in each group. In the group using condoms, four people become infected, while in the other group, 16 people become infected. Then we estimate that $p_1 = 0.04$, $p_0 = 0.16$, and that $TPR_I = 0.25$. Suppose that instead of collecting information on contacts with infectives, we collect only time-of-event data and person-time-at-risk data, and use the incidence rate ratio. If the study is randomized and people do not change their behavior after randomization except to use condoms,

the contact rates, prevalence of infection, and infectiousness in the sexual partners of the two groups might be equal. Then

$$IR(t) = \frac{I_1(t)}{I_0(t)} = \frac{c_1\, p_1.\, P^1(t)}{c_0\, p_0.\, P^0(t)} = \frac{p_{1.}}{p_{0.}} = 0.25.$$

In this simple case, we would get a similar estimate from both the TPR_I and the IR.

Suppose that the study is observational and that people using condoms have a three times higher contact rate than people not using condoms, $c_1 = 3c_0$. However, we do not collect information on the relative contact rates in the groups. Then the expected estimate of $IR(t)$ would be

$$IR(t) = \frac{I_1(t)}{I_0(t)} = \frac{c_1\, p_1.P^1(t)}{c_0\, p_0.P^0(t)}$$
$$= \frac{3c_0(0.25 p_0)}{c_0\, p_0.} = 0.75.$$

Interpretation of the estimate 0.75 would be difficult without further information. If we falsely assumed that the behavior of the two groups was similar, then the results suggest that condom use reduces transmission by less than a factor of two, rather than by a factor of four.

If the contact rate were the same in the two groups, but people who asked their partners to use condoms chose their sexual partners from a partner pool in which prevalence was five times higher, then $P^1(t) = 5P^0(t)$. The expected estimate would be

$$IR(t) = \frac{I_1(t)}{I_j(t)} = \frac{c_1\, p_1.P^1(t)}{c_0\, p_0.P^0(t)}$$
$$= \frac{(0.25 p_0)5p^0(t)}{p_0.P^0(t)} = 1.25.$$

It would appear that condom use actually increases incidence. Thus there could be a difference in the incidence rates of two groups for a variety of reasons.

Under what circumstances could we interpret a difference in the incidence rates in two groups as due to a difference in susceptibility? First, the risk factor (e.g., age) or intervention (e.g., vaccination) in question would have to be associated with the study individual's susceptibility, not exposure to infection. Second, the exposure to infection in the comparison groups would have to be the same. Under randomization, and assuming nothing changed postrandomization, we would expect exposure to infection to be equal in the two groups. Since several factors contribute to exposure to infection, it may be that not each of the factors is the same in each group, but the overall exposure to infection is the same. If exposure to infection in the groups is not the same, however, just as with any confounder, stratifying on a surrogate measure for exposure to infection can improve the estimates of the effects on susceptibility. To stratify by surrogates or risk factors for exposure to infection is not the same as conditioning on actual contacts with infectives.

In designing and interpreting studies, it is important to distinguish risk factors for exposure to infection from risk factors for susceptibility. For any particular risk factor or intervention, one must give thought to the component of the dependent happening expression to which it corresponds. It should then be clear whether the risk factor corresponds to exposure to infection or to susceptibility. Behavioral interventions could affect the contact rate, the transmission probability, or the probability that a given contact is infectious (Halloran et al. 1994). Randomization can help interpretation of the results. With randomization and masking, on the average, the comparison groups should be similar in the absence of intervention. Although estimating the transmission probability ratio requires more information than the unconditional measures, it has clear advantages. Estimates of the transmission probability ratio can be more directly interpreted as evaluating relative infectiousness and susceptibility (Koopman et al. 1991). In fact, estimation of the relative infectiousness is generally not possible except by using the transmission probability ratio. Also, by controlling for contacts between

susceptibles and infectives and exposure to infection, the transmission probability ratio is more robust than the unconditional measures to deviations from randomization.

Population and Community Level Relative Risks

Because of the dependent happenings in infectious diseases, interventions often have effects not only on the people receiving the intervention but also on people not receiving the intervention. The indirect effects are defined not only with regard to a kind of intervention, such as vaccination, but for the allocation of the intervention in the entire population. Although outcomes will still be measured on individuals, evaluation of indirect effects of an intervention in a population involves comparison of populations or communities, not just individuals. The primary unit of analysis and inference is the population.

We define three different types of effects at the population level (Fig. 5–1). Indirect effects are benefits, or detriments, from an intervention program in a population to individuals not directly receiving the intervention, compared to their hypothetical experience if their population had not had the intervention program. Total effects are the combined direct effect in individuals actually receiving the intervention and the benefits due to the indirect effects of the intervention program as a whole. The overall effect of an intervention program is the effect on the population as a whole, including both those receiving and those not receiving the intervention.

Vaccination programs are a common example in which individuals receive the intervention but its widespread application can have indirect effects on those who were not vaccinated. The indirect effects in the unvaccinated people may be different from those in the vaccinated people, which is why we define both indirect and total effects. For example, the average age of first infection may be shifted in both the vaccinated and the unvaccinated people. However, it may be shifted even more in the vaccinated people because of the protection directly conferred

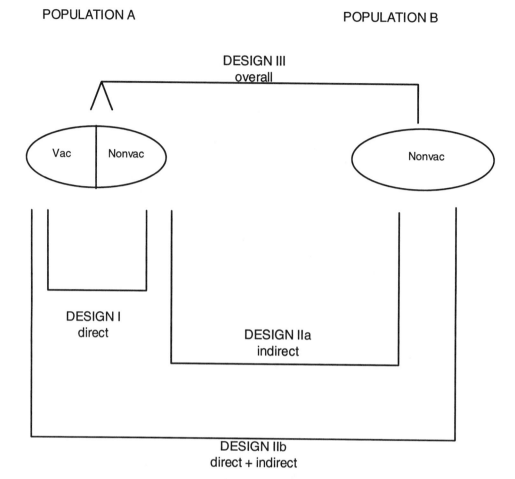

Figure 5–1. Types of effects of interventions against infectious disease and different study designs based on comparison populations for their evaluation.
Source: Halloran and Struchiner 1991.

by the vaccine. As an example of estimating overall effects, Hayes and colleagues (1995) studied the effect of improved treatment of sexually transmitted disease on HIV infection in rural Tanzania with a community randomized controlled trial. Bed net studies for protecting against malaria infection can also be evaluated for their effect on population level incidence. Some interventions are not applied at the level of the individual and have only overall effects. For example, draining mosquito breeding sites is intended to reduce transmission of malaria by reducing the abundance of mosquitoes. Introducing wells for obtaining water is supposed to reduce Guinea worm infection (dracunculiasis).

In Figure 5–1, the assumption is that some individuals in population A received the intervention program and population B did not receive the intervention program. The different kinds of effects are measured by comparing different subpopulations in population A to population B. For indirect effects, individuals in population A not receiving the intervention are compared to individuals in population B, all of whom did not receive the intervention. To measure total effects, the subpopulation in A composed of individuals receiving the intervention is compared to population B. For the overall public health benefits, the average outcome in the entire population A is compared to that in B. The comparison of different subgroups from population A to population B are designated study designs IIA, IIB, and III, respectively They are called the study designs for dependent happenings (Struchiner et al. 1990, Halloran and Struchiner 1991,1995). Different strata within the subpopulations such as age groups or gender can also be compared.

The bottom right portion of Table 5–2 contains examples of possible comparisons using the unconditional estimators to estimate the indirect, total, and overall effects. For example, if the incidence rate ratio is used to measure the indirect effects, then $IR_{IIA}(t) = I_{A0}(t)/I_{B0}(t)$, where $A0$ and $B0$ denote those not receiving the intervention in A and B, respectively. The total effects are estimated from $IR_{IIB}(t) = I_{A1}(t)/I_{B0}(t)$. The proportional hazards parameter is not included in that portion of the table, because the assumption that the baseline hazard rate in the comparison groups is equal would presumably be violated. A change in the basic reproductive number R_0 or shift in age distribution could also be used for comparison of the overall or indirect effects.

Study designs of type I measure those direct effects discussed previously with unconditional parameters and compare people receiving the intervention with people not receiving the intervention within the same population. One important difference to noninfectious disease epidemiology can be made explicit here. In noninfectious diseases, the prevented fraction in a covariate group is generally measured by comparing the incidence proportion in a group with a particular covariate value with that in a group with another covariate value in the same population. The actual number of prevented cases can be calculated by knowing what fraction of the population has the covariate of interest and the relative difference in the two incidence proportions. However, in infectious disease, because of the indirect effects of intervention, this would not be the appropriate comparison. For example, if many people were vaccinated, then the incidence proportion would be lower in both the vaccinated and the unvaccinated groups

than it would have been without vaccination. The number of prevented cases is larger than would be estimated by the comparison used in noninfectious diseases. The appropriate comparison would use a study design IIB. However, generally, use of study design IIB is not possible to estimate the prevented number of cases. If study design type I is used, then the estimated prevented fraction will generally underestimate the total number of cases prevented by the covariate or intervention. This should be kept in mind when interpreting the results.

STUDY DESIGNS

Many study designs are the same for infectious diseases as for noninfectious diseases. Here we focus on concepts relating to these study designs that are specific to infectious diseases, such as the interaction of the study cohorts with the population at large, designs that allow estimation of the transmission probability ratio, and the role of assumptions about population mixing structures in the use and interpretation of data. Other books such as Rothman and Greenland (1998) describe principles of study designs to estimate the unconditional relative risks.

Cohort Studies

In cohort studies, usually the investigator identifies a group of disease-free people and follows them over time to see how their disease outcome depends on varying levels of risk factors or interventions. The question of interest is how the different levels of risk factor affect the time to onset of infection or disease or whether they are infected or not by the end of the study. Cohort studies are generally used to estimate the unconditional relative risks such as incidence rate ratio, hazard rate ratio, or incidence proportion ratio. With information on contacts between infectives and susceptibles, cohort studies can also be used to estimate the transmission probability ratio. The unit composed of the susceptible, the infective, and the contact between them is the irreducible element in the study of transmission. In the infectious disease setting, the cohort may be composed of small transmission units, such as partnerships, households, or schools. The small transmission units can be considered independent of one another and analyzed as minicohorts. Alternatively, the small transmission units may be thought of as embedded within a larger community in which members of the small units mix with one another. The contact patterns of the cohort members either with one another or with the population at large can influence the transmission dynamics and the interpretation of the study results. In this section, we present some of these different study designs.

A *fixed* cohort is assembled at one time and followed, with no new additions to the cohort. If a fixed cohort does not lose people during follow up, it is a *closed* cohort. A closed population in an epidemic is a closed cohort. If people leave a cohort before experiencing an event or they do not experience an event before the end of a study, their event times are not observed. Their event times are said to be *right censored*. *Dynamic* cohorts can have people entering and leaving the risk set during the period of observation. Natural history studies describe the course of infection, disease, mortality, and infectiousness within the human host. *Longitudinal* studies in which several readings are obtained on the same individual are quite common. Since the observations within an individual are correlated, longitudinal studies usually require special methods of analysis (Diggle et al. 1994). *Baseline studies* observe cohorts before an intervention to learn about the feasibility of doing an intervention and to estimate preintervention incidence of infection. For example, a baseline study will yield information on retention rates and how large the study population needs to be.

The cohort may be composed of people who are infected, with the goal being to estimate disease progression or infectiousness based on parasite shedding. Ideally, people will enter the study cohort at the time they are infected. However, sometimes study cohorts are recruited among people who were infected before they entered the study. A cohort of people recruited after they were infected is called a *prevalent* cohort. At the beginning of the HIV epidemic, of necessity, cohorts of already infected people were assembled. Brookmeyer and Gail (1987) discuss biases in risk ratios estimated in prevalent cohorts.

Cohort within a population

We can assemble either a fixed or a dynamic cohort of susceptibles within a larger dynamic population and follow them as in a usual cohort study. The transmission process in the population at large outside the cohort under study can affect incidence within the cohort. If we enroll a cohort of susceptibles and follow them as they become infected, we will observe an epidemic within the cohort. If the contacts made by the cohort members are made at random predominantly with people outside the cohort, the prevalence of infection in the contacts will be similar to the prevalence in the population at large. Prevalence in the population at large may be changing rapidly over time or it may be fairly constant.

Suppose data are collected on the infection status of the cohort members and the number of contacts made by them. Assume also that an estimate of the prevalence, P, of infection in the pool of potential contacts is available, either from the study itself or from other sources. The expression for the infection probability from a contact with unknown infection status can be used to estimate the transmission probability. The probability of infection after n total contacts is $\rho_n = 1 - (1 - Pp)^n$. In this case, the actual infection status of the contacts does not need to be known to estimate the per contact infection probability with someone of unknown infection status. If some estimate of prevalence P is available, then the expression can be used to estimate the transmission probability p. In one study, Hooper and colleagues (1978) used the number of contacts made by men, the number of men who became infected, and an estimate of gonorrhea prevalence in sex workers to estimate the transmission probability of gonorrhea per sex act from women to men. Hudgens and associates (2001) used an estimate of

HIV prevalence in injection drug users, the number of needle sharing acts and the number of injections, and the number of infections to estimate the transmission probability of HIV per needle sharing. If the contacts are predominantly with other members of the initially susceptible study cohort, then in the early phase of the study there will be few infectious contacts. However, the number of infectious contacts will increase as the epidemic within the study cohort spreads as in an epidemic process. If contacts are made with other members of the cohort, then it is likely the infection status will be known.

Transmission probability and contact studies

To estimate the transmission probability or the transmission probability ratio we generally need information on contacts between susceptibles and infectives. The concept of a *contact* is very broad and must be defined in each particular study. The microbe's transmission mode determines what types of contact are potentially infectious. Contacts can be defined between two individuals, or an individual and a vector. More generally, contacts can also be defined within small *transmission units*, such as households, child care centers, school classes, or retirement homes. Within small transmission units, mixing is often assumed to be random. A small transmission unit can also be defined as two individuals, such as a steady sexual partnership or a household with just two susceptible people. The definition of a contact within a study can depend on the definition of the transmission units. The small transmission unit can also be thought of as a minicohort.

Different definitions of a potentially infective contact and transmission unit are possible for the same microbe, and even within the same study. In a study of chickenpox transmission, a potentially infective contact could be defined as being in the same school on one day with someone with chickenpox. Alternatively, it could be defined as living in the same house during the presumed infectious period of the person with chickenpox. In the first case, the transmission unit is the school, and in the latter, it is the household.

In the first case, the contact is defined over one day, and in the latter, it is defined over the entire infectious period. In tuberculosis, a contact could be defined as riding on the same bus with someone with open tuberculosis, or as being in the same prison with someone with tuberculosis. In the former case, the transmission unit is the bus, and in the latter, it is the prison.

There could be different definitions of a contact for one definition of transmission unit. In an HIV study, a potentially infective contact could be defined as each sex act between two sexual partners in a steady relationship, one of whom is infected with HIV. Alternatively, the partnership over its entire duration or over the duration of the study could be defined as one potentially infective contact.

In Chapter 4, we discussed transmission units in the contexts of chain binomial models and of nonrandom mixing. Here we further discuss the implications of thinking about transmission units and contacts within populations for study design and analysis.

Identification of infectives

In one approach to ascertaining transmission units or contacts, infectious individuals are identified, then their transmission units or contacts are identified. The initially identified infectious person in each unit is called the *primary* or *index case*. The transmission probability or secondary attack rate is estimated by observing the proportion of the people in the transmission unit who become infected. Alternatively, a cohort of susceptible individuals could be recruited and followed over time. As individuals become infected the transmission units or contacts might be ascertained. As mentioned in the discussion on observational studies, ascertainment bias can be substantial when ascertaining transmission units by infectives. The latter method of ascertainment of transmission units would be less prone to ascertainment bias.

To estimate the conventional household SAR, data on the time of onset of disease for each case in the household as well as knowledge of who is susceptible are required. Also needed are estimates or assumptions about the minimum and maximum incubation periods, the latent period, and the maximum time that a person remains infectious. Using this information, one then needs to define the time interval after the occurrence of the index case that would include the secondary cases. Based on the time of onset data within each household or transmission unit, each case is defined as being either a secondary case or not. In the measles study in Senegal presented earlier, assumptions about all of these factors were made to define the secondary cases presented in Table 5–3. The estimated household secondary attack rate is the total number of secondary cases in all households divided by the total number of at-risk susceptibles in all households. A generalized estimating equation (GEE) (Liang and Zeger 1986) approach can be used to deal with clustering effects that may occur. In some cases, tertiary or higher generation cases may be included in the analysis by calling the secondary cases the index case. Note that the index cases are not included in the analysis, nor are any coprimaries. *Coprimaries* are people who developed disease too soon after the index case to have been infected by the index case. The assumption is that the households or other small transmission units are independent of one another.

Similar to the household secondary attack rate is the *case-contact* approach. In the case-contact approach, an index case is identified, then the people who have made contact with the index case are identified. For example, in tuberculosis or HIV, through contact tracing the people who have made contact with the infective person might be identified and their infection status ascertained. One difficulty in estimating the transmission probability from such a study is in determining the temporal order of infection in the contacts. Difficulties in estimating the conventional SAR and case-contact rates include determination of the latent and incubation periods, ascertainment of onset times of cases, and determining when an exposure to infection has taken place. The actual value of the estimated SAR

can depend on the choice of the transmission unit and the definition of contact. For example, in a study of measles transmission in Senegal, the SARs estimated in schools, at homes, and in huts differed (Cisse et al. 1999). Kemper (1980) discusses biases in conventional SAR estimation.

Susceptibles exposed to infective contacts
Another study design approach to estimate the transmission probability is to assemble a cohort of susceptibles. The study then follows the susceptibles and collects information on their contacts with infectives or potential infectives. Study subjects might give information on the average number of contacts rather than the exact number of contacts they each make per unit time. From this, the expected number of contacts during the study period can be estimated. The binomial model is probably the most commonly used model for estimating the transmission probability when susceptibles make more than one potentially infectious contact. It can take on very complicated forms, depending on assumptions about variability in the transmission probability, time-varying covariates, and the amount and quality of data available. The model can be embedded in complex Markov or survival models. The principles of the binomial model were discussed in Chapter 4. One approach to including covariate effects as multiplicative factors on the transmission probability was discussed previously in the section on the transmission probability ratio. The data required are infection outcome, number of potentially infective contacts, and covariate status for each person in the study. Parameter estimates are obtained using numerical methods. Unfortunately, only limited software is available for estimating transmission probabilities using the binomial model. Software is usually written for particular situations.

The secondary attack rate can also be defined based on the binomial model for several contacts. For example, let m be the number of sexual contacts between two partners over the course of a study, where one of the partners is infected. Then the probability of being infected after m contacts is $1 - (1 - p)^m$, the per partnership SAR over the study interval.

Studies in a community of transmission units

In the study designs to estimate the transmission probability ratios described before, the transmission units such as houses or partnerships were assumed to be independent of each other. The susceptibles in the transmission unit were assumed to be exposed to infection only by the index case, who had somehow become infected. In Chapter 4, we discuss having small transmission units within a larger community. If the small transmission units (e.g., households or partnerships) are part of a community in which individuals from different transmission units interact, then the individuals can become infected either within the transmission unit or in the community at large.

The model developed by Longini and Koopman (1982) for transmission in a community of households takes into account both sources of infection. Two parameters are estimated. One is the SAR, the probability of being infected within the transmission unit from one infective. The other is the community probability of infection (CPI), the probability of being infected in the community at large over the course of the study or during an epidemic. Thus the model allows estimation of parameters from two different levels. The SAR is a conditional parameter from level I of Table 5–2. The CPI is an unconditional parameter from level IV of Table 5–2, and is closely related to the incidence proportion. The simplest version of the model assumes that mixing is random within the small transmission units and random within the community outside of the transmission units.

In the simplest study design the data requirements to fit the model are to know for each individual his transmission unit and his infection status at the beginning and the end of the study or epidemic. That is, simple final value data and the distribution of susceptibles and infected people within the transmission units are sufficient to estimate the SAR and the CPI. For any particular person, there would be uncertainty about the source of infection. The community could be a town, and the transmission units be households, schools, or other units. This method can be used to study transmission of diseases such as measles, influenza (Longini and Koopman, 1982), or dengue (Dantes et al. 1988). Alternatively, the community could be composed of sexually active people, with nonmonogamous partnerships forming the transmission units.

Table 5–4 presents data from an Asian influenza epidemic from households with three initially susceptible people in them, which we assume to be the whole community. The data are the number of households that had either 0, 1, 2, or all 3 people infected by the end of the epidemic. Using the model developed by Longini and Koopman, the estimated SAR is 0.166, and the estimated CPI is 0.114. The interpretation is that the probability of being infected from one infective in a household is 0.166, while the probability of being infected in the community at large, allowing for transmission within households, is 0.114. We emphasize that the two estimates have very different meanings. The SAR is conditional on being exposed to infection, while the CPI is an unconditional measure related to the incidence proportion.

In fact, we can estimate the usual incidence proportion from these data by simply ignoring the household structure. That is,

Table 5–4 Observed and Expected Distributions of Asian Influenza Data (Sugiyama 1960) in Households of Size Three as Analyzed by Longini and Koopman (1982)

Number of Cases	Observed of Number Households	Expected Number of Households
0	29	29.17
1	9	7.87
2	2	3.62
3	2	1.34
Total	42	42.00

suppose we do not have information on households. There are 42 households with three people each, so the total population is 126 people. From Table 5–4, we can calculate that 19 people became infected. The incidence proportion is $R = 19/126 = 0.151$. The incidence proportion is interpreted as the probability of becoming infected within the population without any further assumptions about the dynamics of interaction. Note that the incidence proportion, R, is higher than the estimate of community probability of infection, CPI. The simple incidence proportion is higher than the community probability of infection, because the incidence proportion includes the portion of the infected individuals who, under the model that included the SAR, were estimated to have been infected within households. This simple example illustrates the importance of considering the mixing assumptions within a population when developing models for estimating meaningful population parameters in infectious disease epidemiology.

At the other extreme, we could fit the Reed-Frost model, presented in Chapter 4, to these data. That model assumes that households are independent of one another. The probability of becoming infected from the community would be 0 and the estimated transmission probability within the household would be higher than that estimated with the model of Longini and Koopman. The Reed-Frost analysis would also not include the 29 households in Table 5–4 in which no one was infected. The Reed-Frost model, similar to the conventional SAR approach, assumes that there is at least one index case in each transmission unit included in the analysis. Note that in this influenza example, we do not have the information required to estimate the conventional SAR, because we have no data on the time of onset of infection, and we have made no assumptions about the latent, incubation, or infectious periods. Also, we have not made assumptions about who became infected from inside the household or outside in the community. We have partially replaced our data requirements with model assumptions.

Covariates are easily incorporated into the model to estimate the effect of risk factors on both the SAR and the CPI (Longini et al. 1988, Haber et al. 1988, Magder and Brookmeyer 1993, O'Neill et al. 2000). In a study of dengue transmission, Dantes and associates (1988) used the model to estimate the relative risk of transmission at both the individual and the household level.

The general principle of modeling transmission in small units embedded within a community can be extended in many different ways. Time can be incorporated into the model and time-to-event data used (Addy et al. 1991, Rampey et al. 1992). We can collect information from study participants on their number of sexual contacts both within their partnerships and with other people in the community (Longini et al. 1999). The parameters of the model to be estimated are then the transmission probability per sexual contact within the partnership and the probability of infection with a person of unknown infection status in the community at large. If an estimate of prevalence of infection in the population is available, then the transmission probability in the community at large can also be estimated (Hudgens et al. 2001).

The *augmented* study design is another extension of the idea of small transmission units within a community (Longini et al. 1996, Datta et al. 1998). In the augmented study design, individuals are recruited and possibly randomized to intervention. The individual recruitment and randomization is similar to standard randomized studies that aim to estimate relative risks based on one of the unconditional measures, such as incidence rate. However, then individuals with whom the primary study participants make contact, such as in a household or partnership, are also recruited. That is, the transmission unit of the participant is recruited into the study and augments the original primary study. The augmented participants may or may not be also randomized to intervention. In this way, the design is similar to that discussed under the conventional SAR studies. The advantage of the augmented design over conventional individual recruitment with randomization is that it permits estimation of the transmission probability ratios and, in particular, the effect of risk factors or interventions on infectiousness.

Comparison of Assumptions and Data Structures

There are more variants of study designs that incorporate information and assumptions about contact structures and transmission units than those presented here, but they will follow the same principles. To estimate the transmission probability and effects of risk factors on susceptibility and infectiousness, generally some information about contacts between susceptibles and infectives is required. Assumptions about how a population mixes in small transmission units and how the transmission units interact influence the transmission model that is developed. This in turn determines how data are analyzed, and ultimately what the parameter estimates are and how we interpret them.

In conventional SAR studies, the assumption is that the households or transmission units are independent, while in the model of households within communities, infection can take place both within and outside the small transmission unit. If the transmission probability or SAR is estimated without taking into account the opportunity to become infected outside of the transmission unit, it will overestimate the actual probability of becoming infected per contact. In general, ratio measures are less biased by this problem. The drawback in using a model such as that developed by Longini and Koopman is that it contains strong modeling assumptions about the mixing in the community. It also requires that the transmission units in fact are part of a community. An advantage of the conventional SAR studies or case-contact study designs is that the minicohorts or transmission units do not need to be within a single community. The minicohorts are assumed to be independent of one another.

The data requirements and use of the data are different in the different approaches. While in the conventional SAR studies, the index cases are excluded from the analysis, in the approach assuming transmission units within a community, all cases are included in the analysis. We leave it as an exercise for the reader to create a hypothetical community composed of small transmission units. Assign to each individual a covariate status $(0,1)$ and also an infection time and infection status at the end of an epidemic. Consider the various approaches for estimating the effect measures, such as the conventional SAR, the SAR and the CPI simultaneously, and the simple incidence proportion. How do the data being used for each approach differ? What parameters can be estimated? What is the interpretation of the measures under each approach?

Case-Control Studies

Case-control studies can produce good estimates of either the incidence rate ratio or the incidence proportion ratio (Greenland and Thomas 1982). In case-control studies, cases are ascertained from the population of interest, or source population. Rather than following an entire cohort or gathering information on the entire source population, however, controls are sampled from the source population to estimate the relative person-time at risk or the relative proportions of the source population in the different treatment or covariate groups. In infectious disease epidemiology, case-control studies can also be used to estimate the transmission probability ratio and for preliminary etiologic studies in outbreak investigations. If properly conducted, case control studies are important, efficient alternatives to cohort studies as well as randomized trials (Smith 1982, 1987, Smith et al. 1984, Rodrigues and Smith 1999).

A case-control study might be conducted within the cohort that is under study (i.e., a nested case-control study), or at least within a well-defined population. Thinking of the case-control study as being nested within a cohort or a well-defined source population enables clearer formulation of assumptions about the underlying dynamics and covariate distributions. This, in turns, aids in choosing the appropriate sampling method and method of analysis for estimating the incidence rate ratio, the incidence proportion ratio, or the transmission probability ratio. We consider first estimating the incidence rate ratio of two covariate groups with a case-control study. The *odds ratio*, OR, is

$$OR = \frac{(A_1 / A_0)}{(B_1 / B_0)} = \frac{A_1 B_0}{A_0 B_1},$$

where A_0 and A_1 are the number of cases in the two different covariate groups, and B_0 and B_1 are the number of controls selected in the two groups. To estimate the incidence rate ratio using the odds ratio, the goal in sampling the controls is to estimate the relative person-time at risk in the two groups.

There are two main ways to sample the controls that give a consistent and unbiased estimate of the incidence rate ratio under certain conditions if the incidence rate ratio is constant in time (Greenland and Thomas 1982). One approach is density sampling, also called risk set sampling. In this approach, controls are selected from the population at risk at the time of onset of each case. By selecting the controls matched on time with the cases, density sampling samples the relative distribution of person-time in the two covariate groups. Another approach to sample controls does not match the sampling on time with the cases. In time-unmatched sampling, controls are selected so that the expected ratio of the number of controls in one covariate group to the number in the other covariate group equals the expected ratio of the total person-time at risk in one covariate group to the person-time at risk in the other covariate group over the entire case ascertainment period. Thus the probability that any control is selected should be proportional to the amount of time that he or she is at risk in the study to become a case.

The underlying cohort can be a dynamic cohort as long as the assumptions are satisfied. If people enter and leave the group at risk so that individuals have different person-time at risk, then the probability of being sampled should be proportional to the person-time at risk. This will occur as a consequence of time-matched sampling, but

would need to be computed with time-unmatched sampling. In both the time-matched and the time-unmatched sampling schemes, controls should be sampled independently of the covariates of interest.

If controls are sampled matched on time with cases using the density sampling, then the odds ratio can be computed using either a time-unmatched or a time-matched analysis. If the odds ratio is computed using an unmatched analysis of the time-matched cases and controls, then it is a consistent estimator of the constant incidence rate ratio if the proportion of the population at risk that has a particular covariate value is constant. This assumption would be violated, for instance, if a vaccination program were beginning so that the proportion of people who were vaccinated increased over the course of the study. If the odds ratio is calculated using a matched pair or discordant pair analysis that is matched on time, then it is a consistent estimator of the constant incidence rate ratio with no further assumptions. That is, if vaccine coverage were increasing, density sampling with a time-matched analysis could still be used to estimate the incidence rate ratio, and thus, the vaccine efficacy. In both of these situations, as long as the incidence rate ratio is constant, the baseline incidence rate may vary. For instance, there could be seasonal variation over the course of the study, such as in malaria, or there could be an epidemic, as with influenza.

If controls are sampled without matching on time, then the analysis cannot be matched on time. The odds ratio computed from the unmatched sampling scheme is a consistent estimator of a constant incidence rate ratio if either (1) the baseline incidence rate or (2) the proportion of those at risk who are in each of the covariate groups is constant. For example, if people were all vaccinated before the influenza season, then the time-unmatched approach could be used to estimate the incidence rate ratio.

If the incidence ratio is not constant, then there is no unique effect to estimate with the odds ratio. A useful illustration of these principles is found in Struchiner and colleagues

(1990). Using the example of malaria vaccination and seasonal transmission of malaria, they compare the three different odds ratio estimators of the incidence rate ratio.

To estimate the relative incidence proportion ratio using a case-cohort study, the controls are used to estimate the relative proportions of the population in each covariate group. That is, the goal is to use the ratio B_1/B_0 to estimate the distribution of the covariate among the cohort members rather than among the person-time at risk. The controls in the cohort are sampled regardless of their person-time at risk (Wacholder 1991, Rothman and Greenland 1998). Individuals who become cases may also be sampled as controls. Again, the controls should be selected independently of their covariate groups.

Case-control studies in infectious diseases need to satisfy the same assumptions as case-control studies in noninfectious diseases. The assumptions underlying many types of case-control studies may, however, be dramatically violated in studies of infectious diseases. Stationarity (i.e., dynamic equilibria of the human and parasite populations) assumptions commonly do not apply, the incidence rate ratio may change with time if the effect of an intervention wanes, and the proportion of the population with a particular covariate value can change quickly (Struchiner et al. 1990). Thus the underlying assumptions should be examined closely for their applicability.

To estimate the transmission probability ratio for susceptibility, cases are those people in the population for whom information on exposure to infection is available. Controls are selected conditional on being exposed to infection, possibly matched on a similar level of exposure, to estimate the odds of having a particular covariate status. The use of case-control studies to estimate the transmission probability ratio needs more formal research.

The preceding sampling designs do not rely on the rare disease assumption for the odds ratio to be a consistent estimator of the effect measure of interest (Rothman and Greenland, 1998). However, a study design frequently used in infectious diseases does rely on the rare disease assumption for the odds ratio estimator to be a good approximation to the incidence rate ratio or the incidence proportion ratio. In outbreak investigations where a point source epidemic is suspected, the potential controls are usually considered to be those people who did not get the illness. Sampling of controls generally takes place after the outbreak has occurred, so it is not matched on time. In this situation, if a large portion of the population became ill, the odds ratio could differ substantially from the population parameter of interest. However, in such studies, the main interest may be in simply identifying that people in one covariate group have a higher risk of being ill than those in the other covariate group. For example, it may be of interest to determine that people who ate potato salad had a higher risk of being ill than those who did not. An unbiased estimate of the underlying relative incidence rate or relative incidence proportion is probably not important.

Two-stage case control studies and studies with validation sets

Exposure to infection is often difficult to measure accurately. Also, definitive diagnosis of a case of a particular infectious disease can be expensive or difficult. For example, in influenza studies the case definition in a study might be a set of symptoms such as coughing, fever, aches, or sore throat, but not include culture-positive confirmation. In either case, with poorly measured exposure to infection or a nonspecific case definition, estimates of effects could be very biased and, in particular, attenuated. Study designs have been developed in nutritional and cancer epidemiology that have potential use in infectious disease epidemiology. The general idea is to measure an inexpensive or easily available covariate or outcome measure on everyone in the study. In a smaller subsample of the study, called a validation set, the more accurate exposure or outcome measure that is somehow correlated with the poorer value is measured. Statistical methods have been developed to combine the two levels of information (Pepe and Fleming 1991, Carroll and Wand 1991, Reilly and Pepe 1995, Robins et al. 1994, 1995). The small group with the good measurement helps to get more accurate effect estimates, while the larger study helps to have smaller variance in the estimate. Case-control studies can be done as two-stage studies (Cain and Breslow 1988, Breslow and Cain 1988, Flanders and Greenland 1991, Zhao and Lipshitz 1992, Breslow and Holubkov 1997), where the more accurate measures or additional covariates are collected on a sample of the cases and controls. Golm and associates (1998, 1999) showed the potential for using two levels of exposure to infection information for good estimates of vaccine efficacy for susceptibility and infectiousness in HIV vaccine trials. Increased use of validation sets and two-stage case-control methods could greatly improve the design of efficient studies in infectious disease epidemiology (Halloran and Longini 2000).

OTHER TYPES OF STUDIES

Cross-Sectional Studies

A cross-sectional study takes place within a short time window and includes all people or a sample of the people in the population at that time. *Prevalence* studies using a cross-sectional study design are used to estimate the current status of infection in a population. Similarly, *seroprevalence* studies measure the prevalence of immune response to an infectious agent and give information on the history of infection in a population. Estimating incidence rates, also age-specific incidence rates, from prevalence data is possible, assuming that the conditions of disease transmission have remained fairly stable and that immunity does not wane (i.e., once infected, the serologic test remains positive) (Grenfell and Anderson 1985, Keiding 1991).

As shown in Chapter 4, seroprevalence can be used as a measure of herd immunity. Seroprevalence can also be used for a simple method to estimate the basic reproductive number, R_0, if the transmission system is assumed to be in dynamic equilibrium, that is, not changing a lot over time. The under-

lying idea is that when the average incidence rate and prevalence of disease are not changing, an infectious case produces on average one other infectious case, so the reproductive number $R = 1$. From the relation $R = R_0 x = 1$, the proportion susceptible at equilibrium would be $x = 1/R_0$. Assuming random mixing, then R_0 is roughly estimated by the reciprocal of the proportion susceptible. In the study of hepatitis A and E in Vietnam (Hau et al. 1999), seroprevalence of anti-HAV IgG was 0.97 and of anti-HEV IgG was 0.09. The proportion susceptible to each is then 0.03 and 0.91, respectively. The estimate of R_0 for hepatitis A in this population is $R_0 = 1/0.03 = 33$ and for hepatitis E is $R_0 = 1/0.91 = 1.1$. Hau and colleagues (1999) express concern that conditions such as flooding or poor hygiene could favor the epidemic spread of hepatitis E. Essentially, a worsening of conditions would increase the R_0 of hepatitis E.

Spatial mapping and GIS systems

Spatial studies of infectious diseases, including vector-borne diseases, are becoming more common. These studies often include the use of geographical information systems (GIS). For instance, they may be used to map the mosquito breeding grounds in relation to houses.

Community level studies

As mentioned previously, estimation of the indirect, total, and overall effects of interventions using the study designs for dependent happenings requires comparison of populations, not just individuals. Such community trials fall into the category of cluster or group randomized trials where whole social units, rather than independent individuals are randomly assigned to treatment groups (Hayes et al. 2000, Koepsell et al. 1992, Donner 1998, Prentice and Sheppard 1995, Klar et al. 1995, Murray 1998). Observational studies in which the community is the level of observation are called ecologic studies. In choosing the communities or populations to include in a study, it is important to assure that they are separated as much as possible in every way that is relevant for transmission. If the populations are not transmission dynamically separated, then the intervention in one population will affect transmission in the other population. The indirect effects might be similar in the two populations. A study that compares nonseparate populations will yield an attenuated estimate of the potential indirect effects of intervention. Transmission patterns that differ greatly among communities can also mask the indirect effects of intervention. Matching by transmission characteristics is an option to consider (Hayes et al. 1995). In selecting communities, some thought is required about the transmission patterns and sources of exposure to infection in a population. These transmission patterns will greatly influence the magnitude of the indirect effects.

Analysis needs to be by unit of observation. For population-level studies, the unit of observation and level of analysis is the population, not the individual, so sample size calculations must be done accordingly. That is, if a study takes place in two populations each with 10,000 people and the comparison is how population A compares to population B, then the sample size is two, not 20,000.

ESTIMATION AND INFERENCE

For estimation of incidence rate ratios or hazard rate ratios, Poisson regression or stratified survival analysis is used most often. Special to infectious disease epidemiology is the possibility of using the dependent happening relation (1) to incorporate information on people who are infected in any given time interval to model the shape of the baseline hazard (Longini and Halloran 1996). The proportional hazards model (Cox 1972) is often used to estimate the regression parameters when time-to-event data are available. In the proportional hazards model, the baseline hazard rate need not be estimated, but just the ratio of the two hazard rates. For example, in malaria, with the high variability of mosquito densities as the seasons change, it is possible to estimate the hazard rate ratio of two covariate groups without having to estimate the actual sea-

sonal variation in transmission. However, if using the proportional hazards model, it is important to check whether the assumption of proportionality holds. These methods of analysis are discussed in detail elsewhere (Cox and Oakes 1984, Andersen et al. 1993).

In the discussion of the incidence rate ratio as the ratio of two dependent happening expressions, we made some strong assumptions without making them explicit. By writing the expressions as we did, there is an implicit assumption that within each of the covariate groups, everyone is the same. That is, each covariate group is assumed homogeneous with respect to the contact rate, transmission probability, and the prevalence of infection in their contacts. However, it is likely there will be unmeasured heterogeneities within study groups. Then, even if the effect of the risk factor in question does not change over time, the effect may appear to change. Some people may be exposed to infection more than others. Some may be more susceptible to infection than others. Those people with the higher susceptibility or higher exposure tend to develop the disease first. The estimated relative risk will change with time. If the estimated relative risk changes with time, the question is whether it is a true time-varying effect or an artifact of the unmeasured heterogeneities. If the effect is truly changing over time, then models for time-varying effects should be used (Schoenfeld 1982, Durham et al. 1998). If it is possible to measure the heterogeneities, then the analysis can be stratified accordingly. It is generally not possible to measure all heterogeneities, however. If the effect seems to vary because of unmeasured heterogeneities, frailty models can be tried. These are random effects models for time-to-event data (Vaupel et al. 1979, Longini and Halloran 1996).

Logistic regression is often used to analyze data obtained on whether an event occurs because the outcome data are binary, not time dependent. The model allows incorporation of covariates. In a cohort study, the estimates of the logistic regression parameters can be transformed to obtain an estimate of the incidence proportion ratio. Logistic regression can also be used to analyze some case-control data.

Little standard software exists for estimating transmission probabilities or the models that are variants of transmission units within communities. Conventional secondary attack rate ratios can be estimated using logistic regression or generalized estimating equations (Liang and Zeger 1986), for which software is available. Generalized estimating equations take into account clustering within households in the variance estimates.

In this chapter we have primarily discussed questions of estimation. Inference as a general topic goes beyond the scope of this chapter. The epidemiologist is well advised to include a biostatistician in the study team early in the design stage. Statistical inference has to do with predicting what might be expected of further observations or further studies, and quantifying degrees of certainty or uncertainty about the results we have obtained. The design of epidemiologic studies needs to include clear statements about the degree of certainty desired in the results. These have important consequences for sample size and power required in the studies.

There are different approaches to statistical inference, including the frequentist, likelihood, and Bayesian approaches. They differ in their emphasis on use of prior information, whether testing or estimation is more important, whether decision or inference is central, and in their sensitivity to the sampling procedure (Oakes 1990). Because of their emphasis on estimation and inference, rather than on testing and decision making, likelihood and Bayesian approaches to inference are more natural than frequentist approaches for epidemiologic studies. Bayesian approaches are being used increasingly as the complex computational methods they require become more feasible. The Bayesian approach allows integration of information from different sources in a natural way, and thus is particularly useful for observational studies. In epidemiology, inference using confidence intervals is preferred over using p-values. The usual confidence intervals depend on a normal approximation. Bootstrap confidence intervals do not require a normal approximation (Efron and Tibshirani 1993) and should be considered for use in the analysis. Clayton and Hills (1993) provide a readable book on statistical models in epidemiology.

SUMMARY

Because of the fundamental role of transmission of the infectious agent and dependent happenings, epidemiologic measures of interest in infectious disease epidemiology include the transmission probability, the contact rate, infectiousness, the basic reproductive number, R_0, as well as direct and indirect effect measures. The key dependent happening relation is that the incidence rate is a function of the contact rate, the transmission probability, and the prevalence of infectives in the population. The dependent happening relation helps distinguish risk factors for susceptibility from risk factors for exposure to infection. Measures such as the transmission probability that condition on contact between infectives and susceptibles are called conditional parameters. Measures of disease frequency that do not, such as incidence rate and incidence proportion, are unconditional measures. Association and causal effects differ under most circumstances. Study designs in infectious disease epidemiology include several that enable estimation of the transmission probability ratio. These generally include information on contacts between individuals or within small transmission units. In estimation of indirect and overall effects of an intervention program, the unit of analysis is the population. The dynamics of infection and transmission units within a population need to be taken into account when designing and interpreting studies in infectious disease epidemiology.

Dr. Halloran was partially supported in writing this chapter by NIH grants RO1-AI32042 and RO1-AI40846.

REFERENCES

Addy CL, Longini IM, and Haber MS. A generalized stochastic model for the analysis of infectious disease final size data. Biometrics. 47:961–974, 1991.

Andersen PK, Borgan O, Gill RD, and Keiding N. Statistical Models Based on Counting Processes. New York: Springer-Verlag, 1993.

Breslow NE, and Cain KC. Logistic regression for two-stage case-control data. Biometrika. 75:11–20, 1988.

Breslow NE, and Holubkov R. Maximum likelihood estimation of logistic regression parameters under two-phase, outcome dependent sampling. J. R. Stat. Soc. B. 59:447–461, 1997.

Brookmeyer R, and Gail MH. Biases in prevalent cohorts. Biometrics. 43:739–749, 1987.

Cain KC, and Breslow NE. Logistic regression analysis and efficient design for two-stage studies. Am. J. Epidemiol. 128:1198–1206, 1988.

Carroll RJ, and Wand WP. Semiparametric estimation in logistic measurement error models. J. R. Stat. Soc. B. 53:573–585, 1991.

Cisse B, Aaby P, Simondon F, et al. Role of schools in the transmission of measles in rural Senegal: implicationsn for measles control in developing countries. Am. J. Epidemiol. 149:295–301, 1999.

Clayton D, and Hills M. Statistical Models in Epidemiology. Oxford: Oxford University Press, 1993.

Cox DR. Regression models and life-tables (with discussion). J. R. Stat. Soc. 30(Series B):284–289, 1972.

Cox DR. Planning of Experiments. New York: John Wiley & Sons, 1958.

Cox DR, and Oakes D. Analysis of Survival Data. London: Chapman and Hall, 1984.

Dantes HG, Koopman JS, Addy CL, et al. Dengue epidemics on the Pacific Coast of Mexico. Int. J. Epidemiol. 17:178–186, 1988.

Datta S, Halloran ME, and Longini IM. Augmented HIV vaccine trial designs for estimating reduction in infectiousness and protective efficacy. Stat. Med. 17:185–200, 1998.

Diggle PJ, Liang K-Y, and Zeger SL. Analysis of Longitudinal Data. Oxford: Oxford University Press, 1994.

Donner A. Some aspects of the design and analysis of cluster randomization trials. Appl. Stat. 47:95–114, 1998.

Durham LK, Longini, IM, Halloran ME, et al. Estimation of vaccine efficacy in the presence of waning: application to cholera vaccines. Am. J. Epidemiol. 147:948–959, 1998.

Efron B, and Tibshirani RJ. An Introduction to the Bootstrap. New York: Chapman and Hall, 1993.

Evans AS. Causation and disease: The Henle-Koch postulates revisited. Yale J. Biol. Med. 49:175–195, 1976.

Fine PEM, Clarkson JA, and Miller E. The efficacy of pertussis vaccines under conditions of household exposure: further analysis of the 1978–80 PHLS-ERL study in 21 area health authorities in England. Int. J. Epidemiol. 17(3):635–642, 1988.

Flanders WD, and Greenland S. Analytic methods for two-stage case-control studies and other stratified designs. Stat. Med. 10:739–747, 1991.

Freeman J, and Hutchison GB. Prevalence, incidence, and duration. Am. J. Epidemiol. 112:707–723, 1980.

Gail MH. Adjusting for covariates that have the same distribution in exposed and unexposed cohorts. In: Moolgavkar SH, and Prentice RL, eds. Modern Statistical Methods. New York: Wiley, 1986: 3–18.

Gail MH. The effect of pooling across strata in perfectly balanced studies. Biometrics. 44:151–162, 1988.

Gail MH, Tan WY, and Piantadosi S. The effect of omitting covariates on tests for no treatment effect in randomized clinical trials. Biometrika. 75:57–64, 1988.

Gail MH, Wieand S, and Piantadosi S. Biased estimates of treatment effect in randomized experiments with non-linear regressions and omitted covariates. Biometrika. 71:431–444, 1984.

Glynn JR, Vynnycky E, and Fine PEM. Influence of sampling on estimates of clustering and recent transmission of mycobacterium tuberculosis derived from DNA fingerprinting techniques. Am. J. Epidemiol. 149:366–371, 1999.

Golm GT, Halloran ME, and Longini IM. Semiparametric models for mismeasured exposure information in vaccine trials. Stat. Med. 17:2335–2352, 1998.

Golm GT, Halloran ME, and Longini IM. Semiparametric methods for multiple exposure mismeasurement and a bivariate outcome in HIV vaccine trials. Biometrics. 55:94–101, 1999.

Greenland S. Interpretation and choice of effect measures in epidemiologic analyses. Am. J. Epidemiol. 125:761–768, 1987.

Greenland S, and Robins JM. Identifiability, exchangeability, and epidemiologic confounding. Int. J. Epidemiol. 15:412–418, 1986.

Greenland S, Robins JM, and Pearl J. Confounding and collapsibility in causal inference. Stat. Sci. 14:29–46, 1999.

Greenland S, and Thomas DC. On the need for the rare disease assumption in case-control studies. Am. J. Epidemiol. 116(3):547–553, 1982.

Grenfell BT, and Anderson RM. The estimation of age-related rates of infection from case notifications and serological data. J. Hyg. Cam. 95:419–436, 1985.

Haber M, Longini IM, and Cotsonis GA. Models for the statistical analysis of infectious disease data. Biometrics. 44:163–173, 1988.

Halloran ME, and Longini IM. Using validation sets for outcomes and exposure to infection in vaccine field studies. Am J Epidemiol (in press) 2001.

Halloran ME, Longini IM, Struchiner CJ, Haber MJ, and Brunet RC. Exposure efficacy and change in contact rates in evaluating prophylactic HIV vaccines in the field. Stat. Med. 13:357–377, 1994.

Halloran ME, and Struchiner CJ. Study designs for dependent happenings. Epidemiology. 2:331–338, 1991.

Halloran ME, and Struchiner CJ. Causal inference for infectious diseases. Epidemiology. 6:142–151, 1995.

Halloran ME, Struchiner CJ, and Longini IM. Study designs for different efficacy and effectiveness aspects of vaccination. Am. J. Epidemiol. 146:789–803, 1997.

Hau CH, Hien TT, Tien NTK, et al. Prevalence of enteric hepatitis A and E viruses in the Mekong River Delta region of Vietnam. Am. J. Trop. Med. Hyg. 60:277–280, 1999.

Hayes RJ, Mosha F, Nicoll A, et al. A community trial of the impact of improved sexually transmitted disease treatment on HIV epidemic in rural Tanzania: 1. Design. AIDS. 9:919–926, 1995.

Hayes RJ, Alexander NDE, Bennett S, Cousens SN. Design and analysis issues in cluster-randomized trials of interventions against infectious diseases. Stat. Methods Med. Res. 9:95–116, 2000.

Holland PW. Statistics and causal inference. J. Am. Stat. Assoc. 81:945–960, 1986.

Hooper RR, Reynolds GH, Jones OG, et al. Cohort study of venereal disease. I: The risk of gonorrhea transmission from infected women to men. Am. J. Epidemiol. 108:136–144, 1978.

Hudgens MG, Longini IM, Halloran ME, et al. Estimating the transmission probability of human immunodeficiency virus in injecting drug users in Thailand. Appl. Stat. 50:(Part 1), 2001.

Keiding N. Age-specific incidence and prevalence: A statistical perspective. J. R. Stat. Soc. A. 154(3):371–412, 1991.

Kemper JT. Error sources in the evaluation of secondary attack rates. Am. J. Epidemiol. 112:457–464, 1980.

Klar N, Gyorkos T, and Donner A. Cluster randomization trials in tropical medicine: a case study. Trans. R. Soc. Trop. Med. Hyg. 89:454–459, 1995.

Koepsell TD, Wagner EH, Cheadle AC, et al. Selected methodological issues in evaluating community-based health promotion and disease prevention programs. Annu. Rev. Public Health. 13:31–57, 1992.

Koopman JS, Longini IM, Jacquez JA, et al. Assessing risk factors for transmission of infection. Am. J. Epidemiol. 133:1199–1209, 1991.

Liang KY, and Zeger SL. Longitudinal data analysis using generalized linear models. Biometrika. 73:13–22, 1986.

Lipsitch M. Vaccination against colonizing bacteria with multiple serotypes. Proc. Natl. Acad. Sci. USA. 94:6571–6576, 1997.

Longini IM, Datta S, and Halloran ME. Measuring vaccine efficacy for both susceptibility to infection and reduction in infectiousness for prophylactic HIV-1 vaccines. J. Acquir. Immune Defic. Syndr. Hum. Retrovirol. 13:440–447, 1996.

Longini IM, and Halloran ME. A frailty mixture model for estimating vaccine efficacy. Appl. Stat. 45:165–173, 1996.

Longini IM, Hudgens MG, Halloran ME, and Sagatelian K. A Markov model for measuring vaccine efficacy for both susceptibility to infection and reduction in infectiousness for prophylactic HIV-1 vaccines. Stat. Med. 18:53–68, 1999.

Longini IM, and Koopman JS. Household and community transmission parameters from final distributions of infections in households. Biometrics. 38(1):115–126, 1982.

Longini IM, Koopman JS, Haber M, and Cotsonis GA. Statistical inference for infectious diseases: Risk-specified household and community transmission parameters. Am. J. Epidemiol. 128(4):845–859, 1988.

Magder L, and Brookmeyer R. Analysis of infectious disease data from partners studies with unknown source of infection. Biometrics. 49:1110–1116, 1993.

Murray DM. Design and Analysis of Group-Randomized Trials. New York: Oxford University Press, 1998.

Oakes M. Statistical Inference. Chestnut Hill: Epidemiology Resources, Inc., 1990.

O'Neill, POD, Balding DJ, Becker NG, Eerola M, and Mollison D. Analyses of infectious disease data from household outbreaks by Markov chain Monte Carlo methods. Appl. Stat. 49:517–542, 2000.

Orenstein WA, Bernier RH, and Hinman AR. Assessing vaccine efficacy in the field: further observations. Epidemiol. Rev. 10:212–241, 1988.

Pepe MS, and Fleming TR. A nonparametric method for dealing with mismeasured covariate data. J. Am. Stat. Assoc. 86:108–113, 1991.

Prentice R, and Sheppard L. Aggregate data studies of disease risk factors. Biometrika. 82: 113–125, 1995.

Rampey AH, Longini IM, Haber MJ, and Monto AS. A discrete-time model for the statistical analysis of infectious disease incidence data. Biometrics. 48:117–128, 1992.

Reilly M, and Pepe MS. A mean score method for missing and auxiliary covariate data in regression models. Biometrika. 82:299–314, 1995.

Rhodes PH, Halloran ME, and Longini IM. Counting process models for differentiating exposure to infection and susceptibility. J. R. Stat. Soc. B. 58:751–762, 1996.

Robins JM, Hsieh F, and Newey W. Semiparametric efficient estimation of a conditional density with missing or mismeasured covariates. J. R. Stat. Soc. Ser. B. 57:409–424, 1995.

Robins JM, Rotnitzky A, and Scharfstein DO. Sensitivity analysis for selection bias and unmeasured confounding in missing data and causal inference models. In: Halloran ME and DA Berry, eds. Statistics in Epidemiology, Environment and Clinical Trials. New York: Springer-Verlag, 1999.

Robins JM, Rotnitzky A, and Zhao LP. Estimation of regression coefficients when some regressors are not always observed. J. Am. Stat. Assoc. 89:846–866, 1994.

Rodrigues L, and Smith P. Case-control approach to vaccine evaluation. Epidemiol. Rev. 21: 56–72, 1999.

Rosenbaum P. Observational Studies. Berlin: Springer-Verlag, 1995.

Ross R. An application of the theory of probabilities to the study of a priori pathometry, Part 1. Proc. R. Soc. Series A. 92:204–230, 1916.

Rothman K, and Greenland S. Modern Epidemiology. Philadelphia: Lippincott-Raven, 1998.

Rubin DB. Bayesian inference for causal effects. The role of randomization. Ann. Stat. 7: 34–58, 1978.

Rubin DB. Comment: Neyman (1923) and causal inference in experiments and observational studies. Stat. Sci. 5:472–480, 1990.

Schoenfeld D. Partial residuals for the proportional hazards regression model. Biometrika. 69:239–241, 1982.

Small PM, Hopewell PC, Singh SP, et al. The epidemiology of tuberculosis in San Francisco: A population-based study using conventional and molecular methods. N. Engl. J. Med. 330:1703–1709, 1994.

Smith PG. Retrospective assessment of the effectiveness of BCG vaccination against tuberculosis using the case-control method. Tubercle. 62:23–35, 1982.

Smith PG. Evaluating interventions against tropical diseases. Int. J. Epidemiol. 16(2):159–166, 1987.

Smith PG, Rodrigues LC, and Fine PEM. Assessment of the protective efficacy of vaccines against common diseases using case-control and cohort studies. Int. J. Epidemiol. 13(1): 87–93, 1984.

Struchiner CJ, Halloran ME, Robins JM, and Spielman A. The behavior of common measures of association used to assess a vaccination program under complex disease transmission patterns—a computer simulation study of malaria vaccines. Int. J. Epidemiol. 19:187–196, 1990.

Sugiyama H. Some statistical contributions to the health sciences. Osaka City Med. J. 6:141–158, 1960.

Vaupel JW, Manton KG, and Stallard E. The impact of heterogeneity in individual frailty on the dynamics of mortality. Demography. 16:439–454, 1979.

Wacholder S. Practical considerations in choosing between the case-cohort and nested case-control design. Epidemiology. 2:155–158, 1991.

Zhao LP, and Lipsitz S. Designs and analysis of two-stage studies. Stat. Med. 11:769–782, 1991.

Part II

DATA SOURCES AND MEASUREMENT

6

Sources of Data

D. PETER DROTMAN and MARC A. STRASSBURG

> It is error to argue in front of your data. You find yourself
> insensibly twisting them around to fit your theories.
>
> Sherlock Holmes (Sir Arthur Conan Doyle)

WHAT ARE DATA?

Data are defined as "factual information (as measurements or statistics) used as a basis for reasoning, discussion, or calculation" (Webster's 1990). In a broader sense, data are the lifeblood of research, regardless of the discipline. Obtaining, analyzing, interpreting, evaluating, and communicating data are major activities of all scientists, not just those who concentrate on the epidemiology of infectious diseases. Arguably, thanks to computerization, data are now more readily available to researchers and the public alike than at any time in history. Why then include a chapter on data sources in a text called *Epidemiologic Methods for the Study of Infectious Diseases*? The reasons are manifold. First, attention to the judicious collection and evaluation of data is the major determinant of the quality of research, as opposed to the quantity of data collected. Second, even though data can be easily accessed or attractively presented (for instance in publications or on the Internet), this alone is no indicator of their reliability,

accuracy, or veracity. One needs only to recall the caveat of Sir Josiah Charles Stamp, the British economist, who pointed out a century ago that, "The government are [*sic*] very keen on amassing statistics. They collect them, add them, raise them to the *n*th power, take the cube root and prepare wonderful diagrams. But you must never forget that every one of these figures comes in the first instance from the village watchman, who just puts down what he damn well pleases" (Stamp 1929). The contemporary way of expressing this observation is "garbage in, garbage out." A more sophisticated statement might be that "the inherent bias in the collection instrument can lead to erroneous conclusions based upon subsequent analysis of the data." A major goal of this chapter is to provide the means to recognize and avoid such hazardous situations.

Surveillance efforts for infectious diseases clearly depend on the medical care system, the main purposes of which are to diagnose and treat human illnesses, not necessarily to generate or gather data. Nevertheless, when an individual contracts an infectious disease and comes to the attention of a health care provider, almost inevitably a large number of "official" documents or records are created during the diagnostic workup and the course of treatment. Such documents not only serve as a clinical record of the illness and the medical management but also have a legal basis. Examples of commonly generated records and reports, in addition to the medical record (or clinician's notes), include laboratory test results, radiographs and pathology reports, prescription and pharmacy records, and insurance and billing records. Some infectious diseases are reportable, meaning that clinicians who make the diagnosis or laboratories that report the diagnostic findings are required to notify public health officials (Table 6–1). The degree of compliance is far from complete and is highly influenced by such disparate factors as disease severity, social stigmatization associated with the diagnosis (such as sexually transmitted diseases), local reporting practices, and many other factors, a number of which are covered within this chapter. Depending upon the infectious agent involved and the quality of the data, relevant information may be used by epidemiologists

Table 6–1   Nationally Notifiable Infectious Diseases, United States, 1999*†

Acquired immunodeficiency syndrome (AIDS)	Malaria
Anthrax	Measles
Botulism	Meningococcal disease
Chancroid	Mumps
Chlamydia trachomatis, genital infections	Pertussis
Cholera	Plague
Coccidioidomycosis (regional)	Poliomyelitis, paralytic
Cryptosporidiosis	Psittacosis
Cyclosporiasis	Rabies, animal
Diphtheria	Rabies, human
Ehrlichiosis, human granulocyctic	Rocky Mountain spotted fever
Ehrlichiosis, human monocytic	Rubella
Encephalitis, California serogroup	Rubella, congenital
Encephalitis, Eastern equine	Salmonellosis
Encephalitis, St. Louis	Shigellosis
Encephalitis, Western equine	Streptococcal disease, invasive, group A
Escherichia coli, O157:H7	Streptococcal toxic-shock syndrome
Gonorrhea	*Streptococcus pneumoniae*, a drug resistant invasive
Haemophilus influenzae, invasive disease	disease
Hansen's disease (leprosy)	Syphilis
Hantavirus pulmonary syndrome	Syphilis, congenital
Hemolytic uremic syndrome, postdiarrheal	Tetanus
Hepatitis A	Toxic-shock syndrome
Hepatitis B	Trichinosis
Hepatitis C/non A, non B	Tuberculosis
HIV infection, pediatric	Typhoid fever
Legionellosis	Varicella deaths
Lyme disease	Yellow fever

*Although varicella is not a notifiable disease, the Council of State and Territorial Epidemiologists (CSTE) recommends reporting of cases via the Nationally Notifiable Disease Surveillance System (NNDSS).

†At its 1999 meeting, CSTE voted to add listeriosis, Q fever, and tularemia to this list.

and researchers to reveal modes of transmission and causal pathways, or to identify risk factors related to the disease. The amount of information obtained may range from a very limited frequency count (incidence or prevalence number) to detailed clinical and demographic information, which can be used to help determine a source of infection or test a hypothesis. The latter is especially useful when dealing with newly identified or emerging infectious diseases.

This chapter describes the principal sources of data for infectious diseases. Although the data sources are similar at the local, state, and national (and even global) levels, the analyses of such data may differ considerably from one jurisdiction to the next. Epidemiologists at each level attempt to create a picture of disease occurrence in the community under their purview. Each level has unique strengths and weaknesses. This chapter focuses on the main sources of infectious disease data, which usually originate at the local level. Challenges in extrapolating and combining primary data sources to create larger databases (sometimes to carry out meta-analyses) and the role of information systems, including data warehousing, are introduced.

HISTORY OF INFECTIOUS DISEASE DATA

Although the germ theory of disease was not established until the nineteenth century, infectious disease data sources can trace their origins to at least the seventeenth century. The year 1662 was notable for two important events in England. First, John Graunt published his *Natural and Political Observations Mentioned in a Following Index and Made Upon the Bills of Mortality*, in which he clearly demonstrated the usefulness of mortality data. Basing his analysis on the number of weekly burials, he attempted to categorize causes of death into those resulting from "acute" and "chronical diseases" (Lilienfeld 1994). That same year, the Royal Society of London was founded and provided a forum for the reporting of scientific progress. During this period, the communi-

cability of diseases such as smallpox, measles, and cholera was being considered (*contagium vivum* theory). For many years, the reporting of infectious diseases occurred only indirectly. Major progress occurred first in England in 1836, when William Farr, a physician, became the director of the Registrar-General's Office (Humphries 1985). The concept of mortality surveillance was born when death information began to be routinely collected and analyzed to discern changes in the health of the population. This was soon followed by the founding of the Office of Population Censuses and Surveys, which proved a critical step in eventually providing data to generate population-based rates. When Dr. John Snow, the acknowledged "father" of epidemiology and friend of Farr, investigated the cholera outbreaks in London in 1854, he had to collect much of the data himself. His successful efforts, resulting in the implication of water as the vehicle for whatever caused cholera, were so thorough and compelling that he stimulated not only the improvement of water supplies but also the collection of key demographic information by registrars on persons who died of cholera (Shephard 1995).

The United States Constitution, ratified in 1787, makes no mention of health, but does call for a national census (by "actual enumeration") every 10 years. The first was carried out in 1790. While accomplished for the specific purpose of apportioning congressional representation among the states, the data gathered in the census have proved extraordinarily useful for many economic, social, health, and epidemiologic purposes. Whereas notifications and reports of infectious diseases provide us with the numerators, census data—with their age, race, sex, and geographically specific population statistics—generally provide the denominators that are needed for the calculation of rates, which are the most commonly presented health statistics after crude or raw numbers. The U.S. Census Bureau, whose mission is "to be the preeminent collector and provider of timely, relevant, and quality data about the people and economy of the United States," maintains an extensive Internet website at: http://www.census.gov. Accessing census data via the Internet is far more user-friendly than wading through the Census Bureau's voluminous publications.

An epidemic of yellow fever in 1793 may have resulted in the deaths of as many as 20% of the 50,000 inhabitants of Philadelphia, then the capital of the United States, but there was no public health department or similar resource to assess the disaster accurately. The sketchy data and estimates we have are derived from contemporary newspaper accounts (Estes 1997). The 1878 Quarantine Act marked the beginning of national disease surveillance in the United States, including publication of the "Bulletin" (Mullan 1989), the first issue of which reported two cases of yellow fever on ships harbored in Key West, Florida. That periodical, which was short-lived, was the forerunner of the *Morbidity and Mortality Weekly Report* (*MMWR*), which began publication under that name in 1952 by an agency that became the National Center for Health Statistics (NCHS). Responsibility for publishing the *MMWR* was transferred to the Centers for Disease Control (CDC) in Atlanta in 1961, and NCHS itself became part of CDC (even though it did not move from its Maryland headquarters) in the mid-1980s. *MMWR* remains the official organ for weekly and annual publication of reportable diseases in the United States. Access to current and some historical data is freely available through CDC's extensive Internet site at http://www.cdc.gov. CDC itself was established as the Communicable Disease Center in Atlanta in 1946, as a direct outgrowth of its predecessor agency's successful malaria control efforts, which were focused on the southeastern states. Although its name and mission have expanded over the years, CDC has retained both its acronym (now standing for the Centers for Disease Control and Prevention) and its primacy as the national infectious diseases data collection and public health agency (Etheridge 1992).

The well-established public health data collection and dissemination systems in place today use several disease notification and registration processes. Some of these systems are relatively new, most having been developed during the twentieth century. By 1928, all 48 states (plus Hawaii, Puerto Rico, and Washington, DC) were reporting infectious disease to the U.S. Public Health Service, mainly via weekly telegrams. Recognizing the need for close coordination among the state health departments and the federal government in the early 1950s, CDC's pioneering epidemiologist, Dr. Alexander Langmuir, helped form a consortium of infectious disease epidemiologists representing each state, a group now known as the Council of State and Territorial Epidemiologists (CSTE; whose website address is: http://www.cste.org). CSTE is the organization that by vote at its annual meeting determines which conditions will be designated as reportable nationally by the states to CDC for publication weekly or at other intervals in the *MMWR*. As public health prevention and control programs have become increasingly important and sophisticated, the corresponding scope of data collected has been widened and improved. For example, one only need look at the reporting of acquired immunodeficiency syndrome (AIDS) cases, which began as a basic case count and evolved into an extensive information-gathering effort, resulting in one of the most comprehensive public use databases and surveillance reports available on any infectious disease (Centers for Disease Control and Prevention 1998).

Globally, only four infectious diseases are required to be reported to the World Health Organization (WHO; http://www.who.int) under the International Health Regulations: cholera, plague, yellow fever, and smallpox, the last of which was eradicated in 1979. Virtually every nation is a member state of WHO and has a listing of nationally notifiable diseases, but the lists vary from nation to nation and the capability to carry out national data collection varies even more greatly. The United States is a founding member of the Pan American Health Organization (PAHO; http://www.paho.org), which serves as the WHO Regional Office for the Americas.

IDENTIFYING DATA SOURCES

For any given disease or condition, a large number of data sources may be available; however, the key lies in knowing where to find the data sources and, more important, how to access them. Some are public, others privately owned; some contain actively gathered data, others contain only passively collected reports; some are obvious, others obscure; some quantitative, others qualitative; some mundane, others limited only by the creativity of their seeker. Sources of data can be categorized as either "ongoing" programs, which collect data routinely, or "ad hoc" efforts to collect data for a particular purpose or nonrecurring event, or from a unique opportunity (for example, when students collect data for a project, or when a special project for some other purpose has collected useful information that provides new unexpected data). Routinely collected and publicly available data on infectious diseases usually are collected by local governments and support a variety of community and disease control surveillance systems. Ad hoc data generally are obtained in special studies, during investigations of outbreaks, or from the study of specific public health problems.

Routinely collected data may be obtained from systems such as reportable disease registries, vital records (defined as records of births, deaths, marriages, and divorces) departments, special registries (such as for cancer or conditions of special interest such as the Gulf War syndrome), dedicated (sometimes referred to as sentinel) surveillance systems, ongoing or recurrent health surveys (such as the National Health and Nutrition Examination Surveys carried out by CDC's NCHS), and hospital (or managed care organization)-based data collection systems.

Notifiable disease reporting systems operate in virtually all public health jurisdictions the world over in some form or other and generally are based on legal mandates. In the United States, such mandates are generated by states, but authorize local (county or city) public health officials to carry them out.

Table 5–1 lists the infectious diseases that are reportable in all states. Many states mandate that additional infectious and non-infectious diseases be reported by clinicians or laboratories to health officials. These conditions vary from infectious diseases of regional importance such as coccidioidomycosis (common in desert regions of the western United States) to toxic exposures such as pesticide or lead poisonings to conditions such as diabetes or epilepsy that might disqualify a patient from maintaining a driver's license.

How to Access Data on Notifiable Diseases

Traditionally, researchers, writers, clinicians, or those simply curious about infectious disease data could take several somewhat cumbersome alternative approaches to obtaining data from public health officials: subscribe to official newsletters in which the data are published, pay a personal visit to the health department, or contact the keeper of the data by phone or letter. Those options still exist, but the advent of the Internet has been a boon for those who wish to access public data sources. Websites now exist for many health departments, and a view of the reports and data they post is literally a few clicks away from anyone with Internet access and minimal search skills. CDC maintains links to all state health department Internet home pages at: http://www.cdc.gov/other.htm. Virtually every state health department posts data on reportable infectious diseases on the Internet.

Judging the Quality of Data Sources

The hallmarks of a good data collection system are ultimately reflected by its scientific worth, the care with which data are collected, and how well the procedures used are documented. The ideal data source has ongoing and in-depth quality control procedures in place, a high degree of clarity (concise and clear documentation), and accessibility (i.e., user-friendliness) (Centers for Disease Control and Prevention 1988). In addition, there should be a reasonable degree of completeness of reporting (or a known fraction of underreporting), consistency in reporting levels (or reporting fraction) over time, a sufficient period over which the data have been collected to allow for secular trend analysis, standardized case definitions that are well defined and comparable to other systems (Centers for Disease Control and Prevention 1997b), and carefully crafted and maintained safeguards for confidentiality of both patients and the individual clinicians who do the reporting. Custodians or owners of data sources should be able to list the ways they adhere to these data system attributes so that users can judge the integrity of the system. Failure to do so should prompt skepticism on the part of data users.

Classification of Infectious Diseases

Several informal classification systems exist for infectious diseases. Some are based on the agents themselves and others on routes of transmission. The following broad categories are generally utilized: bacterial diseases (e.g., salmonellosis, tuberculosis, syphilis), viral infections (e.g., smallpox, measles, chickenpox, poliomyelitis, HIV), fungal infections (e.g., histoplasmosis, coccidioidomycosis), protozoan (e.g., cryptosporidiosis, malaria) and metazoan infections (e.g., hookworm, onchocerciasis), and rickettsial diseases (e.g., typhus and Rocky Mountain spotted fever). Classifications of routes of transmission typically include sexually transmitted diseases (e.g., chlamydia), food- and waterborne diseases (e.g., *Escherichia coli* H7:O157, hepatitis A), bloodborne infections (e.g., hepatitis B and C), nosocomial infections (infections transmitted in health care settings, such as surgical wound infections), infections transmitted through the respiratory route (e.g., TB and influenza), zoonotic infections (infections transmitted from animals to humans, such as rabies), and vector-borne infections, such as Lyme disease. Sometimes vaccine preventable diseases (rubella, mumps, and pertussis) and antibiotic-resistant bacterial infections (such as methicillin-resistant *Staphylococcus aureus*) are regarded as unique categories. Recently, infectious agents with the potential

to be used in bioterrorism or as biological weapons threats have been listed (including smallpox virus, anthrax spores, botulinum toxin) (Kortepeter 1999).

The major official codification of all diseases, health conditions, and injuries is the International Statistical Classification of Diseases and Related Health Problems, which has gone through many revisions and editions. The Tenth Revision (ICD-10) is the latest in a series that originated in 1893 as the Bertillon Classification or International List of Causes of Death (see: http://www.who.int/whosis/icd10/). The ICD is continually being revised as new conditions, including emerging infections, are described. Every infectious and noninfectious disease of humans is assigned a unique three-digit number (plus multiple decimal places) in the ICD system. The numbers are used in many medical and public health records, such as hospital discharge reports, billing records, and death certificates. The widely available and standard American Public Health Association handbook, *Control of Communicable Diseases Manual*, lists ICD codes for each of the several hundred infectious diseases it describes in its alphabetically arranged chapters (Chin 2000).

Hospital Data Used to Measure Morbidity

Hospital records are voluminous and vary greatly in their usefulness from place to place and from diagnosis to diagnosis. Furthermore, data based on hospital admissions or discharges can provide a biased picture of certain diseases in the community. Hospital visits may be limited to only the more severe forms of a disease, and therefore cases and or controls that are selected from a hospital base may suffer from "Berkson's bias"; that is, admission practices are selective, being influenced by such factors as access, finances, availability of beds, policies, physician acumen, and culture (Berkson 1946). Although there have been improvements in the standardization of data collection, no uniform mechanism has yet been accepted nationally for collection and utilization of epidemiological data from hospitals. Attempts to standardize hospital reporting by a number of states have met with only modest success. Initially, these data sets included hospital discharge diagnoses, but the explosive growth of outpatient surgery and home health care has prompted extension of such systems to outpatients visits as well. Such data sets are by their nature very large and require considerable "data cleaning" prior to being made available for research use. In addition, they may have confidential patient information sections and may not be available to the general public. Of particular interest for infectious disease studies are separate hospital internal reporting or monitoring systems of infectious diseases. Such systems are generally maintained by Communicable Disease Committees or staff in charge of nosocomial infections. In response to major cost-cutting efforts in hospitals, some have become "data entrepreneurs" by packaging and selling their databases, usually through vendors with considerable computing expertise and always after removal of individual identifiers. Purchasers have included both public health and economic researchers. Paying close attention to the data system's quality parameters is very important for purchasers.

Hospital emergency room data can serve as a sensitive indicator to monitor both new and existing community infections. However, medical records in emergency venues are not the best or most legible. Problems often arise with the way the information is maintained, which is generally in log books that are not computerized. Sometimes, the best emergency room data are the billing records or laboratory results.

Disease Registries

Some jurisdictions have created specific disease registries. A registry is defined as a system that keeps track of individuals with specific diseases or conditions. These may include tuberculosis, typhoid carriers, leprosy (Hansen's disease), congenital syphilis, and pregnant women with HIV. Such registries help provide follow-up and can be used to elucidate the natural history of a disease in a given area. Some registries are population-based, while others are more narrowly focused. They are often useful in doing cohort studies and in determining case fatality rates. Users of data from registries must pay careful attention to the degree of ascertainment of these systems (i.e., how sensitive and specific they are), which often depends on how confidentially they maintain their reports (particularly true for potentially stigmatizing diseases).

Morbidity Surveys

Disease-specific surveys are especially valuable in obtaining the prevalence of nonreportable diseases. Point prevalence surveys, however, tend to be most useful for those infectious diseases that are more chronic in nature such as hepatitis C and coccidioidomycosis (valley fever), where long-term damage to the liver and lungs, respectively, can be detected years after primary infection. For example, the National Health and Nutrition Examination Survey, conducted by CDC's NCHS during 1988 through 1994, revealed the national prevalence of hepatitis C to be about 1.8% (2.7 million chronic active infections) (Alter 1999).

The NCHS conducts a variety of ongoing and special surveys of high quality. The National Health Survey provides a continuing source of information about the nation's health status but may not contain much on infectious diseases, or may not be specific enough for local jurisdictions to use the data. However, this survey can be useful for immunization coverage rates and some self-reported history data on infectious diseases. Without good documentation, parental memory may not correlate well with actual disease occurrence (e.g., "measles" could be recalled and recorded as any number of viral or even noninfectious exanthems). The Health Interview Survey similarly lacks medical confirmation of diagnoses. The Health Examination Survey includes physical exams. The Health Records Survey incorporates institution-based sampling. The National Survey of Family Growth reveals fertility patterns. Information on these surveys and data reports from them can be found on the Internet. Some of the data sets are quite large.

National Surveillance Data Sets

Many infectious diseases are chronically underreported for a variety of reasons including social stigmatization of patients with AIDS and other sexual transmitted diseases, improper diagnosis, lack of laboratory support, inconvenience to the clinician, and ignorance of the requirements. On the other hand, reporting may be essentially complete for infections that are severe, infrequent, and easy to recognize. CDC publishes an annual summary of notifiable diseases as well as Surveillance Summaries at irregular intervals as supplements to its *MMWR* (Centers for Disease Control and Prevention 1997a). Some reflect data on reportable diseases, such as malaria (Centers for Disease Control and Prevention 1999a). Others reflect special analyses of data collected for other reasons, such as the extraction of trends in opportunistic infections derived from AIDS case reports (Centers for Disease Control and Prevention 1999c). The sexually transmitted diseases surveillance data are published annually as a free-standing volume (Division of STD Prevention 1998), as are HIV/AIDS surveillance data (Centers for Disease Control and Prevention 1998).

Linked Health Records

Some countries, such as Finland and Sweden, have advanced medical record linkage systems. The possibility of integrating all recorded information into one record system has long been a dream of health researchers. Such linked records could provide a means to correlate vital statistics with health events, or they could help link immunization coverage with the incidence of vaccine preventable diseases. The ability to link preventive services, primary clinical care, and inpatient care records has obvious clinical and research utility, but linking such systems in the United States has proved insurmountably difficult so far. Concerns have related to fears of discrimination, loss of confidentiality, and misuse of the data as well as financing and portability of records. Where

the systems exist, mainly in geographically demarcated managed care organizations, they are quite useful.

CENSUS DATA

Census data are key to providing information about the size and composition of the population one is studying. There are two principal methods for enumerating a population: "de facto"—at time of enumeration or survey (this might be better for studies involving migrant or homeless populations) and "de jure"—usual place of residence (this is a better indication of permanent population and household composition of a study area). The U.S. Census Bureau defines and numbers census tracts (the basic unit of enumeration, roughly equivalent to a neighborhood) and Metropolitan Statistical Areas (MSAs). These are urban areas with a population of 50,000 or more. Although many of the census data are confidential, aggregate data are available by census tract and zip-code groupings. However, not all data are summarized and available by these geographic designations. Small numbers are suppressed if individuals could be identified from the data.

VITAL EVENTS

Deaths, births, fetal deaths, marriages, and divorces are all considered "vital events." In every state, registration systems are legally mandated to collect and compile such information on a routine basis. Registration systems were incrementally implemented. For example, in the United States, death registration was begun in some states in 1902, but it was not until 1933 that all states adhered to a system. The information included on birth, fetal death, and death certificates can be viewed in Figures 6–1, 6–2, and 6–3.

Mortality Data

Death is one of the "vital" records required for legal and demographic purposes in almost every country. Although there are differences among states, most locales in the United States use the standard death certifi-

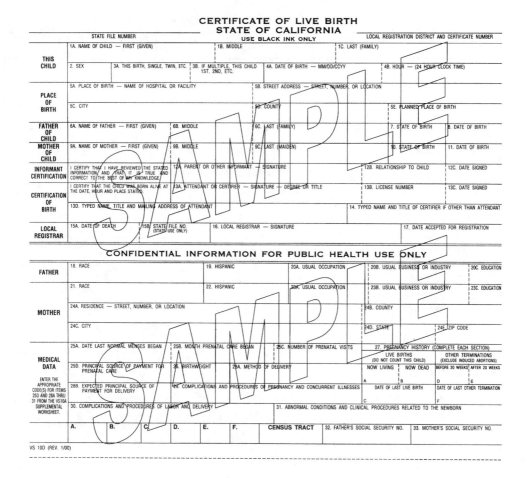

Figure 6–1. State of California birth certificate.

cate format developed by the NCHS. Although most variables (demographic and causal) have remained constant over the years, some have varied, and comparisons between years and between locales must therefore be made with caution. As mentioned in the section of this chapter titled History of Infectious Disease Data, death registration formed the rudiments of early infectious disease surveillance systems. It is still useful as a source for case ascertainment of diseases with high case fatality rates, such as rabies, botulism, and AIDS in the 1980s. Where case fatality rates are low or decreas-

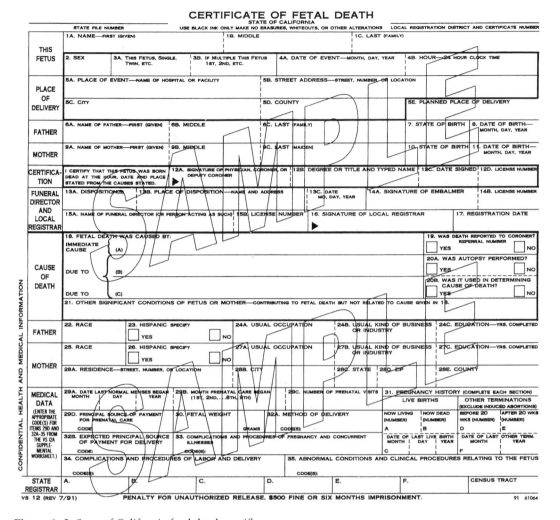

Figure 6–2. State of California fetal death certificate.

ing, however, using death data alone can be misleading. Another consideration is the interval between onset of the disease and death; for pneumonia and influenza, the leading infectious cause of death in the United States, the interval is very short, while for rabies it may be long and variable.

Although death registration is nearly complete in most Western countries, in many developing countries it tends to be biased. Ascertainment in these countries is better in urban than rural areas and for persons who have been hospitalized or can afford the care of a health professional.

Regardless of location, the coding of the cause of death on the certificate is also highly variable, particularly for infectious diseases, where the laboratory support for any diagnosis may be critical or the diagnosis stigmatizing (as with AIDS). Deaths that are unexpected or that occur in undiagnosed patients or under unusual circumstances are usually handled by the medical examiner, who provides autopsy findings. These are important for classifying some infectious diseases, which are sometimes not recorded on the certificate (but may be added as an amendment later and included in the database). The accuracy of diagnosis may vary with the specific diagnosis, level of laboratory support, or host characteristics. In addition, coding may be complex, as may clas-

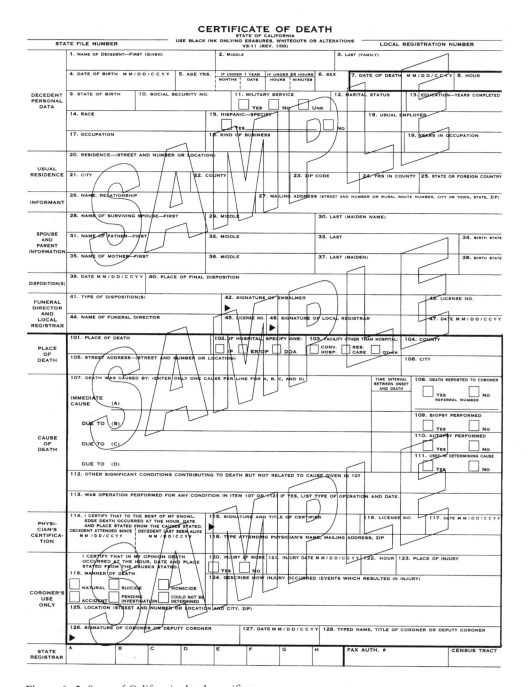

Figure 6–3. State of California death certificate.

sification of the disease itself. Further, many systems only code a single underlying cause of death rather then include multiple causes of death, although this trend has been changing in recent years. The system of death cod-

ing is revised periodically by the WHO, and is known as the ICD. A good example is pneumonia, which might be specified as an immediate cause but not coded as such if the underlying cause was considered to be cardiovascular disease. To further complicate things, different countries use different methods for selecting an underlying disease.

Occasionally, crude death rates (nonspecific causes) can be useful in monitoring infectious disease events that have great impact on the community. Gauging the impact of severe influenza epidemics is frequently cited as an example, where both the total deaths and cause-specific influenza death rates are clearly elevated during pandemics. In the future, improved linkages from death certificates to other clinical and epidemiologic databases may provide more complete ascertainment of case fatality rates and outcomes for a variety of infectious diseases.

Autopsy records can serve as a source of mortality data. Although such data sources may provide a wealth of details not generally found on the death certificate, such data are subject to selection bias: autopsy data may not be representative of the population from which the data are drawn because unusual deaths tend to be overrepresented.

Natality Data (Birth Certificates)

Another vital record is certification of birth. For infectious diseases, birth certificates offer a more limited arena of case ascertainment than death certificates. But a number of perinatal conditions may be recorded. During the 1960s, many jurisdictions added sections to the certificate to include information on complications of pregnancy and abnormalities of the infant. Although not always filled out completely, this section has been a source of case ascertainment for a variety of congenital conditions, including congenital rubella syndrome, HIV infection, and congenital syphilis. Alone, however, the birth certificate is inadequate for surveillance of these infectious diseases, because the diagnoses are often confirmed well after the birth is certified.

Fetal Deaths

Fetal deaths are not complete in their registration. Most jurisdictions only require reporting of abortions that occur after 20 or more weeks of gestation. Information related to infectious diseases of the mother may

not be coded but can sometimes be found in other sections of the certificate, for example, in the "contributing conditions" section. Despite incomplete reporting, fetal deaths are important. If such deaths are included in a study, a visual review of the certificates may be necessary. Given the relatively low reported rate of fetal deaths (usually 1 per 1000 live births), visual review is not a difficult task in most local jurisdictions. Completeness of reporting varies considerably by location, time period, and population group. Nevertheless, such reports have been used to identify a number of infectious diseases associated with fetal demise, such as listeriosis. A problem common to all vital records systems is the delays between registration (which usually occurs reasonably soon after the event) and availability of the preliminary data, and the generation of a final report. Sometimes the interval can be several years. However, it is not uncommon for localities to set up a "hand-review" system in which clerks and registrars involved in the process of registration are on the lookout for certain birth, death, or fetal death certificates and send copies as soon as they receive them to the appropriate public health units for further analysis. NCHS publishes monthly (*National Vital Statistics Reports*) and more comprehensive annual reports of vital statistics, the most useful of which for disease researchers are those summarizing annual mortality. For example, NCHS published final mortality data for 1997 in mid-1999 (Hoyert 1999). Reports are available on the Internet (see: http://www.cdc.gov/nchs/) as well as in print.

LABORATORY DATA

Louis Pasteur, the nineteenth-century French scientist and founding father of microbiology, called laboratories "temples of the future" (Valdiserri 1993). The ever-increasing number, speed, and types of laboratory assays available seem to support Pasteur's metaphor. The variety of biomedical laboratories is great, as are the populations they serve. Some laboratories are public, others privately owned; some operate for profit, others do not; some serve specific hospitals and thus reflect the patients admitted there, while others are large corporate networks that serve a national clientele via express interstate transportation of specimens. Some laboratories specialize in selected infectious diseases such as sexually transmitted diseases or tuberculosis, while others serve special functions, such as blood bank laboratories, that have a specific mission to screen donations of blood and plasma for seven infectious agents: hepatitis B and hepatitis C viruses, human immunodeficiency virus (HIV)-1 and HIV-2, human T-lymphotropic virus (HTLV)-1 and HTLV-2, and the bacteria that cause syphilis. Data from each of these types of laboratory are useful for study purposes, but only if the population that is the source of the specimens can be described epidemiologically.

The characteristics of laboratory data generally include personal identifiers in addition to test results and sometimes include disease-specific clinical information, although not always. In general, laboratory data specify the results of specific tests and the source of the specimen (e.g., blood, urine, cerebrospinal fluid, throat swab), not clinical conclusions. Test results are often viewed as "hard data," but many laboratory test results may require additional interpretation in a clinical or epidemiologic context, and their utility for surveillance purposes varies from disease to disease. For some diseases, a laboratory result essentially defines a case (e.g., positive culture from normally sterile sites for invasive bacterial pathogens). For others, such as syphilis, hepatitis B, or toxoplasmosis, serologic antibody test results alone fail to distinguish between recent and past infections and must be supplemented by clinical information or more specific tests.

Laboratory data can be useful in many areas of infectious disease epidemiology, including case confirmation and identification, detection of outbreaks or epidemics, monitoring changes in infectious agents (e.g., antibiotic resistance), defining a clinical spectrum (ranging from asymptomatic to fatal cases), facilitating epidemiologic

studies (both prospective and retrospective studies, which may rely on stored laboratory specimens), and evaluating diagnostic methods. In many situations, knowing negative test results may be as valuable as knowing positive ones.

Obtaining access to clinical laboratory results, however useful they may be, can be difficult. Access may depend on the type of laboratory and the purpose of the research. The institutional review board may play a role in facilitating access to data collected by the laboratory.

Distinguishing laboratory from surveillance data is important because they are not always the same, although many infectious disease surveillance systems rely on clinical data from both the laboratory and the physician. Both paper and electronic laboratory data can support surveillance systems but rarely provide surveillance independently.

CDC, CSTE, and the Association of Public Health Laboratories convened a Working Group on Electronic Laboratory Surveillance (ELS), which drafted a set of recommendations on electronic reporting of laboratory data. Despite many past improvements, the review panel agreed that "laboratory reporting to public health lags behind other applications of state-of-the-art technology." The experts cited the lack of standardized and connected electronic formats, and noted that many laboratories still rely mainly on paper to communicate results. Electronic reporting of clinical laboratory data is a worthy goal advocated by many in the public health community (Centers for Disease Control and Prevention 1999b).

MANAGED CARE DATA

The health care system in the United States is in a major state of flux because of the rapid growth of managed care plans. The impetus for this growth is not medical or scientific, but economic. Yet one rationale for economies of scale, that is the "managed" part of managed care plans, is that findings from the analysis of huge data warehouses created by the plans will result in efficiencies not otherwise achievable. The plans' unique ability to generate and store thousands of data elements derived from a known population of patients is a potential boon to data users. Some managed care or other health insurance plans make their information available. For example, with Blue Cross/Blue Shield of Tennessee, more than 200 users can log on to review quality management, Health Plan Employer Data and Information Set (HEDIS) reporting, managed care contracting, provider profiling, utilization management, product management, and forecasting information. Specific infectious disease information may not be easy to obtain from such databases, but some indirect measures can be, such as trends in outpatient visits for otitis media.

A major measurement of quality of medical care provided by managed care plans is the HEDIS, which is somewhat like a "report card" in that it represents a standard set of criteria that the plan is "graded" on. Because the data are generated by a variety of different systems, data sets are not always easy to compare, however. HEDIS was developed by the National Committee for Quality Assurance (NCQA), which expected that such data would be used for performance measures to ensure that health care providers give consumers information they need to evaluate managed care plans, including effectiveness of care, access to/availability of care, satisfaction with the experience of care, informed health care choices, health plan descriptive information, cost of care, health plan stability, and use of services. HEDIS is widely used by health and consumer organizations and state and federal regulators, less for its quality or utility than for its availability as one of the few standard measurement tools. HEDIS uses a standardized method to the integrity of the collection and calculation process that consists of four major components: data capture and processing verification, system verification and review, specification and source code verification, and validation of data derived from medical records and administrative sources.

The vision for HEDIS 3.0 (see: http://www.outcomes-trust.org/srcpages/pm12.htm)

and future versions of HEDIS is of an integrated measurement broad enough to respond to the range of issues that matter to all who make choices about health plans—public as well as private purchasers and all consumers. Although most measures relate to noninfectious diseases, many managed care health plans use HEDIS procedures to measure childhood immunization rates. HEDIS data can serve as very useful sources for adult and childhood immunizations in appropriate populations. An important limitation of HEDIS and other managed care, plan-based studies is the substantial turnover in plan membership over time.

PURCHASING DATA

Managed care plans, insurance companies, pharmaceutical and laboratory companies, and vendors of various sorts have seen untapped value in the data they collect. Exercising their entrepreneurial spirit and seeking to derive "added value" from their products, many have begun to market databases or to perform searches and reviews for fees. *Caveat emptor* (buyer, beware) applies. Some of these data sources are highly reputable, science based, quality controlled, and peer reviewed. One such example is the Cochrane Collaboration, based in England, which gathers and synthesizes evidence from controlled clinical trials in all fields of medicine. Subscriptions to its findings may be purchased in several ways, including over the Internet. Other vendors simply sell whatever they have, often results of billing, admission, or laboratory records, sometimes from large, but epidemiologically uncharacterized, populations. Some vendors can customize outputs for purchasers, such as printouts of hospital discharge diagnoses over a set time period, for a set of states, by race or age or sex. Purchasers should be careful how they phrase the questions they buy the answers to, because changes are likely to add to the costs. Such data tend to be more useful for common infectious diseases like pneumonia and sepsis, but less useful for conditions rarely diagnosed in the United States such as malaria, leprosy, measles, and Chagas' disease. Some purchased data sources are in entirely new arenas of infectious disease concern, such as those sold by laboratory or pharmaceutical companies reporting isolates or summarizing findings related to antibiotic resistance. Their usefulness and representativeness are typically unknown.

DATA AND COMPUTER SECURITY

Just as data recorded on paper should be held securely—as in a locked filing cabinet in a locked room in a locked building—so as to limit unauthorized access, so should data maintained in a computer or other electronic storage system be secured, albeit the system of limiting access is altogether different. Several products and methods are commonly used to protect computer data against threats to confidentiality, reliability, and integrity. Such threats may be in the form of human error or deliberate sabotage (including intrusion by computer hackers), as well as from power outages and natural disasters. With increased use of networks and remote access via the Internet, the need to protect data has increased by degrees of magnitude. Categories of measures include authorization, attribution, and data interface, while specific measures include authentication, firewalls, encryption, antiviral software, power protection, and approaches to disaster recovery.

Authentication

The most commonly used authentication technique is use of a password. Passwords may be either software or hardware coded, such as by requiring the user to insert a readable "smart card" with or without a PIN (personal identification number). Other authentication techniques include biometrics, which employs stored facial, fingerprint, or cornea scans of authorized users. For businesses, a popular method is the Secure Sockets Layer, which requires both the server and the client to communicate with a third site, which, at least initially, holds the key for access.

Firewalls

Firewalls, as the name implies, are barriers that control access to networks. Firewalls are set up by many public and private organizations to help keep the "open" or public portions of their Internet site segregated from their internal networks. They are also used to separate internal networks from one another (for example, a university's library catalog may be open to the public, but its payroll records and students' grades are not). The firewall consists of both hardware and software, allowing only authorized "traffic" to pass.

Encryption

Cryptography involves encoding messages so their content can only be understood by the intended recipient. Use of cryptography dates back to ancient times. Currently, encryption is used to transmit sensitive data across computer networks or internally to keep sensitive computer files private. The messages are changed from readable to unreadable and back again by using complex mathematical algorithms and keys.

Antiviral Software

Computer virus protection is a basic security measure. Viruses, or viral bugs, are computer programming instructions that, when attached to various computer programs and documents sometimes intentionally by criminals, pranksters, or terrorists, can damage the "infected" computer's software. Viruses can be spread via floppy disks, downloaded files, e-mail, e-mail attachments, or by macro files. Antivirus software protects against viruses by scanning the computer for known malicious signatures, or strings of zeroes and ones. Such software is highly recommended.

Security Administration Tools

Security management tools can help network administrators to manage user permissions and sign-ons and to monitor activities. Special monitoring software helps to identify security breaches. These tools are typically found in larger networks like those maintained in universities and government agencies and thus go beyond the purview of individual researchers and users.

Power Protection

Electrical power outages, current variation, blackouts, and line noise all pose potential threats to hardware and data. Damage can be prevented from such unpredictable events as lightning, downed power lines, and peak-period electricity demands. Surge suppressors, power conditioners, and uninterruptible power supplies (UPSs) assist in maintaining an even power supply, and any network or individual researcher should have such safeguards in place. Some computers have such protections built in by manufacturers.

Disaster Recovery

Most organizations should have a clearly defined disaster recovery plan. Mission-critical systems need to have provisions for data replacement and access in case of a natural disaster, fire, or other disruptive act. Regular data backups and redundant storage are necessary and may even include complete duplicates of systems software, data, and hardware. Individuals would be well advised to maintain a frequently updated, secure, and backed-up version of any data they would be hard-pressed to reproduce.

Epi Info

Epi Info is a software program developed by CDC in collaboration with WHO. This program is widely used by public health professionals, with over 100,000 copies distributed in over 100 countries. Described as "A Word-Processing, Database, and Statistics Program for Public Health on IBM-Compatible Microcomputers," the software is provided without cost and can be downloaded from the CDC Internet site (http://www.cdc.gov/epiinfo).

Epi Info has a full range of tools including the capability to develop questionnaires and data entry forms, customize the data entry process, and analyze routines for databases. Epidemiologic statistics, graphs, and tables can be produced with user-friendly basic commands. A particular strength of Epi Info is its ability to aggregate and summarize data, for example, by generating stratified 2-by-3 tables. A component called Epi Map generates and displays geographic maps with data from Epi Info.

A strength of Epi Info has been its portability. The previous DOS versions could easily run on most basic computer systems. Epi Info 2000 has additional resource requirements in terms of both operating systems and memory. Regardless, either system can be installed on computer laptops and therefore maintains its usefulness in field operations. Data entry can be carried out either directly in the field or later back in the office. The number of variables that can be created is virtually unlimited; however, close attention should be paid to collecting only that information needed to answer specific study questions. Otherwise, data entry can overwhelm the researcher. Although Epi Info provides reasonably good-looking graphics, they are not up to the quality of a professional graphics program such as PowerPoint or Freelance. Epi Info 2000 does have export capability, however, which allows the user to create files that can be used by such graphics programs.

Many versions of Epi Info have been disseminated, but only the one titled Epi Info 2000 is compatible with Microsoft Windows 95, 98, NT, and 2000. Written in Visual Basic, Version 5, Epi Info 2000 data are stored in Microsoft Access files, but many other file types can be accessed and analyzed. Output is transferred to the user's browser in HTML-compatible files. A useful feature is that CDC supports the Epi Info Hotline, offering free technical help to Epi Info users during normal East Coast working hours. The hotline can be reached by telephone at (770) 488-8440, FAX (770) 488-8456, and e-mail at epiinfo@cdc.gov. CDC maintains a LISTSERVer for users of Epi Info. Users who send an e-mail to subscribe to the List will receive an e-mail with instructions in return, and then will automatically receive messages submitted by other users to the List.

PUBLIC HEALTH INFORMATICS

Information resources are becoming larger, more dynamic, and more numerous, making public health information widely accessible via computer and electronic media. With the advent of the Internet, a new field combining both communications and information is rapidly evolving. Referred to as informatics, data-source-related applications of the new discipline generally aim to improve mechanisms for: (1) finding and retrieving information, (2) querying and analyzing data files, (3) entering data on-line as well as transmitting surveillance and other data files, (4) electronic messaging (subscribing to and exchanging electronic mail as well as being able to communicate via discussion groups with one's peers on a myriad of topics, and (5) disseminating state and local health information and data. "Paperless" medical records, telemedicine, and extensive educational and training applications are among the many uses of health informatics.

A topic that often appears in conjunction with informatics is data visualization, one major aspect of which is geographic information systems (GIS). Combining mapping, public health data, and graphics with computer science, GIS can simultaneously depict and analyze such variables as disease occurrence, infectious disease exposure and risk, morbidity and mortality, health-inducing behavior, and access to preventive care and services. GIS may allow for increased cost-effective use of scarce disease prevention resources in regional and localized settings.

Enterprise-wide information systems have proliferated in recent years. Such systems tend to provide a uniform and one-stop approach for almost all of an individual's data needs in a certain area. Despite the proliferation of these systems in the business environment, few government organizations have developed them. One of the lead agencies for disease resource and health information retrieval tools is CDC. Many of CDC's systems cover a specific disease (e.g., HIV infection and AIDS) or a public health practice area (e.g., surveillance or training).

For both public and private data sources, the ease of information retrieval varies, as does the complexity of the technology required at the user's end, ranging from telephone, to stand-alone microcomputer, to microcomputer-plus-modem, to the Internet. Additionally, information retrieval is not always cost-free to the user.

DATA WAREHOUSING

Simply put, a data warehouse is a place, not necessarily a physical place, where users can access data. Data warehouses typically combine data from a variety of sources into a single Internet site or other access point from which an individual can query a number of different systems. Sometimes, the systems consist of a variety of personal, mini, and mainframe computers. Many are considered to be "legacy" systems, that is, systems that employ older programming languages or depend on older (possibly obsolete) technology. The copying and moving of data sets into the warehouse generally focus on the development of subject-oriented tables, accessed via networked computers (which may include the Internet).

Users of data warehouses, who usually must obtain security clearance beforehand, can retrieve and manipulate data. These data may be accessed and analyzed by using either prepackaged reports or software tools available to the user for reporting, assessing, and planning functions. Usually, the data available in warehouses are copies of original data sets, and may even be a smaller subset with certain information removed (such as confidential identifiers). Generally, such systems are updated periodically.

Data warehouses became major features of information system architectures in the 1990s. Generally, the building of a data warehouse takes a step-by-step approach. One of the key attributes of a data warehouse is that the data standards must be integrated throughout the system. The integration appears in a variety of ways: in naming conventions, in measurement of variables, in encoding structures, and in the attributes of the data. For example, a local health department with a well-integrated data warehouse in place would have standardized race fields for death and morbidity data.

Ultimately, data warehouses will improve researchers' ability to obtain and analyze data, tasks that previously required expensive mainframe computers and specialized software and training to use it properly. In addition, data warehouses facilitate timely retrieval of data directly by end users as well as provide increased flexibility for mixing and matching variables and fields from different data sets, all at a single location.

CHALLENGES FOR THE FUTURE

The generation of data is perhaps less of an issue for the future than access is. Computer-based data systems exist or are in development that can track and link everything from consumer purchases to patient health information to financial and government records. Many individuals are concerned that those with access to some or all of these databases will not always have their best interests at heart. The debate is under way on how individual rights to privacy can be sustained in an era when information is so rapidly and widely generated and disseminated. Public health data are a small but important part of the debate involving researchers, public health officials, medical care providers, insurers, and consumers.

Some issues researchers face today will surely remain challenges in the future, such as knowing how representative any particular database is. Ascertainment bias, reporting bias, and access to care will all continue to need attention, but perhaps differently than in the past. Electronic reporting of notifiable diseases may increase the speed and efficiency of collection of such data, but measuring completeness of reporting will remain an important factor in determining the usefulness of a system and in analyzing trends.

Evolving bioethical issues, while sometimes administratively challenging, must not be overlooked by database users and managers. If individuals and their health care providers do not have assurance that the data they supply or rely on are generated and maintained in confidence and applied fairly (e.g., genetic screening information is not used to "label" a particular population, resulting in discrimination), no one can expect such systems to thrive or even survive. Informed consent for data-gathering efforts, institutional review board oversight, and prevention of discriminatory uses of data are among the challenges data source managers and users will face.

The future is bright for databases, largely because of major advances in hardware and software development and communications capabilities, but preventing misapplications and frank abuse will be more important than ever. And we must still pay attention to that "village watchman, who just puts down what he damn well pleases."

The internet addresses cited in this chapter were correct at the time that the chapter was written but they are subject to change.

REFERENCES

Alter MJ, Kruszon-Moran D, Nainan OV, et al. The prevalence of hepatitis C virus infection in the United States, 1988 through 1994, N. Engl. J. Med. 341:556–562, 1999.

Berkson J. Limitations of the application of four-fold analysis to hospital data. Biometrics Bull. 2:47–53, 1946.

Centers for Disease Control and Prevention. CDC Surveillance Summaries: Malaria surveillance—United States, 1995. MMWR. 48 (No. SS-1):1–23, 1999a.

Centers for Disease Control and Prevention. Summary of notifiable diseases, United States, 1997. MMWR. 46(54):1–87, 1997a.

Centers for Disease Control. Guidelines for evaluating surveillance systems. MMWR. 37 (suppl. no. S-5):1–18, 1988.

Centers for Disease Control and Prevention. Case definitions for infectious conditions under public health surveillance. MMWR. 46 (No. RR-10):1–55, 1997b.

Centers for Disease Control and Prevention. Summary: Electronic Reporting of Laboratory Data for Public Health: Meeting Report and Recommendations. Updated 08-24-99 posted at: http://www.phppo.cdc.gov/DLS/pdf/elr1030.pdf as [PFP#280807883], 1999b.

Centers for Disease Control and Prevention. HIV/AIDS Surveillance Report. 10(No. 2): 1–43, 1998.

Centers for Disease Control and Prevention. CDC Surveillance Summaries: Surveillance for AIDS-definining opportunistic illnesses, 1992–1997. MMWR. 48(No. SS-2):1–22, 1999c.

Chin J, ed. Control of Communicable Diseases Manual. 17th ed. Washington, DC: American Public Health Association 2000.

Division of STD Prevention. Sexually Transmitted Disease Surveillance, 1997. Department of Health and Human Services, U.S. Public Health Service, Centers for Disease Control and Prevention, September 1998.

Estes JW, and Smith BG, eds. A Melancholy Scene of Devastation: The Public Response to the 1793 Philadelphia Yellow Fever Epidemic. Canton, MA: Science History Publications/USA, 1997.

Etheridge EW. Sentinel for Health: A History of the Centers for Disease Control. Berkeley, CA: University of California Press, 1992.

Hoyert DL, Kochanek KD, and Murphy SL. Deaths: Finala Data for 1997. National Vital Statistics Reports. 47(No. 19). Hyattsville, MD: National Center for Health Statistics, 1999.

Humphries N, ed. Vital Statistics: A Memorial Volume of Selections from the Reports and Writings of William Farr. London: Office of Sanitary Institute, 1985: 343–351.

Kortepeter MG, and Park GW. Potential biological weapons threats. Emerg. Infect. Dis. 5:523–527, 1999.

Lilienfield DE, and Stolley PD. Foundations of Epidemiology. 3rd ed. New York: Oxford University Press, 1994.

Mullan F. Plagues and Politics: The Story of the United States Public Health Service. New York: Basic Books, 1989: 26.

Shephard DAE. John Snow: Anaesthetist to a Queen and Epidemiologist to a Nation: A Biography. Cornwall, PE, Canada: York Point Publishing, 1995:204.

Stamp JC. Some Economic Factors in Modern Life. London: King and Sons, 1929:258–259.

Valdiserri RO. Temples of the future: an historical overview of the laboratory's role in public health practice. Annu. Rev. Public Health. 14:635–648, 1993.

Webster's Ninth New Collegiate Dictionary. Springfield, MA: Merriam-Webster Inc., 1990.

7

Disease Surveillance

TERENCE L. CHORBA

In 1348, the Republic of Venice erected its first quarantine station at which all travelers from plague stricken ships were detained to monitor for signs of disease (Moro 1988). The term "surveillance" was introduced into English at the time of the Napoleonic wars, and in public health terms was restricted until 1949 to such monitoring of contacts of persons with serious communicable diseases (Langmuir 1971). As numerous disease surveillance systems have evolved in many cultures, various definitions have been offered for surveillance in its application to human morbidity and mortality data.

Epidemiologic data may be gathered through time-limited cross sectional or longitudinal studies or through surveillance systems that function continuously. In *A Dictionary of Epidemiology*, J.M. Last (1983) defines surveillance of disease as "the continuing scrutiny of all aspects of occurrence and spread of a disease that are pertinent to effective control." He also includes the systematic collection and evaluation of morbidity and mortality data, special reports of field investigations and epidemics and of in-

dividual cases, laboratory findings, data regarding use of vaccines and other substances used in control and their sequelae, information regarding immunity levels in the population, and other relevant epidemiological data. In this chapter we address these varied and important elements.

The definition of disease surveillance that is most frequently applied in the United States has evolved over many years of epidemiological research at the World Health Organization (WHO) (Raska 1996, 1983) and the Centers for Disease Control and Prevention (CDC) (Thacker 1988): surveillance is the ongoing, systematic collection, analysis, and interpretation of health data used in the planning, implementation, and evaluation of public health programs. As with any set of information systems, disease surveillance systems pertaining to the occurrence of specific diseases need to be designed to support decision making and action, and to assess the effectiveness of intervention programs. Hence, the final links in the surveillance chain are the timely dissemination of aggregated and analyzed data to those who have contributed information to the system and those who need to know, and the subsequent application of the processed information to disease control and prevention. Analysis and distribution of data in a timely and systematic manner is integral to the goal of a surveillance system to determine priorities, identify and evaluate control measures, generate and evaluate hypotheses, determine strategies, monitor changes in infectious agents, identify and target populations at high risk, and implement and evaluate programs (Kaslow 1997).

As noted by Thacker and Berkelman (1988), surveillance systems are usually designed to monitor trends, to detect and describe problems, and to establish hypotheses to be tested in more refined research designs. The similarity has been noted between the feedback cycle of public health surveillance and the basic element of total quality management (TQM), the "Shewhart Cycle for learning and improvement" (Halperin 1996). This cycle consists of four stages: (1) plan a change or test aimed at improvement, (2) carry out the change or the test, (3) study the results, and (4) adopt the change, or abandon it, or run through the cycle again.

Classically, publicly financed surveillance systems concerned with infectious diseases have focused on monitoring mortality, and to lesser extent, morbidity. The determination of what diseases, conditions, or risk factors should come under surveillance should reflect how the information will influence decision making, especially in a resource-constrained environment. Indeed, a disease or condition must be important enough to warrant time and effort of surveillance. In many countries, lack of interest, lack of feedback, and the voluminousness of the list of reportable diseases have greatly impeded surveillance activities (Anon 1976). At a national and regional level, Canada has taken the lead in developing criteria in a rational system for setting priorities in determining the relative importance of surveillance for specific infectious diseases (Carter 1992). The criteria developed are predicated on the goals of facilitating the prevention and control of the diseases under surveillance, and

satisfying the needs of government, health care professionals, voluntary agencies, and the public for information on risk patterns and trends in the occurrence of communicable disease. The criteria include WHO interest, Agriculture Canada and federal food regulatory agency interest, incidence, morbidity, mortality, case fatality rate, communicability and potential for outbreaks, socioeconomic impact, public perception of risk, vaccine preventability, and necessity for an immediate public health response (Carter 1992). In considering developing a surveillance system of any size for infectious diseases, inclusion of these or similar criteria should be considered, depending upon the goals of the surveillance system proposed.

ELEMENTS OF A GOOD SURVEILLANCE SYSTEM

To be useful, an infectious diseases surveillance system has attributes for which it should be periodically evaluated as useful performance criteria (Centers for Disease Control 1988):

- Simplicity of design
- Flexibility and acceptability
- Timeliness
- Sensitivity
- Positive predictive value
- Representativeness
- Cost

Simplicity of Design
The simplicity of a surveillance system refers to both its structure and ease of operation. Often, in the interest of gathering as much data as possible, infectious diseases surveillance systems become very complex in terms of the amount of information gathered on each and every case of infectious disease, with multiple layers of reporting involved, much time required to collect case information, and many individuals involved in maintaining the system. In developing systems, there are often significant duplication of effort and greater possibility of error introduction in multiple entry and transmission

of data. It is also intuitive that as data are aggregated at higher and higher levels of a centralized disease surveillance system, the ability to detect clusters of localized outbreaks may be lost.

Flexibility and Acceptability

Flexibility describes the extent to which a surveillance system can adapt to changing information needs or operating conditions with little additional cost in time, personnel, or allocated funds. For example, when penicillinase-producing *Neisseria gonorrhoeae* (PPNG) appeared in the United States in 1976, it was detected by the state-based system for the surveillance of gonorrhea (Centers for Disease Control 1976). The same system was subsequently used to monitor the spread of the disease in the United States, direct prevent programs, and assess the impact of intervention procedures (Thacker 1988).

Acceptability reflects the willingness of individuals and organizations to participate in the surveillance system. In the United States, the consistent variations from disease to disease seen in reporting of notifiable diseases in the National Notifiable Diseases Surveillance System (NNDSS) may in part be disease-specific variations in acceptability of this surveillance system. The acceptability of a largely voluntary system depends on the perceived public health importance of the events under surveillance, minimization of the burden of time and effort in participating, and feedback for the individual's contribution to the system in which the value of the contribution can be recognized.

Timeliness

The timeliness of a surveillance system should be evaluated in terms of availability of information for disease control—either for immediate control efforts or for long-term planning. Notification of certain conditions within hours of suspicion of a diagnosis provides for rapid implementation of control and prevention measures by public health authorities. Prompt reporting permits rapid case investigation and early detection of epidemics. Thus if an ill person seeks medical attention promptly, there is a minimum amount of time between onset of symptoms and the report of the event to the public health agency responsible for instituting control and prevention measures. There have been published cases in which failure to report certain conditions in a timely fashion has delayed the identification of disease clusters, thus hindering the initiation of prevention measures (Anon 1989). A few studies have examined the timeliness of reporting and its potential impact on disease prevention (Birkhead 1991, Rosenberg 1977, Centers for Disease Control 1968, Thacker 1986, Bernier 1974). In a study of disease reports to the NNDSS in the United States, the timeliness of reporting was found to vary widely by type of disease (Fig. 7–1) and by state (Birkhead, 1991).

In settings where there is a common practice to self-medicate, as in the developing world, timeliness of reporting of diseases will be problematic. When cholera entered Peru in 1991, it spread through the existing sanitation and water systems, resulting in more than 3000 deaths and estimated losses of $770 million in one year to the Peruvian economy because of seafood export embargoes and decreased tourism (Heymann 1998). Because reporting of cholera cases was often delayed, the scope of the epidemic was initially unclear. Thus there can be both burden of disease and financial considerations that merit attending to the timeliness of reporting.

Sensitivity

Sensitivity is the measure of the system's ability to account for all incidents of a condition that occur. An alternative measure of sensitivity is the ability of the system to detect clusters or epidemics. The sensitivity depends on the proportion of disease detected, correctly diagnosed, and reported. Quantitatively, sensitivity is the ratio of the total number of cases or health events detected by a system over the total number of true cases or health events as determined by some "gold standard." Lack of sensitivity is a classic shortcoming of infectious diseases surveillance systems, a frequently cited example of which was the finding that, during the smallpox eradication program, only 1%–10% of cases were reported, and that due to loss of data, only about 25% of the cases reported by first-line providers were registered nationally (Henderson 1976). To increase the likelihood that gathering surveillance data will result in timely application of effective interventions, increasing the sensitivity of surveillance systems often takes priority over increasing positive predictive value.

Positive Predictive Value

Positive predictive value is the likelihood that a case report of a disease does, in fact, constitute a true case of that disease. Quantitatively, it is the ratio of the number of all persons detected by the surveillance system who truly are cases, as determined by some "gold standard," over the total number of persons identified by the system as being cases. If a system encourages reporting of suspected cases as well as reporting of confirmed cases of disease, the positive predictive value of suspected case reporting could be evaluated, based on what percentage of suspected cases is later confirmed. However, the positive predictive value of preliminary reports would be of little concern, except where expensive and labor-intensive control measures are routinely instituted immediately upon receipt of a suspected case report. Relative lack of laboratory confirmation of diagnosis and reliance on physician diagnosis as to what constitutes a case may result in substantial variation in the positive predictive value of data reported. Where there is lack of codification of case definitions and lack of "gold standards" for diagnosis, the evaluation of the positive predictive value of a surveillance system is difficult. For well-functioning infectious disease surveillance systems, there is a need for identifying, developing, and agreeing on the use of standardized case definitions for surveillance.

Representativeness

A surveillance system that is representative accurately describes (1) the occurrence of a

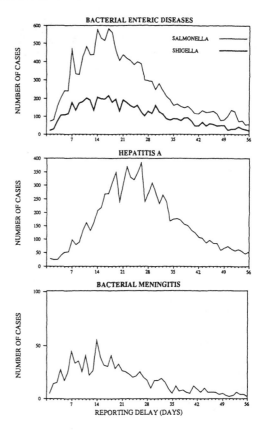

Figure 7–1. Reporting delay by type of disease 1987 NNDSS data.
Source: Birkhead 1991.

health event, and (2) its distribution in the population by place and person. Where completeness of reporting is high, data tend to be representative, for example, measles reporting in the United States. A major concern is that nonrepresentativeness of reporting in a surveillance system may direct prevention activities away from populations at risk (Kimball 1980).

Cost

As with any health information system, surveillance systems for infectious conditions and diseases should be minimized with respect to number of diseases reported and frequency of reporting in the interest of meeting the goals of the surveillance system within the budget allocated. The cost of routine reporting systems is thought to be substantial: in seven countries in Latin America in 1987, the cost of the routine health information system was estimated to range from 10% to 25% of the total wage bill of the ministries of health (Ledogar 1988).

Costs should be judged relative to benefits, but unfortunately few evaluations of surveillance systems have included cost-benefit analyses. In a 1985 report from Kentucky, the economic benefits from health department–initiated surveillance of hepatitis A far exceeded the costs (Hinds 1985). As a more sophisticated model, the reader is referred to an analysis of the costs and benefits of a computerized system of notification and analysis of infectious diseases in Sheffield, England, in which the hours invested in developing the system were offset by a continuing saving of those hours every two years (Payne 1992). The marginal utility of data that are gathered should drive decisions with respect to what disease events are deemed reportable. It is technically inefficient if the desire to collect data exceeds the ability to act on those data.

The attributes just discussed can be developed into specific criteria for surveillance program development and evaluation (Centers for Disease Control 1988). Using these specific criteria, surveillance systems should also be reviewed periodically and modified as needed.

USES AND NEEDS

Surveillance is necessary for effective public health practice, which requires accurate assessment of the public health problems at hand, definition of specific public health priorities, development and implementation of research and control programs to improve health, and evaluation of these programs. Surveillance data should provide the factual basis for appropriate policy decisions and allocation of scarce resources, health services, and infrastructure; analyses of these data should also contribute to the redefinition of public health priorities as problems are resolved and new needs arise, and enable researchers to identify areas of interest for further investigation (Thacker 1992).

Conceptually, the importance of surveillance is not limited to infectious disease problems. Valid data, in an accessible and understandable form, are the foundation of any effective program in public health, whether the problem be one of infectious disease, environmental exposures, injury control, nutrition, chronic disease, or any of a host of other problems that concern the health practitioner. Standardized data are essential for identifying problems, factors associated with these problems, and emerging issues, as well as for evaluating the effectiveness of interventions and making informed judgments about where to invest limited resources.

In the world of infectious diseases, effective surveillance is necessary to halt the spread of communicable disease. In most countries, the reporting of cases of infectious diseases has been and remains a vital step in controlling and preventing the spread of infectious diseases. These reports are useful in many ways, including assurance of provision of appropriate medical therapy and determination of resource allocation (e.g., tuberculosis), determination of a baseline for detection of epidemic activity (e.g., human immunodeficiency virus [HIV]), early detection of common-source outbreaks (e.g., food-borne outbreaks) and epidemics, and planning and evaluating prevention and control programs (e.g., vaccine preventable diseases). Renewed interest in the surveillance of infectious diseases has occurred in response to the HIV/AIDS epidemic, emergence of drug-resistance complicating infections with common bacterial pathogens and tuberculosis, reemergence of malaria as a health threat to travelers, and the spread of dengue fever to Australia (Hall 1991) and its potential spread to the continental United States.

HISTORICAL BACKGROUND

The control and prevention of infectious disease has traditionally been a primary public health mandate, and in most developed countries, notifiable disease reporting systems have evolved as the basis of infectious disease surveillance (Moro 1988, Valleron

1986, Thacker 1983). Records of vital events were preserved in many European towns beginning in the sixteenth century, as local governments assumed responsibility for rudimentary health concerns of the population (Hartgerink 1976). In the seventeenth century, John Graunt attempted to define the basic laws of "natality and mortality," estimated the population of London and the numbers that died from specific causes, and advocated the use of numerical data to study the causes of disease (Eylenbosch 1988). In the eighteenth century, William Farr, the superintendent of the Statistical Department of the General Registry in London, analyzed and disseminated vital statistics with the purpose of controlling and preventing infectious diseases, hazardous work conditions, and occupational diseases and injuries (Eylenbosch 1988).

In the United States, a publisher and bookseller, Lemuel Shattuck, produced the Report of the Massachusetts Sanitary Commission in 1850, relating deaths, infant and maternal mortality, and communicable diseases (scarlet fever, typhus, typhoid fever, diphtheria, and tuberculosis) with living conditions. Shattuck recommended a decennial census, standardization of nomenclature of causes of disease and death, and the collection of health data by age, sex, occupation, socioeconomic level, and locality (Trask 1915). As an outgrowth of the work of Shattuck, systematic reporting of various diseases in the United States began in 1874 when the State Board of Health of Massachusetts inaugurated a plan for the weekly voluntary reporting of prevalent diseases by physicians. A model disease reporting postcard was designed to "reduce to the minimum the expenditure of time and trouble" entailed in reporting (Bowditch 1915). Because many aspects of communicable disease control were more appropriately addressed from a national perspective, the federal Quarantine Act of 1878 authorized the United States Public Health Service (USPHS) to collect morbidity data for use in quarantine measures against cholera, smallpox, and yellow fever.

In 1883, Michigan became the first U.S. jurisdiction to mandate the reporting of specific infectious diseases, and the Quarantine Act of 1893 authorized the USPHS to collect morbidity information each week from state and local public health authorities throughout the United States. By 1901, all states required notification of selected communicable diseases to local health authorities. The poliomyelitis epidemic in 1916 and the influenza pandemic of 1918–1919 heightened interest in reporting requirements, resulting in the participation of all states in national morbidity reporting by 1925.

In the United States, the concept of surveillance evolved further under the National Poliomyelitis Surveillance Program, which was established at CDC in 1955 in response to six cases of paralytic polio following the use of Salk vaccine (the "Cutter incident"); the cases had been reported through state and local health departments. The intent of the program was to monitor polio trends, measure the effectiveness of polio immunization programs, and detect potential vaccine-associated cases (Nathanson 1963). In 1957, the Asian influenza surveillance system was created at CDC as a fundamental part of the national efforts to control an influenza pandemic. CDC and the Council of State and Territorial Epidemiologists (CSTE), an affiliate of the Association of State and Territorial Health Officers (ASTHO), have continued to evolve other ongoing systems of reporting, usually in response to national emergencies, for example, shellfish-associated hepatitis A in 1961, toxic shock syndrome in 1980, identification of the HIV/AIDS epidemic in the early 1980s, and eosinophilia-myalgia syndrome in 1990.

In the United States, CDC has also had responsibility since 1961 for operating the NNDSS, for the purpose of tabulating and disseminating summary morbidity data. Personal identifiers are not included in the NNDSS. All states and territories of the United States participate in this system, reporting on a weekly basis to CDC the aggregate or case-specific data for a set list of infectious diseases and related conditions. CSTE determines the list of diseases in collaboration with CDC, revising it annually as needed; the list includes those infectious diseases for which data can provide a basis for state and local agencies to plan more effective programs for disease prevention and control (Roush 1999).

In recent years, the specter of bioterrorism has attracted the attention and resources of governments (Henderson 1999), and has heightened awareness of the need for infectious disease reporting systems that maximally meet the performance criteria outlined earlier in this chapter (McDade 1998, Hughes 1998).

ELEMENTS OF INFECTIOUS DISEASE SURVEILLANCE AND DATA SOURCES

Fundamental Variables and Case Definitions

In assembling epidemiological information on an infectious disease problem, for example, ascertaining who is affected with a disease or condition and the circumstances surrounding the event, two descriptive variables referent to personal characteristics are almost universally collected: age and gender. Other descriptive variables referent to personal characteristics are often routinely gathered: age, marital status and measures referent to race, ethnic group (e.g., Hispanic vs. non-Hispanic), socioeconomic status, and occupation. Other important variables that would be integral to interpretation of data with respect to the incidence or prevalence of any infectious disease include the relevant place (place of domicile, place of occupation, place of death, etc.) and time (as in date of onset or date of exposure).

Issues of the use of different clinical, laboratory, and epidemiological criteria to define cases are also of paramount importance, as the use of different diagnostic criteria have a great impact on the comparability of disease data reported from different geographic areas or in different years. Before 1990, lack of uniformity among states regarding the case definitions for many diseases made comparisons between states difficult. For example, some states have required any person with a culture positive for *Salmonella* to

be reported whereas other states have required reporting of culture-positive individuals only if they were symptomatic (Moro 1988). To facilitate comparison of surveillance data among states, standardized case definitions for the nationally notifiable diseases were developed by CDC and CSTE, approved by CSTE in 1989 (Centers for Disease Control 1990) and revised in 1997 (Centers for Disease Control and Prevention 1997). Standardized case definitions have also recently been revised in Canada (Advisory Committee on Epidemiology and Bureau of Infectious Diseases 2000). It is hoped that these definitions will also facilitate interstate and interprovincial reciprocal notification of disease. In general, in developing case definitions for a disease surveillance system, criteria should allow for characteristics of person, time, and place, as well as clinical and/or laboratory diagnostic criteria, and epidemiological features. Case definitions need to be simple, acceptable, understandable, and to have diagnostic criteria that are unambiguous and easy to comprehend or obtain (Declich 1994). During periods in which epidemics, outbreaks, or clusters are being monitored, cases that are epidemiologically linked may satisfy a case definition, whereas in nonepidemic periods, a more strict case definition may require serologic or other specific criteria (Teutsch 1995).

Vital Records Registration

Morbidity registration is the oldest form of disease reporting and has the advantages of being the only health-related data available in a standard format in most countries, being legally required and having a high order of completeness. Most infectious diseases of sufficient severity to cause death exhibit characteristic clinical findings that allow diagnosis. The possibility of an autopsy also contributes to the accuracy of identification of the disease process. In the United States, about 90,000 deaths per year are attributed to infectious diseases (McGinnis 1993).

Mortality registration is useful only for diseases that result in fatalities. If the case fatality rate is too low, then mortality statistics may not provide an accurate assessment of the occurrence of the disease. For example, most viral diseases are not fatal, and as a result, mortality data have limited usefulness in surveillance of the occurrence of most viral diseases.

The quality of mortality data depends on numerous factors, including completeness of registration, relevance of categories used for diseases, injuries, or other conditions, accuracy of demographic data and diagnoses provided on death certificates, and the computerization and accessibility of these data (Stroup 1994). Unfortunately, there is often a long delay in the tabulation and publication of mortality data. Although birth and death certificates are filed shortly after the event occurs, the process of producing final vital statistics at a national level from these data can take several years (Stroup 1994).

Vital statistics data regarding infectious diseases can be used to monitor long-term trends (Chorba 1994, Brzezinski 1986) and monitor deaths that are generally considered to be preventable (Lew 1991, Weiss 1990, Sutter 1990). An example of such use of death data for assessing the impact of HIV/AIDS on mortality among persons with hemophilia is given in Figure 7–2. Another example of the use of mortality data for surveillance is the collection of pneumonia and influenza weekly mortality reports from American cities. The USPHS has published pneumonia and influenza deaths in a large group of U.S. cities on a weekly basis since 1925 (Collins 1930). To maintain national surveillance of influenza, 121 urban jurisdictions representing about one-third of all deaths in the United States voluntarily participate in CDC's Mortality Reporting System, often known as the "121 Cities Surveillance System" (Centers for Disease Control 1978). Weekly counts for all deaths and for deaths from pneumonia or influenza in each reporting jurisdiction are reported by age group to CDC by local vital statistics registrars located in health departments or vital records offices. Published CDC procedures for reporting of an influenza death to this system specify that an influenza death should be reported if a diagnosis of influenza appears anywhere on the death certificate (Manual of Procedures for National Morbidity Reporting and Public Health Surveillance Activities 1985). Death certificates filed in each city for each one-week period are tabulated by age group and published weekly in the *Morbidity and Mortality Weekly Report* (*MMWR*). Total deaths due to pneumonia and influenza for each city are also presented in the *MMWR*. Evaluations of trends in mortality from all causes and from pneumonia and influenza have demonstrated that such data are useful for estimating overall U.S. mortality trends (Collins 1932, Serfling 1963, Barker 1981, Choi 1981a, b, c, Lui 1987, Baron 1988, Stroup 1988). Weekly data on deaths from influenza and pneumonia in 121 cities are compared to the average number of deaths in the same week of the five previous years, and when two consecutive weeks occur in which influenza and pneumonia deaths exceed the 95% confidence limits of the historical values, the deaths that exceed this "epidemic threshold" are attributed to influenza. Because the cyclic nature of influenza activity is such that long-term data on mortality are important supports to the inexact science of epidemic prediction, data from the 121 Cities Surveillance System can also be used to supplement other surveillance systems, such as the U.S. Vital Records or the National Hospital Discharge Survey, in studying long-term trends in influenza morbidity and mortality.

To serve these purposes, data from the 121 Cities Surveillance System must be sensitive and specific enough to detect the majority of outbreaks with reasonable accuracy. This does not require that all pneumonia and influenza deaths be detected by the system. However, those deaths that are detected must be representative of all deaths on demographic characteristics. If substantial bias were to occur in detection of pneumonia and influenza deaths as a proportion of all deaths, excess mortality from these causes would either be submerged in background noise or would appear to be more dramatic than it is. Fortunately, seasonal excess mortality based on the 121 Cities Sur-

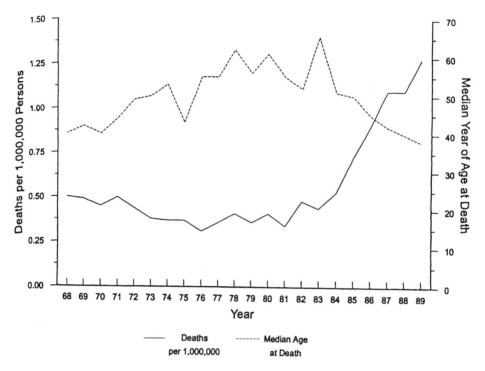

Figure 7–2. Hemophilia A death rates and median age at death by year, United States, 1968–1989.
Source: Chorba 1994.

veillance System correlates well with national data, and can be used for the timely assessment of the severity of future influenza epidemics and pandemics (Simonsen 1997). The timeliness of this system is a great advantage, because these are the only influenza data in the United States that are widely available within a few weeks of occurrence of the case.

Passive Morbidity Reporting

Most infectious disease surveillance systems rely primarily on receipt of case reports from physicians or other health care providers. Such passive reporting systems have variability and incompleteness as major deficiencies. There are substantial differences among states as to the specific list of diseases for which reporting is required. Similar differences exist for the lists of reportable diseases in other countries as well, including the various Canadian provinces and territories (Carter 1988). In agreement with CSTE, CDC provides forms to state health depart-

ments for reciprocal notification for (1) cases of all diseases having onset in one state but hospitalized or transferring to another state, (2) cases of reportable diseases having onset within the state, but presumably infected in another state, and (3) cases regarding which epidemiological information or other public health action may be needed, for example, contact tracing (Centers for Disease Control 1985).

Case reports provided to state and local health departments by physicians and other health care providers usually contain incomplete data and may not be representative for certain populations; completeness of reporting varies greatly for many of the common notifiable diseases (Moro 1988) and is affected by the severity of the disease in question (Thacker 1983). For example, an analysis in 1977 of the completeness of reporting of 570 cases of notifiable communicable diseases from 11 hospitals in Washington, DC, revealed an overall reporting rate of 35%, with considerable variation from disease to disease (Marier 1977). Similarly, an analysis of the completeness of reporting of 364 cases of eight notifiable communicable diseases from 16 hospitals in Vermont for 1982–83 revealed an overall reporting rate of 35%, with considerable variation from disease to disease, but with gonorrhea as the disease most frequently reported (Vogt 1986). Hypotheses that have been advanced to explain the phenomenon of underreporting in passive disease surveillance systems include lack of importance or saliency of the case, patient interference, violation of the physician-patient relationship, insufficient incentives, and excessive administrative costs to the reporter (Rothenberg 1980). However, if the level of completeness is consistent over time, case reports provided to state and local health departments by physicians and other health care providers usually are the best source of information about the temporal and geographic trends and the characteristics of the persons affected. Clinician-based surveillance has also been useful in identifying common-source outbreaks of diseases, for example, hepatitis A (Lowry 1989), hepatitis B (Centers for Disease Control 1986, Reingold 1982), and hepatitis non-A, non-B (Centers for Disease Control 1989).

One of the strengths of the NNDSS as a surveillance system in the United States is its timeliness. Reports of cases received in state health departments are forwarded to CDC and disseminated to epidemiologists, clinicians, and other health professionals within a week of receipt (Stroup 1989). The CDC reports surveillance data weekly in the *MMWR* and annually in its Summary of Notifiable Diseases. To encourage partnership with those physicians or other health professionals who report, most state health departments also use newsletters to provide feedback of data to the health care professionals who contribute to the notifiable diseases surveillance database.

Active Morbidity Reporting

Surveillance activities are often strengthened when the disease in question is given a high priority, such as when primary preven-

tion of most or all cases is feasible (e.g., measles) or when the disease is targeted for eradication (e.g., dracunculiasis, poliomyelitis), when the disease is targeted for elimination (e.g., neonatal tetanus, leprosy), or when the disease is severe and newly emerging (e.g., AIDS, toxic shock syndrome). These activities frequently include working closely with hospitals to identify cases, reviewing hospital discharge records, and working closely with physicians who are likely to diagnose and treat patients. Such active surveillance systems can validate the representativeness of passive reports, assure more complete reporting of conditions, or be used in conjunction with specific epidemiologic investigations (Teutsch 1994). Examples of such increased surveillance activities include those to estimate rates of occurrence and to describe the epidemiology of toxic shock syndrome (Todd 1985) and non-A non-B hepatitis (Alter 1987), to determine the adequacy of treatment of gonorrhea in a community (Eisenberg 1976), and to monitor the occurrence of Reye syndrome following public warning to avoid use of salicylates in young febrile children (Centers for Disease Control 1982).

Some active surveillance systems are unique, being designed to fit the specific needs of the disease or condition of particular importance, and because resources are often limited, active systems are often used only briefly and for discrete purposes. For example, nationwide surveillance for Guillain-Barré syndrome following the initiation of the National Influenza Immunization Program in October 1976 was conducted and accomplished through a network of neurologists (Centers for Disease Control 1980). Recently, population-based active surveillance has been used in four U.S. areas to determine the incidence of cryptococcosis and its risk factors among HIV-infected persons (Hajjeh 1999). Additional active surveillance systems are the three that are activated and used by CDC for tracking influenza morbidity and mortality on an acute basis in addition to the 121 Cities Surveillance described earlier in this chapter: state epidemiologists telephone a weekly assessment of influenza activity (none, sporadic, regional, widespread) to CDC; CDC receives weekly reports of influenza isolates and the number of specimens submitted from the WHO Collaborating Laboratories; and CDC receives weekly reports of office visits for influenzalike illness from about 150 family practitioners (Centers for Disease Control 1991). Data from these three systems are published in periodic *MMWR* reports or in annual summaries.

Epidemic or Outbreak Reporting

Centralized disease surveillance systems are usually of little use for the detection and control of outbreaks. Frequently, there is quantitative improvement of reporting when clusters of cases occur. A cluster is defined as a set of events occurring unusually close to each other in time, space, both time and space, or within demographic characteristics, for example, persons in the same occupation (Thacker 1989). Single cases of salmonellosis or shigellosis may go unreported, but if there is an epidemic, then most or all cases meeting a case definition may be reported during the epidemic. A major use of infectious disease surveillance data is the determination of whether increases in the number of cases with a given infection represents an outbreak or epidemic meriting immediate attention and intervention. The recognition and identification of epidemic infectious diseases are commonly more accurate than individual case reports, because public health officials and laboratory facilities are usually involved. For example, this is true of outbreaks of yellow fever, influenza, rubella, rubeola, hepatitis, and arbovirus infections. Thus, surveillance systems can serve as early warning systems for public health officials (Cates 1994). Increases in numbers of cases of hepatitis B among U.S. military recruits provided a stimulus to intervene with drug-prevention programs (Cowan 1984). In the United States, monitoring of regional trends in rubella and congenital rubella resulted in the identification of outbreaks among the Amish in 1989–1990 (Centers for Disease Control 1991).

Unfortunately, outbreaks of infection for some communicable agents with potentially life-threatening consequences for some members of the population may go unrecognized because they produce primarily mild or unapparent infection in the majority of persons infected (Chorba 1986).

Laboratory-, Clinic-, and Hospital-Based Surveillance Systems

There is growing interest in surveillance systems for infectious diseases that need not rely on mandatory reporting by clinicians; many states have developed reporting requirements for laboratories and/or hospitals, especially for those diseases requiring specific laboratory results for confirmation. Others have used special provider-based surveillance systems (Valleron 1986, Vogt 1983), periodic reviews of hospital discharge summaries for selected infectious diseases (Vogt 1986), laboratory-based surveillance systems (Sacks 1985, Reichelderfer 1987, Godes 1982), and other nonprovider-based systems (Francis 1984). These systems can complement and improve on the coverage and timeliness of clinicians' reporting.

Isolation and/or serological identification of the causative agent is necessary for the etiological diagnosis of individual cases of viral diseases, with the exception of poliomyelitis and some viral exanthems that have characteristic clinical features (Kaslow 1997). In the developing world, the absence of appropriate infrastructure makes epidemic surveillance difficult, as it often requires trained personnel, specialized equipment, availability of resources such as clean water and reagents including standardized antigens and antiserum, and reliable electricity sources for refrigeration. Gastroenteritis is another example of a disease with multiple etiologies that cannot always be differentiated on the basis of clinical or epidemiologic data, and for which microbiologic data are routinely gathered by state health departments, independent of data gathered from clinicians, and for which the time-person-place links among cases might go unrecognized by individual practitioners (Berkelman 1991). In the United States, multistate epidemics of infection with *Salmonella newport* (Van Beneden 1999), *Salmonella enteritidis* (St. Louis 1988), and *Shigella sonnei* (Centers for Disease Control 1987) have been detected through laboratory-based surveillance systems. Information routinely collected through hospital claims, emergency department claims, outpatient claims, and automated pharmacy dispensing records can be the basis of an efficient passive surveillance system for identifying surgical site infections occurring after hospital discharge (Sands 1999). Unfortunately, for some pathogens, laboratory reports provide little clinical information and rarely distinguish between new and old cases of some diseases, as in the case of a positive test for hepatitis B surface antigen.

National health care plans and prepaid health insurance groups may include morbidity and mortality information in their computerized record systems that can be used for infectious disease surveillance. For example, the Kaiser Permanente Plan in California and the Cooperative Group Health Insurance Plan in Seattle have been used for these purposes (Kaslow 1997). Unfortunately, notifiable disease surveillance based solely on International Classification of Diseases (ICD) diagnosis codes (International Classification of Diseases 1980) from hospital discharge summaries does not appear to be very sensitive (Watkins 1991).

In recent years, increases in antimicrobial resistance among common pathogens has affected treatment and control of important diseases, resulting in prolonged illness and duration of epidemics, and in increases in morbidity and mortality. The monitoring and management of antimicrobial resistance is an important laboratory function that has to be pursued at the local level, as the movement of resistance genes and strains through the populations of a community, a hospital, an intensive care unit, or even a single patient, may be more complex than the movement of a strain of influenza virus throughout the world (O'Brien 1997). De-

tailed surveillance can guide antimicrobial choices and aid in limiting the spread of pathogens (Stelling 1997).

Sentinel Surveillance Systems

Because of the prohibitive expense and effort required to conduct active surveillance on complete populations, networks of sentinel health care providers are active in many European countries, Australia, New Zealand, Israel, Canada, and the United States (Van Casteren 1991, Freedman 1999). In most networks, primary care physicians report a minimum amount of information, usually at weekly intervals, on a select group of health events that are relatively common in general practice (Stroup 1994, Monto 1995).

In some areas, networks of cooperating physicians record morbidity data intended to address broader needs, which can also provide valuable information with respect to infectious diseases. For example, the National Disease and Therapeutic Index is the result of the cooperative efforts of over 1500 participating U.S. physicians providing data on the frequency of different diagnoses and drug prescribing patterns throughout the United States (National Disease and Therapeutic Index 1969).

Although they can give more timely information on infectious disease occurrence and may yield more detailed information, one provider's patients may not be representative of the general population. However, although one may not be able to infer population-based rates, these systems do provide relatively constant denominator (clinic clientele) data, allowing one to infer fluctuations in morbidity at the population level. Since 1982, CDC has conducted intensive surveillance of hepatitis in four sentinel counties (Denver County, CO; Jefferson County, AL; Pierce County, WA; Pinellas County, FL) (Centers for Disease Control 1988). Through this system, changes were identified in the 1980s and corroborated in terms of the principal modes of transmission of hepatitis B infection in the United States: the numbers of persons citing homosexual behavior as a risk factor decreased; the numbers of persons citing intravenous drug use or heterosexual behavior as a risk factor increased; and approximately 30% of hepatitis patients had no known source of infection (Alter 1987, Centers for Disease Control 1988). In addition, this system has heightened awareness that those who are at the greatest risk of infection—intravenous drug users, persons acquiring disease through heterosexual exposure, and homosexual men—often are not reached by hepatitis B vaccine programs.

Surveillance of the number of patients with acute respiratory infection in emergency rooms, outpatient clinics, and pediatric clinics combined with prospective virologic surveillance can provide sensitive and specific indicators of influenza outbreaks (Kaslow 1997). It is the level of acute respiratory tract illness reported in student health clinics of a number of universities in North Carolina that serves each winter to monitor influenza activity in the state. There is a general assumption that such sentinel surveillance systems for certain infectious diseases, for example, influenza and hepatitis, are cost-effective. Unfortunately, demonstrations of the cost-effectiveness of sentinel surveillance systems of this type do not exist in the indexed literature for infectious diseases, although use of hospital discharge records has been found to be a cost-effective system for accomplishing prevention-related goals with respect to silicosis surveillance under the Sentinel Event Notification System for Occupational Risks (SENSOR), a state/federal system for the surveillance and intervention of occupational conditions (Watkins 1991).

Existing databases such as computerized hospital discharge summaries are useful in surveillance of infectious diseases, but a lack of timeliness often precludes the computerized hospital database from being the primary source of data. In addition, diagnostic serology can be costly and may not be routinely drawn for all suspected cases of some notifiable diseases, and laboratory reports may select only those atypical cases where the diagnosis is uncertain. There also remain diseases (e.g., Lyme disease) for which there is no sensitive and specific laboratory test (Brown 1999) and, although serious, may be treated on an outpatient basis and thus would not be captured by many of these alternate data sets (Young 1998).

Vaccine-Related Injury Surveillance

A unique system was created by the National Childhood Vaccine Injury Act of 1986 (NCVIA) that required that health care providers who administer certain vaccines and toxoids record permanently certain information and report to the U.S. Department of Health and Human Services (DHHS) selected adverse events occurring after vaccination. Events occurring after receipt of publicly purchased vaccines were reported through local, county, and/or state health departments to CDC; events occurring after receipt of a privately purchased vaccine usually were reported directly to the Food and Drug Administration (FDA) by the health care provider or the manufacturer (Smith 1988).

The enactment of the NCVIA was an attempt to reduce threats to the stability of the immunization program and to compensate persons who may have been injured by a vaccine. DHHS has since determined that a Vaccine Adverse Event Reporting System (VAERS) be established to provide a single system for the collection and the analysis of reports on all adverse events associated with the administration of any U.S. licensed vaccine in all age groups (Centers for Disease Control 1990). To meet CDC's responsibilities for control of vaccine preventable diseases and for providing financial and technical assistance to public sector vaccine programs, and to meet FDA's responsibilities for licensing and regulating vaccines, CDC and FDA have worked together since 1988 to develop and implement VAERS (Centers for Disease Control 1990), and, in 1990, VAERS became fully operational for reporting vaccine adverse events in the United States (Chen 1994). The VAERS form is designed to permit description of the adverse event, as well as type of vaccine(s) received, timing of vaccination and adverse event, demographic information about the recipient, concurrent medical illness or medications, and prior history of adverse events following vaccination. The form is pre-addressed and postage-paid; copies of the form are mailed annually to physicians in the United States who are likely to administer vaccines. These include approximately 200,000 physicians in the specialties of pediatrics, family practice, general practice, internal medicine, obstetrics/gynecology, and emergency medicine. Copies of the form are also available through the state health departments to public health clinics that administer vaccines.

Reports to VAERS may initiate additional clinical, epidemiologic, or laboratory investigation to assess whether there is a causal association. Reports of adverse outcomes to vaccine prior to VAERS have triggered investigations of possible associations of poliomyelitis with administration of inactivated polio vaccine (Nathanson 1963) and oral polio vaccine (Henderson 1964); sudden infant death syndrome following vaccination for diphtheria, pertussis, and tetanus (Bernier 1982, Mortimer 1987); meningoencephalitis following mumps vaccination (McDonald 1989, Cizman 1989, Miller 1993); and Guillain-Barré syndrome following influenza vaccine administration (Schonberger 1979, Chen 1992). Such investigations may reveal that the associations were unsubstantiated (Mortimer 1987), statistically impossible to assess due to small sample sizes (Bernier 1982, Wentz 1991), or indeed causal (Nathanson 1963, Henderson 1964, McDonald 1989, Schonberger 1999). While VAERS has many methodological limitations intrinsic to such systems, it has been important in helping to monitor vaccine safety and maintain public confidence in immunizations (Chen, 1994).

Other Data Sources

Additional sources of data may be useful to supplement routine surveillance data (Kaslow 1997):

1. *Biologics and drug utilization data.* The use of biologics and drugs for treatment or prophylaxis of a disease may potentially be used to monitor disease occurrence. The most dramatic example of this was unusual clustering of five cases of *Pneumocystis carinii* pneumonia among young males at three hospitals in Los Angeles and the resulting increase in requests to CDC to provide pentamidine to treat this rare entity that led to the identification of the HIV/AIDS epidemic in 1981 (Centers for Disease Control 1981). One might expect that in the face of a diarrheal disease outbreak, there would be local increased sales of antidiarrheal medications, or during influenza season there would be increased sales of over-the-counter cold medicines. A similar application of monitoring the use of biologics is the use of cluster sampling techniques to assess immunization coverage by WHO's Expanded Programme on Immunization (EPI), the goal being elimination of lack of immunization as a risk factor for disease (Cutts 1993).

2. *Animal-reservoir and vector-distribution studies.* Animal-reservoir and vector-distribution studies are important in surveillance of diseases acquired from animals or of diseases in which the vector is arthropod-borne (Li 1998). For example, knowledge of rabies in animal reservoirs is important in determining treatment regimens for persons bitten by unidentified animals, seroconversion of sentinel chickens has been used for monitoring St. Louis encephalitis activity (Reisen 1990), and the occurrence of plague in rodents can be helpful in diagnosing human plague. Integration of veterinary and epidemiologic activities is often necessary for adequate approaches to surveillance for zoonoses such as leptospirosis and anthrax, as well as dengue and the hemorrhagic fevers. Entomological services are valuable for surveillance and understanding of various vectors such as ticks in the case of Rocky Mountain spotted fever and mosquitoes for yellow fever, malaria, and arbovirus infection (Reisen 1990).

3. *Media and news broadcasting reports.* News media often identify and report outbreaks of disease before they have been detected by disease reporting mechanisms, and many state health departments use news-clipping services as a supplement to their

disease surveillance activities. News media may also report outbreaks of nonreportable diseases that have an infectious etiology. Media coverage driven by community interest and medical interest in newly emerging diseases or conditions may also improve reporting. For example, a significant increase in reporting of toxic shock syndrome was observed after media publicity first appeared (Davis 1982).

4. *Disease registries and specialized surveillance systems for medical research*. Registries designed to collect information on a specific topic and specialized surveillance systems developed for research purposes can have great public health application, although they are usually limited in scope. For example, Virus Watch Programs in New York City and Seattle involve the systematic sampling of a population of families for enteric and respiratory viruses, antibody testing, and analyses of coincident illness patterns (Cooney 1970, Fox 1966). Similarly, human population laboratories such as the one intended for the study of gastrointestinal illnesses in Dacca, Pakistan, have served as valuable sources of information in the diagnosis, treatment, and prevention of infectious diseases (Black 1982). Similarly, routine surveillance systems targeted at infectious diseases can serve as a catalyst for further epidemiological, clinical, or behavioral research.

Technological Improvements in Surveillance

The tools for surveillance are improving. Telephone notification, provision of preaddressed prestamped forms, and computer-based telecommunication have improved the efficiency of disease reporting. With the use of computers and the Internet, databases may be better managed and analyzed.

In the United States, NETSS is a computer-based telecommunications system initiated in 1984 for reporting the NNDSS data from the states to CDC (Graitcer 1987). This computerized system allows more efficiency, case detail, and analytic capability than previously available with only summary reports available by telephone; disease distribution

can be mapped by county, onset dates of disease can be examined more precisely, and comparative information on age, race, and sex distribution is available.

Specific technological applications for computer-based infectious disease surveillance are developing rapidly. For example, WHO has now developed WHONET, a computer program for microbiology laboratories to facilitate the management of antibiotic susceptibility test results from routine clinical isolates (Stelling 1997), and it is envisioned that the network of national microbiology laboratories using WHONET will allow ongoing surveillance of antimicrobial resistance at the regional and global levels (Leduc 1994) as well as locally (Stelling 1997). There is also an increasing sophistication of statistical methods for evaluating surveillance data (e.g., to estimate completeness of reporting) and for analysis (e.g., to detect spatial and temporal trends) (Stroup 1989, 1993).

As computer-based infectious disease surveillance systems have enjoyed rapid technological advances, confidentiality concerns have arisen that have necessitated the development of confidentiality procedures and protections including computer encryption of data, physical security, limited access, and penalties for abuse (Chorba 1989). All states and many localities have legal safeguards of confidentiality for government-held data, and these laws tend to provide greater protection than laws protecting the confidentiality of health information held by private health care providers. Most states also have specific statutory protections for public health data related to HIV (Chorba 1989).

DATA ANALYSIS AND APPLICATIONS

The usefulness of surveillance data and the programs to which the data are applied vary with the disease, but generally such data are used to monitor short- and long-term trends, to identify epidemics, to alert health professionals to important changes in trends, and to estimate the magnitude of morbidity and mortality. Surveillance facilitates epidemiologic and laboratory research both by providing cases for more detailed investigation or a case-control study, and by directing which research avenues are most important. More specifically, all individuals reported with selected diseases (e.g., tuberculosis, syphilis) are routinely followed up by health departments either directly or through their physicians to assure initiation of appropriate therapy of the individual. Health departments also provide diagnostic tests and prophylactic therapy, as needed, for contacts of persons with infectious conditions such as hepatitis and tuberculosis. Counseling and partner notification activities may be provided to persons such as those infected with HIV, so that those who test positive may appreciate the significance of that fact and know how to protect others from infection. Reports of unusual clusters of disease are often followed by an epidemic investigation to identify and remove any common-source exposure or to reduce other associated risks of transmission. For example, of 307 domestic epidemic assistance requests received by CDC in fiscal years 1985 through 1988, 134 (44%) were for problems related to specific diseases reportable in the requesting jurisdictions (Centers for Disease Control 1999). With advances in epidemiologic expertise and ability to analyze large quantities of data rapidly, the majority of infectious disease epidemics identified in the United States are now handled at the state or county level.

Surveillance data have been used to identify and characterize previously unidentified syndromes. As noted earlier, the HIV/AIDS epidemic was first detected because of increases in requests for pentamidine, the distribution of which was being overseen by CDC (Centers for Disease Control 1981). Surveillance data also provide the basis for determining public health priorities, planning, and implementing prevention and control programs. Policymakers use these data to determine overall priorities for resources for public health programs; and, in certain instances, these data may be the basis for geographic distribution of funds for treatment (e.g., federal reimbursement to states for zidovudine therapy in individu-

als with severe disease due to HIV infection). In addition to directing resources, surveillance data are the basis for evaluating the success or failure of prevention and control programs; for example, the success of immunization initiatives can be inferred from the decreases in the numbers of cases of vaccine preventable diseases. Thus through participation in surveillance systems, physicians and other health care providers are integral to assuring that public health resources are used most effectively. Because of the discriminating climate and stigma that surround infection with HIV, acknowledgment should also be given here of the important surveillance function that is served by access to confidential and/or anonymous counseling and testing (Kegeles 1990).

Time, Person, Place

In the planning of any surveillance system, there are several fundamental considerations, including the enumeration of variables necessary to address the questions that are relevant to the goals of disease prevention and control. It is customary that following an assessment of the crude numbers of cases and rates (incidence rates, attack rates, prevalence rates), one evaluates the period in which the cases occurred (time), the geographic distribution in which the cases occurred (place), and the population in which the disease occurred (person). Considerations of these basic analyses dictate what information needs to be systematically collected and at what level of detail.

Time

In considering issues of time relative to surveillance systems for infectious disease, several intervals need to be kept in mind because there are delays that occur between disease exposure, expression of symptoms, diagnosis of the problem, and report of the illness to health authorities. Analyses of surveillance data by time necessitate consideration of four types of time trends:

1. *Secular trends.* Secular trends refers to the occurrence of disease over a prolonged period of time such as years. The long-term or secular trend of diphtheria is one of grad-

ually decreasing incidence. A decreasing secular trend of an infectious disease is usually the result of specific and nonspecific immunity and improved hygiene among the involved population, as was the situation with tuberculosis in the United States before the HIV/AIDS epidemic began. Changes in the case definition used for surveillance, changes in methods of diagnosis including diagnostic criteria, and changes in reporting requirements or practices can cause perturbations in secular trends that merit understanding and explanation when conveying data to wider audiences. For example, the 1987 revision of the surveillance case definition for AIDS resulted in an increase in the number of reported cases among heterosexual drug abusers that required interpretation for those monitoring trends in the epidemic (Selik 1990). Understandably, another increase in the reported incidence of AIDS was observed when the AIDS case definition was further expanded in 1993 to include persons infected with HIV who had low T-lymphocyte counts, pulmonary tuiberculosis, recurrent pneumonia, or invasive cervical cancer (Singleton 1996).

2. *Periodic trends.* Periodic trends refers to temporary variations from the secular trend. For example, in the case of pertussis in the United States, periodic increases in incidence occur approximately every five years, superimposed on a background of a secular trend of decreasing incidence. The periodic trends represent variations in the level of immunity to the etiological agent as reflected either by natural infection or vaccination of the population or by changes in the antigenic composition of the agent.

3. *Annual variation.* Annual variation frequently represents seasonal patterns. Foodborne diseases are associated with seasonal increases in the late summer and fall. Respiratory illnesses are associated with seasonal increases in the late fall and winter. Vector-borne illnesses are associated with exposure during the summer months when people are most inclined to engage in outdoor recreation.

4. *Epidemic occurrence.* An epidemic may be detected by analysis of surveillance data, especially when cases are scattered over several health jurisdictions. For example, *Salmonella*-contaminated food may result in the occurrence of cases over the distribution route of the food. It is customary to graph the number of cases of an outbreak, using a histogram; if the histogram is used to portray the duration of an epidemic, it is referred to as an epidemic curve.

Person
Person factors to be defined in analyzing surveillance data may include age, sex, race, nationality, level of immunity, nutrition, life style, socioeconomic status, and occupation. If a single or special attribute can be ascribed to the majority of cases, it may indicate the group at risk, the source of exposure, or the mode of spread. The use of race and ethnicity in reporting systems has been largely hampered by inaccuracies and misclassification (Hahn 1992), as well as by lack of scientific consensus on the nature of race and ethnicity and on the measurement of these variables (Hahn 1999). However, the identification of patterns of health and disease among subpopulations is integral with surveillance. Although flawed, the use of race and ethnic variables in public health surveillance remains a cornerstone in identifying and targeting groups at risk and in addressing differential racial health status.

Place
The concept of place in the context of surveillance refers both to the geographic location of the source and reservoir of the organism, and to the location of the patient at the time infection occurred and at the time of onset of clinical disease. The development of effective control and prevention measures depends on carefully defining each of these areas, as the place of exposure and the place of onset are often different. Control measures directed at the site where the host came into contact with the agent can lead to control of additional similar cases immediately related to the initial case, but may not prevent future cases if there are multiple sources of the organism that can be brought into contact with other susceptible hosts.

For example, *Salmonella* contamination of food at the factory level and exposure of the host in a restaurant will not prevent further cases from occurring in association with another restaurant that obtained contaminated food from the same factory.

Other Practical Considerations

The frequency with which data from a surveillance system need to be analyzed is dependent on the use of the summary data. Routinely, surveillance programs may require analyses at monthly intervals, but in epidemic situations, analysis at weekly and even daily intervals may be necessary. Attention must also be paid to how carefully and systematically data are analyzed, interpreted, and presented for understanding.

For further illustration of the concepts and applications described previously, the reader is directed to Disease Surveillance On-Line, Canada's Laboratory Centre for Disease Control's Interactive web-based tool for easy access to surveillance data, at http://www.hc-sc.gc.ca/hpb/lcdc/webmap/. This is a new tool that allows visitors to use LCDC's website to access notifiable disease data over a range of years, and to customize the data for their specific needs. Data can be generated according to choice of parameters, for example, disease type, geographic area (provinces, territories, and all of Canada), period of time, type of data to be viewed (cases, rates, ratios) and choice of presentation mode, that is, tables, maps, or charts (multiline graphs, pie charts, bar graphs). With growing use of the Internet, it is anticipated that access to national data sets will result in a much broader understanding of epidemiologic principles, including surveillance issues, in the general population.

ISSUES IN UNDERREPORTING

During the training of clinicians, little attention has been given to the legal requirements or the importance of reporting. A study of New York City physicians demonstrated that many do not know the requirements or methods for reporting in their state; reasons given by physicians for underreporting include not knowing which diseases are required to be reported, not knowing how it should be reported, concerns about confidentiality and perceptions that the list of reportable diseases is too extensive (Konowitz 1984). A more recent study in Vermont concluded that physicians often failed to report because they assumed that the laboratory would have reported the case (Schramm 1991). For many diseases, the laboratory is a vital component, but the physician and other primary health care providers are still integral to the notifiable disease reporting systems. Indeed, there are a number of reportable diseases, such as *Haemophilus influenzae* disease and meningococcal infections, for which timeliness of reporting is important and waiting for laboratory reports is not practical (Davis 1984).

Although surveillance systems do not need complete reporting to be useful, underreporting may adversely affect public health efforts by distorting trends observed in incidence of disease (Kimball 1980, Alter 1987); distorting attributable risk estimates for disease acquisition (Todd 1985, Alter 1987); preventing accurate assessment of potential benefits or impact of control programs (Chalker 1988); preventing timely identification of disease outbreaks (Kimball 1980, Anon. 1989); distorting observed periods at risk and geographic distribution of cases (Kimball 1980); and undermining the success of prevention and control programs for tuberculosis, sexually transmitted diseases, and immunization programs (Thacker 1983, Eisenberg 1976, Hinman 1982).

DISSEMINATION OF SURVEILLANCE

Reports/Publications

In the first section of this chapter, it was noted that the working definition of disease surveillance in the United States includes the timely dissemination of aggregated and analyzed data to those who have contributed information to the system and those who need to know, and the subsequent application of the processed information to disease control and prevention. The effective communication of data, analyses, and interpretation to those who are responsible for action is integral to the purpose of surveillance. The recent Hong Kong outbreak of an avian influenzalike virus, with 18 confirmed human cases, many of which were severe or fatal, underscores the need for health facilities to communicate in a timely fashion at local and national levels, and at international levels when warranted (Snacken 1999).

The effective communication of data, analyses, and interpretation to those who have participated in providing data has the added effect of encouraging continued participation in the system of data collection. Several weekly publications have a very wide readership in the epidemiologic community and provide valuable surveillance information that in turn is made available to a much wider audiences through secondary publication and communication in print and broadcast media. These include the *WHO Epidemiological Record*, the *PAHO Weekly Epidemiological Report*, and the *MMWR*.

In the United States, surveillance data, analyses, and reports are disseminated through the *MMWR* series of publications, monthly public health bulletins in states, and special reports in peer-reviewed journals. Since 1961, CDC has had responsibility for publication of the *MMWR*. As noted previously, data from the 121 Cities Surveillance System are published in the *MMWR* within a week of receipt by CDC. Also as noted before, CDC has had the responsibility of operating the NNDSS since 1961 for the purpose of tabulating and disseminating summary morbidity data. Since 1990, all reporting states and localities have transmitted data electronically to CDC through NETSS (Centers for Disease Control 1991). National case counts for most notifiable diseases are published in the *MMWR* in provisional form in the week after they are reported to CDC and are made available to epidemiologists, clinicians, and other public health professionals in a timely manner. Since December 1989, the *MMWR* has also published on a weekly basis a graph that uses horizontal bars to indicate the ratio of the current level of disease to the previous five-year average, an example of which is presented in Figure 7–3. This graph is intended to facilitate interpretation of routine notifiable-disease data. Striping in the bars indicates whether the number of reported cases during the most recent four-week interval was higher or lower than the expected based on the mean and two standard deviations of the four-week totals. Numbers of cases in the current four-week period are listed to facilitate interpretation of instability caused by small numbers. Using this approach, changes in the occurrence of disease can be identified that merit more detailed scrutiny of the data.

Annual summaries are also prepared and published in the last issue of each volume of the *MMWR*. Other public health publications such as the CDC Surveillance Summaries, provide detailed in-depth analyses and interpretations of data (Centers for Disease Control 1983). Journals aimed at health care providers also serve as conduits for surveillance data, for example, JAMA regularly reprints articles from the *MMWR* to facilitate the access of the readership to this information.

CONCLUSION

The intent of this chapter has been to describe the methods for conducting disease surveillance in the context of its practice in the United States and Canada. Numerous topics have been presented, but for more in-depth reading on infectious disease surveillance issues, the reader is referred to several excellent texts (Teutsch 1994, Gregg 1996, Halperin 1992). One principle that will change despite the technological changes is the fact that infectious diseases surveillance systems must be useful, and to that end, surveillance systems must be reassessed on a routine basis according to the concepts and criteria discussed above.

The use of computers and the potential of the Internet are rapidly changing every aspect of our lives, including how we engage in disease surveillance. Not only are data more manageable and accessible, but record

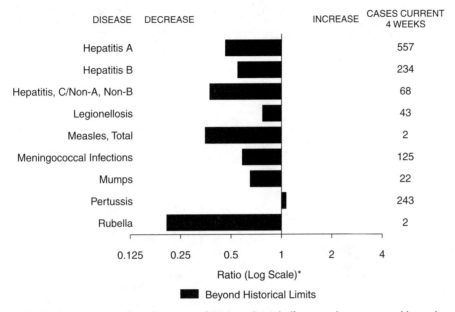

DISEASE	DECREASE	INCREASE	CASES CURRENT 4 WEEKS
Hepatitis A			557
Hepatitis B			234
Hepatitis, C/Non-A, Non-B			68
Legionellosis			43
Measles, Total			2
Meningococcal Infections			125
Mumps			22
Pertussis			243
Rubella			2

0.125   0.25   0.5   1   2   4

Ratio (Log Scale)*

■ Beyond Historical Limits

*Ratio of current 4-week total to mean of 15 4-week totals (from previous, comparable, and subsequent 4-week periods for the past 5 years). The point where the hatched area begins is based on the mean and two standard deviatons of these 4-week totals.

Figure 7–3. Selected notifiable disease reports, comparison of provisional 4-week totals ending March 11, 2000, with historical data—United States.
Source: *MMWR* March 2000.

linkages and epidemiologic and statistical analyses are greatly facilitated, and more sophisticated analyses can now be applied to detect changes in patterns of disease occurrence. Although in the past two decades we have seen great improvements in the analysis of surveillance data and dissemination of written reports published periodically by state and federal agencies, the use of electronic media is revolutionizing the access and speed with which information can be reported, analyzed, and disseminated. More importantly, the use of microcomputers has provided many levels with the opportunity to reconsider needs and to reevaluate the utility of the data gathered (Sandiford 1992). Laboratory techniques will continue to improve, also facilitated by computer-based improvements. Surveillance systems that are currently in use will be improved upon or replaced by more efficient methodologies, and public health officials will have to grapple with many ethical and legal issues

raised by the burgeoning technology and information access. In all of this, surveillance principles will have broader application to emerging areas of public health practice and newly identified diseases, risk factors, and other public health issues.

REFERENCES

Advisory Committee on Epidemiology and Bureau of Infectious Diseases, Laboratory Centre for Disease Control. Case definitions for diseases under national surveillance. Canada Communicable Disease Report 26 (Suppl): S3, 2000

Alter MJ, Mares A, Hadler SC, Maynard JE. The effect of underreporting on the apparent incidence and epidemiology of acute viral hepatitis. Am. J. Epidemiol. 125:133–139, 1987.

Anon. Epidemiological surveillance. Int. J. Epidemiol. 5:4–6, 1976.

Anon. Hepatitis A cluster: the need to report disease occurrence. Delaware Monthly Surveillance Report 89(1):1–2, 1989.

Barker WH, and Mullooly JP. Underestimation of the role of pneumonia and influenza in causing excess mortality. Am. J. Public Health 71:643–645, 1981.

Baron RC, Dicker RC, Bussell KE, and Herndon JL. Assessing trends in mortality in 121 U.S. cities, 1970–79, from all causes and from pneumonia and influenza. Public Health Rep. 103:120–128, 1988.

Berkelman RI, and Buehler JW. Surveillance. In: Holland WW, Detels R, Knox G, eds. Oxford Textbook of Public Health. 2nd ed. Vol 2: Methods of Public Health. Oxford: Oxford University Press, 1991: 161–176.

Bernier RH. Viral hepatitis reporting in greater New Haven. New Haven, CT: Yale University School of Medicine, Department of Epidemiology and Public Health, 1974. Thesis.

Bernier RH, Grank JA, Dondero TJ, and Turner P. Diphtheria-tetanus-toxoids-pertussis vaccination and sudden infant deaths in Tennessee. J. Pediatr. 101:419–421, 1982.

Birkhead G, Chorba TL, Root S, Klaucke DN, and Gibbs NJ. Timeliness of national reporting of communicable diseases: the experience of the National Electronic Telecommunications System for Surveillance. Am. J. Public Health 81:1313–1315, 1991.

Black RE, Brown KH, Becker S, Abdul Alim ARM, and Huq I. Longitudinal studies of infectious diseases and physical growth of children in rural Bangladeshi. Am. J. Epidemiol. 115:315–324, 1982.

Bowditch HI, Webster DL, Hoadley JC, et al. Letter from Massachusetts State Board of Health to physicians. Public Health Rep. Suppl 12:31, 1915.

Brown SL, Hansen SL, and Langone JJ. Role of serology in the diagnosis of Lyme disease. JAMA. 282:62–66, 1999.

Brzezinski ZJ. Mortality indicators and health-for-all strategies in the WHO European region. World Health Stat. Q. 39:365–378, 1986.

Carter AO. Notifiable diseases in Canada. Can. Med. Assoc. J. 139:645–648, 1988.

Carter AO. Setting priorities: the Canadian experience in communicable disease surveillance. MMWR 41 Suppl: 79–84, 1992 Dec.

Cates W Jr, and Williamson GD. Descriptive epidemiology: analyzing and interpreting surveillance data. In: Teutsch SM, Churchill RE, eds. Principles and Practice of Public Health Surveillance. Oxford: Oxford University Press, 1994; 96–135.

Centers for Disease Control. Review of the mechanics of influenza surveillance. In: Influenza—Respiratory Disease Surveillance. Report no. 84. September 1968:2–9.

Centers for Disease Control. Penicillinase-producing Neisseria gonorrhoeae. MMWR 25:261, 1976.

Centers for Disease Contro. Influenza—United States. MMWR 27:472–474, 1978.

Centers for Disease Control. Guillain-Barré Syndrome Surveillance Report, January 1978–March 1979. Atlanta: Centers for Disease Control, 1980.

Centers for Disease Control. Pneumocystis pneumonia–Los Angeles. MMWR 30:250–252, 1981.

Centers for Disease Control. National surveillance for Reye syndrome, 1981: Update—Reye syndrome and salicylate usage. MMWR 31:53–56,61, 1982.

Centers for Disease Control. Surveillance summaries. MMWR 32:1SS–43SS, 1983.

Centers for Disease Control. Manual for Procedures for National Morbidity Reporting & Public Health Surveillance Activities. Atlanta: Centers for Disease Control, 1985.

Centers for Disease Control. Hepatitis B associated with jet gun injection—California. MMWR 35:373–376, 1986.

Centers for Disease Control. Nationwide dissemination of multiply resistant Shigella sonnei following a common-source outbreak. MMWR 36:633–634, 1987

Centers for Disease Control. Changing patterns for groups at high risk for hepatitis B in the United States. MMWR 39:429–432, 437, 1988.

Centers for Disease Control. Guidelines for evaluating surveillance systems. MMWR 37 (suppl. no. S-5):1–18, 1988.

Centers for Disease Control. Non-A, non-B hepatitis—Illinois. MMWR 38:529–562, 1989.

Centers for Disease Control. Case definitions for public health surveillance. MMWR Recommendations and Reports 39(RR-13):1–43, 1990.

Centers for Disease Control. Vaccine Adverse Event Reporting System—United States. MMWR 39:730–733, 1990.

Centers for Disease Control. Influenza activity—United States, 1991–92. MMWR 40:809–810, 1991.

Centers for Disease Control. National electronic telecommunications system for surveillance—United States, 1990–1991. MMWR 40:502, 1991.

Centers for Disease Control. Outbreak of rubella among the Amish—United States, 1991. MMWR 40:264–265, 1991.

Centers for Disease Control and Prevention. Case definitions for infectious diseases under surveillance. MMWR Recommendations and Reports 46(RR-10):1–57, 1997.

Centers for Disease Control and Prevention. Guidelines for National Human Immunodeficiency Virus Case Surveillance, Including Monitoring for Human Immunodeficiency Virus Infection and Acquired Immunodeficiency Syndrome. MMWR Reports and Recommendations 48(RR13):1–28, 1999.

Chalker RB, and Blaser MJ. A review of human salmonellosis. III. Magnitude of Salmonella infection in the United States. Rev. Infec. Dis. 10:111–124, 1988.

Chen RT, Kent J, Simon P, Schonberger L, and the GBS investigation team. Investigation of a possible association between influenza vaccination and Guillain-Barré syndrome in the United States, 1990–91 (abstract). Postmarket Surv. 6:5–6, 1992.

Chen RT, Rastogi SC, Mullen JR, et al. The Vaccine Adverse Event Reporting System (VAERS). Vaccine. 12:542–550, 1994 May.

Choi K, and Thacker SB. An evaluation of influenza mortality surveillance, 1962–1979. I. Time series forecasts of expected pneumonia and influenza deaths. Am. J. Epidemiol. 113:215–226, 1981a.

Choi K, and Thacker SB. An evaluation of influenza mortality surveillance, 1962–1979. II. Percentage of pneumonia and influenza deaths as an indicator of influenza activity. Am. J. Epidemiol. 113:215–226, 1981b.

Choi K, and Thacker SB. Improved accuracy and specificity of forecasting deaths attributed to pneumonia and influenza. J. Infect. Dis. 144:606–608, 1981c.

Chorba T, Coccia P, Holman RC, et al. The role of parvovirus B19 in aplastic crisis and erythema infectiosum (fifth disease). J. Infect. Dis. 154:383–393, 1986.

Chorba TL, Berkelman RL, Safford SK, Gibbs NP, and Hull HF. Mandatory reporting of infectious diseases by clinicians. JAMA. 262:3018–3026, 1989.

Chorba TL, Holman RC, Strine TW, Clarke MJ, and Evatt BL. Changes in longevity and causes of death among persons with hemophilia A. Am. J. Hematol. 45:112–121, 1994.

Cizman M, Mozetic M, Radescek-Rakar R, Pleterski-Rigler D, and Susec-Michieli M. Aseptic meningitis after vaccination against measles and mumps. Pediatr. Infect. Dis. J. 8:302–308, 1989.

Collins SD. Influenza-pneumonia mortality in a group of about 95 cities in the United States, 1920–1929. Public Health Rep. 45:361–406, 1930.

Collins SD. Excess mortality from causes other than influenza and pneumonia during influenza epidemics. Public Health Rep. 47:2159–2180, 1932.

Cooney MK, Hall CE, and Fox JP. The Seattle Virus Watch Program. I. Infection and illness experience of Virus Watch families during a community-wide epidemic of echovirus 30 aseptic meningitis. Am. J. Public Health 60:1456–1465, 1970.

Cowan DN, and Prier RE. Changes in hepatitis morbidity in the United States Army, Europe. Milit. Med. 149:260–265, 1984.

Cutts FT, Waldman RJ, and Zoffman HMD. Surveillance for the Expanded Programme on Immunization. Bull. World Health Organ. 71(5):633–639, 1993.

Davis JP, and Vergeront JM. The effect of publicity on the reporting of toxic-shock in Wisconsin. J. Infect. Dis. 145:449–457, 1982.

Davis JP, and Bohn MJ. The extent of underreporting of meningococcal disease in Wisconsin, 1980–82. Wisc. Med. J. 83:11–14, 1984.

Declich S, and Carter AO. Public health surveillance: historical origins, methods and evaluation. Bull. World Health Organ. 72:285–304, 1994.

Eisenberg MS, and Wiesner PJ. Reporting and treating gonorrhea: results of a statewide survey in Alaska. J. Am. Venereal Dis. Assoc. 3(2):79–83, 1976.

Eylenbosch WJ, and Noah ND. Historical aspects. In: Surveillance in Health and Disease. Oxford: Oxford University Press, 1988:3–8.

Fox J, Elveback LR, Spigland I, et al. The Virus Watch Program: a continuing surveillance of viral infections in metropolitan New York families. 1. Overall plan, methods of collecting and handling information and a summary report of specimens collected and illnesses observed. Am. J. Epidemiol. 83:389–412, 1966.

Francis DP, Hadler SC, Prendergast TJ, et al. Occurrence of hepatitis A, B, and non-A/non-B in the United States: CDC sentinel county hepatitis study I. Am. J. Med. 76:69–74, 1984.

Freedman DO, Kozarsky PE, Weld LH, and Cetron MS. GeoSenitnel: the global emerging infections sentinel network of the International Society of Travel Medicine. J. Travel Med. 6:94–98, 1999.

Godes JR, Hall WN, Dean AG, and Morse CD. Laboratory-based disease surveillance. A survey of state laboratory directors. Minn. Med. 65:762–764, 1982.

Graitcer PL, and Burton AH. The epidemiologic surveillance project: a computer-based system for disease surveillance. Am. J. Prev. Med. 3:123–127, 1987.

Gregg MB, ed. Field Epidemiology. Oxford: Oxford University Press, 1996.

Hahn RA. The state of federal health statistics on racial and ethnic groups. JAMA. 267:268–271, 1992.

Hahn RA. Why race is differentially classified on U.S. birth and infant death certificates: an examination of two hypotheses. Epidemiology. 10:108–111, 1999.

Hajjeh RA, Conn LA, Stephens DS, et al. Cryptococcosis: population-based multistate active surveillance and risk factors in human immunodeficiency virus-infected persons. Infect. Dis. 179:449–454, 1999.

Hall R. Surveillance of communicable diseases. Med. J. Aust. 154(12):787–788, 1991.

Halperin W, and Baker EL Jr, eds. Public Health Surveillance. New York: Van Nostrand Reinhold, 1992.

Halperin WE. The role of surveillance in the hierarchy of prevention. Am. J. Ind. Med. 29: 321–323, 1996.

Hartgerink MJ. Health surveillance and planning for health care in the Netherlands. Int. J. Epidemiol. 5:87–91, 1976.

Henderson DA. Surveillance of smallpox. Int. J. Epidemiol. 5:19–28, 1976.

Henderson DA. The looming threat of bioterrorism. Science. 283:1279–1282, 1999.

Henderson DA, Witte JJ, Morris L, and Langmuir AD. Paralytic disease associated with oral polio vaccines. JAMA. 190:153–160, 1964.

Heymann DL, and Rodier GR. Global surveillance of communicable diseases. Emerg. Infect. Dis. 4:362–365, 1998.

Hinds M, Skaggs JW, and Bergeisen GH. Benefit-cost analysis of active surveillance of primary care physicians for hepatitis A. Am. J. Public Health. 75:176–177, 1985.

Hinman AR, Eddins DL, Kirby CD, et al. Progress in measles elimination. JAMA. 247: 1592–1595, 1982.

Hughes JM. The emerging threat of bioterrorism. Emerg. Infect. Dis. 4:494–495, 1998.

International Classification of Diseases, 9th Revision, Clinical Modification (ICD-9-CM), Volume 1: Diseases: Tabular List. Hyattsville, MD: National Center for Health Statistics, 1980.

Kaslow RA, and Evans AS. Surveillance and seroepidemiology. In: Evans AS, Kaslow RA, eds. Viral Infections. New York: Plenum Medical Book Company, 1997: 89–115.

Kegeles SM, Catania JA, Coates TJ, Pollack LM, and Lo B. Many people who seek anonymous HIV-antibody testing would avoid it under other circumstances. AIDS 4:585–588, 1990.

Kimball AM, Thacker SB, and Levy ME. Shigella surveillance in a large metropolitan area: assessment of a passive reporting system. Am. J. Epidemiol. 70:164–166, 1980.

Konowitz PM, Petrossian GA, and Rose DN. The underreporting of disease and physicians' knowledge of reporting requirements. Public Health Rep. 99:31–35, 1984.

Langmuir AD. Evolution of the concept of surveillance in the United States. Proc. R. Soc. Med. 64:681–689, 1971.

Last JM, ed. A Dictionary of Epidemiology. New York: Oxford University Press, 1983:101.

Ledogar R, et al. Monitoring and evaluation for child survival and development: report of a subregional workshop, 13–15 October 1987. Guatemala, UNICEF, 1988.

Leduc JW, and Tikhomirov E. Global surveillance for recognition and response to emerging diseases. Ann. NY Acad. Sci. 740:341–345, 1994.

Lew JF, Glass RI, Gangarosa RE, et al. Diarrheal deaths in the United States, 1979 through 1987. JAMA. 265:3280–3284, 1991.

Li X, and Rossignol PA. Probability model on the use of sentinel animal monitoring for arbovirus. Epidemiology. 9:446–451, 1998.

Lowry PW, Levine R, Stroup DF, et al. Hepatitis A outbreak on a floating restaurant in Florida, 1986. Am. J. Epidemiol. 129:155–164, 1989.

Lui KJ, and Kendal AP. Impact of influenza epidemics on mortality in the USA from October 1972 to May 1985. Am. J. Public Health. 77:712–716, 1987.

Manual of Procedures for National Morbidity Reporting and Public Health Surveillance Activities. Centers for Disease Control. March 1985.

Marier R. The reporting of communicable diseases. Am. J. Epidemiol. 105:587–590, 1977.

McDade JE, and Franz D. Bioterrorism as a public health threat. Emerg. Infect. Dis. 4:493–494, 1998.

McDonald JC, Moore DL, and Quennec P. Clinical and epidemiologic features of mumps meningoencephalitis and possible vaccine-related disease. Pediatr. Infect. Dis. J. 8:751–755, 1989.

McGinnis JM, and Foege WH. Actual causes of death in the United States. JAMA. 270:2207–2212, 1993.

Miller E, Goldacre M, Pugh S, et al. Risk of aseptic meningitis after measles, mumps, and rubella vaccine in UK children. Lancet. 341: 979–982, 1993.

Monto AS, Ohmit SE, Margulies JR, and Talsma A. Medical practice-based influenza surveillance: viral prevalence and assessment of morbidity. Am. J. Epidemiol. 141(6):502–506, 1995.

Moro ML, and McCormick A. Surveillance of communicable disease. In: Eylenbosch WJ, Noah ND, eds. Surveillance in Health and Disease. Oxford: Oxford University Press, 1988: 166–182.

Mortimer EA Jr. DTP and SIDS: when data differ. Am. J. Public Health. 77:925–926, 1987.

Nathanson N, and Langmuir AD. The Cutter incident. Am. J. Hyg. 78:16–81, 1963.

National Disease and Therapeutic Index. Ambler, PA: Lea Associates, 1969.

O'Brien TF. The global epidemic nature of antimicrobial resistance and the need to monitor and manage it locally. Clin. Infect. Dis. 24 (Suppl 1):S2–S8, 1997.

Payne JN. The introduction of a computerized system for notification and improved analysis of infectious diseases in Sheffield. J. Public Health Med. 14:62–67, 1992.

Raska K. Epidemiological surveillance in the control of infectious diseases. Rev. Infect. Dis. 6:1112–1117, 1983.

Raska K. National and international surveillance of communicable diseases. WHO Chron. 20:313–321, 1996.

Reichelderfer PS, Kappus KD, and Kendal AP. Economical laboratory support system for influenza virus surveillance. J. Clin. Microbiol. 25:947–948, 1987.

Reingold AL, Kane MA, Murphy BL, et al. Transmission of hepatitis B by an oral surgeon. J. Infect. Dis. 145:262–268, 1982.

Reisen WK, Hardy JL, Reeves WC, et al. Persistence of mosquito-borne viruses in Kern County, California, 1983–1988. Am. J. Trop. Med. Hyg. 43:419–437, 1990.

Rosenberg ML, Gangarosa EJ, Pollard RA, Wallace M, and Bolinsky O. Shigella surveillance in the United States, 1975. J. Infect. Dis. 136:458–460, 1977.

Rothenberg R, Bross DC, and Vernon TM. Reporting of gonorrhea by private physicians: a behavioral study. Am. J. Public Health. 70:983–986, 1980.

Roush S, Birkhead G, Koo D, Cobb A, and Fleming D. Mandatory reporting of diseases and conditions by health care professionals and laboratories. JAMA. 282:164–170, 1999.

Sacks JJ. Utilization of case definitions and laboratory reporting in the surveillance of notifiable communicable diseases in the United States. Am. J. Public Health. 75:1420–1422, 1985.

Sandiford P, Annett H, and Cibuslkis R. What can information systems do for primary health care? An international perspective. Soc. Sci. Med. 34:1077–1087, 1992.

Sands K, Vineyard G, Livingston J, Christiansen C, and Platt R. Efficient identification of postdischarge surgical site infections: use of automated pharmacy dispensing information, administrative data, and medical record information. J. Infect. Dis. 179:434–441, 1999.

Schonberger LB, Bregman DJ, Sullivan-Bolyai JZ, et al. Guillain-Barré syndrome following vaccination in the national influenza immunization program, United States, 1976–1977. Am. J. Epidemiol. 110:105–123, 1979.

Schramm MM, Vogt RL, and Mamolen M. The surveillance of communicable disease in Vermont: who reports? Public Health Rep. 106 (1):95–97, 1991.

Selik RM, Buehler JW, Karon JM, Chamberland ME, and Berkelman RL. Impact of the 1987 revision of the case definition of acquired immune deficiency in the United States. J. Acquir. Immune Defic. Syndr. 3:73–82, 1990.

Serfling RE. Methods for current statistical analysis of excess pneumonia-influenza deaths. Public Health Rep. 78:494–506, 1963.

Simonsen L, Clarke MJ, Stroup DF, et al. A method for timely assessment of influenza-associated mortality in the United States. Epidemiology. 8(4):390–395, 1997.

Singleton JA, Tabnak, F, Kuan J, and Rutherford GW. Human immunodeficiency virus disease in California. Effects of the 1993 expanded case definition of the acquired immunodeficiency syndrome. West. J. Med. 164:122–129, 1996.

Smith MH. National Childhood Vaccine Injury Compensation Act. Pediatrics. 82:264–269, 1988.

Snacken R, Kendal AP, Haaheim LR, and Wood JM. The next influenza pandemic: lessons from Hong Kong, 1997. Emerg. Infect. Dis. 5: 195–203, 1999.

Stelling JM, and O'Brien TF. Surveillance of antimicrobial resistance: the WHONET Program. Clin. Infect. Dis. 24 (Suppl 1):S157–S168, 1997.

St. Louis ME, Morse DL, Potter ME, et al. The emergence of grade A eggs as a major source of *Salmonella enteritidis* infections: new implications for the control of salmonellosis. JAMA. 259:2103–2107, 1988.

Stroup DF, Thacker SB, and Herndon JL. Application of multiple time series analysis to the estimation of pneumonia and influenza mortality by age, 1962–1983. Stat. Med. 7: 1045–1059, 1988.

Stroup DF, Williamson GD, Herndon JL, and Karon JM. Detection of aberrations in the occurrence of notifiable diseases surveillance data. Stat. Med. 8:323–332, 1989.

Stroup DF, Wharton M, Kafadar K, and Dean AG. Evaluation of a method for detecting aberrations in public health surveillance data. Am. J. Epidemiol. 137:373–380, 1993.

Stroup NE, Zack MM, and Wharton M. Sources of routinely collected data for surveillance. In: Teutsch SM, Churchill RE, eds. Principles and Practice of Public Health Surveillance. Oxford: Oxford University Press, 1994: 31–85.

Sutter RW, Cochi SL, Brink EW, and Sirotkin BI. Assessment of vital statistics and surveillance data for monitoring tetanus mortality, United States, 1979–1984. Am. J. Epidemiol. 131: 132–142, 1990.

Teutsch S. Considerations in planning a surveillance system. In: Teutsch SM, Churchill RE, eds. Principles and Practice of Public Health Surveillance. Oxford: Oxford University Press, 1994: 18–30.

Teutsch SM, and Churchill RE, eds. Principles and Practice of Public Health Surveillance. Oxford: Oxford University Press, 1994.

Teutsch SM, and Thacker SB. Planning a public health surveillance system. Epidemiol. Bull./ PAHO. 16:1–16, 1995.

Thacker SB, Choi K, and Brachman PS. The surveillance of infectious diseases. JAMA. 249: 1181–1185, 1983.

Thacker SB, Redmond S, Rothenberg RB, et al. A controlled trial of disease surveillance strategies. Am. J. Prev. Med. 2:345–350, 1986.

Thacker SB, and Berkelman RL. Public health surveillance in the United States. Epidemiol. Rev. 10:164–190, 1988.

Thacker SB, Parrish RG, Trowbridge FL, and Surveillance Coordination Group. A method for evaluating systems of epidemiological surveillance. World Health Stat. Q. 41(1):11–18, 1988.

Thacker SB, Berkelman RL, and Stroup DF. The science of public health surveillance. J. Public Health Policy. 10:187–03, 1989.

Thacker SB. Les principes et la practique de la surveillance en sante publique: l'utilisation des donnees en sante publique. Sante Publique. 4:43–49, 1992.

Todd JK, Wiesenthal AM, Ressman M, Caston SA, and Hopkins RS. Toxic shock syndrome. II. Estimated occurrence in Colorado as influenced by case ascertainment methods. Am. J. Epidemiol. 122:857–867, 1985.

Trask JW. Vital statistics: A discussion of what they are and their uses in public health administration. Public Health Rep. Suppl 12, 1915.

Valleron A-J, Bouvet E, Garnerin P, et al. A computer network for the surveillance of communicable diseases: the French experiment. Am. J. Pub Health. 76:1289–1292, 1986.

Van Beneden CA, Keene WE, Strang RA, et al. Multinational outbreak of *Salmonella enterica* serotype Newport infections due to contaminated alfalfa sprouts. JAMA. 281(2): 158–62, 1999.

Van Casteren V. Inventory of sentinel health information systems with GPs [general practitioners] in European countries. Eurosentinel. Brussels, Belgium: Institute of Hygiene and Epidemiology, January 1991.

Vogt RL, Clark SW, and Kappel S. Evaluation of the state surveillance system using hospital discharge diagnoses, 1982–1983. Am. J. Epidemiol. 123:197–198, 1986.

Vogt RL, LaRue D, Klaucke DN, and Jillson DA. Comparison of an active and passive surveillance system of primary care providers for hepatitis, measles, rubella, and salmonellosis in Vermont. Am. J. Public Health. 73:795–797, 1983.

Watkins M, Lapham S, and Hoy W. Use of a medical center's computerized health care data base for notifiable disease surveillance. Am. J. Public Health. 81:637–639, 1991.

Weiss KB, and Wagener DK. Asthma surveillance in the United States: a review of current trends and knowledge gaps. Chest. 98:179S–184S, 1990.

Wentz KR, and Marcuse EK. Diphtheria-tetanus-pertussis vaccine and serious neurologic illness: an updated review of the epidemiologic evidence. Pediatrics. 87:287–297, 1991.

Young D. Underreporting of Lyme disease. N. Engl. J. Med. 338:1629, 1998.

8

Microbial Molecular Techniques

LOREEN A. HERWALDT, MICHAEL A. PFALLER, and STEFAN WEBER

An avalanche of new molecular typing tests has recently overwhelmed hospital epidemiologists, field epidemiologists, and infectious disease clinicians. The plethora of new acronyms confuse even experts in the field, many of whom have given up following each development unless it is related to their own research. In a letter published in the *Journal of Clinical Microbiology*, Achtmann coined several acronyms to describe the current state of the art: YATM (Yet Another Typing Method), TBCA (Totally Boring Clonal Analysis), and TATBSTM (Tried And True But Stodgy Typing Method) (Achtmann 1996). The extremely rapid pace of development is illustrated by the fact that a review of molecular typing methods published in December, 1989 referred to polymerase chain reaction (PCR) and ribotyping as "newer methods" but did not mention pulsed field gel electrophoresis (PFGE), which is now one of the most commonly used typing methods (John, 1989). Even a cursory review of the literature documents that the number of published manuscripts describing molecular typing methods has grown exponentially.

When used properly in conjunction with classical epidemiologic studies or appropriate clinical evaluations, molecular typing methods facilitate the epidemiologist's and the infectious diseases clinician's work. When used inappropriately, molecular typing methods will at best add substantial cost to an investigation or clinical evaluation and at worst could lead the epidemiologist or clinician to incorrect conclusions.

The purpose of this chapter is to review typing methods that have been used successfully in the practice of hospital epidemiology, field epidemiology, and infectious diseases. We explain the basic principles of these methods and describe their strengths and weaknesses. In addition, we cite published studies and our own experience in hospital epidemiology and clinical medicine to demonstrate how epidemiologists and clinicians can use these methods to solve problems. We hope that our approach will allow readers to use these methods wisely so that they do not stray into a morass of YATMs and TBCAs.

HOW EPIDEMIOLOGISTS AND CLINICIANS USE TYPING METHODS

Hospital epidemiologists often want to determine whether isolates causing a cluster of infections are all the same strain (i.e., an outbreak exists) or are unrelated strains (i.e., there is no outbreak). This step is particularly important if the etiologic agent is a common environmental contaminant or if it is a member of the normal microbial flora. In addition, hospital epidemiologists must identify either the reservoir or the mode of transmission (or both) for the epidemic strain so that they can terminate the current outbreak and prevent similar outbreaks in the future.

Like their counterparts in hospitals, epidemiologists in the field or the community often must determine whether an outbreak exists and if one exists, they must identify the reservoir or mode of transmission. However, the populations about which they are concerned are larger and more difficult to define than those evaluated by hospital epidemiologists. In addition, epidemiologists in the community may conduct population-based surveillance studies over a long period of time to determine whether particular strains, especially those with known virulence factors or those with specific antimicrobial resistance genes, are spreading within a population. Epidemiologists can use such studies to identify appropriate preventive strategies, to assess the efficacy of interventions, and to identify emerging or re-emerging pathogens.

Clinicians, in contrast to epidemiologists, are more interested in the fate of individual patients. Clinicians often must determine whether an infection represents a reinfection with a different strain or is a relapse caused by a strain that caused a previous infection. In the latter case, the clinician must ask whether:

- the prior treatment did not eradicate the first infection because the treatment was inadequate,
- the patient has a metastatic focus of infection that persisted after the first infection (e.g., osteomyelitis after a *Staphylococcus aureus* blood stream infection),
- a foreign body is persistently infected, or
- the infecting organism acquired resistance to the antimicrobials used to treat the first infection. (Wendt et al. 1999)

Thus, epidemiologists and clinicians often ask questions that routine epidemiologic, clinical, and microbiological investigations cannot answer. Epidemiologic typing techniques may help epidemiologists and clinicians answer these tough questions. However, to be a useful epidemiologic or clinical tool, a typing system must meet several criteria. The method must:

- provide an unambiguous result for each isolate (typeability),
- provide the same result each time an isolate is tested (reproducibility),
- differentiate among epidemiologically unrelated strains (discriminatory power).

Occasionally, methods that are used for routine microbiological purposes such as antimicrobial susceptibility testing or biotyping can fulfill these criteria adequately. However, antibiotic susceptibility profiles (i.e., antibiograms) frequently lack discriminatory power. Modern molecular typing methods are more likely to discriminate among strains, but some methods have limited typeability and others are not reproducible. At present, no typing system fulfills all criteria for the perfect method. Epidemiologists and clinicians must remember this fact whenever they use typing methods or evaluate results produced by these methods.

In many instances, simple species identification and antimicrobial susceptibility testing can be used to determine whether isolates from a possible outbreak are all the same strain or to track a particular strain over time. However, if the infection of interest is caused by organisms such as *Esche-*

richia coli, Staphylococcus epidermidis, or *Pseudomonas aeruginosa*, which are frequent or universal members of the normal flora or often contaminate the environment, additional tests might be required to determine whether the isolates are related. The additional tests are done to determine whether members of a microbial species can be further delineated into subgroups known as strains or subtypes. Isolates that give the same result or "fingerprint" with one or more typing tests are considered to be indistinguishable and represent the same strain, and isolates that give different results to these tests are considered to be unrelated or different strains. If the same strain is isolated from a group of patients, the strain may have been transmitted among patients from a common source or by a common mechanism. Similarly, if the same strain is repeatedly isolated from a single patient, the organism most likely is infecting or colonizing the patient, not just contaminating the cultures (Herwaldt et al. 1990).

The earliest typing methods used for epidemiologic purposes evaluated phenotypic characteristics, such as antimicrobial susceptibility, biochemical reactions, bacteriophage susceptibility, and surface proteins (e.g., multilocus enzyme electrophoresis [MLEE], and immunoblotting) (Tables 8–1 and 8–2). Phenotypic methods detect characteristics expressed by microorganisms in response to antibiotics or other inhibitors, as a product of one of their enzymes, or as a protein on their cell surface. Phenotypic characteristics are not as stable as the organism's genetic material. Thus the results of phenotypic methods may vary depending on the test conditions, the number of times the organism is passaged, and environmental stresses. Phenotypic methods often are labor intensive. In addition, these methods tend to lump isolates together in large groups, and thus do not discriminate between strains as well as DNA-based methods.

Today, investigators often use typing methods that evaluate genetic material (i.e., plasmid or chromosomal DNA) to discriminate among strains. Consequently, we will review only a few phenotypic methods that have been used successfully in epidemiologic studies. Our primary purpose is to describe how epidemiologists and clinicians can use genotypic methods to enhance their understanding of hospital-acquired or community-acquired infections, to identify trends in antimicrobial susceptibility, and to determine whether a patient has a relapsing infection. Before describing the methods, we present two scenarios to illustrate the power of molecular typing methods in some situations and the limitations of these same methods in other situations.

Scenario 1

Back et al. (1993) reported two outbreaks caused by erythromycin-resistant *S. aureus* (ERSA) in the well-baby nursery of a 700-bed university teaching hospital. The first outbreak, which occurred in April 1990, affected 15 babies. The investigators obtained cultures from 45 health care workers to determine the source of the outbreak. Nineteen health care workers carried *S. aureus*, and in four of them it was an erythromycin-resistant isolate. The antibiogram of three isolates matched that of the epidemic strain. An epidemiological investigation identified a nursing assistant (nursing assistant A) as the most likely source of the epidemic. She was removed from the nursery, treated, and allowed to return to work only after several follow-up cultures were negative. No ERSA infections were identified while the nursing assistant was on furlough. After she returned to work, two additional ERSA infections occurred but each time the nursing assistant's cultures were negative. The nursing assistant subsequently retired in October 1990.

In September 1991, 11 infants became infected with ERSA. The isolates all had similar antibiograms that matched the antibiogram of the previous epidemic strain. The investigators obtained cultures from 57 health care workers, 12 of whom carried *S. aureus*. Six of these isolates were ERSA. By plasmid pattern analysis and pulsed-field gel electrophoresis (PFGE), all isolates obtained from infected infants were identical,

Table 8–1 Epidemiological Typing Systems*

Typing System	Typeability	Reproducibility	Discriminatory Power	Advantages	Disadvantages
Phenotypic Methods					
Biotyping	Excellent	Fair	Poor	Inexpensive, readily available, unique pattern may be a marker	Not stable, detects enzyme function, designed for taxonomic purposes, not validated for some organisms
Susceptibility testing	Excellent	Good	Poor	Easy to perform, inexpensive, useful for most bacteria, readily available, unique pattern may be a marker, method/interpretation standardized	May not be stable, limited sensitivity for highly susceptible or resistant strains, question how many and which antibiotics to test, question how many differences distinguish unrelated strains
Phage typing	Variable	Fair	Variable	Standardized for *S. aureus*, useful for *S. aureus* and *S. epidermidis*	Not standardized for most organisms, not time-efficient, not readily available, many organisms untypeable
Serotyping	Variable	Good	Variable	Rapid, long established, reagents for some species widely available, e.g., *Salmonella, Shigella, Legionella*	Standardized reagents lacking for most species, many isolates are not typeable
PAGE/Immunoblot (Polyacrylamide gel electrophoresis)	Excellent	Good	Unknown	All organisms should be typeable, relatively simple, inexpensive	Few data, patterns very complex, immunoblot sera not standardized, scanning equipment expensive, method/interpretation not standardized
MLEE (Multilocus enzyme electrophoresis)	Excellent	Excellent	Good	Stable profiles, phenotype reflects genotype, detects variation in enzyme structure, profiles reflect differences in electrophoretic mobility of enzymes	Few data, time/labor intensive, requires specialized equipment expensive enzymes and reagents
Genotypic Methods					
Plasmid analysis	Variable	Fair	Variable	Technically simple, inexpensive, types numerous organisms, can digest DNA with restriction enzymes	Technical factors may affect results, Detects possibly unstable extrachromosomal element, few data on some organisms, interpretation not standardized

(continued)

Table 8–1—Continued

REA of chromosomes (Restriction enzyme analysis)	Excellent	Variable	Variable	Many organisms typeable, genomic DNA relatively stable	Limited data, patterns very complex, question which enzymes are the best, question how many enzymes to use, interpretation not standardized, scanning equipment very expensive
Ribotyping	Excellent	Excellent	Good	Ribosomal genes highly conserved, completely automated device available	Automated method very expensive, limited data, interpretation not standardized
PFGE (Pulsed-field gel electrophoresis)	Excellent	Excellent	Excellent	Less hands-on time, many organisms typeable, fewer bands so patterns are easier to interpret, no probes required but may be included, efforts to standardize method/interpretation have been made	Limited data, high start-up costs, may need two gels to visualize upper and lower molecular weight ranges, level of standardization is still low
PCR (Polymerase chain reaction)	Excellent	Excellent	Unknown	Rapid, relatively inexpensive, universally applicable when non-specific primer used; types organisms that grow slowly or not at all, are nonviable, are in tissues, are hazardous to grow; can use sheared/single stranded DNA, needs only nanograms of DNA, equipment can be used for diagnostic-tests	Amplifies any contaminating DNA, sensitive to conditions (Mg^{+2}-content, temperature), method/ interpretation not standardized, difficult to find the right primers, each primer pair requires a new gel, limited data

Source: Weber S, Pfaller MA, and Herwaldt LA. Role of molecular epidemiology in infection control. Infect. Dis. Clin. North Am.

*The rankings reflect the opinions of the authors and are primarily based on how the tests function when bacteria are typed.

but isolates obtained during the first epidemic from staff, including nursing assistant A, were different strains. In contrast, three of six isolates obtained from health care workers during the second outbreak had the same plasmid pattern as the epidemic strain. By PFGE two of these isolates were identical to the epidemic strain.

Nursing assistant B and an attending physician carried the epidemic strain. The nursing assistant was present during the two outbreaks and also continuously during the 15-month interval between the epidemics. The physician was attending at the onset of both outbreaks but was not present continuously between the epidemics. The attending physician had contact with most of the cases and she remembered a "boil" on her face at the time of the second epidemic. She did not remember any similar lesions during the first epidemic. The nursing assistant's follow-up culture was negative so she was not treated.

Table 8–2   Utility of Typing Systems for Different Organisms*

Typing System[†]	Bacteria	Fungi	Viruses
Biotyping	++	+	na
Susceptibility testing	++	−	−
Phage typing	+	−	na
Serotyping	+	+	+
PAGE* Immunoblot	++	++	na
MLEE	++/+++	++	na
Plasmid analysis	++/+++	−	na
Chromosomal REA	++/+++	+++	++
Southern blot/Ribotyping	++/+++	++/+++	−
PFGE	++++	++/+++	−
PCR	+++/++++	+++	+++/++++

Source: Weber S, Pfaller MA, and Herwaldt LA. Role of molecular epidemiology in infection control. Infect. Dis. Clin. North Am.

*The rankings reflect the opinions of the authors and are primarily based on how the tests function when bacteria are typed.

++++Considered the best method for an organism. A high degree of discriminatory power and typeability.

+++Method has been used for a variety of organisms in the group, acceptable degree of discriminatory power or typeability.

++Method has been used for a variety of organisms in the group, fair to moderate degree of discriminatory power or typeability.

+Method has been used for only few organisms in the group. Except for some special cases (e.g., serotyping of *Salmonella* spp., *Legionella pneumophila* or *Streptococcus pneumoniae*) only limited discriminatory power.

−Method not recommended, because of insufficient data.

Na Method not applicable for this organism group.

[†]PAGE = Polyacrylamide gel electrophoresis; MLEE = Multilocus enzyme electrophoresis; REA = Restriction enzyme analysis; PFGE = Pulsed-field gel electrophoresis; PCR = Polymerase chain reaction.

The physician, who was already off the service, was treated with mupirocin.

In this scenario, antibiograms and classical epidemiological methods identified the wrong person as the source of the initial outbreak. If the investigators had used molecular typing methods during the first outbreak, they could have identified and treated the actual source of the epidemic strain, thereby preventing both the second outbreak and the emotional trauma experienced by nursing assistant A who was identified incorrectly as the source.

Scenario 2
Torrea et al. (1996) probed restriction fragment length polymorphisms (RFLP) with IS6110 to type *Mycobacterium tuberculosis* isolates obtained from 105 patients who were hospitalized during 1993, in three hospitals in Paris, France. Eighty-eight patients were infected with genetically different isolates. IS6110 typing identified six clusters. Persons involved in clusters 1 and 2 were relatives and the patients in cluster 3 were HIV seropositive friends, two of whom lived together. The authors could not identify epidemiologic links between the patients in the remaining three clusters. Further RFLP analysis with two different probes (i.e., small fragments of DNA) and with polymerase chain reaction (PCR) could not separate the isolates in these clusters. Alland et al. (1994) conducted a similar study in a highly endemic area of New York City. In contrast to the investigators in France, Al-

land and colleagues successfully used epidemiological and molecular typing methods to identify the routes by which *M. tuberculosis* was transmitted.

The second scenario demonstrates that molecular typing methods do not always discriminate among epidemiologically unrelated isolates. This can occur for several reasons: (1) the species may have minimal strain variation, (2) the method may lack discriminatory power, or (3) a particular strain may have become endemic in a community. Thus investigators should interpret the results of molecular typing methods cautiously if they do not have epidemiologic evidence for transmission. In addition, this scenario illustrates that a method may be useful in some settings but not in others.

PHENOTYPIC METHODS

Biotype

The genus and species of an organism can be identified by its reactions to a panel of biochemical reagents. Because biotyping methods were developed to identify organisms to species level, these tests aggregate isolates into large groups. Therefore, biotyping methods do not discriminate well between strains of the same species. However, biotyping methods are available in all clinical microbiology laboratories and they are inexpensive. If the laboratory identifies a cluster of organisms that has an unusual biotype, the epidemiology team would be wise to investigate further to determine whether the organisms were transmitted in the hospital (Perl et al. 1999). In fact, several investigators have used biotyping to detect important outbreaks, including a nationwide epidemic of bacteremia caused by *Enterobacter amnigenus* (Maki et al. 1976). Investigators suspected a common-source outbreak when the Centers for Disease Control (CDC) received reports of numerous nosocomial infections caused by an unusual species (biotype) of *Enterobacter*. Subsequently, the investigators determined that intrinsically contaminated intravenous fluid was the source of the epidemic (Maki et al. 1976).

Antimicrobial Susceptibility Patterns

Like biotyping methods, antimicrobial susceptibility testing is routinely performed for most bacteria by staff in clinical microbiology laboratories. In fact, antimicrobial susceptibility testing is the only widely available typing method that has standardized methods and interpretation. However, many important nosocomial pathogens such as methicillin-susceptible *S. aureus* and vancomycin-susceptible *Enterococcus* spp. exhibit little variability in their antimicrobial susceptibility patterns. Thus, like biotypes, antibiograms are not very discriminatory. Antibiotic susceptibility patterns also can change over time. For example, several bacterial genera including *Pseudomonas* spp. and several species of *Enterobacteriaceae* can acquire or lose antimicrobial resistance rapidly.

On occasion, epidemiologists can identify an outbreak if they identify a cluster of organisms that has a distinctive susceptibility pattern (Perl et al. 1999). Some laboratories use computer software programs that track antimicrobial susceptibility patterns. Such programs may allow the epidemiology staff to identify a possible epidemic strain amidst the many sporadic or endemic strains. However, antibiograms rarely provide enough information. Therefore epidemiologists often must conduct additional studies to fully evaluate a possible cluster identified by antimicrobial susceptibility testing. Investigators at the Miriam Hospital in Providence, Rhode Island have published reports of several investigations in which they used antibiotic susceptibility patterns to identify the outbreaks. Subsequently, these investigators conducted meticulous epidemiologic and molecular epidemiologic studies to identify the source and mode of transmission (Boyce et al. 1990, 1992, 1993). One of these outbreaks was caused by an *S. epidermidis* strain that was resistant to penicillin, oxacillin, gentamicin, and trimethoprim-sulfamethoxazole and susceptible to erythromycin, clindamycin, tetracycline, chloramphenicol, and vancomycin (Boyce et al. 1990). The surgeon implicated by the epidemiologic study carried a strain of *S. epidermidis* that had the same susceptibility pattern and plasmid pattern (Boyce et al. 1990).

Other Phenotypic Methods

Phenotypic methods such as phage typing and serotyping were used extensively in the past. Phage typing has been used primarily to investigate the epidemiology of *S. aureus* but has also been used to study other organisms including *Salmonella* spp. Serotyping has been used to study the epidemiology of organisms such as *Salmonella* spp. (DuPont 1991, Paton et al. 1991), *Legionella pneumophila* (Helms et al. 1983, Meenhorst et al. 1985), and *Streptococcus pneumoniae* (Grandsen et al. 1985, Smart et al. 1987). In addition, serotyping identified *Escherichia coli* O157:H7 as a subspecies that causes outbreaks of hemorrhagic colitis with hemolytic uremic syndrome (Whittam et al. 1988). Neither phage typing nor serotyping are very discriminatory and both have poor typeability. Thus most reference laboratories in the United States no longer keep phage stocks, and serotyping data usually must be supplemented with data from molecular typing studies.

Some investigators have used polyacrylamide gel electrophoresis (PAGE) of cellular proteins with or without immunoblotting as typing methods for epidemiologic investigations (Mulligan et al. 1988a,b). Other investigators have used multilocus enzyme electrophoresis (MLEE) as an epidemiologic typing method (Arthur et al. 1990). MLEE is a very powerful tool for studying populations of bacteria (Cookson et al. 1998, Blackall et al. 1998, Tomayko 1995), but it has only limited applicability for epidemiologic analysis of clinical isolates. For example, Arthur and associates (1990) showed that many virulent *E. coli* isolated from patients with pyelonephritis have the same MLEE pattern although they are epidemiologically unrelated. Like most phenotypic methods, PAGE, immunoblotting, and MLEE are generally more useful for identifying species rather than for discriminating among isolates of the same species.

Furthermore, these methods are rarely performed outside of research laboratories. Investigators who use these methods to study microbial pathogens are usually those who use these methods in their research or they have a colleague who does the typing.

GENOTYPIC METHODS

Background Information

Investigators have used a variety of DNA-based methods to genotype microbial pathogens (Tables 8–1 and 8–2). All of these methods use electric fields to separate pieces of DNA, including whole chromosomes, plasmids, restriction endonuclease digestion fragments of chromosomal or plasmid DNA, and amplified DNA fragments. The unique patterns or "fingerprints" are visualized by staining the DNA with ethidium bromide or by hybridizing the DNA with labeled probes. In the future, improved methods of genomic analysis, including automated nucleic acid sequencing and DNA chip technology, may allow epidemiologists to detect and characterize organisms in clinical specimens. Such methods could improve significantly the speed and sensitivity of molecular typing methods.

DNA-based typing methods can also be categorized into comparative methods and library typing methods (Struelens et al. 1998). Investigators use comparative methods most often in outbreak investigations to determine whether a single strain was transmitted in a hospital or a community. In this setting, the investigator uses the typing method to compare a limited number of isolates collected during a limited time period (e.g., days to months). The typing methods appropriate for this application must be reproducible within a single assay, have a high index of discrimination (>0.95), and have full typeability (provide results for each organism) (Struelens et al. 1998). Methods shown to be effective for this purpose include PFGE analysis of large genomic restriction fragments and PCR fingerprinting including arbitrarily primed [AP]-PCR, randomly amplified polymorphic DNA (RAPD), and interrepetitive element PCR typing (rep-PCR) (Struelens et al. 1998). In general, the specific DNA patterns produced by comparative typing systems are relevant only to a particular investigation.

Library typing methods can be used in long-term prospective epidemiologic surveillance studies to evaluate the efficacy of preventive strategies, to detect and monitor emerging and reemerging pathogens, and to track the development of antimicrobial resistance. In a surveillance study, a typing system enables the investigator to map the spread of specific organisms and to determine whether the prevalence of epidemic and endemic clones changes over time (Struelens et al. 1998). The investigators must balance the discriminatory power of the method against the evolutionary stability of the organism of interest if they want to study the dispersion of specific clones over prolonged periods of time (i.e., high number of infection cycles) (Struelens et al. 1998). Such studies typically involve hundreds to thousands of organisms collected over months to years. Thus the typing methods must be standardized, provide highly reproducible results over time and in different laboratories, and allow the investigator to evaluate numerous isolates quickly. The patterns generated by these methods must also be amenable to computer-based storage and analysis. Methods appropriate for this purpose include: analysis of RFLPs of the chromosomal DNA (e.g., ribotyping, insertion sequence [IS] probe fingerprinting), repetitive elements PCR spacer typing (e.g., $^{16-23}$S rDNA, inter-IS elements) [for references pertaining to repetitive PCR spacer typing, see Appendix, section A], selective amplification of genome restriction fragments, multilocus allelic sequence-based typing (e.g., PCR-RFLP, PCR sequencing), and assessment of high density oligonucleotide hybridization patterns (DNA chip) (Struelens et al. 1998).

Investigators can adapt molecular typing methods so that they identify specific genes rather than produce nonspecific banding patterns or fingerprints. For example, researchers have used hybridization with probes or DNA amplification techniques to detect various genes that encode for antimicrobial resistance factors, thus providing an antimicrobial resistance genotype (Arlet 1992, Persing et al. 1996, Tenover et al. 1995). Antimicrobial resistance genotyping is not highly discriminatory (Tenover et al. 1994), however, when combined with other genotyping methods, it is an excellent means for characterizing the epidemiology of antimicrobial resistance among nosocomial- and community-acquired pathogens (Persing et al. 1996, Bergeron 1998, Jones et al. 1997, Marshall et al. 1998). Moreover, microbiologists can use methods that detect antimicrobial resistance genes to calibrate conventional susceptibility tests (Cormican et al. 1996, Che et al. 1998). In the future, clinicians might consider the results of such tests when choosing antimicrobial therapy so they use agents that are least likely to select resistant organisms given the isolate's genetic background (Bergeron et al. 1998).

DNA-based typing methods have enabled investigators to study the relationship between colonizing and infecting isolates in individual patients, distinguish contaminating from infecting strains, document cross-infection among hospitalized patients, evaluate reinfection versus relapse in patients being treated for an infection, and to follow the spread of specific antimicrobial resistant strains within and among different hospitals over time. [Numerous references pertaining to these methods are listed in the Appendix, section B, DNA typing methods used to study the relationship between colonizing and infecting isolates in individual patients; section C, DNA typing methods used to distinguish between contaminating and infecting strains; section D, DNA typing methods used for documenting cross-infection among hospitalized patients; section E, DNA typing methods used for evaluating reinfection versus relapse in patients; section F, DNA typing methods used in surveillance of resistant pathogens within and among hospitals over time.]

All laboratory tests have limitations, and the genotypic typing methods are no exceptions. Epidemiologists and clinicians must understand these limitations so that they do not misinterpret the test results. The DNA patterns generated by these techniques are often highly complex and difficult to analyze. Thus investigators must become well versed in the basic principles of molecular biology and epidemiology and must learn the art of reading the patterns. Computer-assisted systems can help investigators compare complex banding patterns (Struelens et al. 1998, Pfaller et al. 1998, 1996); however, these systems are not entirely automated and the user must do considerable editing. The banding patterns may vary if the DNA is not extracted and digested properly, if the conditions of amplification (PCR-based methods) or electrophoresis are not consistent, or if the DNA undergoes rearrangements over time (Echeita et al. 1998). Consequently, isolates can be compared only if they were typed under identical conditions. The laboratory ideally should assess all isolates from a particular study simultaneously. This is often not possible for large outbreaks or for prospective surveillance studies. Investigators then either must use a highly standardized molecular library typing method or must repeat the typing several times so that critical isolates can be processed and evaluated simultaneously.

To date, investigators have not developed standardized methods for processing DNA or for interpreting the results for most molecular epidemiologic tests. Flexible and sophisticated computer-based analysis systems such as Dendron (Solltech, Iowa City, IA) and fully automated molecular typing systems such as the RiboPrinter (Qualicon, Wilmington, DE) have helped standardize some of the molecular typing methods and quantify analysis of the results (Jones et al. 1997, Marshall et al. 1998, Pfaller et al. 1998, 1996, Schmid et al. 1990, Struelens et al. 1996). In addition, groups of investigators are developing standards and guidelines for the use of DNA-based typing methods, but more work remains to be done in this area (Struelens et al. 1996, Arbeit et al. 1997, Tenover et al. 1995).

Investigators can use many DNA-based methods to study microbial infections, but particular methods may be easier to perform or may be more useful for specific studies. Several excellent and comprehensive reviews provide more detailed information on each technique and discuss the practical applications, strengths, and weaknesses of each method. [For references pertaining to DNA-typing methods, see Appendix, section G.]

Analysis of Plasmid DNA

Plasmids are mobile genetic elements that can be exchanged within a bacterial species and between species. Investigators have shown that some plasmids carry one or more genes that code for antibiotic resistance or virulence factors. Other plasmids are known as cryptic plasmids because their functions have not been ascertained. Members of some bacterial species (e.g., *S. epidermidis*) frequently carry several plasmids, whereas, some bacteria (e.g., *S. aureus*) usually carry only one plasmid, and others (e.g., *P. aeruginosa* and streptococci) rarely or never carry plasmids.

Plasmid pattern analysis can be used to type many bacterial pathogens. The technique is easy to perform, and the methods have been well described (Meyers et al. 1976). At present, several companies market kits that substantially simplify the method for isolating plasmid DNA and decrease the amount of time needed to do the procedure. For example, the conventional miniprep method for isolating plasmid DNA takes eight hours but a method that incorporates a commercial kit takes only four hours. With either method the electrophoresis step requires four hours. Thus an investigator who uses the commercial kit could have the results at the end of one work day. Furthermore, most of the equipment (e.g., incubator, centrifuge, pipetters, etc.) required for plasmid pattern analysis is already present in a standard clinical microbiology laboratory. The additional equipment, including the electrophoresis apparatus, ultraviolet light box, and camera, is relatively inexpensive.

The primary limitation of plasmid pattern analysis is that some bacteria do not carry plasmids and are, therefore, not typeable by this method. Another limitation of plasmid pattern analysis is that plasmids exist in different conformations (i.e., supercoiled, closed circular, and linear). Thus, the same plasmid can migrate to one or more locations, depending on the conditions under which the gel is run. Consequently, the same strain could produce several different patterns. The laboratory can easily overcome this limitation by digesting the plasmid DNA with a restriction enzyme. This modification, known as restriction endonuclease analysis of plasmid DNA (REAP), is also useful when a bacterium such as *S. aureus* has a single large plasmid that migrates only a short distance into the gel.

Another limitation of typing methods that assess plasmid DNA is that these genetic elements are mobile and they can be shared with organisms that are not related at the genomic level. Because plasmids may be gained or lost over time, plasmid patterns or REAP patterns may not remain stable. The frequency with which plasmids are gained or lost depends on the bacterial species and on the antibiotic pressure in the environment. An epidemiologist who is trying to track an epidemic strain over a long period of time may be misled if the strain has gained or lost plasmids or if the plasmid has been shared with epidemiologically and genetically unrelated members of the same species. At times epidemiologists can turn this disadvantage into an advantage. For example, O'Brien et al. (1980) described an outbreak in which a plasmid carrying the gene for 2″ aminoglycoside nucleotidyltransferase spread within their hospital. The investigators identified a particular susceptibility pattern (gentamicin, chloramphenicol, sulfonamides, ampicillin, and carbenicillin) that was "epidemic" in their hospital. This susceptibility pattern was identified in isolates from *Klebsiella pneumoniae*, *Serratia marcescens*, *E. coli*, *Enterobacter* spp., *Citrobacter* spp., and *Proteus morganii*. Regardless of their species designation, all isolates that had this antibiogram carried the same or "epidemic" plasmid. If the investigators thought of an outbreak only in traditional terms—a single pathogen spreading over time in a particular geographic area—

they would have missed the outbreak. Prodinger et al. (1996) obtained similar results when they investigated an outbreak caused by *K. pneumoniae* that produced SHV-5-β-lactamase. In both outbreaks, plasmid pattern analysis allowed the investigators to track the real culprit—a transmissible resistance determinant.

Despite the limitations inherent in assessing plasmid DNA, many investigators have used these techniques successfully to solve outbreaks and to elucidate the epidemiology of bacterial pathogens. A humorous example is the multistate outbreak of gastroenteritis caused by *Salmonella muenchen* that was described by Taylor et al. (1982). The investigators found an epidemiologic link between illness and smoking marijuana. They confirmed this observation by identifying the same plasmid in isolates obtained from patients and marijuana samples but not in control isolates (Taylor et al. 1982).

Boyce and colleagues (1992) used antibiograms and plasmid pattern analysis to study a putative outbreak of ampicillin-resistant enterococci in their hospital. These investigators determined that rates of infection increased because one strain spread among 19 patients and because the incidence of infections caused by unrelated strains of *Enterococcus faecium* also increased. Arroyo and associates (1987) used plasmid pattern analysis to determine that an apparent outbreak of *Achromobacter xylosoxidans* infections was caused by unrelated strains and did not result from transmission of a single strain. The investigators used whole cell polypeptide analysis to confirm the results of plasmid pattern analysis.

Typing methods that evaluate plasmid DNA were once the molecular typing methods of choice for epidemiologic and clinical investigations. Subsequently, techniques that evaluate the chromosomal DNA have assumed this role. However, we think that plasmid pattern analysis and REAP are still useful techniques. In general, we think these methods are used best either as screening tests with which to identify the isolates that should be subjected to genomic-based typing methods or as methods for subtyping isolates that have been evaluated by a genomic method. In some instances, plasmid pattern analysis or REAP alone may be adequate.

Investigators have used plasmid pattern analysis or REAP to study many nosocomial pathogens. We refer readers who are interested in further information to two excellent manuscripts that review the use of those methods for infection control purposes (Hawkey 1987, Wachsmuth 1986).

Restriction Endonuclease Analysis of Chromosomal DNA (REA)

Like plasmids, chromosomal DNA can be digested with restriction enzymes and the fragments can be separated by agarose gel electrophoresis. The number of bands depends on the recognition sequence of the enzyme and the composition of the DNA. Restriction endonuclease digestion of whole chromosomal DNA usually creates so many small DNA fragments that the patterns produced by conventional gel electrophoresis look to an untrained eye like smears of DNA (Fig. 8–1A). Because the banding patterns are too complex to be compared easily, this technique has either been modified by hybridizing the chromosomal DNA with probes or has been supplanted by other genotypic typing methods. The banding patterns generated by this and other methods that distinguish between organisms on the basis of the number and size of the fragments are called RFLPs.

Use of Probes

One way to simplify the RFLP generated by digesting chromosomal DNA is to transfer the DNA fragments onto a nitrocellulose membrane (Southern blot) and then incubate the membrane with a probe labeled with an isotope, a chemiluminescent substance, or an enzyme such as horseradish peroxidase. The probe will bind only to areas of complementary DNA. After unbound probes are removed, the bound probe is visualized by exposing the membrane to a photographic film or by adding the enzyme's substrate. The result is a simplified banding pattern that can be assessed

visually or by scanning equipment. The more highly related the organisms are, the more likely it is that the sequences identified by the probe are distributed similarly over their genomes and will produce identical or similar banding patterns after digestion with endonucleases. This highly reproducible technique can type all organisms that have regions in their chromosomal DNA that are complementary to the probe. However, the discriminatory power of the technique is affected by the probe; probes that detect a region that is repeated numerous times in the chromosome will produce more bands on the gel and will have a greater discriminatory power than probes that detect a region that occurs infrequently.

Ribotyping

Ribotyping assesses the RFLPs within the genes coding for ribosomal RNA (Fig. 8–1B). These sequences are highly conserved (i.e., are quite similar from species to species), and thus, probes such as *E. coli* rRNA can be used to type most bacterial pathogens (Stull et al. 1988). Furthermore, the results usually are highly reproducible, and isolates from outbreaks typically have the same ribotype. The discriminatory power of this method is comparable to MLEE (Arthur et al. 1990, Tenover et al. 1995a). Ribotyping works well for a number of different nosocomial pathogens; however, its discriminatory power is usually less than that achieved by PFGE (Pfaller et al. 1996, Gordillo et al. 1993, Prevost et al. 1992). Our own experience and that of other investigators indicate that one must use two different restriction enzymes to achieve discriminatory power similar to that provided by PFGE (Widmer et al. 1992, Gustaferro 1993).

The RiboPrinter produced by Qualicon (Wilmington, DE) automates ribotyping (Pfaller et al. 1996). The system, which can be applied to virtually all bacteria, types and analyzes a batch of eight isolates within eight hours. New batches can be started every two hours so that 32 isolates can be analyzed in one day. The advantages of this system include a high level of automation and standardization, use of chemilumines-

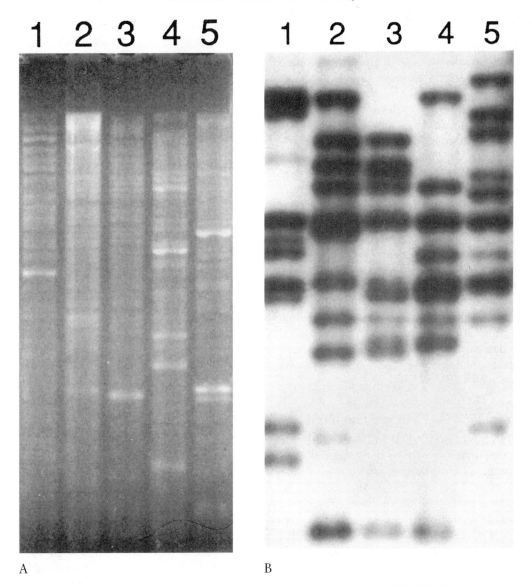

A   B

Figure 8–1A and B. A: Restriction endonuclease analysis of chromosomal DNA. Whole chromosomal DNA from five isolates of coagulase-negative staphylococci digested with *Hind* III and separated by conventional agarose gel electrophoresis. The bright bands are plasmid DNA. **B:** Ribotyping. The Southern blot of the DNA shown in Figure 7–1A was probed with the *E. coli* ribosomal RNA gene that was labeled with ^{32}P. The patterns in lanes 2 and 3 are similar but not identical. All other patterns are unique.

cent labels rather than isotopes to detect bands, and a sophisticated computerized imaging system that digitizes and normalizes the banding patterns. An extensive computer database allows the laboratory to compare stored banding patterns both within a gel and between gels and to identify clusters of related isolates. This system appears to be a major step toward standardization of molecular typing. Given the high cost of the equipment, few hospitals will be able to buy it. However, reference laboratories could use this equipment to screen organisms so that the staff can determine which isolates should be evaluated by tests that are more discriminatory.

Insertion Sequence Typing

Insertion sequences (IS), mobile genetic elements usually present in numerous copies within a bacterial genome, can also be used as probes. Because the number and location of IS elements vary, each strain has a unique banding pattern. This method has been used to type methicillin-resistant *S. aureus*, *Candida* spp., *M. tuberculosis*, and *Salmonella typhimurium* (Soria et al. 1994). Insertion sequence typing in which IS6110 was used as the probe has helped elucidate the epidemiology of *M. tuberculosis* and is currently the typing method of choice for this organism (van Embden et al. 1993). The discriminatory power of this method depends on the number of copies of the IS element that are present. One major advantage of IS6110 typing is that the entire process, including interpretation, has been carefully standardized to ensure that results obtained in different laboratories can be compared (van Embden et al. 1993).

Pulsed-Field Gel Electrophoresis (PFGE)

DNA fragments larger than 20–25 kilobases are separated poorly by conventional agarose gel electrophoresis, which uses a unidirectional current. PFGE separates large fragments of 40–1000 kilobases (mega base sized DNA) in agarose gels by varying the duration of the electrical pulse and shifting the direction of the current frequently (Schwartz 1984). To ensure that the PFGE patterns are reproducible, the genomic DNA must be isolated in a manner that minimizes damage from shearing or crushing. This is accomplished by embedding a suspension of the organism in agarose before the cell wall is lysed and the DNA is digested. The number of DNA fragments is limited by using restriction enzymes with recognition sites that occur infrequently in the genome. The choice of the restriction enzyme is critical because each enzyme produces a different number of fragments and particular enzymes work best for certain species. Readers who want to know which enzymes have been useful for specific organisms are referred to the reviews by Maslow and Mulligan (1996), Maslow et al. (1993), and Pfaller et al. (1992). We

have also included references to 27 studies in which the investigators used PFGE successfully (for references pertaining to PFGE, see Appendix, section H). Figure 8–2 illustrates a variety of RFLP produced when *S. aureus* chromosomal DNA was digested with *Sma* I and the fragments were separated by PFGE.

PFGE has several important advantages compared with techniques that use conventional electrophoresis such as REA of chromosomal DNA, ribotyping, and IS typing. Because the chromosomal DNA is digested with restriction enzymes that cut only in a few places, PFGE patterns have only 15–20 well-separated bands. Consequently, investigators can assess the patterns of a limited number of isolates without using scanning equipment and without simplifying the patterns with probes. PFGE patterns are highly reproducible and the discriminatory power of this method is excellent. In special situations, investigators may want to increase the discriminatory power of the test by digesting the DNA with two enzymes.

The main disadvantages of PFGE are the cost of the equipment and the time that the procedure requires. The equipment required for PFGE costs $15,000 to $20,000, which may prohibit many clinical laboratories from acquiring a system. Moreover, the entire PFGE protocol takes about one week. Although one week is adequate turn-around time for most epidemiologic investigations, there may be situations in which it would be advantageous or even essential to have the results within 24 to 48 hours. Some PFGE protocols allow laboratory staff to decrease the amount of time required for various steps. Despite these shortcuts, PFGE cannot produce results as quickly as plasmid pattern analysis or PCR-based methods. Furthermore, certain organisms such as *Clostridium difficile* and *Aspergillus* spp. may not be typeable by PFGE because their DNA cannot be extracted intact.

Tenover et al. (1995a) published recommendations that stipulate how PFGE patterns should be interpreted. They recommended that isolates be considered the same strain if all bands match, closely related strains if the patterns differ by one to three

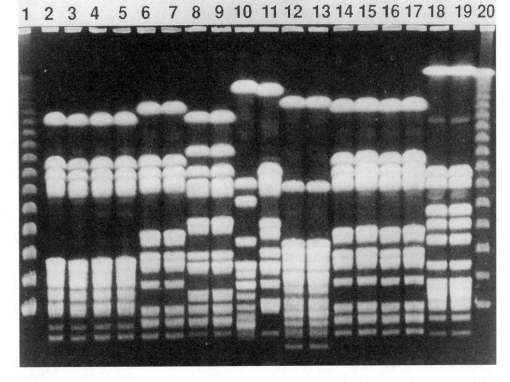

Figure 8–2. Pulsed-field gel electrophoresis. Pulsed-field electrophoresis of 18 *S. aureus* isolates. Lanes 1 and 20 contain the molecular weight standard. Lanes 2 to 5 contain chromosomal DNA from isolates obtained from a patient who carried one strain during the course of the study. Lanes 6 to 9 contain chromosomal DNA from isolates obtained from a patient who carried two different strains. Lanes 10 to 13 contain chromosomal DNA from isolates obtained from a patient who carried three different strains over time. Lanes 14 to 17 contain chromosomal DNA from a patient who carried one strain during the course of the study. Lanes 18 and 19 contain chromosomal DNA from a patient who carried one strain during the course of the study.

bands, possibly related strains if the patterns differ by four to six bands, and unrelated strains if the patterns differ by more than six bands. These recommendations are very important, because they represent the first attempt to standardize the interpretation of results obtained by a molecular typing technique. To date, no one has recommended a standardized procedure for performing PFGE.

Polymerase Chain Reaction (PCR)

Polymerase chain reaction is another molecular method that has become increasingly important for epidemiological purposes. Investigators have developed many different PCR methods, most of which have similar advantages and disadvantages. The primary advantage of PCR is that it detects and amplifies minuscule amounts of DNA. Theoretically, PCR could be done with only one copy of the template. In reality, 10 to 100 copies of the template DNA must be present in the sample. Thus PCR can be used to type organisms that either grow slowly on laboratory media (e.g., *M. tuberculosis*) (Hance et al. 1989) or do not grow in vitro (e.g., *Mycobacterium genavense*, *Pneumocystis carinii*) (Boettger et al. 1992, Kitada et al. 1991). PCR can also be used to detect and type pathogens in patients treated with antimicrobial agents before cultures were obtained. Moreover, PCR can be used to amplify the DNA of organisms that are present in tissues preserved in formalin (Sung et al. 1993, von Weizsacker et al. 1994). These advantages may on occasion be of use to epidemiologists if they must investigate outbreaks caused by fastidious organisms or if they are informed of problems after the fact. Unlike other typing methods, PCR may allow epidemiologists, clinicians, and laboratory personnel to salvage samples and, consequently, to solve seemingly insoluble epidemiologic and clinical problems.

Unfortunately, PCR's biggest advantage is also its biggest disadvantage. Because PCR amplifies minute amounts of DNA, any bit of contaminating DNA, of which there is an endless supply in a clinical microbiology laboratory, can produce inaccurate results. To minimize contamination, PCR should be conducted in a laboratory that is dedicated to that procedure (McCreedy and Calloway 1993). In addition, minor deviations from the ideal temperature or from the ideal concentrations of particular cations (e.g., magnesium) can alter the results (Persing 1993).

Conventional PCR

In conventional PCR, the test organism's genomic DNA (template) is denatured, two oligonucleotide probes are hybridized to the complementary DNA strands, and a DNA polymerase replicates the template from the points at which the primers are attached. The process is repeated about 20 to 30 times (cycles). After several cycles, only the DNA between the insertion sites of the two primers is replicated. During this process, the number of copies of the DNA between the two primers is exponentially multiplied.

To use conventional PCR methods, the investigator must know the DNA sequence to which the primers are annealed, because unique primer pairs must be created for each species. Investigators have successfully used these methods to assess the epidemiology of nosocomial pathogens.

PCR-RFLP

Amplified DNA segments of a known region in the bacterial genome can be digested with a restriction enzyme and the resulting fragments can be separated by agarose gel electrophoresis. If the DNA fragments from two isolates produce different patterns, the organisms are not likely to be related. PCR-RFLP has been used to subtype slow growing or fastidious bacteria like *Rochalimaea henselae*, (now *Bartonella henselae*), which causes cat-scratch fever (Norman et al. 1995), the etiologic agent of Whipple's disease (Relman et al. 1992), and *Neisseria meningitidis* (Kertesz et al. 1993, McLaughlin et al. 1993, Zhu et al. 1995). This method has also been used to type viruses such as cytomegalovirus and herpes simplex virus. PCR-RFLP has some advantages over methods that assess RFLPs of the whole chromosomal DNA, because additional Southern blotting is not necessary and the amplification product is cleaved more efficiently than genomic DNA. However, it may be difficult to amplify a fragment that is large enough to be digested, and the method is not very discriminatory. We include three additional references for readers who wish to know more about PCR-RFLP (Desai et al. 1998, Nachamkin et al. 1993, Goh et al. 1992).

Random Amplified Polymorphic DNA (RAPD)

Random amplified polymorphic DNA, also known as arbitrarily primed PCR (AP-PCR), has increased the applicability of PCR for epidemiologic purposes. The basic principle of RAPD is that short primers, which are not complementary to known genetic sites, hybridize randomly in the genome. If two such sites are located close enough (i.e., within a few kilobases) then the intervening sequences will be amplified and can be visualized by gel electrophoresis. In general, the investigator must assess each isolate with several PCR reactions, each of which uses a different primer. For each primer, the investigator compares where the amplified fragments from each isolate migrate in the gel, to determine whether the isolates are closely related.

In theory, this technique has several attractive features. One can generate a fingerprint from very little DNA and the template DNA can be quite crude. In addition, one does not need to know the sequence of particular genes, and the same primer set could be used to type most organisms. Moreover, some primer sets (e.g., Operon random primer kits) are commercially available.

Investigators have used this technique to type numerous species, including fungi such as *Aspergillus fumigatus* (Cohen et al. 1992, Loudon et al. 1993). In some instances, RAPD has provided useful molecular epidemiologic data when other methods, such as PFGE, did not (Villanueva et al. 1997). However, current data indicate that RAPD is fraught with many problems, the chief of which are poor reproducibility and lower discriminatory power than other methods. We include two additional references for those readers who would like to know more about RAPD (Lai et al. 1998, van Belkum et al. 1997).

PCR of Repetitive Chromosomal Elements (Rep-PCR)

PCR of repetitive chromosomal elements is another modification of the PCR technique that is more suitable for epidemiologic purposes than is conventional PCR. In this case, the primers are directed toward repetitive chromosomal elements (rep-PCR) such as IS6110 in *M. tuberculosis* and the Enterobacterial repetitive intergenic consensus (ERIC) sequences in other bacteria (Versalovic et al. 1991). If two sequences are close enough to each other, the genomic sequence between those elements is amplified. Because IS and other repetitive elements are present in more than one copy, rep-PCR produces several bands of different size. As with RAPD, organisms that are related have similar banding patterns. The reproducibility of this technique is high and the discriminatory power is comparable to MLEE (Woods et al. 1992). This technique has also been applied to higher organisms like fungi and amoeba (Niesters et al. 1993, van Belkum et al. 1992). We include two additional references for readers who would like to know more about rep-PCR (Cimolai et al. 1997, Lessing et al. 1995).

Other Amplification Methods

The literature is replete with reports of new amplification methods including cleavase fragment length polymorphism (Olive and Bean 1999), amplified fragment polymorphism (Olive and Bean 1999), DNA sequencing (Olive and Bean 1999), ligase chain reaction, self-sustaining sequence replication, Qβ replicase, and strand displacement amplification. At present, these methods are used primarily for research and are most useful as detection methods. However, when they are developed further, these methods could have a role in epidemiologic studies. In the future, rapid detection methods could allow the laboratory to quickly identify organisms that carry genes for methicillin or vancomycin resistance or that are likely to be resistant to numerous antimicrobial agents. For example, amplification of the mycobacterial gene rpoB by PCR followed by a DNA conformation–dependent method such as single–stranded conformational polymorphism (SSCP) is the most rapid method available for identifying *M. tuberculosis* isolates that are resistant to numerous antimicrobial agents (Telenti et al. 1993). Furthermore, some newer techniques may allow epidemiologists to study the transmission of organisms that are difficult to grow or do not grow in culture. For example, Yusof et al. (1994) used PCR followed by SSCP to study transmission of hepatitis B virus. The amplification techniques could have many applications in the future; however, most of them are not readily available for routine use in epidemiologic or clinical investigations at the present time.

Choosing the Right Method— Mission Impossible?

Tables 8–1 and 8–2 summarize basic characteristics of several phenotypic and genotypic typing techniques used to study nosocomial pathogens. Even our short list of typing methods resembles a confusing conglomerate. After reviewing such information, epidemiologists and clinicians are often left asking which method is best for their setting, in general, or which is best for the current outbreak, endemic situation, or a particular patient.

In an earlier section on how epidemiologists and clinicians use typing methods, we discussed several criteria for assessing typing methods—typeability, reproducibility, and discriminatory power. Although these criteria are important, the ideal typing method for epidemiologic and clinical purposes should also have several other characteristics. The test should be rapid, reliable, and inexpensive. Furthermore, the method should allow epidemiologists and clinicians to answer the questions they commonly ask:

- Are the isolates from numerous patients the same?
- Are the isolates from the environment the same as the patients' isolates?
- Does the patient have a relapsing infection with the same organism or reinfection with a different one?

As the reader has surmised already, no single typing system fulfills all these characteristics or can answer every question. The answer to the question of which method is the best will vary with:

- the organism of interest,
- the goals of the particular investigation,
- the situation—epidemic investigation vs. prospective surveillance system, and
- the available resources.

A one-size-fits-all approach does not work when applied to molecular epidemiologic typing. We have included for interested readers references to 45 additional studies that illustrate how these methods are used in real life situations. [For references pertaining to molecular methods used in outbreak investigations, see Appendix, section I.] In addition, the review by Olive and Bean compares several molecular techniques and describes situations in which they have been useful (Olive and Bean 1999).

A review of the literature shows that investigators routinely use only a few techniques to assess the epidemiology of clinically important pathogens (Table 8-2). (See John 1989, Struelens et al. 1998, 1996, Arbeit 1997, 1995, Tenover et al. 1995a, Maslow et al. 1996, 1993, Pfaller et al. 1997, Sader et al. 1995, Olive and Bean 1999, Farmer 1988, Jarvis 1994, Falkiner 1988). Currently, REAP, PFGE, PCR-RFLP, and RAPD (or AP-PCR) are the most frequently used techniques. REAP often is considered to be an old-fashioned method.

However, commercially available kits standardize the process for extracting plasmid DNA and simplify the method. In addition, commercial kits may allow clinical laboratories to do REAP analysis as an adjunct to an epidemiologic investigation or as a screening test.

PCR is the technique of choice whenever the suspected agent grows slowly or does not grow in culture. Thus investigators frequently use PCR to study the epidemiology of viral diseases. With bacterial diseases the choice of methods is between REAP, variations on PCR, and PFGE. The authors have used PFGE when investigating the epidemiology of common bacterial pathogens, because PFGE provides excellent typeability, reproducibility, and discriminatory power. In many instances, PFGE has been superior to PCR in terms of reproducibility and discriminatory power (Liu 1997a, De Gheldre et al. 1997). However, we acknowledge that the equipment and supplies for PFGE are more expensive than those for PCR, and the cost of equipment is often very important for the laboratory. Furthermore, PFGE takes about five days to perform, whereas PCR techniques require only one to two days (Table 8-3, also reviewed by Olive and Bean [1999]).

Epidemiologists or directors of clinical laboratories who wish to start doing molecular typing must remember that they cannot introduce these techniques instantaneously. Even if the procedural aspects go well, personnel also must learn how to interpret the results. We would recommend that individuals who wish to implement molecular techniques should spend time in a laboratory that is already using these methods. In this manner, novices can learn both the technical aspects of the methods and also the art of interpreting the results.

Molecular Epidemiology at the University of Iowa Hospitals and Clinics

The University of Iowa Hospitals and Clinics has benefited for years from a symbiotic relationship between the infection control program and the microbiology laboratory. Although we realize that our approach can-

Table 8-3   Comparison of the Costs and Time Required for Genotypic Typing Methods*

	Plasmid Pattern Analysis	Pulsed-Field Gel Electrophoresis	Polymerase Chain Reaction
Supplies ($/run)	8	17	8
Hands-on time (min)	120	125	90
Overall time (days)	1.5	5	1
Equipment costs ($)	2,000–4,000	15,000–20,000	8,000–10,000

Source: Weber S, Pfaller MA, and Herwaldt LA. Role of molecular epidemiology in infection control. Infect. Dis. Clin. North Am.

*We calculated the costs and times based on our experience with doing PCR or PFGE on a batch of 18 strains or with doing plasmid pattern analysis on a batch of 10 strains.

not be generalized to all hospitals, we think that personnel in other hospitals may benefit from our experience. Since 1984, staff from the infection control program and the clinical microbiology laboratory have collaborated closely on numerous investigations of nosocomial infections. To facilitate this collaboration, the laboratory banks all isolates from normally sterile sites and all isolates obtained from documented nosocomial infections. The laboratory saves these isolates for five years. The laboratory also facilitates the infection control effort by processing surveillance cultures and cultures of the environment when the hospital epidemiologist and the laboratory director deem that these cultures are necessary. A team of personnel from both the clinical microbiology laboratory and a research laboratory perform molecular typing in the clinical microbiology laboratory.

In general, we do not conduct full-scale epidemiologic investigations before typing the isolates. We usually screen the organisms by their antibiograms and gather basic demographic and epidemiologic data. If these basic data suggest the possibility of nosocomial transmission, we assess the isolates by automated ribotyping to determine whether they are the same or different. If the ribotypes are all different, we do not type the isolates further. If the ribotypes are all identical or very similar and if the epidemiologic and clinical situation warrants, we do additional typing with PFGE. Moreover, we immediately begin an appropriate epidemiologic investigation and implement interventions while we wait for the typing results if the outbreak includes serious infections.

Over the years, we have saved countless hours, which would have been spent doing case-control studies, by first determining whether isolates were related genetically. We often find that all of the isolates are different and conclude that further epidemiologic investigation is not warranted. For example, we detected an unusual cluster of S. aureus infections in patients on our neurosurgery service. The organisms had similar antibiograms but PFGE demonstrated that each isolate was a unique strain. Therefore we reminded the staff about infection control precautions and the pseudooutbreak disappeared. In contrast, if we find that all of the isolates are the same strain, we carefully determine whether we should conduct a case-control study to identify the source or whether cultures of possible carriers or of potential environmental reservoirs are likely to identify the source more quickly (Meier et al. 1996, Berrouane et al. 1996, Weber et al. 1996). Thus we save time and optimize our resources by tailoring our approach to each cluster or endemic problem.

CONCLUSION

Epidemiologists and clinicians should use typing methods wisely in a hierarchic manner, which entails first using readily available, inexpensive tests and proceeding with more sophisticated typing tests only if the results of the simple tests and the basic epidemiologic investigation indicate that more extensive molecular typing is warranted. We recommend that epidemiologists read several articles to see how a hierarchic approach to typing works in real situations. [For references pertaining to the hierarchic approach to molecular typing methods, see Appendix, section J.]

Epidemiologists also must remember that no individual typing method is ideal. At times, epidemiologists, clinicians, and laboratory staff must combine the results of two or more methods to answer the question at hand. Even more important, molecular typing methods, regardless of their sophistication, cannot replace epidemiologic studies in the arsenal of weapons used by epidemiologists. To be efficient and effective in the twenty-first century, epidemiologists must use both traditional epidemiologic methods and molecular typing methods, choosing their weapons on the basis of what is required to end the current skirmish or battle. At times, one or the other method might suffice; at other times, a combination of both may be required. Even in the situations that require both epidemiologic and molecular epidemiologic studies, the balance of power may shift between battles—some may require more traditional epidemiology and others may require more molecular epidemiology.

REFERENCES

Achtmann M. A surfeit of YATMs? J. Clin. Microbiol. 34:1870, 1996.

Alland D, Kalkut GE, Moss AR, et al. Transmission of tuberculosis in New York City: An analysis by DNA fingerprinting and conventional epidemiological methods. N. Engl. J. Med. 330:1710–1716, 1994.

Arbeit RD, Goering RV, Tenover FC, et al. How to select and interpret molecular strain typing methods for epidemiologic studies of bacterial infections: A review for health care epidemiologists. Infect. Control Hosp. Epidemiol. 18:426–439, 1997.

Arbeit RD. Laboratory procedures for the epidemiologic analysis of microorganisms. In: Murray PR, Baron EJ, Pfaller MA, Tenover FC, Yolken RH, eds. Manual of Clinical Microbiology. 6th ed. Washington, DC: American Society for Microbiology, 1995:190–208.

Arlet G, and Philippon A. PCR-based approaches for the detection of bacterial resistance. In: Erlich HA, ed. PCR Technology: Principles and Applications for DNA Amplification. New York: WH Freeman & Co., 1992:665–687.

Arroyo JC, Jordan W, Lema MW, et al. Diversity of plasmids in *Achromobacter xylosoxidans* isolates responsible for a seemingly common-source nosocomial outbreak. J. Clin. Microbiol. 25:1952–1955, 1987.

Arthur M, Arbeit RD, Kim C, et al. Restriction fragment length polymorphisms among uropathogenic *Escherichia coli* isolates: Pap-related sequences compared with rrn operons. Infect. Immun. 58:471–479, 1990.

Back NA, Linnemann CC, Pfaller MA, and Staneck JL. Recurrent epidemics caused by a single strain of erythromycin-resistant *Staphylococcus aureus*. The importance of molecular epidemiology. JAMA. 270:1329–1333, 1993.

Bergeron MG, and Oullette M. Preventing antibiotic resistance using rapid DNA-based diagnostic tests. Infect. Control Hosp. Epidemiol. 19:560–564, 1998.

Berrouane YF, McNutt LA, Buschelman BJ, et al. An outbreak of severe *P. aeruginosa* infections caused by a contaminated whirlpool tub drain. Abstract SHEA, Washington, DC, April, 1996.

Blackall PJ, Fegan N, Chew GT, and Hampson DJ. Population structure and diversity of avian isolates of *Pasteurella multocida* from Australia. Microbiology. 144 (Pt 2):279–289, 1998.

Boettger EC, Teske A, Kirschner P, et al. Disseminated infections with "*Mycobacterium genavense*" in patients with AIDS. Lancet. 340:76–80, 1992.

Boyce JM, Opal SM, Potter-Bynoe G, et al. Emergence and nosocomial transmission of ampicillin-resistant enterococci. Antimicrob. Agents Chemother. 36:1032–1039, 1992.

Boyce JM, Opal SM, Potter-Bynoe G, and Medeiros AA. Spread of methicillin–resistant *Staphylococcus aureus* in a hospital after exposure to a health care worker with chronic sinusitis. Clin. Infect. Dis. 17:496–504, 1993.

Boyce JM, Potter-Bynoe G, Opal SM, Dziobek L, and Medeiros AA. A common-source outbreak of *Staphylococcus epidermidis* infections among patients undergoing cardiac surgery. J. Infect. Dis. 161:493–499, 1990.

Chen Y-S, Marshall SA, Winokur PL, et al. Use of molecular and reference susceptibility testing methods in a multicenter evaluation of MicroScan dried overnight gram-positive MIC panels for detection of vancomycin and high-level aminoglycoside resistances in enterococci. J. Clin. Microbiol. 36:2996–3001, 1998.

Cimolai N, Trombley C, Wensley D, and LeBlanc J. Heterogeneous *Serratia marcescens* genotypes from a nosocomial pediatric outbreak. Chest. 111:194–197, 1997.

Cohen J, and Holden DW. Use of randomly amplified polymorphic DNA markers to distinguish isolates of *Aspergillus fumigatus*. J. Clin. Microbiol. 30:2991–2993, 1992.

Collier MC, Stock F, DeGirolami PC, Samore MH, and Cartwright CP. Comparison of PCR-based approaches to molecular epidemiologic analysis of *Clostridium difficile*. J. Clin. Microbiol. 34:1153–1157, 1996.

Cookson ST, Corrales JL, Lotero JO, et al. Disco fever: Epidemic meningococcal disease in northeastern Argentina associated with disco patronage. J. Infect. Dis. 178:266–269, 1998.

Cormican MG, Wilke WW, Barrett MS, Pfaller MA, and Jones RN. Phenotypic detection of mec A-positive staphylococcal bloodstream isolates: High accuracy of simple disk diffusion tests. Diagn. Microbiol. Infect. Dis. 25: 107–112, 1996.

De Gheldre Y, Maes N, Rost F, et al. Molecular epidemiology of an outbreak of multidrug-resistant *Enterobacter aerogenes* infections and in vivo emergence of imipenem resistance. J. Clin. Microbiol. 35:152–160, 1997.

Desai M, Tanna A, Wall R, et al. Fluorescent amplified-fragment length polymorphism analysis of an outbreak of group A streptococcal invasive disease. J. Clin. Microbiol. 36:3133–3137, 1998.

Echeita MA, and Usera MA. Chromosomal rearrangements in *Salmonella enterica* serotype typhi affecting molecular typing in outbreak investigations. J. Clin. Microbiol. 36:2123–2126, 1998.

Falkiner FR. Epidemiological typing: A user's view. J. Hosp. Infect. 11(suppl A):303–309, 1988.

Farmer JJ. Conventional typing methods. J. Hosp. Infect. 11(suppl A):309–314, 1988.

Goh SH, Byrne SK, Zhang JL, and Chow AW. Molecular typing of *Staphylococcus aureus* on the basis of coagulase gene polymorphisms. J. Clin. Microbiol. 30:1642–1645, 1992.

Gordillo ME, Singh KV, and Murray BE. Comparison of ribotyping and pulsed-field gel electrophoresis for subspecies differentiation of strains of *Enterococcus faecalis*. J. Clin. Microbiol. 31:1570–1574, 1993.

Grandsen WR, Eykyn SJ, and Phillips I. Pneumococcal bacteremia: 325 episodes diagnosed at St. Thomas's Hospital. Br. Med. J. 290:505–508, 1985.

Gustaferro CA. Chemiluminescent riobotyping. In: Persing DH, et al., eds. Diagnostic Molecular Microbiology: Principles and Applications. Washington, DC: American Society for Microbiology, 1993:584–589.

Hance AJ, Grandchamp B, Lévy-Frébault V, et al. Detection and identification of mycobacteria by amplification of mycobacterial DNA. Mol. Microbiol. 3:843–849, 1989.

Hawkey PM. Molecular methods for the investigation of bacterial cross-infection. J. Hosp. Infect. 9:211–218, 1987.

Helms CM, Massanari M, Zeitler R, et al. Legionnaires' disease associated with a hospital water system: A cluster of 24 nosocomial cases. Ann. Intern. Med. 99:172–178, 1983.

Herwaldt LA, Boyken LD, and Pfaller MA. Biotyping of coagulase-negative staphylococci: 108 isolates from nosocomial bloodstream infections. Diagn. Microbiol. Infect. Dis. 13:461–466, 1990.

Jarvis WR. Usefulness of molecular epidemiology for outbreak investigations. Infect. Control Hosp. Epidemiol. 15:500–503, 1994.

John JF. Molecular analysis of nosocomial epidemics. Infect. Dis. Clin. North Am. 3:683–700, 1989.

Jones RN, Marshall SA, Pfaller MA, et al. Nosocomial enterococcal blood stream infections in the SCOPE Program: Antimicrobial resistance, species occurrence, molecular testing results, and laboratory testing accuracy. Diagn. Microbiol. Infect. Dis. 29:95–102, 1997.

Keller DW, Hajjeh R, DeMaria A, et al. Community outbreak of Legionnaires' disease: An investigation confirming the potential for cooling towers to transmit Legionella species. Clin. Infect. Dis. 22:257–261, 1996.

Kertesz DA, Byrne SK, and Chow AW. Characterization of *Neisseria meningitidis* by polymerase chain reaction and restriction endonuclease digestion of the porA gene. J. Clin. Microbiol. 31:2594–2598, 1993.

Kitada K, Oka S, Kimura S, et al. Detection of *Pneumocystis carinii* sequences by polymerase chain reaction: Animal models and clinical application to noninvasive specimen. J. Clin. Microbiol. 29:1985–1990, 1991.

Lai KK, Brown BA, Westerling JA, et al. Long-term laboratory contamination by *Mycobacterium abscessus* resulting in two pseudo-outbreaks: Recognition with use of random amplified polymorphic DNA (RAPD) polymerase chain reaction. Clin. Infect. Dis. 27:169–175, 1998.

Lessing MP, Jordens JZ, and Bowler IC. Molecular epidemiology of a multiple strain outbreak of methicillin-resistant *Staphylococcus aureus* amongst patients and staff. J. Hosp. Infect. 31:253–260, 1995.

Liu PY, Ke SC, and Chen SL. Use of pulsed-field gel electrophoresis to investigate a pseudo-outbreak of *Bacillus cereus* in a pediatric unit. J. Clin. Microbiol. 35:1533–1535, 1997a.

Liu PY, and Wu WL. Use of different PCR-based DNA fingerprinting techniques and pulsed-field gel electrophoresis to investigate the epidemiology of *Acinetobacter calcoaceticus-Acinetobacter baumannii* complex. Diagn. Microbiol. Infect. Dis. 29:19–28, 1997b.

Loudon KW, Burne JP, Coke AP, and Matthews RC. Application of polymerase chain reaction to fingerprinting *Aspergillus fumigatus* by random amplification of polymorphic DNA. J. Clin. Microbiol. 31:1117–1121, 1993.

Louie L, Louie M, and Simor AE. Investigation of a pseudo-outbreak of Nocardia asteroides infection by pulsed-field gel electrophoresis and randomly amplified polymorphic DNA PCR. J. Clin. Microbiol. 35:1582–1584, 1997.

Louie M, Jayaratne P, Luchsinger, et al. Comparison of ribotyping, arbitrarily primed PCR, and pulsed-field gel electrophoresis for molecular typing of *Listeria monocytogenes*. J. Clin. Microbiol. 34:15–19, 1996.

Maki DG, Rhame FS, Mackel DC, and Bennett JV. Nationwide epidemic of septicemia caused by contaminated intravenous products. I. Epidemiologic and clinical features. Am. J. Med. 60:471–485, 1976.

Marshall SA, Wilke WW, Pfaller MA, and Jones RN. *Staphylococcus aureus* and coagulase-negative staphylococci from bloodstream infections: Frequency of occurrence, antimicrobial susceptibility, and molecular (mec A) characterization of oxacillin resistance in the SCOPE program. Diagn. Microbiol. Infect. Dis. 30:205–214, 1998.

Maslow J, and Mulligan ME. Epidemiologic typing systems. Infect. Control Hosp. Epidemiol. 17:595–604, 1996.

Maslow J, Slutsky AM, and Arbeit RD. The application of pulsed field gel electrophoresis to molecular epidemiology. In: Persing DH, et al., eds. Diagnostic Molecular Microbiology: Principles and Applications. Washington, DC: American Society for Microbiology, 1993:563–572.

Maslow JN, Mulligan ME, and Arbeit RD. Molecular epidemiology: the application of contemporary techniques to typing bacteria. Clin. Infect. Dis. 17:153–164, 1993.

McCreedy BJ, and Callaway TH. Laboratory design and work flow. In: Persing DH, et al., eds. Diagnostic Molecular Microbiology: Principles and Applications. Washington, DC: American Society for Microbiology, 1993: 149–159.

McLaughlin GL, Howe DK, Bigg DR, et al. Amplification of rDNA loci to detect and type *Neisseria meningitidis* and other eubacteria. Mol. Cell Probes. 7:7–17, 1993.

Meenhorst PL, Reingold AL, Groothuis DG, et al. Water-related nosocomial pneumonia caused by *Legionella pneumophila* serogroups 1 and 10. J. Infect. Dis. 152:356–364, 1985.

Meier PA, Carter CD, Wallace SE, et al. Eradication of methicillin–resistant *Staphylococcus aureus* from the burn unit at a tertiary medical center. Infect. Control Hosp. Epidemiol. 17:798–802, 1996.

Meyers JA, Sanchez D, Elwell LP, and Falkow S. Simple agarose gel electrophoretic method for the identification and characterization of plasmid deoxyribonucleic acid. J. Bacteriol. 127:1529–1537, 1976.

Moro ML, Gori A, Errante I, et al. An outbreak of multidrug-resistant tuberculosis involving HIV-infected patients of two hospitals in Milan, Italy. Italian Multidrug-Resistant Tuberculosis Outbreak Study Group. AIDS. 12:1095–1102, 1998.

Mulligan ME, Kwok RYY, Citron DM, John JF Jr, and Smith PB. Immunoblots, antimicrobial resistance, and bacteriophage typing of oxacillin–resistant *Staphylococcus aureus*. J. Clin. Microbiol. 26:2395–2401, 1988a.

Mulligan ME, Peterson LR, Kwok RYY, Clabots CR, and Gerding DN. Immunoblots and plasmid fingerprints compared with serotyping and polyacrylamid gel electrophoresis for typing *Clostridium difficile*. J. Clin. Microbiol. 26:41–46, 1988b.

Nachamkin I, Bohachick K, and Patton CM. Flagellin gene typing of *Campylobacter jejuni* by restriction fragment length polymorphism analysis. J. Clin. Microbiol. 31:1531–1536, 1993.

Niesters HGM, Goessens WHF, Meis JFMG, and Quint WGV. Rapid, polymerase chain reaction-based identification assays for *Candida* species. J. Clin. Microbiol. 31:904–910, 1993.

Norman AF, Regnery R, Jameson P, Greene C, and Krause DC. Differentiation of bartonella-like isolates at the species level by PCR-restriction fragment length polymorphism in the citrate synthase gene. J. Clin. Microbiol. 33:1797–1803, 1995.

O'Brien OJ, Ross DG, Guzman MA, et al. Dissemination of an antibiotic resistance plasmid in hospital patient flora. Antimicrob. Agents Chemother. 17:537–543, 1980.

Olive DM, and Bean P. Principles and applications of methods for DNA-based typing of microbial organisms. J. Clin. Microbiol. 37: 1661–1669, 1999.

Paton S, Nicolle L, Mwongera M, et al. *Salmonella* and *Shigella* gastroenteritis at a public teaching hospital in Nairobi, Kenya. Infect. Control Hosp. Epidemiol. 12:710–717, 1991.

Perl TM, Kruger W, Houston A, et al. Investigation of suspected nosocomial clusters of *Staphylococcus haemolyticus* infections. Infect. Control Hosp. Epidemiol. 20:128–131, 1999.

Persing DH, Relman DA, and Tenover FC. Genotypic detection of antimicrobial resistance. In: Persing DH, ed. PCR Protocols for Emerging Infectious Diseases. Washington, DC: American Society for Microbiology, 1996:33–57.

Persing DH. Target selection and optimization of amplification reactions. In: Persing DH, et al., eds. Diagnostic Molecular Microbiology: Principles and Applications. Washington, DC: American Society for Microbiology, 1993: 88–104.

Pfaller MA, and Herwaldt LA. The clinical microbiology laboratory and infection control: Emerging pathogens, antimicrobial resistance and new technology. Clin. Infect. Dis. 25:858–870, 1997.

Pfaller MA, Hollis RJ, and Sader HS. Chromosomal restriction fragment analysis by pulsed-field gel electrophoresis. In: Isenberg HD, ed. Clinical Microbiology Procedures Handbook. Washington, DC: American Society of Microbiology, 1992:10.5c.1–10.6.3.

Pfaller MA, Lockhart SR, Pujol C, et al. Hospital specificity, region specificity, and fluconazole resistance of *Candida albicans* bloodstream isolates. J. Clin. Microbiol. 36:1518–1529, 1998.

Pfaller MA, Wendt C, Hollis RJ, et al. Comparative evaluation of an automated ribotyping system versus pulsed-field gel electrophoresis for epidemiological typing of clinical isolates of *Escherichia coli* and *Pseudomonas aeruginosa* from patients with recurrent gram-negative bacteremia. Diagn. Microbiol. Infect. Dis. 25:1–8, 1996.

Prevost G, Jaulhac B, and Piemont Y. DNA fingerprinting by pulsed-field gel electrophoresis is more effective than ribotyping in distinguishing among methicillin–resistant *Staphylococcus aureus* isolates. J. Clin. Microbiol. 30: 967–973, 1992.

Prodinger WM, Fille M, Bauernfeind A, et al. Molecular epidemiology of *Klebsiella pneumoniae* producing SHV-5 beta-lactamase. Parallel outbreaks due to multiple plasmid transfer. J. Clin. Microbiol. 34:564–568, 1996.

Relman DA, Schmidt TM, MacDermott RP, et al. Identification of the uncultured bacillus of Whipple's disease. N. Engl. J. Med. 327:293–301, 1992.

Sader HS, Hollis RJ, and Pfaller MA. The use of molecular techniques in the epidemiology and control of infectious diseases. Clin. Lab. Med. 15:407–431, 1995.

Schmid J, Voss E, and Soll DR. Computer-assisted methods for assessing strain relatedness in *Candida albicans* by fingerprinting with the moderately repetitive sequence Ca3. J. Clin. Microbiol. 28:1236–1243, 1990.

Schwartz DC, and Cantor CR. Separation of yeast chromosome-sized DNAs by pulsed-field gradient gel electrophoresis. Cell. 37: 67–75, 1984.

Smart LE, Dougall AJ, and Girdwood RWA. New 23-valent pneumococcal vaccine in relation to pneumococcal serotypes in systemic and non-systemic disease. J. Infect. 14:209–215, 1987.

Soria G, Barbe J, and Gibert I. Molecular fingerprinting of *Salmonella typhimurium* by IS200-typing as a tool for epidemiological and evolutionary studies. Microbiologia. 10:57–68, 1994.

Struelens MJ and the Members of the European Study Group on Epidemiological Markers of the European Society for Clinical Microbiology and Infectious Diseases. Consensus guidelines for appropriate use and evaluation of microbial epidemiologic typing systems. Clin. Microbiol. Infect. 2:2–11, 1996.

Struelens MJ, DeGheldre Y, and Deplano A. Comparative and library epidemiological typing systems: Outbreak investigations versus surveillance systems. Infect. Control Hosp. Epidemiol. 19:565–569, 1998.

Stull TL, LiPuma JJ, and Edlind TD. A broad-spectrum probe for molecular epidemiology of bacteria: ribosomal RNA. J. Infect. Dis. 157:280–286, 1988.

Sung KG, Kim SB, Choi JH, et al. Detection of Mycobacterium leprae DNA in formalin-fixed, paraffin-embedded samples from multibacillary and paucibacillary leprosy patient by polymerase chain reaction. Int. J. Dermatol. 32:710–713, 1993.

Taylor DN, Wachsmuth IK, Shangkuan Y-H, et al. Salmonellosis associated with marijuana: A multistate outbreak traced by plasmid fingerprinting. N. Engl. J. Med. 306:1249–1253, 1982.

Telenti A, Marchesi F, Balz M, et al. Rapid identification of Mycobacteria to the species level by polymerase chain reaction and restriction enzyme analysis. J. Clin. Microbiol. 31:175–178, 1993.

Tenover FC, Arbeit RD, Archer G, et al. Comparison of traditional and molecular methods of typing isolates of *Staphylococcus aureus*. J. Clin. Microbiol. 32:407–415, 1994.

Tenover FC, Arbeit RD, Goering RV, et al. Interpreting chromosomal DNA restriction patterns produced by pulsed-field gel electrophoresis: Criteria for bacterial strain typing. J. Clin. Microbiol. 33:2233–2239, 1995a.

Tenover FC, Popovic T, and Olsvik O. Genetic methods for detecting antibacterial resistance genes. In: Murray PR, Baron EJ, Pfaller MA, Tenover FC, Yolken RH, eds. Manual of Clinical Microbiology. 6th ed. Washington, DC: American Society for Microbiology, 1995b: 1368–1378.

Tomayko JF, and Murray BE. Analysis of *Enterococcus faecalis* isolates from intercontinental sources by multilocus enzyme electrophoresis and pulsed-field gel electrophoresis. J. Clin. Microbiol. 33:2903–2907, 1995.

Torrea G, Offredo C, Simonet M, et al. Evaluation of tuberculosis transmission in a community by 1 year of systematic typing of *Mycobacterium tuberculosis* clinical isolates. J. Clin. Microbiol. 34:1043–1049, 1996.

van Belkum A, De Jonckheere J, and Quint WGV. Genotyping *Naegleria fowleri* isolates by interrepeat polymerase chain reaction. J. Clin. Microbiol. 30:2595–2598, 1992.

van Belkum A, Melchers WJ, Ijsseldijk C, et al. Outbreak of amoxicillin-resistant *Haemophilus influenzae* type b: Variable number of tandem repeats as novel molecular markers. J. Clin. Microbiol. 35:1517–1520, 1997.

van Embden JDA, Cave MD, Crawford JT, et al. Strain identification of *Mycobacterium tuberculosis* by DNA fingerprinting: Recommendations for a standardized methodology. J. Clin. Microbiol. 31:406–409, 1993.

Versalovic J, Koeuth T, and Lupski JR. Distribution of repetitive DNA sequences in eubacteria and application to fingerprinting of bacterial genomes. Nucleic Acids Res. 19:6823–6831, 1991.

Villanueva A, Calderon RV, Vargas BA, et al. Report on an outbreak of postinjection abscesses due to *Mycobacterium abscessus*, including management with surgery and clarithromycin therapy and comparison of strains by random amplified polymorphic DNA polymerase chain reaction. Clin. Infect. Dis. 24:1147–1153, 1997.

von Weizsacker F, Blum HE, and Wands JR. Polymerase chain reaction analysis of Hepatitis B virus DNA in formalin-fixed, paraffin-embedded liver biopsies from alcoholics using a simplified and standardized amplification protocol. J. Hepatol. 20:646–649, 1994.

Wachsmuth K. Molecular epidemiology of bacterial infections: Examples of methodology and of investigations of outbreaks. Rev. Infect. Dis. 8:682–692, 1986.

Weber S, Barr BA, Delius, RE, et al. Outbreak of methicillin-susceptible *Staphylococcus aureus* mediastinitis and high frequency of nasal carriage among staff on a pediatric cardiothoracic surgery service. SHEA, Washington, DC, April, 1996.

Wendt C, Messer SA, Hollis RJ, et al. Molecular epidemiology of gram-negative bacteremia. Clin. Infect. Dis. 28:605–610, 1999a.

Wendt C, Messer SA, Hollis RJ, et al. Recurrent gram-negative bacteremia: Incidence and clinical patterns. Clin. Infect. Dis. 28:611–617, 1999b.

Whittam TS, Wachsmuth IK, and Wilson RA. Genetic evidence of clonal descent of *Escherichia coli* O157:H7 associated with hemorrhagic colitis and hemolytic uremic syndrome. J. Infect. Dis. 157:1124–1133, 1988.

Widmer AF, Boyken LA, Hollis RJ, et al. Evaluation of three molecular typing methods for *Staphylococcus aureus* for clinical microbiology laboratories. Abstract 32th ICCAC, Anaheim, CA, 1992.

Woods CR, Versalovic J, Koeuth T, and Lupski JR. Analysis of relationships among isolates of *Citrobacter diversus* by using DNA fingerprints generated by repetitive sequence-based primers in the polymerase chain reaction. J. Clin. Microbiol. 30:2921–2929, 1992.

Yusof JHM, Flower AJE, and Teo CG. Transmission of Hepatitis B virus analysed by conformation dependent polymorphisms of single stranded viral DNA. J. Infect. Dis. 169:62–67, 1994.

Zhu P, Hu X, and Xu L. Typing *Neisseria meninitidis* by analysis of restriction fragment length polymorphisms in the gene encoding the class 1 outer membrane protein: Application to assessment of epidemics throughout the last 4 decades in China. J. Clin. Microbiol. 33:458–462, 1995.

APPENDIX

A. Library Typing Methods: Repetitive PCR Space Typing

Arthur M, Arbeit RD, Kim C, et al. Restriction fragment length polymorphisms among uropathogenic *Escherichia coli* isolates: Pap-related sequences compared with rrn operons. Infect. Immun. 58:471–479, 1990.

Grandsen WR, Eykyn SJ, Phillips I. Pneumococcal bacteremia: 325 episodes diagnosed at St. Thomas's Hospital. Br. Med. J. 290:505–508, 1985.

Helms CM, Massanari M, Zeitler R, et al. Legionnaires' disease associated with a hospital water system: a cluster of 24 nosocomial cases. Ann. Intern. Med. 99:172–178, 1983.

Meenhorst PL, Reingold AL, Groothuis DG, et al. Water-related nosocomial pneumonia caused by *Legionella pneumophila* serogroups 1 and 10. J. Infect. Dis. 152:356–364, 1985.

Mulligan ME, Kwok RYY, Citron DM, John JF Jr, Smith PB. Immunoblots, antimicrobial resistance, and bacteriophage typing of oxacillin-resistant *Staphylococcus aureus*. J. Clin. Microbiol. 26:2395–2401, 1988a.

Mulligan ME, Peterson LR, Kwok RYY, Clabots CR, Gerding DN. Immunoblots and plasmid fingerprints compared with serotyping and polyacrylamid gel electrophoresis for typing *Clostridium difficile*. J. Clin. Microbiol. 26:41–46, 1988b.

Smart LE, Dougall AJ, Girdwood RWA. New 23-valent pneumococcal vaccine in relation to pneumococcal serotypes in systemic and non-systemic disease. J. Infect. 14:209–215, 1987.

Whittam TS, Wachsmuth IK, Wilson RA. Genetic evidence of clonal descent of *Escherichia coli* O157:H7 associated with hemorrhagic colitis and hemolytic uremic syndrome. J. Infect. Dis. 157:1124–1133, 1988.

B. DNA Typing Methods: Distinguishing between Colonizing and Infecting Isolates in Individual Patients

Reagan DR, Pfaller MA, Hollis RJ, Wenzel RP. Nosocomial candidemia: Characterization of the sequence of colonization and infection using DNA fingerprinting and a DNA probe. J. Clin. Microbiol. 28:2733–2378, 1990.

Swaminathan B, Matar GM. Molecular typing methods: definitions, applications, and advantages. In: Persing DH, Smith TF, Tenover FC, White TJ, eds. Diagnostic Molecular Microbiology: Principles and Applications. Washington, DC: American Society for Microbiology, 1993:26–50.

Voss A, Hollis RJ, Pfaller MA, Wenzel RP, Doebbeling BN. Investigation of the sequence of colonization and candidemia in non-neutropenic patients. J. Clin. Microbiol. 32:975–980, 1994.

C. DNA Typing Methods: Distinguishing between Contaminating and Infecting Strains

Herwaldt LA, Boyken LD, Pfaller MA. Biotyping of coagulase-negative staphylococci: 108 isolates from nosocomial bloodstream infections. Diagn. Microbiol. Infect. Dis. 13:461–466, 1990.

Tenover FC. Plasmid fingerprinting: A tool for bacterial strain identification and surveillance of nosocomial and community acquired infections. Clin. Lab. Med. 5:413–436, 1985.

D. DNA Typing Methods: Documenting Cross-Infection among Hospitalized Patients

Back NA, Linnemann CC, Pfaller MA, Staneck JL. Recurrent epidemics caused by a single strain of erythromycin-resistant *Staphylococcus aureus*. The importance of molecular epidemiology. JAMA 270:1329–1333, 1993.

Bingen EH, Weber M, Dorelle J, et al. Arbitrarily primed polymerase chain reaction as a rapid method to differentiate crossed from independent *Pseudomonas cepacia* infections in cystic fibrosis patients. J. Clin. Microbiol. 31:2589–2593, 1993.

Boyce JM, Potter-Bynoe G, Opal SM, Dziobek L, Medeiros AA. A common-source outbreak of *Staphylococcus epidermidis* infections among patients undergoing cardiac surgery. J. Infect. Dis. 161:493–499, 1990.

Diekema DJ, Barr J, Boyken LD, et al. A cluster of serious Escherichia coli infections in a neonatal intensive-care unit. Infect. Control Hosp. Epidemiol. 18:774–776, 1997a.

Diekema DJ, Messer SA, Hollis RJ, Wenzel RP, Pfaller MA. An outbreak of *Candida parapsilosis* prosthetic valve endocarditis. Diagn. Microbiol. Infect. Dis. 29:147–153, 1997b.

Meier PA, Carter CD, Wallace SE, et al. Eradication of methicillin-resistant *Staphylococcus aureus* from the burn unit at a tertiary medical center. Infect. Control Hosp. Epidemiol. 17:798–802, 1996.

Pfaller MA, Lockhart SR, Pujol C, et al. Hospital specificity, region specificity, and fluconazole resistance of *Candida albicans* bloodstream isolates. J. Clin. Microbiol. 36:1518–1529, 1998.

Sader HS, Pignatari AC, Leme I, et al. Epidemiologic typing of multiply drug-resistant *Pseudomonas aeruginosa* isolated from an outbreak in an intensive care unit. Diagn. Microbiol. Infect. Dis. 17:13–18, 1993.

E. DNA Typing Methods: Evaluating Reinfection Versus Relapse in Patients

Arbeit RD, Slutsky A, Barber TW, et al. Genetic diversity among strains of *Mycobacterium avium* causing monoclona and polyclonal bacteremia in patients with AIDS. J. Infect. Dis. 167:1384–1390, 1993.

Maslow JN, Whittam T, Wilson RA, et al. Clonal relationship among bloodstream isolates of *Escherichia coli*. Infect. Immun. 63:2409–2417, 1995.

Pfaller MA, Wendt C, Hollis RJ, et al. Comparative evaluation of an automated ribotyping system versus pulsed-field gel electrophoresis for epidemiological typing of clinical isolates of *Escherichia coli* and *Pseudomonas aeruginosa* from patients with recurrent gram-negative bacteremia. Diagn. Microbiol. Infect. Dis. 25:1–8, 1996.

Wendt C, Messer SA, Hollis RJ, et al. Molecular epidemiology of gram-negative bacteremia. Clin. Infect. Dis. 28:605–610, 1999a.

Wendt C, Messer SA, Hollis RJ, et al. Recurrent gram-negative bacteremia: Incidence and clinical patterns. Clin. Infect. Dis. 28:611–617, 1999b.

F. DNA Typing Methods: Surveillance of Resistant Pathogens within and among Hospitals Over Time

Back NA, Linnemann CC, Pfaller MA, Staneck JL. Recurrent epidemics caused by a single strain of erythromycin-resistant *Staphylococc-*

cus aureus. The importance of molecular epidemiology. JAMA 270:1329–1333, 1993.

Jones RN, Marshall SA, Pfaller MA, et al. Nosocomial enterococcal blood stream infections in the SCOPE Program: Antimicrobial resistance, species occurrence, molecular testing results, and laboratory testing accuracy. Diagn. Microbiol. Infect. Dis. 29:95–102, 1997.

Marshall SA, Wilke WW, Pfaller MA, Jones RN. *Staphylococcus aureus* and coagulase-negative staphylococci from bloodstream infections: Frequency of occurrence, antimicrobial susceptibility, and molecular (mec A) characterization of oxacillin resistance in the SCOPE program. Diagn. Microbiol. Infect. Dis. 30:205–214, 1998.

Pfaller MA, Lockhart SR, Pujol C, et al. Hospital specificity, region specificity, and fluconazole resistance of *Candida albicans* bloodstream isolates. J. Clin. Microbiol. 36:1518–1529, 1998.

Sader HS, Pignatari AC, Leme I, et al. Epidemiologic typing of multiply drug-resistant *Pseudomonas aeruginosa* isolated from an outbreak in an intensive care unit. Diagn. Microbiol. Infect. Dis. 17:13–18, 1993.

G. DNA Typing Methods: Reviews

Arbeit RD, Goering RV, Tenover FC, et al. How to select and interpret molecular strain typing methods for epidemiologic studies of bacterial infections: A review for health care epidemiologists. Infect. Control Hosp. Epidemiol. 18:426–439, 1997.

Arbeit RD. Laboratory procedures for the epidemiologic analysis of microorganisms. In: Murray PR, Baron EJ, Pfaller MA, Tenover FC, Yolken RH, eds. Manual of Clinical Microbiology. 6th ed. Washington, DC: American Society for Microbiology, 1995:190–208.

Maslow J, Mulligan ME. Epidemiologic typing systems. Infect. Control Hosp. Epidemiol. 17:595–604, 1996.

Pfaller MA, Herwaldt LA. The clinical microbiology laboratory and infection control: Emerging pathogens, antimicrobial resistance and new technology. Clin. Infect. Dis. 25:858–870, 1997.

Struelens MJ and the Members of the European Study Group on Epidemiological Markers of the European Society for Clinical Microbiology and Infectious Diseases. Consensus guidelines for appropriate use and evaluation of microbial epidemiologic typing systems. Clin. Microbiol. Infect. 2:2–11, 1996.

Struelens MJ, DeGheldre Y, Deplano A. Comparative and library epidemiological typing systems: outbreak investigations versus surveillance systems. Infect. Control Hosp. Epidemiol. 19:565–569, 1998.

Tenover FC, Arbeit RD, Goering RV, et al. Interpreting chromosomal DNA restriction patterns produced by pulsed-field gel electrophoresis: Criteria for bacterial strain typing. J. Clin. Microbiol. 33:2233–2239, 1995.

H. Examples of Pulsed-Field Gel Electrophoresis

Ackers ML, Mahon BE, Leahy E, et al. An outbreak of *Escherichia coli* 0157:H7 infections associated with leaf lettuce consumption. J. Infect. Dis. 177:1588–1593, 1998.

Ackman D, Marks S, Mack P, et al. Swimming–associated haemorrhagic colitis due to *Escherichia coli* 0157:H7 infection: evidence of prolonged contamination of fresh water lake. Epidemiol. Infect. 119:1–8, 1997.

Beall B, Cassiday PK, Sanden GN. Analysis of *Bordetella pertussis* isolates from an epidemic by pulsed-field gel electrophoresis. J. Clin. Microbiol. 33:3083–3086, 1995.

Brett MS, Short P, McLauchlin J. A small outbreak of listeriosis associated with smoked mussels. Int. J. Food Microbiol. 43:223–229, 1998.

Cody SH, Glynn MK, Farrar JA, et al. An outbreak of *Escherichia coli* 0157:H7 infection from unpasteurized commercial apple juice. Ann. Intern. Med. 130:202–209, 1999.

Dib JC, Dube M, Kelly C, Rinaldi MG, Patterson JE. Evaluation of pulsed-field gel electrophoresis as a typing system for *Candida rugosa*: Comparison of karyotype and restriction fragment length polymorphisms. J. Clin. Microbiol. 34:1494–1496, 1996.

Diekema DJ, Messer SA, Hollis RJ, Wenzel RP, Pfaller MA. An outbreak of *Candida parapsilosis* prosthetic valve endocarditis. Diagn. Microbiol. Infect. Dis. 29:147–153, 1997b.

DuPont HL. Nosocomial salmonellosis and shigellosis. Infection Control & Hospital Epidemiology 1991; 12(12):707–709.

Edmond MB, Hollis RJ, Houston AK, Wenzel RP. Molecular epidemiology of an outbreak of meningococcal disease in a university community. J. Clin. Microbiol. 33:2209–2211, 1995.

Isaac-Renton JL, Cordeiro C, Sarafis K, Shahriari H. Characterization of *Giardia duodenalis* isolates from a waterborne outbreak. J. Infect. Dis. 167:431–440, 1993.

Izumiya H, Terajima J, Wada A, et al. Molecular typing of enterohemorrhagic *Escherichia coli* 0157:H7 isolates in Japan by using pulsed-field gel electrophoresis. J. Clin. Microbiol. 35:1675–1680, 1997.

Jelfs J, Jalaludin B, Munro R, et al. A cluster of meningococcal disease in western Sydney, Australia, initially associated with a nightclub. Epidemiol. Infect. 120:263–270, 1998.

Jochimsen EM, Frenette C, Delorme M, et al. A cluster of bloodstream infections and pyrogenic reactions among hemodialysis patients traced to dialysis machine waste-handling option units. Am. J. Nephrol. 18:485–489, 1998.

Kool JL, Fiore AE, Kioski CM, et al. More than 10 years of unrecognized nosocomial transmission of legionnaires' disease among transplant patients. Infect. Control Hosp. Epidemiol. 19:898–904, 1998.

La Scola B, Fournier PE, Musso D, Tissot-Dupont H. Pseudo-outbreak of listeriosis elucidated by pulsed-field gel electrophoresis. Eur. J. Clin. Microbiol. Infect. Dis. 16:756–760, 1997.

Liu PY, Ke SC, Chen SL. Use of pulsed-field gel electrophoresis to investigate a pseudo-outbreak of Bacillus cereus in a pediatric unit. J. Clin. Microbiol. 35:1533–1535, 1997a.

Luzzaro F, Perilli M, Migliavacca R, et al. Repeated epidemics caused by extended-spectrum beta-lactamase–producing Serratia marcescens strains. Eur. J. Clin. Microbiol. Infect. Dis. 17:629–636, 1998.

Mahalingam S, Cheong YM, Kan S, et al. Molecular epidemiologic analysis of Vibrio cholerae O1 isolates by pulsed-field gel electrophoresis. J. Clin. Microbiol. 32:2975–2979, 1994.

Miranda G, Kelly C, Solorzano F, et al. Use of pulsed-field gel electrophoresis typing to study an outbreak of infection due to Serratia marcescens in a neonatal intensive care unit. J. Clin. Microbiol. 34:3138–3141, 1996.

Puohiniemi R, Heiskanen T, Siitonen A. Molecular epidemiology of two international sproutborne Salmonella outbreaks. J. Clin. Microbiol. 35:2487–2491, 1997.

Sarafis K, Isaac-Renton J. Pulsed-field gel electrophoresis as a method of biotyping of Giardia duodenalis. Am. J. Trop. Med. Hyg. 48:133–144, 1993.

Sobel J, Cameron DN, Ismail J, et al. A prolonged outbreak of Shigella sonnei infections in traditionally observant Jewish communities in North America caused by a molecularly distinct bacterial subtype. J. Infect. Dis. 177:1405–1409, 1998.

Stephens CP, On SL, Gibson JA. An outbreak of infectious hepatitis in commercially reared ostriches associated with Campylobacter coli and Campylobacter jejuni. Vet. Microbiol. 61:183–190, 1998.

Thong KL, Puthucheary S, Pang T. Outbreak of Salmonella enteritidis gastroenteritis: Investigation by pulsed-field gel electrophoresis. Int. J. Infect. Dis. 2:159–163, 1998.

Van Beneden CA, Keene WE, Strang RA, et al. Multinational outbreak of Salmonella enterica serotype newport infections due to contaminated alfalfa sprouts. JAMA 281:158–162, 1999.

Vigeant P, Loo VG, Bertrand C, et al. An outbreak of Serratia marcescens infections related to contaminated chlorhexidine. Infect. Control Hosp. Epidemiol. 19:791–794, 1998.

Welbel SF, McNeil MM, Kuykendall RJ, et al. Candida parapsilosis bloodstream infections in neonatal intensive care unit patients: Epidemiologic and laboratory confirmation of a common source outbreak. Pediatr. Infect. Dis. J. 15:998–1002, 1996.

I. Outbreak Investigation: Examples Using Molecular Methods

Authors Anonymous. Multistate outbreak of listeriosis—United States. MMWR 47:1085–1086, 1998.

Bevanger L, Bergh K, Gisnas G, Caugant DA, Froholm LO. Identification of nasopharyngeal carriage of an outbreak strain of Neisseria meningitidis by pulsed-field gel electrophoresis versus phenotypic methods. J. Med. Microbiol. 47:993–998, 1998.

Bingen E, Bonacorsi S, Rohrlich P, et al. Molecular epidemiology provides evidence of genotypic heterogeneity of multidrug-resistant Pseudomonas aeruginosa serotype O:12 outbreak isolates from a pediatric hospital. J. Clin. Microbiol. 34:3226–3229, 1996.

Brian MJ, Van R, Townsend I, et al. Evaluation of the molecular epidemiology of an outbreak of multiple resistant Shigella sonnei in a daycare center by using pulsed-field gel electrophoresis and plasmid DNA analysis. J. Clin. Microbiol. 31:2152–2156, 1993.

Burns DN, Wallace RJ Jr, Schultz ME, et al. Nosocomial outbreak of respiratory tract colonization with Mycobacterium fortuitum: Demonstration of the usefulness of pulsed-field gel electrophoresis in an epidemiologic investigation. Am. Rev. Respir. Dis. 144:1153–1159, 1991.

Castellani Pastoris M, Ciceroni L, Lo Monaco R, et al. Molecular epidemiology of an outbreak of Legionnaires' disease associated with a cooling tower in Genova-Sestri Ponente, Italy. Eur. J. Clin. Microbiol. Infect. Dis. 16:883–892, 1997.

Cheng K, Smyth RL, Govan JR, et al. Spread of beta-lactam–resistant Pseudomonas aeruginosa in a cystic fibrosis clinic. Lancet. 348:639–642, 1996.

Chetoui H, Melin P, Struelens MJ, et al. Comparison of biotyping, ribotyping, and pulsed-field gel electrophoresis for investigation of a common-source outbreak of Burkholderia pickettii bacteremia. J. Clin. Microbiol. 35:1398–1403, 1997.

Farmer JJ. Conventional typing methods. J. Hosp. Infect. 11(suppl A):309–314, 1988.

Fiore AE, Nuorti JP, Levine OS, et al. Epidemic Legionnaires' disease two decades later. Old sources, new diagnostic methods. Clin. Infect. Dis. 26:426–433, 1998.

Georghiou PR, Hamill RJ, Wright CE, et al. Molecular epidemiology of infections due to *Enterobacter aerogenes*: Identification of hospital outbreak–associated strains by molecular techniques. Clin. Infect. Dis. 20:84–94, 1995.

Gibson JR, Fitzgerald C, Owen RJ. Comparison of PFGE, ribotyping and phage-typing in the epidemiological analysis of *Campylobacter jejuni* serotype HS2 infections. Epidemiol. Infect. 115:215–225, 1995.

Hartmann FA, West SE. Utilization of both phenotypic and molecular analyses to investigate an outbreak of multidrug–resistant Salmonella anatum in horses. Can. J. Vet. Res. 61:173–181, 1997.

Hlady WG, Mullen RC, Mintz CS, et al. Outbreak of Legionnaire's disease linked to a decorative fountain by molecular epidemiology. Am. J. Epidemiol. 138:555–562, 1993.

Jorgensen M, Givney R, Pegler M, Vickery A, Funnell G. Typing multidrug-resistant *Staphylococcus aureus*: Conflicting epidemiological data produced by genotypic and phenotypic methods clarified by phylogenetic analysis. J. Clin. Microbiol. 34:398–403, 1996.

Keller DW, Hajjeh R, DeMaria A, et al. Community outbreak of Legionnaires' disease: An investigation confirming the potential for cooling towers to transmit *Legionella* species. Clin. Infect. Dis. 22:257–261, 1996.

Kluytmans J, Berg H, Steegh P, et al. Outbreak of *Staphylococcus schleiferi* wound infections: strain characterization by randomly amplified polymorphic DNA analysis, PCR ribotyping, conventional ribotyping, and pulsed-field gel electrophoresis. J. Clin. Microbiol. 36:2214–2219, 1998.

Knippschild M, Ansorg R. Epidemiological typing of *Alcaligenes xylosoxidans* subsp. Xylosoxidans by antibacterial susceptibility testing, fatty acid analysis, PAGE of whole-cell protein and pulsed-field gel electrophoresis. Zentralblatt fur Bakteriologie 288:145–157, 1998.

Laconcha I, Lopez-Molina N, Rementeria A, et al. Phage typing combined with pulsed-field gel electrophoresis and random amplified polymorphic DNA increases discrimination in the epidemiological analysis of *Salmonella enteritidis* strains. Int. J. Food Microbiol. 40:27–34, 1998.

Lindenmayer JM, Schoenfeld S, O'Grady R, Carney JK. Methicillin-resistant *Staphylococcus aureus* in a high school wrestling team and the surrounding community. Arch. Intern. Med. 158:895–899, 1998.

Louie L, Louie M, Simor AE. Investigation of a pseudo-outbreak of *Nocardia asteroides* infection by pulsed-field gel electrophoresis and randomly amplified polymorphic DNA PCR. J. Clin. Microbiol. 35:1582–1584, 1997.

Louie M, Jayaratne P, Luchsinger I, et al. Comparison of ribotyping, arbitrarily primed PCR, and pulsed-field gel electrophoresis for molecular typing of *Listeria monocytogenes*. J. Clin. Microbiol. 34:15–19, 1996.

Luk WK. An outbreak of pseudobacteraemia caused by *Burkholderia pickettii*: The critical role of an epidemiological link. J. Hosp. Infect. 34:59–69, 1996.

Navarro F, Llovet T, Echeita MA, et al. Molecular typing of *Salmonella enterica* serovar typhi. J. Clin. Microbiol. 34:2831–2834, 1996.

Neuwirth C, Siebor E, Lopez J, Pechinot A, Kazierczak A. Outbreak of TEM-24-producing *Enterobacter aerogenes* in an intensive care unit and dissemination of the extended-spectrum beta-lactamase to other members of the family Enterobacteriaceae. J. Clin. Microbiol. 34:76–79, 1996.

Nicolle LE, Bialkowska-Hobrzanska H, Romance L, Harry VS, Parker S. Clonal diversity of methicillin-resistant *Staphylococcus aureus* in an acute-care institution. Infect. Control Hosp. Epidemiol. 13:33–37, 1992.

Nocera D, Altwegg M, Martinetti Lucchini G, et al. Characterization of Listeria strains from a foodborne listeriosis outbreak by rDNA gene restriction patterns compared to four other typing methods. Eur. J. Clin. Microbiol. Infect. Dis. 12:162–169, 1993.

Obayashi Y, Fujita J, Ichiyama S, et al. Investigation of nosocomial infection caused by arbekacin-resistant, methicillin-resistant *Staphylococcus aureus*. Diagn. Microbiol. Infect. Dis. 28:53–59, 1997.

On SL, Nielsen EM, Engberg J, Madsen M. Validity of SmaI-defined genotypes of *Campylobacter jejuni* examined by SalI, KpnI, and BamHI polymorphisms: Evidence of identical clones infecting humans, poultry, and cattle. Epidemiol. Infect. 120:231–237, 1998.

Patterson JE, Madden GM, Krisiunas EP, et al. A nosocomial outbreak of ampicillin-resistant *Haemophilus influenzae* type b in a geriatric unit. J. Infect. Dis. 157:1002–1007, 1988.

Ratto P, Sordelli DO, Abeleira E, Torrero M, Catalano M. Molecular typing of *Acinetobacter baumannii-Acinetobacter calcoaceticus* complex isolates from endemic and epidemic nosocomial infections. Epidemiol. Infect. 114:123–132, 1995.

Ridell J, Bjorkroth J, Eisgruber H, et al. Prevalence of the enterotoxin gene and clonality of

Clostridium perfringens strains associated with food-poisoning outbreaks. J. Food Protection 61:240–243, 1998.

Savor C, Pfaller MA, Kruszynski JA, et al. Comparison of genomic methods for differentiating strains of *Enterococcus faecium*: Assessment using clinical epidemiologic data. J. Clin. Microbiol. 36:3327–3331, 1998.

Schumacher-Perdreau F, Jansen B, Seifert H, Peters G, Pulverer G. Outbreak of methicillin-resistant *Staphylococcus aureus* in a teaching hospital—epidemiological and microbiological surveillance. Zentralblatt fur Bakteriologie 280:550–559, 1994.

Seifert H, Gerner-Smidt P. Comparison of ribotyping and pulsed-field gel electrophoresis for molecular typing of *Acinetobacter* isolates. J. Clin. Microbiol. 33:1402–1407, 1995.

Skibsted U, Baggesen DL, Dessau R, Lisby G. Random amplification of polymorphic DNA (RAPD), pulsed-field gel electrophoresis (PFGE) and phage-typing in the analysis of a hospital outbreak of *Salmonella enteritidis*. J. Hosp. Infect. 38:207–216, 1998.

Smith DL, Gumery LB, Smith EG, et al. Epidemic of *Pseudomonas cepacia* in an adult cystic fibrosis unit: Evidence of person-to-person transmission. J. Clin. Microbiol. 31:3017–3022, 1993.

Stanley J, Desai M, Xerry J, et al. High-resolution genotyping elucidates the epidemiology of group A streptococcus outbreaks. J. Infect. Dis. 174:500–506, 1996.

Thompson CJ, Daly C, Barrett TJ, et al. Insertion element IS3-based PCR method for subtyping *Escherichia coli* O157:H7. J. Clin. Microbiol. 36:1180–1184, 1998.

Tram C, Simonet M, Nicolas MH, et al. Molecular typing of nosocomial isolates of *Legionella pneumophila* serogroup 3. J. Clin. Microbiol. 28:242–245, 1990.

Traub WH, Eiden A. Leonhard B, Bauer D. Typing of nosocomial strains of *Serratia marcescens*: Comparison of restriction enzyme cleaved genomic DNA fragment PFGE analysis with bacteriocin typing, biochemical profiles and serotyping. Zentralblatt fur Bakteriologie 284:93–106, 1996.

VanCouwenberghe CJ, Cohen SH, Tang YJ, Gumerlock PH, Silva J Jr. Genomic fingerprinting of epidemic and endemic strains of *Stenotrophomonas maltophilia* (formerly *Xanthomonas maltophilia*) by arbitrarily primed PCR. J. Clin. Microbiol. 33:1289–1291, 1995.

van der Zee A, Verbakel H, van Zon JC, et al. Molecular genotyping of *Staphylococcus aureus* strains: Comparison of repetitive element sequence-based PCR with various typing methods and isolation of a novel epidemicity marker. J. Clin. Microbiol. 37:342–349, 1999.

van Dijck P, Delmee M, Ezzedine H, Deplano A, Struelens MJ. Evaluation of pulsed-field gel electrophoresis and rep-PCR for the epidemiological analysis of *Ochrobactrum anthropi* strains. Eur. J. Clin. Microbiol. Infect. Dis. 14:1099–1102, 1995.

Weber S, Pfaller MA, Herwaldt LA. Role of molecular epidemiology in infection control. Infectectious Disease Clinics of North America 1997; 11(2):257–78.

J. Hierarchic Approach to Choosing a Molecular Typing Method

Bale M, Sanford M, Hollis RJ, Pfaller MA. Application of a biotyping system and DNA restriction fragment analysis to the study of *Serratia marcescens* from hospitalized patients. Diagn. Microbiol. Infect. Dis. 16:1–7, 1993.

Boyce JM, Opal SM, Potter-Bynoe G, et al. Emergence and nosocomial transmission of ampicillin–resistant enterococci. Antimicrob. Agents Chemother. 36:1032–1039, 1992.

Boyce JM, Opal SM, Potter-Bynoe G, Medeiros AA. Spread of methicillin-resistant *Staphylococcus aureus* in a hospital after exposure to a health care worker with chronic sinusitis. Clin. Infect. Dis. 17:496–504, 1993.

Boyce JM, Potter-Bynoe G, Opal SM, Dziobek L, Medeiros AA. A common-source outbreak of *Staphylococcus epidermidis* infections among patients undergoing cardiac surgery. J. Infect. Dis. 161:493–499, 1990.

DuPont HL. Nosocomial salmonellosis and shigellosis. Infect. Control Hosp. Epidemiol. 12:707–709, 1991.

Perl TM, Kruger W, Houston A, et al. Investigation of suspected nosocomial clusters of *Staphylococcus haemolyticus* infections. Infect. Control Hosp. Epidemiol. 20:128–131, 1999.

Pfaller MA, Wendt C, Hollis RJ, et al. Comparative evaluation of an automated ribotyping system versus pulsed-field gel electrophoresis for epidemiological typing of clinical isolates of *Escherichia coli* and *Pseudomonas aeruginosa* from patients with recurrent gram-negative bacteremia. Diagn. Microbiol. Infect. Dis. 25:1–8, 1996.

Voss A, Pfaller MA, Hollis RJ, et al. Investigation of *Candida albicans* transmission in a surgical intensive care unit cluster by using genomic DNA typing methods. J. Clin. Microbiol. 33:576–580, 1995.

9

Evaluation of Diagnostic Tests

ROBERT H. FLETCHER and SCOTT B. HALSTEAD

Central attributes of infectious diseases are the enormous number of potential disease-causing organisms, the limited repertoire of acute human responses to invasion of tissues by these organisms, and the wide diversity of late effects that may occur. During the acute phase of infection, many different agents can cause a similar host response syndrome. Diagnostic tests are needed to determine which specific organism is responsible. To complicate matters, some syndromes, such as abdominal abscesses, may be caused not by a single but by a combination of organisms.

The diagnosis of acute infectious disease and its causal organism or organisms, usually proceeds through three stages. The first stage is to describe and identify a clinical syndrome. Here, in addition to physical examination and clinical judgment, the physician requires an understanding of the performance of diagnostic procedures and clinical laboratory tests that measure physiologic manifestations of infectious diseases but not the infecting organism itself. The second stage is to establish a differential di-

agnosis. This requires a basic understanding of the pathogenesis of infection and global epidemiology of the candidate infectious agents. For example, many microbial organisms are opportunistic and may express pathogenicity only when the human host's immune defenses are compromised. Others selectively infect people with a specific genetic inheritance. At the other extreme, at a time when millions of people undertake international travel each year, often over great distances in a very short time, exotic infectious diseases must be considered in the differential diagnosis of nearly every serious infectious disease. The third stage of diagnosis involves the performance and interpretation of laboratory tests designed to establish the specific infectious agents that are causing the syndrome.

Tests to establish etiology may involve a very broad array of techniques from many disciplines, such as the direct visualization of the organism by light or electron microscopy, histology, culture, animal inoculation, identification of amino acid or nucleotide sequences, serology, and clinical laboratory tests such as X-ray, sonography, computerized axial tomography (CAT) scans, and magnetic resonance imaging (MRI). The diagnostic tests of infectious diseases are used by epidemiologic and clinical researchers to study pathogenesis and define causal relationships, by clinicians who base decisions about diagnosis and treatment on the test result, and by public health workers who may design interventions or establish policies based upon the results of diagnostic tests.

Regulatory oversight is provided by the U.S. government for some diagnostic tests. Some tests/diagnostic reagents based on biological products are reviewed and licensed by the U.S. Food and Drug Administration. Information is available on the U.S. FDA website (www.fda.gov), Center for Device and Radiological Health, or at 1–800–532–4440. Many other commercial diagnostic test kits or diagnostic reagents are evaluated informally by various branches of the Center for Infectious Diseases, Centers for Disease Control and Prevention, Atlanta, Georgia. Individuals interested in more information can access the website, www.cdc.gov. A special diagnostic service is available for parasitic diseases: www.dpd.cdc.gov/dpdx/.

Diagnostic tests may not be the most accurate, for practical reasons, such as cost, acceptability, simplicity, or because of the need for a rapid answer. The possibility then arises that the test result is misleading. Therefore a central question—for researchers, clinicians, and public health officials—is the nature and magnitude of misclassification relative to the best possible identification of etiology, and how misclassification can be minimized.

In this chapter, we discuss the conceptual basis for describing the performance of tests that establish the etiology of infectious disease. We begin by outlining the simple case, where the test is considered either normal or abnormal and the disease either present or absent. Next we consider how misclassification arises and can be minimized. We then consider the next level of complexity: when the cut-point between normal and abnormal is varied, when different degrees of abnormality are considered, and when tests are used in combination. Finally, we consider how diagnostic testing fits into technology assessment as a whole, especially studies of the cost and effectiveness of diagnostic testing.

THE DISEASE

Infection and Acute Infectious Disease

Infection can occur with or without overt consequences to the host, so a conceptual distinction should be made between infection and infectious disease. In general, it is easier to establish unambiguously whether infection is present than whether the infection is causing the disease in question. For example, recovery of streptococci from the tonsils of a person with sore throat does not mean this bacterium is causing the symptoms, because asymptomatic carriage of streptococci is common. Similarly, infections with *Mycobacterium tuberculosis* and most of the herpesviruses may be silent for many years but manifest late effects—tuberculosis or fever blisters, genital lesions, and shingles.

A special challenge in deciding whether an infectious disease is present is to sort out whether current infection is causing acute disease or whether the host has evidence of a past infection, a contemporary inapparent infection, or a chronic infection, none being the cause of the acute syndrome. For example, if an individual has a silent, chronic infection, the recovery of an organism from tissues and the identification of specific antibodies circulating in the person's blood may be coincidental and without etiologic relationship to the present illness. The protean nature of infectious disease syndromes and the occurrence of silent infections place stringent requirements on the evidence needed to prove causation of infectious diseases. Recognizing this, the pioneers in the field of microbiology struggled to define rules of evidence for causation. The most famous of these, Koch's postulates, are still useful but are often superseded by other kinds of evidence in this technologically sophisticated era (see Chapter 3 for a fuller discussion of causal criteria).

Infection and Late Effects

One of the most dramatic areas of recent causal research has been the discovery that infectious organisms, after an interval of months or years, may produce pathologic changes that are totally unlike acute phase host responses to infection. Often, these changes are in the form of neoplasia, for example, chronic infection with Epstein-Barr (human gamma herpesvirus type 4) virus and Burkitt's lymphoma or nasopharyngeal carcinoma; chronic infection with hepatitis B and carcinoma of the liver; or chronic infection with *Helicobacter pylori* and peptic ulcer, or gastric cancer. Here, Koch's postulates are of some value if an experimental animal infected with the organism develops the late effects. Otherwise, etiology is based upon evidence of past or chronic infection, such as antibody, but preferably the detection of an organism's genetic material in or near tissues involved in the late disease. When relying on indirect measures of infection, such as antibody, case-control studies are crucial in establishing causal linkage. The complexity of documenting strong evidence on etiology is reflected in the slow pace at which infectious chronic disease causal associations have been identified and the controversy which stills surrounds some of the data.

Gold Standards

The standard used to establish with the greatest certainty possible whether an infection is present has come to be called the "gold standard." Two kinds of evidence, taken together, are regarded as the gold standard: identification of the organism and host reaction.

The first is isolation or specific identification of the organism/antigen in affected tissues, or on mucosal surfaces in the case of infections of the respiratory, gastrointestinal, or genitourinary tracts. As a general rule (with human immunodeficiency virus [HIV] infection as the exception), the success in identifying or recovering microorganisms is a function of the stage of the disease. Organisms are most abundant early in infection. As humoral and cellular immune responses are mounted, invading organisms may be attacked, resulting in death of the organism and loss of diagnostic antigens. The ability to recover living organisms progressively decreases. Even if infecting organisms persist in the tissues, antibodies may block the diagnostic antigens required for identification. Generally, specific nucleic acids remain in tissues after the viability of the invading organism is destroyed. Tests for RNA or DNA may be positive when it is no longer possible to recover organisms or detect specific antigens. However, with time, organism-specific nucleic acids are lost. For research purposes, reisolation in one laboratory or independent isolation in two or more laboratories of causal agents are important evidence against environmental contamination and inadvertent recovery of an infectious agent from biological materials.

The second part of the evidence of cause is a specific, concurrent host response to the organism, usually the identification of specific antibody of the IgM class. After a period of one to three months, the IgM response is terminated and replaced by antibodies of the IgG class. Thus the presence of IgM antibodies is accepted as evidence of a recent infection. In general, there is greater uncertainty in establishing the presence of infection by detecting specific antibodies than by recovering a disease-producing organism. This is best illustrated with the well-known example of serological tests for HIV-1 infections. A large number of screening tests are on the market that have the advantage of high sensitivity, but unacceptable specificity. Even the gold standard Western blot, which measures the existence of antibodies directed against viral subunits, has resulted in false positives and false negatives. Antibody detection is affected by a variety of factors such as the concentration of antibodies in the test sample, concentration and purity of test antigens, the correctness of three-dimensional conformation of test antigens, the test conditions, for example, pH, solutions, observer reliability, and recording reliability.

Increasingly, tests used to document chronic infections are based upon the detection of antigen or organism-specific nucleic acid in appropriate diagnostic specimens.

When there is no gold standard

Many infectious diseases present for diagnosis when the optimal period for direct identification or recovery of the causal organism has ended. Other categories of infectious diseases, such as arthropod-borne viral encephalitis, result in infections of organs that cannot be sampled (e.g., brain—the virus is seldom found in CSF), and if virus circulates in the blood it has done so long before the onset of symptoms. This group of viral diseases, and virtually all other viral diseases observed after the period of fever has ended, must be identified serologically. Here, the IgM test, often applied in an enzyme linked immunosorbent assay (EIA or ELISA), gives excellent evidence that an acute infection has just occurred. But viruses occur in antigenically related families that cannot be discriminated by antibody-based tests. Finding the correct antigen in the laboratory to match the infecting virus is a matter of hit or miss.

Other tests that may exhibit relatively low sensitivity and specificity include skin tests, widely used to detect the existence of infection, present or past, such as systemic mycosis, tuberculosis, leprosy, or leishmaniasis.

Some diseases are believed to be infectious before the causal microorganism has been identified and it is necessary to create a working case definition, for surveillance and studies of risk factors. Examples are the early definitions of toxic shock syndrome (Table 9–1) and acquired immunodeficiency syndrome (AIDS) before HIV was discovered.

DIAGNOSTIC TESTS

Cultures

Recovery of the suspected microorganism from nonsterile body tissues or secretions (such as the gastrointestinal tract or mucous membranes) represents evidence of infection, as long as it can be established that it

---

Table 9–1   Case Definition of Toxic Shock Syndrome

Fever: temperature > 38.9°C

Rash: diffuse macular erythroderma

Desquamation of palms and soles one to two weeks after onset of illness

Hypotension: systolic blood pressure <90 mm Hg for adults or below fifth percentile by age for children below 16 years of age, orthostatic drop in diastolic blood pressure >15 mm Hg from lying to sitting, or orthostatic syncope

Multisystem involvement—three or more of the following:
  Gastrointestinal: vomiting or diarrhea at onset of illness
  Muscular: severe myalgia or creatine phosphokinase level at least twice the upper limit of normal for laboratory
  Mucous membrane: vaginal, oropharyngeal, or conjunctival hyperemia
  Renal: blood urea nitrogen or creatinine at least twice the upper limit of normal for laboratory or urinary sediment with pyuria (>5 white cells per high-power field) in the absence of urinary tract infection
  Hepatic: total bilirubin, SGOT,* or SGPT† at least twice the upper limit of normal for laboratory
  Hematologic: platelets <100,000 per cubic millimeter
  Central nervous system: disorientation or alterations in consciousness without focal neurologic signs when fever and hypotension are absent

Negative results on the following tests, if obtained:
  Blood, throat, or cerebrospinal fluid cultures
  Rise in titer to Rocky Mountin spotted fever, leptospirosis, or rubeola

*SGOT, serum aspartate aminotransferase.

†SGPT, serum alanine aminotransferase.

is not there because of contamination. The organism's presence, however, may represent colonization and not the cause of disease. In normally sterile areas (such as blood or cerebrospinal fluid) recovery of the organism is infection by definition, although the infection may be asymptomatic. Thus pneumococcus would rarely be found in the blood except with an acute pneumococcal infection such as pneumonia, whereas its recovery from a throat culture might simply represent colonization. The case for a true positive test indicating that the organism plays a role in a disease is weakened if other organisms are recovered in the same specimen, such as diphtheroids in a blood culture growing staphylococcus.

Microscopic Identification

Some microorganisms have such a characteristic appearance that they can be identified by microscopy alone with conventional or special stains. Examples include eggs in feces for intestinal parasites, which an experienced examiner can identify with confidence in stool specimens—fresh and concentrated, with and without iodine staining. Similarly, *Pneumocystis pneumonii* organisms in sputum have a characteristic appearance in methenamine silver–stained sputum, and malaria infection, including species differentiation, can be diagnosed reliably by examination of stained blood smear.

Tests for Antibody

The presence of antibodies to microbial antigens circulating in the host's blood is taken as evidence of infection, though not necessarily disease. An example is EIA antiviral antibodies to hepatitis C, which connote recent or chronic infection. The level of antibody is commonly expressed as a titer, the dilution at which the serum still reacts, using a specific laboratory method such as precipitation or agglutination, but does not react at the next dilution. Typically, dilutions are twofold, resulting in titers of 1/2, 1/4, 1/8, 1/16, etc. A common form of antigen-antibody reaction occurs on what is termed a "solid state." In this test,

one of the reagents, antigen or antibody, is adsorbed to the inside surface of a small, plastic well. An appropriate second reagent is reacted with the adsorbed reagent; next, a third reagent is added, usually an anti-antibody (or an antigen). This antibody carries with it an indicator system, often an enzyme that acts on a substrate producing a color reaction. There are many variations on this theme.

Because immunologic reaction to one antigen may cause a rise in antibodies to other related antigens, there is a possibility that a low titer might suggest a specific infection is present when it is not. To diminish the probability of a false positive test, several strategies are used. Small molecules, peptides or polypeptides, may be synthesized and used instead of complete protein antigens. Problems may result with the use of such specific reagents, since the antibodies or antigens that occur in nature are often unpredictably heterogeneous and may not interact at all or interact improperly with highly specific test reagents. The evidence of specific infection is stronger if the level of antibody measured at one point in time after infection is especially high; stronger yet if the level is substantially higher than at a previous time. If the rise is from before to after clinical disease (acute and convalescent sera), and large enough—for example, a fourfold rise—to not be discounted as measurement variation, the evidence is stronger. The evidence is most compelling if the specific class of antibody that rises is one known to respond to the acute phases of disease. For example, simply having a fourfold or greater rise in titer of antibody to hepatitis B is not nearly as convincing evidence that the patient's recent disease is caused by hepatitis B virus than if IgM antibody is present.

Tests for Cell-Mediated Immunity

Skin tests are used to detect the occurrence of infection, usually at some unspecified time in the past. They are convenient but especially prone to inaccuracy. Skin tests can be falsely positive in the presence of infection with a related organism—for example, the reaction to antigen for *Mycobacterium tuberculosis* in a patient who has had an atypical mycobacterial infection. They can be falsely negative if the host has an impaired ability to mount a cellular immune reaction—for example, because of overwhelming infection, chemotherapy, malignancy, or treatment with immunosuppressive drugs.

Detection of Antigen

Examples of antigen detection include identification of specific antigen in blood or body secretions: hepatitis B, malaria, influenza, and other respiratory pathogens in respiratory tract secretions. Microorganisms can also be identified by immunofluorescence staining either of antigens or organisms in tissues or skin lesions; examples include cestodes, nematodes, fungi, protozoa, plasmodia and protista, mycobacteria, certain other bacteria, and viruses (e.g., rabies). Detection of antigens, or of specific organisms in tissues or following culture, requires the use of antibodies. Antibodies are biologic reagents. Antibody-antigen reactions can be exquisitely specific and sensitive. However, "raising" of antibodies, both polyclonal and monoclonal, follows biologic and not biochemical principles and is inherently subject to error. Many antigen-antibody reaction systems require an indicator reaction (i.e., a reaction that indicates in some visible way the presence of a material or organism). For example, in the hemagglutination-inhibition test for rubella antibody, inactivated rubella viruses are adsorbed to the surface of a red blood cell where the viruses serve as ligands binding together several red blood cells forming a visible clump. This reaction is dependent on various conditions such as the composition of the suspension medium, pH, the concentration of antigen, and the precise chemical modification of antigen.

Antigen-antibody interactions may identify heterophile antigens (i.e., unexpected antigenic similarities across species or on proteins with different functions). This may be a source of false positive test results. Occasionally, heterophile antigens have utility, as in the diagnosis of infectious mononucleosis caused by Epstein-Barr virus (human gamma herpesvirus type 4), in which convalescent human antibodies react with beef erythrocytes.

Detection of Nucleotide Sequences

The principle involved in detection of genes is the synthesis of a short, complementary DNA or RNA nucleotide sequence used as a genetic probe. The probe is labeled with a radioisotopic or visible labeling system and applied to a source of DNA or RNA. If the probe sequences are matching and complementary to a sequence to be detected, the probe will bind to the target. The radioisotope or visible indicator permits identification. A common and more sensitive genetic sequence detection method is the extraction of DNA or RNA from the specimen and its amplification through the polymerase chain reaction (PCR). If the test specimen contains RNA this can be transformed to DNA, using the enzyme reverse transcriptase (RT). It is possible to use a short probe to fish out a longer length of gene and then amplify this by PCR. Large amounts of DNA obtained from PCR are gel-electrophoresed then stained, permitting precise identification of the nucleotide sequences that form the genetic code.

PCR or RT-PCR have many applications in the direct identification of microbial genetic material in fluids, secretions, or excretions. Examples include identification of influenza or respiratory syncytial viruses in respiratory secretions; or hepatitis B or HIV-1 in blood, urine, or saliva. Direct genetic probes are used to detect microbial DNA or RNA in tissue specimens obtained at biopsy, surgery, or autopsy. Examples include detection of mycoplasma in swabs of cervical epithelial cells and herpes simplex or varicella in biopsies of herpetic lesions. A source of test nonspecificity is inherent in the uniqueness of the nucleotide sequence of the probe in relation to all sequences found in nature. Because these sequences are virtually infinite, identifications may be expressed as a probability. The probability of correct identification varies directly with uniqueness in composition and the length of the gene probe.

PCR is an enormously sensitive and specific test but it can result in false positives if the specimen is contaminated. Since PCR can identify and amplify as few as several gene copies, incomplete removal of genes from the laboratory environment and their transfer from one test to another test is a common source of false positive results. Great care must be taken to keep test specimens separate, in order to protect against false positive identification. Special isolation facilities are usually dedicated for this purpose.

Gene sequences are surrogates for defined regions of proteins. Direct detection of specific gene sequences or amplification followed by detection of specific sequences are the basis of the most sensitive and reliable methods of detecting infectious agents. Gene probes are short nucleotide sequences, usually synthetic, coupled with a detection system (e.g., radioisotope or enzyme). This probe interacts with a target gene sequence when there is a high degree of complementarity.

Other

During infection some organisms release defensive or excretory products, including proteins. Some, such as *H. pylori* urease, can be used to establish the presence of the organism. Some replicating agents either may not yet have been identified or yield no unique diagnostic antigen. Recognition of the disease may result from the identification of suggestive findings from appropriate clinical diagnostic tests (e.g., EEG patterns in Creutzfeldt-Jakob [prion] disease).

MISCLASSIFICATION

It is common practice to consider a diagnostic test either normal or abnormal and the disease either present or absent. But in fact, both test and disease usually occur over a range of values (i.e., they are continuous variables) and information is lost when they are dichotomized. Epidemiologic studies often forfeit richer data (e.g., continuous measures) for measures that are easily interpreted, such as estimates of the proportion

of people likely to experience a particular outcome.

Figure 9–1 shows the relationship between test and disease when both are dichotomous. There are two opportunities for misclassification. The disease may be present and the test is negative, in which case the test result is called "false negative." Or the disease may be absent and the test is positive, in which case the test is a "false positive." Misclassification can arise for many reasons, both biologic and technical. For example, a PPD skin test for *Mycobacterium tuberculosis* might be falsely negative if the patient has a diminished immune response (as with AIDS, advanced age, treatment with immunosuppressive agents, or in the presence of overwhelming infection), and falsely positive if the patient has been infected with another mycobacterium.

Sensitivity and Specificity

While it is easy to accept that such misclassification can occur, the more important question is the direction and degree of misclassification. This information can be used to estimate the extent to which misclassification leads to misleading conclusions in epidemiologic research, and the consequences of the error (Fletcher et al. 1996, Sackett et al. 1991, Riegelman and Hirsch 1989, Sox 1996, Griner et al. 1981). One kind of question about misclassification is how well a test performs in the presence or absence of disease. Two summary statistics, sensitivity and specificity, are commonly used to describe this kind of misclassification by diagnostic tests (Fig. 9–2). Estimates of sensitivity and specificity are properties of a given test under the specific conditions of the study to which the research question applies. Studies summarize the experience with a group of people, for research and public health purposes, but can be used to estimate the probability of disease in individual patients for clinical purposes.

Sensitivity describes the proportion of people with the disease who have a positive test. It is a measure of how well the test detects disease if it is present, without regard to whether or not it produces false positive

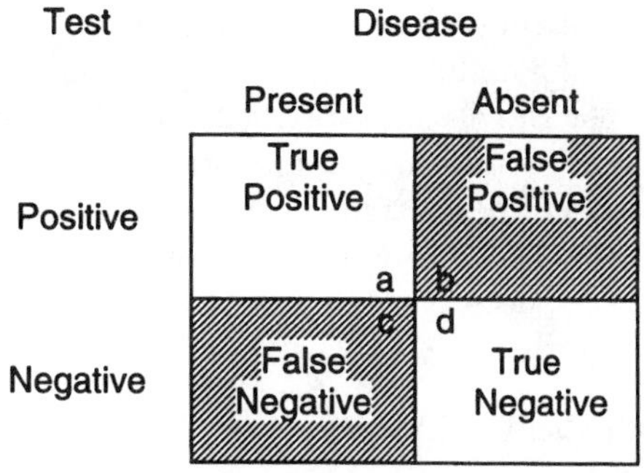

Test   Disease

	Present	Absent
Positive	True Positive	False Positive
Negative	False Negative	True Negative

Figure 9–1. The relationship between a diagnostic test result and the occurrence of disease. There are two possibilities for the test result to be correct (true positive and true negative) and two possibilities for the result to be incorrect (false positive and false negative).

results in the process. Sensitivity is a ratio, with the numerator the number of people with a true positive test and the denominator the number with disease in the sample being described. A synonym is the "true positive rate" (though it is in fact a ratio, not a "rate," which implies a time dimension). Good examples of sensitive tests for infectious disease are those based on polymerase chain reaction, which can in theory react to a single molecule of organism-specific DNA.

The meaning of the term "test sensitivity" in epidemiology should not be confused with another use of the term, sometimes called "analytic sensitivity," in clinical and laboratory studies of infectious diseases: the ability to react to a very small quantity of a biologic entity. The two are related but the epidemiologic "sensitivity" is a summary

statistic describing how well a test picks up disease on average in a group of people, whereas biologic sensitivity refers to how well a laboratory method performs relative to a biologic standard.

Specificity is the proportion of people without disease who have a negative test. It measures the degree to which people without disease are called normal by the test. Specificity is a ratio, with the numerator the number of people in the sample with a true negative test result and the denominator the number of people without disease. Many find it easier to interpret the same concept with its complement, "false positive rate," the proportion of people without disease who are called abnormal by the test, which is [1 - specificity]. Examples of specific tests are the recovery of herpesvirus from brain in

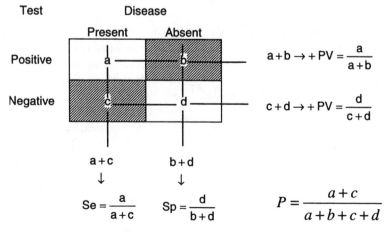

Figure 9–2. Diagnostic test characteristics and definitions. Se = sensitivity; Sp = specificity; +PV = positive predictive value; −PV = negative predictive value; P = prevalence of disease in the sample.

a patient with encephalitis or of onchocerca in skin nodules.

Sensitivity and specificity should be considered as a pair, because for a given test the level of one is traded off against that of the other. Therefore it is not possible to interpret one properly without information on the other.

Predictive Value

Another kind of question concerning misclassification has to do with interpreting the results of a test once it has been performed: how well does the result of the diagnostic test predict the presence or absence of disease? Two summary statistics are used to describe this information.

The *positive predictive value* is the proportion of people with a positive test who actually have the disease. It expresses the degree to which a positive test result represents disease. The numerator is the number of people in the sample with a true positive test and the denominator all people with a positive test. For example, if 120 people in a sample have a positive test and 80 of them actually have the disease, the positive predictive value is 67%. The *negative predictive value* is the comparable statistic for a negative test: the proportion of people with a negative test who are true negatives.

Predictive values depend not only on sensitivity and specificity, which are properties of the test, but also on the overall probability of disease in the group being tested. In a population, this probability is called the point prevalence, the proportion of people in a defined population who have the disease. In samples or individuals, it is common to refer to the same statistic as the "pretest probability."

For a given sensitivity and specificity, positive predictive value declines as the prevalence falls (Fig. 9–3). With the prevalence below about 1 in 100, positive predictive

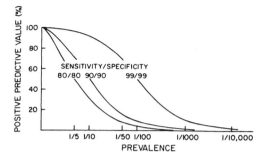

Figure 9–3. The relationship between positive predictive value and prevalence.
Source: From Fletcher RH, Fletcher SW, Wagner EH. Clinical Epidemiology. The Essentials. 3rd ed. Baltimore: Williams & Wilkins, 1996.

values are relatively low, even for highly sensitive and specific tests. Most infectious diseases occur at a much lower prevalence in the general population, but not necessarily in clinical settings with groups of patients who have strong risk factors for disease or clinical evidence that it might be present. A consequence is that false positive tests are a fact of life in most epidemiologic surveys and screening programs. In the case of research, misclassification of variables can affect the validity of the conclusion. In screening programs, false positive and false negative tests have personal consequences to the individuals who are incorrectly classified.

Interrelationships

The definitions and interrelationships of sensitivity, specificity, and predictive value are summarized in Figure 9–3.

The description of the way to think about the probability of disease, given a particular test result and prevalence of disease before the test was conducted, is based on Bayes' theorem, proposed by the Reverend Thomas Bayes in the 1700s. The general formula can be found at the foot of this page. Bayes' theorem is increasingly used in epidemiologic

Positive predictive value =

$$\frac{(sensitivity \times pretest\ probability)}{(sensitivity \times pretest\ probability) + [(1 - pretest\ probability) \times (1 - specificity)]}$$

and clinical research to estimate how predictions change based on new information (e.g., with changes in disease prevalence).

VALIDITY

Misclassification arises because of variation inherent in all measurement. In general terms, variation arises by two processes: bias (systematic error) and chance (random error). To obtain measurements with as little misclassification as possible, it is necessary to know the sources of variation, minimize bias, and have a large enough sample to yield a precise estimate of test performance. It is then necessary to estimate the extent to which random variation and remaining bias might affect the estimate of test performance.

Sources of Variation

Variation in epidemiologic observations, including diagnostic tests for infectious diseases, can be attributed to two general sources: biologic and measurement.

Biologic variation occurs within and among individuals. First, the individual's actual state varies over time. For example, people infected with HIV may be seronegative one week and seropositive the next, as time passes since the onset of infection. Similarly, people with a positive tuberculin skin test may convert to a negative test with overwhelming infection or immunodeficiency (as in AIDS). A survey at any point in time may catch some of the people who ordinarily have a positive test at a moment when their test is negative. Biologic variation among individuals occurs because of differences across individuals in the state of infection.

Measurement variation is partly attributable to the instrument used to make the measurement (culture media, gels, gene probes, and the like). Thus an improperly prepared culture medium for *Neisseria gonorrhoeae* will result in false negative test results, whereas contaminated blood cultures will give false positive results. Some measurement variation can also be attributed to the person making the measurement—for example, the clinician reading the skin test, the patholo-gist reading the tissue stained for specific organisms, or the technician doing the Gram stains.

Biases

Any systematic error in measurement contributes to variation and, in the case of a diagnostic test, increases misclassification so that the information available from the test is diminished (Begg 1987). In an epidemiologic study of infectious disease, all results that are based on faulty measurement are misleading.

Two kinds of observer error tend to create a greater correspondence between the results of the test and the true state of disease than actually exists in nature. The liability for these biases is greater in situations where there is a large element of judgment in either the test interpretation or diagnosis, such as reading of acid fast stains for mycobacteria or silver stains for *Pneumocystic carinii* or assigning a clinical diagnosis of influenza or hantavirus infection.

On the one hand, the person interpreting the test result may be biased if he or she has other information on whether the patient has the disease and takes this information into account when interpreting the test result. On the other hand, the person assigning the diagnosis might know the results of the test and take it into account when making the judgment whether the disease is present. In both instances, the reasoning is circular: the diagnostic test result and disease status are more strongly related to each other under the conditions of the study than they would otherwise be because of a natural tendency to make the test result fit with the diagnosis or the diagnosis fit with the test result. Users of the information are left uncertain about how much additional information the test result really contributes to the diagnosis.

Quality Control

Diagnostic instruments must be continually calibrated. It is important for the laboratorian and user of diagnostic tests alike to understand that gauges and other measuring instruments can err. Quality assurance is an ongoing challenge and failure of quality assurance is a major source of error. Some level of insensitivity and nonspecificity is continually introduced into diagnostic tests due to quality assurance failures. Such events occur as a result of human error and with wear and tear. The manufacturer usually provides gauges, rotor meters, or other sensors that are used routinely for calibrating performance. These in turn must be calibrated. Calibration is often done by the manufacturer's representative or by quality assurance teams from the home institution or government agencies. Instrument performance must be tested against a gold standard and retested at appropriate intervals.

Similar principles apply to questionnaire-based instruments. The properties of the instrument are established through studies of validity, including whether it includes all aspects of the thing being measured (content validity), yields results that are consistent with existing theory (construct validity), and predicts physically verifiable manifestations of the thing being measured (criterion validity). Quality is maintained by training sessions for research assistants and surveillance on how the instruments are being used.

For tests that depend on an observer's judgment, observer error can be reduced by several methods. (1) One can choose an objective outcome, one that involves relatively little judgment, such as the results of a culture or gene probe. However, one would do so only if that measurement were to correspond to the research question; not only to achieve more objective measurements. (2) Researchers can create explicit, detailed "decision rules" for using the data to assign test results and diagnoses. An example is the set of criteria for a research diagnosis of toxic shock syndrome shown in Table 9–1. (3) Researchers can also assure that decision rules are followed uniformly by all who collect and code data by beginning the data collection phase of the study with training sessions and continuing with regular meetings to revise the rules to take into account situations that were not anticipated when the rules were first established. (4) Observers may be masked so that those who interpret the test do not have other information about the diagnosis and those assigning the diagnosis do not have information about the test. (5) In every case, investigators should measure agreement between observers during data collection and institute measures to correct any identified causes of disagreement.

Random Variation

Misclassification can also arise because of random variation. The main issue is the extent to which a sample of people included in a study, even if selected by an unbiased (random) method, misrepresents the situation for the source population as a whole because of random variation in samples. This risk is especially high for small samples of patients and can be reduced by studying large samples. The extent to which random error might account for the observed test performance is estimated by statistical methods and commonly expressed as a confidence interval for the estimate, also called the "statistical precision" of the estimate (Heckerling 1988, Gardner et al. 1989). A 95% confidence interval—for example, of the sensitivity, specificity, or predictive value—is interpreted as having at least a 95% chance of including the true value in the population studied.

For the simple situation, common in epidemiologic studies, in which the measurement (e.g., sensitivity) is expressed as a proportion, the 95% confidence can be approximated by assuming that the results have a binomial distribution. Thus

95% Confidence Interval =

$$p \pm 1.96 \times \sqrt{\frac{p(1-p)}{N}}$$

where ± 1.96 is the proportion of a binomial distribution that includes 95% of the values, p is the observed proportion (e.g., sensitivity or specificity), and N is the number of observations.

In general, the effect of random variation is to decrease the observed relationship between test result and disease, relative to what it is in nature. Even with meticulous methods, such as decision rules, training sessions, and masking, random error in diagnostic test results introduces noise that, if accumulated over measurements of many phenomena, can drown out the signal and result in a negative study.

GENERALIZABILITY

The samples of people with and without an infectious disease that are included in a study of a diagnostic test determine the observed performance of the test (Ransohoff and Feinstein 1978). The characteristics of people in the sample can be strongly related to sensitivity and specificity, and therefore to predictive value. The particular mix of patients with these characteristics has been called the "spectrum" of patients. The question then arises: to whom do the results of the study apply? The answer is called the "generalizability" of the test performance.

The sample of people *with* disease determines the observed sensitivity of the test. Not all patients with a disease have a similar likelihood of having a positive test. In general, those with long-standing, advanced, or classic disease are more likely to have a positive test than those with recent, mild, and atypical disease. If sampling results in a group of patients who are especially likely to have a positive test, sensitivity will be high. For example, sputum smears and cultures for *Mycobacterium tuberculosis* infection are likely to be very sensitive in patients with well-established AIDS and pulmonary disease, a situation in which mycobacteria multiply to massive numbers. On the other hand, the sensitivity is likely to be lower in a sample of patients with a positive skin test and infiltrate but who are not immunocompromised and not coughing.

The sample of people without disease determines the specificity of the test. The more they resemble those with the disease, the more likely are false positive test results (i.e., the lower the specificity). Thus people with a variety of diseases that elevate serum immunoglobulins have false positive reactions on second-generation tests for hepatitis C. These are, unfortunately, the very diseases for which one would want to use the test in order to distinguish people without hepatitis C from patients actually infected with hepatitis C. On the other hand, the more healthy the noncases are, the higher the specificity. It has been shown many times that if normal volunteers are used as the nondiseased controls, few have abnormal tests and specificity is very high.

Although prevalence itself does not affect sensitivity and specificity, there is commonly an association between the two because the settings in which high and low prevalence occurs are also ones in which the spectrum of patients differ. Thus the predictive value for chlamydia tests in a sexually transmitted disease clinic might be higher than in the general population not only because of the high probability of disease in the clinic but also because patients there are more severely affected, and so more likely to produce a positive result, than those with less severe infections in the general population.

The main goal in choosing a sample is to get one that matches the research question. For example, if one wants to know the accuracy of a skin test for tuberculosis among patients with AIDS, cases should be those with AIDS and tuberculosis and noncases those with AIDS and similar symptoms and signs but without tuberculosis.

Data for studies of diagnostic tests usually come from clinical records, not experiments. Often data on the ideal samples of noncases are not available because the process of establishing the gold standard diagnosis is so costly and invasive that it is not acceptable to apply it to patients who do not have evidence, from simpler observations such as epidemiologic risk factors and clinical symptoms and signs, that the disease is likely to be present. Thus a pediatrician in office practice would not obtain blood cultures on children with fever unless there was strong evidence of bacteremia, even though some of the children not cultured might in fact have bacteremia. As a consequence, when data are from clinical practice there is incomplete information about the performance of the test in people without the disease; only those with earlier positive tests, a biased sample of all patients without disease, are included. The result is an inability to determine sensitivity and specificity, and although positive predictive value can be obtained, negative predictive value cannot. This is a major problem; if the data are not available, no amount of analyses can make up for the deficit. Sometimes the problem can be overcome by obtaining consent for testing from people without positive results from preliminary tests or by finding a naturally occurring sample, perhaps in a different setting, in which such testing has been done.

AGREEMENT

When there is no standard of validity for a diagnostic test, it may be useful to summarize the extent to which two observers' observations are concordant, either to arrive at a consensus diagnosis or to describe the level of agreement. Here the observers are on an equal footing; neither is taken as a standard of validity for the other.

If the data are dichotomous, as they are in the usual situation where there are two observers deciding whether disease is present or absent, the data can be placed in a 2 × 2 table and agreement described by the proportion of all cases that falls in the two cells representing agreement. However, this does not take into account the amount of such agreement that might occur by chance alone. To obtain a better view of the extent of agreement beyond chance, the kappa statistic is used (Fleiss 1981).

Two observers may be asked to place people into more than two categories of disease status. An example is when the presence of disease is rated on an ordinal scale: present, probably present, possibly present, probably absent, and absent. There is then the possibility of degrees of disagreement. It would be misleading to rate a near miss (such as one saying probably present and the other present) the same as a wide miss (one says present and the other absent). In this situation it is advisable to present the data for visual inspection in a N × N table, with each patient represented by a dot (or all patients in a cell represented by a number).

One can also obtain a summary statistic for agreement beyond chance (a weighted kappa) by weighting the magnitude of disagreement on the diagnosis in individual cases, giving more credit for near misses than for large ones. This presents a fairer picture of agreement beyond chance than an unweighted kappa but the weighted kappa statistic may be heavily affected by the particular weighting scheme chosen.

If the data are continuous, they can be displayed by a figure. If there are few patients in the study, it is best to represent each case by a data point, allowing the reader to judge the distribution of values for each observer, the number of observations (hence, statistical stability of the observed relationships), observed agreement, and the number and extremity of outliers. The data can also be summarized by a correlation coefficient (r), and a statistical test of whether r exceeds 0 (no association) beyond what might have been expected by chance.

BEYOND DICHOTOMOUS TEST AND DISEASE

Up until this point, test result and disease presence have been discussed as dichotomous variables. Tests for the presence of infection using various methods ranging from culture to molecular diagnosis do in fact yield a present/absent result. However, tests for infectious disease (such as serologic and skin tests) that are based on the host's biologic reaction to the infection are rarely actually dichotomous. Nearly all can take on a range of values, that is, they are expressed as continuous variables. Thus urine cultures (the test) in women with carefully documented urinary tract infection (the disease) can vary over 100,000-fold, from a few organisms to over $10^6/mm^3$. There is usually an overlap in test result values for people with and without infection. Moreover the distribution of values in a population of people with and without the disease usually has no humps or breaks that suggest a biologic reason for deciding where to place a cut-point between normal and abnormal values. For example, while it is clear that urine cultures showing greater than 10^5 bacteria per ml or mm^3 clearly represent urinary tract infection, and that negligible concentrations of bacteria are detected in specimens collected from people who are not infected, there is uncertainty in how to interpret values in the 10^2 to 10^5 range.

Defining Normal and Abnormal

It is common to define a level beyond which a test is considered abnormal. Often a statistical definition of abnormal is used, in which unusual is considered abnormal. This is usually defined as beyond two standard deviations from the mean of a population of apparently healthy people. The statistical definition of abnormal is artificial, from the epidemiologic or clinical point of view. For example, by this definition, the prevalence of all infectious diseases would be 5%. More substantive decisions about what to consider abnormal take into account the range of values that is associated with clinical disease or improvement with treatment.

Choosing a Cut-Point

By whatever means the definition of normal is assigned, creating a dichotomous variable from a continuous one requires a choice about where the cut-point between normal and abnormal is placed in a distribution of test result values. The choice is up to the investigator and necessarily involves a trade-off.

Sensitivity and specificity are inversely related as one moves the cut-point from a low to a high value. It is possible to establish a tuberculin skin test that is highly sensitive for *Mycobacterium tuberculosis* infection (or, alternatively, very specific) by where one places the cut-point. Experience has shown that cut-points of around 5–15 mm provide diagnostically useful information. If one were to set the point at which the test was called positive extremely low, perhaps at 2 mm of induration, the test would detect nearly all cases (i.e., high sensitivity) but would result in many false positive diagnoses. On the other hand, if one were to call positive only those tests resulting in greater than 2.0 cm of induration, few people without tuberculosis would be falsely labeled as having the disease (i.e., high specificity) but there would be many false negatives. Because it is possible to raise sensitivity at the expense of the specificity, and vice versa, seeing one or the other in isolation does not tell one whether the test contributes a net gain in information about the diagnosis. In general, sensitivity and specificity can be traded off against each other for a given test, with no gain in information. To have more information, one must devise a better test, not just move the cut-point.

Epidemiologic information can help investigators or clinicians choose a cut-point that improves both sensitivity and specificity. For example, one might choose to call a PPD with 5 mm of induration a positive test in people with an abnormal chest roentgenogram, a 10 mm PPD positive in a person who has had a recent negative test, and a 15 mm PPD positive in people in whom there is no other reason to suspect tuberculosis.

The relationship between sensitivity and specificity at various cut-points for normal and abnormal is shown graphically as a receiver operating characteristic (ROC) curve. Figure 9–4 shows an example. The test is a culture of clean catch urine, the disease is gram-negative bacterial infection of the urinary tract, confirmed by either catheterization or needle aspiration of the bladder, and the population young women with symptoms suggesting urinary tract infection. A traditional cut-point for infection is 10^5 bacteria per ml or mm^3; it was established in women with pyelonephritis and worked well for them. However, some less severely ill women were infected with counts as low as 10^2. As the cutoff point between normal and abnormal urine culture is raised, sensitivity declines and specificity increases. At the traditional point of 10^5, 48% of infected women are called normal.

In the general case, ROC curves plot sensitivity on the vertical axis against (1 - specificity) on the horizontal axis. The curve shows the sensitivity and (1 - specificity) corresponding to each cut-point. Tests that distinguish well between normal and abnormal occupy the upper left corner of the fig-

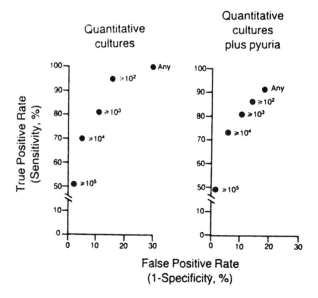

Figure 9–4. A receiver operating characteristic (ROC) curve: quantitative urine culture versus true presence of bacteria in the urine.
Source: Data from Stamm WE, Counts GW, Running KR, et al. Diagnosis of coliform infection in acutely ill dysuric women. N. Engl. J. Med. 307: 463–468, 1982.

ure. Those that contribute no information beyond what was known before the test was applied (the pretest probability) have ROC "curves" on the diagonal. It is possible to characterize the information contributed by a test by the area under the curve and to compare the performance of tests by comparing their areas and seeing if observed differences are beyond chance.

The choice of where to place the cutpoint is driven by the consequences of the resulting misclassification. A test that is intended to be sensitive—because it is important (for the purposes of epidemiologic description, patient care, or research) to discover most cases—should have a low cutoff point, even if this results in a substantial number of false positive test results. On the other hand, a test that should be very specific, because of major consequences of a false positive diagnosis, as is the case with HIV infection, may need to be operated with a high cut-point, even at the expense of sensitivity.

For a given test, the trade-off between sensitivity and specificity is inescapable. However, a new test may be better in both sensitivity and specificity, not requiring as much of a trade-off between the two as its predecessor. On an ROC curve, the new test would be farther in the upper left corner than the old test.

Likelihood Ratios

It is somewhat artificial to consider tests simply normal or abnormal, even taking into account different cut-points. Tests can take on a range of values and it is intuitively obvious (and established by studies) that extremely high values are more likely to represent disease than ones just above the cutpoint. The exact result of the test carries more information, which is discarded when the test is dichotomized. To take into account how different levels of a test represent different probabilities of disease, another summary statistic of test performance, the likelihood ratio, is useful.

A likelihood ratio (LR) is defined as:

$$LR = \frac{\text{Probability of disease in people with a positive test}}{\text{Probability of disease in people with a negative test}}$$

Likelihood ratios carry the same kind of information as sensitivity and specificity together, but for various levels of test results. In addition, they have an attractive mathematical property: it is relatively easy to calculate posttest probability from pretest probability and the test result. However, to take advantage of it, one must first convert probabilities to odds and odds back to probability using the following formulae:

$$\text{Probability} = \frac{\text{odds}}{1 + \text{odds}}$$

$$\text{Odds} = \frac{\text{Probability of event}}{1 - \text{Probability of event}}$$

It is then possible to get posttest odds by simply multiplying pretest odds by the likelihood ratio corresponding to the test result:

$$\text{Posttest odds} = \text{Pretest Odds} \times \text{Likelihood Ratio}$$

Although likelihood ratios have many desirable mathematical and conceptual properties, their meaning is not as intuitively obvious as sensitivity and specificity and so they have not been as widely used for summarizing the information conveyed by a diagnostic test. Many investigators do summarize the performance of a test both ways, however, allowing the reader to choose the methods that suits him or her best.

COMBINATIONS OF TESTS

Single diagnostic tests are rarely sufficient; ordinarily several are used together. The combination of diagnostic tests makes up a diagnostic strategy. Several kinds of strategies are possible, depending on how the tests are combined.

Using Tests in Series

In serial testing if the first test is positive, a second is employed; if the second is positive, a third is done; and so on. This strategy is common for screening for infectious disease. The first test is chosen to be sensitive, so as to miss few cases, to be inexpensive, because it will be applied to many people, and to be safe, because it is not ethical to expose people to risk when they are well. Some (often the majority) of the people with a positive test have false positive results. A second test is chosen to be specific, to avoid labeling people with disease who do not have it, because of the many consequences, financial and human, that accompany a false positive test. If a subsequent test is needed, it may legitimately be more expensive and risky, because it is being applied to relatively few patients and they have an increased probability of having the disease, relative to the original, screened population.

Serologic testing for syphilis is an example of serial testing. Any of several tests based on a lipid nontreponemal antigen (probably present in treponemes but in other tissues as well) is sensitive and inexpensive, and so it is used first. If the reagin test is positive, it is then worth proceeding to a much more specific, sensitive, and expensive test for treponemal antigen, FTA-ABS.

Testing in series tends to decrease the sensitivity and increase the specificity for the strategy as a whole, relative to the individual tests in the series. In effect, it sets a higher standard, with several filters, before a diagnosis is assigned.

Using Tests in Parallel

A second strategy is to test in parallel. One applies several tests together and a positive result for any one of them is considered evidence for disease. If none is positive, this is considered evidence against disease. An example is testing for fungal infections, many of which are difficult to detect, where a clinician might use sputum cultures and stains, skin tests, and serologic testing together to see if any suggests infection. Parallel testing tends to increase the sensitivity and decrease the specificity for the strategy as a whole, relative to any of the individual tests.

Prediction Rules

The information from several tests may be used together to arrive at a single diagnosis. This is a special case of using tests in parallel. For example, one can pool the information contained in the clinical and epidemiologic features of a patient with sore throat (fever, purulence, cervical adenopathy, age, geographic location, season of the year) to predict whether that patient has infection with group A beta-hemolytic streptococcus.

Modern prediction rules are often constructed by using logistic regression to model the relationships between several variables and the presence or absence of disease in a sample of people (Wasson et al. 1985). The model as a whole is the test and its component observations are in effect subtests. The values for a specific patient can be entered into the model, based on data from a sample of similar patients, and his or her probability of disease calculated. The coefficients for each variable are sometimes reduced to whole numbers, to simplify calculations and in recognition of the underlying imprecision of individual components of the model. Even simpler models consider the variables present or absent.

THRESHOLDS FOR DECISION MAKING

Diagnostic tests are a prelude to action. Those using the information must decide on the basis of the test whether to treat or not, report to health officials or not, or enter a research variable as present or absent. Two thresholds for these decisions, defining three courses of action, are diagrammed in Figure 9–5 (Pauker and Kassirer 1975). When the test suggests a low probability of disease one may decide not to act further, on the conviction (based on data) that disease is sufficiently unlikely. At higher probabilities, one reaches a threshold where further testing is warranted, but disease is not likely enough to act on it (e.g., by prescribing antibiotics or entering the patient in a data set as a confirmed case without the results of the test). At a still higher probability of disease, one reaches another threshold where disease is considered sufficiently likely that it is judged present without further testing. The location of these thresholds depends on the disease and test, and also the judgment of the tester and the norms in the setting in which the test is done. For example, in some settings, with few resources, fever alone is sufficient evidence for malaria to begin treatment; in others, the presence of parasites on blood smear, confirmed by a parasitologist, is required. In general, research definitions of disease are more stringent than those used in patient care and public health, because misclassification of variables is cumulative and small decrements in the quality of the data can have large effects on the results of the study, possibly obscuring important relationships in the data.

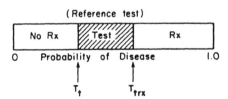

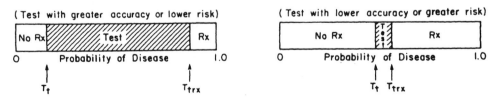

Figure 9–5. Threshold for decision making: The concept of probability at which an infectious disease is considered likely enough to treat (clinical medicine) or code as present (epidemiologic research) or to require further testing to decide. T_t = test. T_{trx} = treat without further testing.
Source: Adapted from Pauker SG, Kassirer JP. The threshold approach to clinical decision-making. N. Engl. J. Med. 302: 1109–1117, 1980.

TECHNOLOGY ASSESSMENT

Diagnostic tests in and of themselves do not help people. To be helpful the information they convey must be used to select effective intervention. Therefore when diagnostic tests are evaluated for practical purposes—to establish public or clinical policy—it is necessary to describe the test's contribution by following through the cascade of events from result of the test to health outcomes (Sox et al. 1988). This process, for tests for infectious and other diseases, has come to be called "technology assessment"; it is a major public policy interest, because of the rising cost of health care and concern that not all care necessarily achieves its main purpose, better outcomes of disease.

First, the test result must be noticed and acted on. Many studies have shown that a distressingly high proportion of tests performed in the care of patients fails to be useful at this level. Additional testing might be necessary to confirm the presence or absence of disease. With the diagnosis confirmed, there must be effective treatment. The treatment must be acceptable to patients and health care providers—because of convenience, comfort, cost, and safety—so that the treatment is actually received. Finally, there must be evidence that the treatment improves the health outcomes.

Health Outcomes

There is a growing consensus that all efforts to improve health should be judged mainly by their effects on clinical outcomes, the sort that could be recognized and valued by the affected people themselves. These health outcomes include: symptoms (e.g., pain, dyspnea, or nausea); disability (e.g., being unable to perform daily activities at work or home); and death (especially if untimely). Biologic outcomes such as negative cultures, fall in antibody titers, or improvement in tests of organ dysfunction, may well be related to health outcomes but this cannot be assumed without strong evidence.

Cost

There is also consensus that cost is a major outcome of health care interventions, certainly including diagnostic tests and their consequences. The cost of diagnostic tests is especially at issue with the advent of new technologies such as computerized tomography, magnetic resonance imaging, and gene probes. Cost analysis is a specialized skill that is not squarely within the discipline of epidemiology, but it is highly relevant to some epidemiologic questions, especially when epidemiologic studies are used to inform public policy decisions.

The total cost attributable to a test includes not only the cost of the test itself but all of the effects that follow from the test. These are commonly divided into two general types: direct and indirect. Direct costs are those directly related to the test and its clinical consequences. Direct medical costs include those that are incurred in the medical setting. Examples for gram-negative sepsis include the cost of diagnostic tests, antibiotics, hospital bed, and physician services. Direct nonmedical costs, which may be a substantial proportion of direct costs, include such things as transportation to a medical facility and food and lodging for family. Indirect costs are the rest, mainly the loss of wages for patient and family either during the illness and its evaluation and treatment until recovery or, if the illness leads to permanent disability or death, lost wages up until the expected time of retirement.

In calculating the costs of a decision to use a diagnostic test, three issues must be borne in mind. First, charges for a service are rarely a fair reflection of its true monetary value because of the widespread accounting practice of charging more than their true costs for some services and less for others. Second, the value of money depends of when it is spent. In general, the present value of money is different in the future because of inflation and the opportunity to invest the money to make it increase in value over time. Therefore analyses of costs that are incurred over many years must discount future costs. Third, the importance of cost depends on who must pay. While many cost analyses are from the perspective of society as a whole, actual costs are often incurred at a more local level—an individual insurance plan, practice, or family.

Cost-Benefit Analysis

Cost-benefit analysis is a way of summarizing the purely monetary consequences of a test. One expression is net cost, the difference between the benefits (in dollars) attributed to the test minus the costs (also in dollars) attributed to the test. Cost-benefit analysis is of limited value in the assessment of health technologies because it fails to take into account nonmonetary aspects of health and disease; it is better suited to commerce.

Cost-Effectiveness Analyses

It is helpful to calculate a number that summarizes the relationship between cost and effect, so that the cost for a given effect for different diagnostic tests can be compared. Cost effectiveness is the ratio of the cost (in dollars or other monetary units) to the effects, such as death averted or disease detected. A common example is the cost per year of life saved. To take into account outcomes of care other than money one can calculate the cost per quality adjusted year of life saved.

SUMMARY

In this chapter, we reviewed the most common quantitative measures for evaluating the validity and reliability of tests used to diagnose infections. We also made brief mention of measures of the utility of tests in terms of their relative costs. Diagnostic tests that are specific to particular infections, such as vector-borne and sexually transmitted infections, are discussed in more detail in Chapters 10–13, addressing the research methods pertaining to the particular types of transmission.

REFERENCES

Begg CB. Biases in the assessment of diagnostic tests. Stat. Med. 6:411–423, 1987.

Fleiss JL. Statistical Methods for Rates and Proportions. 2nd ed. New York: John Wiley & Sons, 1981.

Fletcher RH, Fletcher SW, and Wagner EH. Clinical Epidemiology: The Essentials. 3rd ed. Baltimore: Williams & Wilkins, 1996.

Gardner MJ, and Altman DG. Statistics with confidence—confidence intervals and statistical guidelines. London: British Medical Journal, 1989.

Griner PF, Mayewski RJ, Mushlin AI, and Greenland P. Selection and interpretation of diagnostic tests and procedures. Ann. Intern. Med. 94:553–600, 1981.

Heckerling PS. Confidence in diagnostic testing. J. Gen. Intern. Med. 3:604–606, 1988.

Pauker SG, and Kassirer JP. Therapeutic decision making: A cost-benefit analysis. N. Engl. J. Med. 293:229–234, 1975.

Ransohoff DF, and Feinstein AR. Problems of spectrum and bias in evaluating the efficacy of diagnostic tests. N. Engl. J. Med. 299:926–930, 1978.

Riegelman RK. Studying a Study and Testing a Test. How to Read the Medical Evidence. 4th ed. Philadelphia: Lippincott Williams & Wilkins, 2000.

Sackett DL, Haynes RB, Guyatt GH, and Tugwell P. Clinical Epidemiology. A Basic Science for Clinical Medicine. 2nd ed. Boston: Little, Brown, 1991.

Sox HC, Blatt MA, Higgins MC, and Marton KI. Medical Decision-Making. Boston: Butterworths, 1988.

Sox HC. The evaluation of diagnostic tests: Principles, problems, and new developments. Ann. Rev. Med. 47:463–471, 1996.

Wasson JH, Sox HC Jr, Neff RK, and Goldman L. Clinical prediction rules. Applications and methodological standards. N. Engl. J. Med. 313:793–799, 1985.

Part III

METHODS BY TRANSMISSION TYPE

10

Respiratory Transmission

JACK M. GWALTNEY, JR., and J. OWEN HENDLEY

Richard Riley, a pioneer aerobiologist of the twentieth century, traced concern over respiratory spread of disease back to the time of the ancient Egyptian dynasties (Riley 1980). In fact, early theories of contagion tended to focus on respiratory spread of disease more than subsequent work has shown to be warranted. The nineteenth century discovery of important water and foodborne transmission routes shifted attention away from respiratory mechanisms of spread. Interest in the respiratory area was renewed in the twentieth century by the work of William Wells who proposed the concept of droplet nuclei, small ($<10\mu$) infectious particles that remain suspended in air (Wells 1934). This mode of transmission was subsequently shown to be important in some respiratory diseases such as tuberculosis and measles. The route by which common cold viruses spread remained speculative. More recent work has implicated virus contaminated fingers in the transmission of rhinovirus colds (Hendley et al. 1973). This discovery has shifted attention to direct contact as a method of transmission for some respiratory viruses.

It now appears that not all respiratory pathogens are transmitted in the same manner and that small particle aerosol, large ($>10\mu$) particle aerosol, and direct contact may each have a role. This in turn affects the methodology required for epidemiologic studies of respiratory pathogens. A broad range of microbial pathogens infects the respiratory tract of humans including bacteria, mycobacteria, mycoplasmas, chlamydia, fungi, and viruses. The biological characteristics of these organisms and the environmental and behavioral features that influence risk of infection are so diverse that a comprehensive review of the subject is impractical in one chapter. Consequently, this chapter addresses methodology related to studying the viruses that cause acute respiratory infection.

VIRAL PATHOGENS

A number of viruses are spread by respiratory secretions and/or infect by way of the respiratory tract (Table 10–1). This group is composed of more than 200 antigenically

Table 10–1 Viruses that Are Transmitted in Respiratory Secretions and/or Infect by Way of the Respiratory Tract

Predominant Manifestations of Disease	No. Serotypes
Respiratory	
Upper airway	
Rhinovirus	>100
Coronavirus	4
Upper and lower airways	
Influenza virus	3
Parainfluenza virus	4
Respiratory syncytial virus	2
Adenovirus virus	>33
Nonrespiratory	
Skin	
Measles virus	1
Rubella virus	1
Varicella virus	1
Systemic	
Hantavirus	1*
CNS	
ECHO virus	31
Coxsackie virus	29

*Serotypes Puumala (PUU), Seoul (SEO), Hantaan (HTN), or HTN-like types, and Dobrav.

distinct types and several different virus families. Some of these viruses produce disease that is primarily restricted to the respiratory tract. Others enter by the respiratory tract and then disseminate by way of the blood stream to produce disease elsewhere, such as in skin and the central nervous system. The reservoir of the major respiratory viruses is the respiratory tract of humans. In general, respiratory viruses cause acute self-limited infections. Long-term carriage can occur with some such as adenovirus, but "colonization" as with the respiratory bacteria does not occur. The genome of most of the viruses in Table 10–1 is composed of RNA with the exceptions of adenovirus and varicella virus, which contain DNA. Most of the viruses are surrounded by a lipid-containing envelope or membrane except for rhinovirus, adenovirus, and the enteroviruses (ECHO and Coxsackie A and B). The viruses vary in size from the picornavirus family (25–30 nm) to the myxoviruses and varicella virus (100–300 nm).

Certain biologic characteristics of these viruses appear to be associated with their epidemiologic behavior. The site(s) at which virus replicates in the respiratory tract may influence the route by which virus exits the infected host. For example, replication of virus in the lower respiratory tract coupled with cough would be expected to result in the production of virus-containing aerosols, while viral replication in the nose would be associated with virus in nasal secretions but not in droplet nuclei. Once released into the environment, the virus's duration of survival is an important characteristic that is related to the chemical and physical properties of the viral coat. Enveloped viruses show somewhat less stability on surfaces and in aerosols than viruses that do not have envelopes. For example, rhinovirus, a nonenveloped virus, has been shown to survive at least four days on hard surfaces (Hendley and Gwaltney 1988), while respiratory syncytial virus, an enveloped virus, survived for less than seven hours on nonporous surfaces (Hall et al. 1980). Also, nonenveloped viruses, such as rhinovirus and adenovirus, survive better in relative humidities above 50%, while enveloped viruses, such as influenza and parainfluenza viruses, survive better at low relative humidity (Buckland and Tyrrell 1962, Gwaltney 1984). Humidity affects virus survival both on surface and in aerosols.

Another feature of respiratory viruses that is important in epidemiologic behavior is the capacity to evoke immunity. For example, infection with a rhinovirus serotype usually, but not always, leads to long-lasting immunity to that serotype, while respiratory syncytial virus and coronavirus infections do not usually provide lasting immunity. An important characteristic of influenza virus is its capacity for antigenic change. The antigenic shifts and drifts of influenza virus are clearly associated with its epidemiologic behavior.

POPULATIONS

Acute Respiratory Infections Are Universal

Epidemiologic studies of natural respiratory illness have been conducted in various groups, including industrial populations (Lidwell and Williams 1961, Gwaltney et al. 1966), families (Dingle et al. 1964, Dick et al. 1967,

Hendley et al. 1969), military recruits (Johnson et al. 1962, Voors et al. 1968), and students (Hamre and Procknow 1963, Glezen et al. 1975). Also, following the lead of Dr. Walter Kruse, who originated the method (Kruse 1914), a considerable amount of work has been done with experimentally infected volunteers (Andrewes 1965, Tyrrell 1965, Douglas 1970, Dick et al. 1987, Hayden et al. 1996, Gwaltney In press).

CASE IDENTIFICATION AND MEASUREMENT OF ILLNESS SEVERITY

The clinical features of acute viral respiratory illness, especially of the common cold, are primarily subjective in nature. This influences the methods that have been used in epidemiologic studies to diagnose illness. The methods of case identification used for common colds includes self-diagnosis by the patient, diagnosis by the investigator, and specific diagnostic criteria based on symptom reporting (Monto 1994).

Self-Diagnosis by the Patient

Some of the classic epidemiologic studies of acute respiratory illness, such as the Cleveland (Dingle et al. 1964) and Tecumseh (Monto et al. 1971) studies, used self-diagnosis by the patient for case definition. Identification of illness was based on the individual subject's perception of what he or she believed constituted a common cold or influenzal illness. An adult family member, usually the mother, identified illness in children and sometimes other family members.

Case definition by self-diagnosis has the advantage of simplicity, but variables such as cultural background and age may influence the perception of what constitutes illness. This method can be used to collect nominal data, presence or absence of illness. It also has been used to collect information on individual symptoms, using a diary.

Diagnosis by the Investigator

Diagnosis by the investigator has been used in epidemiologic studies of acute respiratory illness both with natural illness (Hilleman et al. 1962, Selwyn 1990) and in experimental infection (Murphy et al. 1980). Investigator-based diagnosis reduces the individual variation associated with self-diagnosis, but the major disadvantage in the method is that much of respiratory illness is subjective in nature. Objective findings of excessive nasal secretions, sneezing/coughing, and erythema of the mucosa of the upper airways are too episodic and variable to be valid measures of the occurrence of illness. Thus an individual with a severe cold based on symptoms experienced may show only minimal objective evidence of disease at the one point in time when seen by the investigator.

Criteria-Based Diagnosis

In recent decades, epidemiologic studies of acute respiratory illness have moved toward identification of illness based on preestablished criteria. With these methods, subjects use a standardized form to report on the presence or absence of a preselected list of respiratory and general symptoms (Gwaltney et al. 1966). Recording of symptoms is either done by the subject or by a member of the investigative team on a daily basis. This system can provide either nominal data based on presence or absence of symptoms or ordinal data when the severity of symptoms is quantified. Case identification is based on preselected criteria for diagnosis of an illness. Criteria-based diagnosis has the important advantage of yielding data that can be replicated by other investigators, thus providing consistency over space and time.

The Jackson Method

One of the early criteria-based methods was reported in 1958 by Dr. Jackson and colleagues, who used it for identifying the occurrence of acute respiratory illness in volunteers with experimental respiratory infections (Jackson et al. 1958). This method, slightly modified for use with the rhinovirus challenge model, has been widely used and proven to be very useful. With the Jackson method, the subject reports each morning on the occurrence and severity of the following symptoms: sneezing, rhinorrhea, nasal obstruction, sore (or scratchy) throat, cough, headache, malaise, and chilliness. Symptom severity is graded absent (0), mild (1+), moderate (2+), severe (3+). In some studies, a very severe category (4+) has been used.

Baseline symptoms present prior to virus challenge are also collected. Scoring is done by subtracting the score of any symptom present at baseline from the score of that symptom on each day it is present after virus challenge. The daily scores of the individual symptoms are summed and the sums of all symptoms over the five-day observation period added to give a total symptom score. In Jackson's original work, which was with Coxsackie A-21 virus infection, the diagnosis of illness depended on the subject having a total symptom score of ≥ 14 over five days plus the subjective impression (at the end of the study) that he or she had had a cold and/or the presence of rhinorrhea on ≥ 3 of the five days of observation. Because rhinovirus colds are less severe on average than Coxsackie A-21 respiratory illness, the reference standard for the total symptom score was reduced from 14 to 5 or 6 for use with the rhinovirus challenge model (Hendley et al. 1972).

A number of data sets have been collected using the modified Jackson Method for scoring experimental rhinovirus colds. With this method, the mean ($\pm$SD) total symptom score over five days in experimental rhinovirus colds is approximately 16 (Parekh et al. 1992, Gwaltney, Park et al. 1996). The performance characteristics of the rhinovirus challenge model have been examined, and the relationship between effect size, variance, and statistical significance has been defined (Gwaltney, Buier et al. 1996) (Fig. 10–1). Currently, the Jackson Method of case identification (with modification for rhinovirus) is the best validated and most widely used method for diagnosing acute respiratory illness in experimental models. New methods of scoring and diagnosis should be validated against the Jackson Method before they are employed in epidemiologic studies.

The University of Virginia Method
The University of Virginia Method is another criteria-based system for the diagnosis of the acute respiratory illness that has primarily been used with natural colds. In a long-term epidemiologic study of acute respiratory illness, begun in 1963, in a population of insurance company employees, subjects recorded the daily presence or absence of sneezing, runny nose, nasal obstruction, sore (scratchy) throat, cough, headache, malaise, feverishness, and chilliness on symptom record cards that covered a two-week period (Gwaltney et al. 1966). They were visited weekly at their desks by a member of the investigative team to encourage complete and accurate recording of symptoms. Subjects were instructed not to record symptoms that they believed to be of allergic etiology.

The criteria for the diagnosis of an acute respiratory illness was the presence of two or more respiratory symptoms on one or more days or of one or more respiratory symptom(s) on two or more days. Sneezing alone on two or more days was not counted as an illness, because it became apparent that the occurrence of this single symptom was not representative of a common cold. Similar criteria-based methods have been used in other epidemiologic studies, sometimes with quantification of symptom severity to provide ordinal data (Elkhatieb et al. 1993).

Objective measurements of illness severity
Although the features of acute respiratory illnesses are primarily subjective in nature, several objective measurements provide interval data. These include sneeze and cough counts, nasal resistance, nasal mucus weights, eustachian tube function, middle ear pressure, and sinus CT examination.

Sneeze and cough count. Sneeze and cough counts have been manually recorded by subjects in some studies. With the rhinovirus model, good correlations have been observed between the number of sneezes and coughs per day and the subjective severity of these symptoms graded by the Jackson Method (Gwaltney, Park et al. 1996, Gwaltney and Druce 1997). Also, tape recordings of coughs have been used in trials of cough treatments (Kuhn et al. 1982).

Nasal resistance. Nasal resistance has been measured by anterior rhinomanometry (Connell 1982). This measurement has considerable person-to-person variation and is

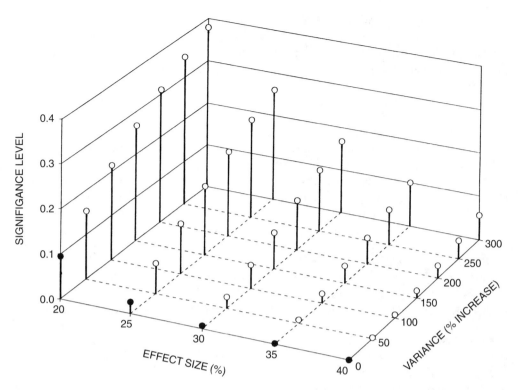

Figure 10–1. The influence of signal variance and treatment effect size on significance level in experimental rhinovirus colds. Student's *t* test was used to evaluate the mean differences in total symptom scores between treatment and control groups. The beginning mean total symptom score (15.9) for the control group and the associated SD (var = 10.7) are from part of the data set (58 young adults) of an earlier clinical trial (Gwaltney, Park et al. 1996). Values represented by ● are based on the amount of variance in the actual data set.

subject to the normal nasal cycle of turbinate engorgement. Measured nasal resistance does not correlate well with severity of the subjective feeling of nasal obstruction. In one study, evidence of swelling of the nasal turbinates or thickening of the nasal walls was present in only 9 of 16 subjects with elevated airway resistance (Gwaltney et al. 1994). Nasal resistance measurement has been used most successfully in clinical trials of nasal decongestants, especially when studies were conducted over short intervals of time and compared sequential changes in the same individual.

Nasal mucus weight. A method of measuring nasal mucus weights in subjects with experimental colds was developed by Knight (Kravetz et al. 1961). With this method, all paper tissues that have been used for nose blowing by a subject are stored in an airtight container. The weight of a 24-hour collection of used nasal tissues is compared to the weight of an equal number of unused tissues to give the mucus weight. In a data set from 151 young adults with experimental rhinovirus colds, the mean (±SD) total mucus weight per subject for five days was 22.6 (±28.2) gm (Parekh et al. 1992). Nasal mucus weights have correlated well with subjective scores of rhinorrhea severity (Parekh et al. 1992, Gwaltney, Park et al. 1996, Gwaltney and Druce 1997) but did not correlate well in multivariant analysis with nasal obstruction or total symptom score (Parekh et al. 1992). Nasal mucus weight measurement is perhaps the best objective measurement of cold severity currently available. Nasal mucus weight is usually performed on subjects who are housed in a research facility or motel room where it is convenient for the subject to collect and store the used tissues.

Eustachian tube function and middle ear pressure. Measurement of eustachian tube function by the nine-step test and middle ear pressure by tympanometry have been adapted to common cold studies. Abnormalities in both parameters occur regularly in experimental (McBride et al. 1989, Buchman et al. 1994) and natural (Elkhatieb et al. 1993) colds and have been used in clinical trials of cold remedies (Sperber et al. 1992). Because of the role of colds in the pathogenesis of middle ear disease, these tests, when appropriate, can provide a useful addition to epidemiologic studies of acute respiratory disease.

Sinus CT scan examination. The recent discovery of sinus involvement in the common cold has provided another objective measurement of illness. The common cold is correctly viewed as a viral rhinosinusitis, with up to 85% of adults showing sinus abnormalities on CT examination (Gwaltney et al. 1994). The abnormalities consist primarily of viscous fluid accumulations in the sinus cavities and drainage passages (Gwaltney 1996, Gwaltney et al. 2000), but the findings are frequently misread as "mucosal thickening." Attempts to develop quantitative scoring systems for determining the degree of sinus abnormality have focused on the amount of "mucosal thickening" and have not been very successful. At present, it is most useful to determine if sinus disease is present or absent in patients with colds and if present, to follow the subject for evidence of clearing. CT measurement of sinus abnormality can be used to study the pathogenesis of viral and bacterial rhinosinusitis and to evaluate the effectiveness of treatments for these diseases.

MEASUREMENT OF INFECTION AND VIRUS IDENTIFICATION

Studies of the epidemiology of acute respiratory illness were greatly facilitated by the development of cell culture techniques for virus propagation. Cell culture remains the criterion standard for the diagnosis of most known respiratory viruses. Serologic diagnosis using acute and convalescent serum specimens has also been a standard method in epidemiologic work. More recently, other techniques including electron microscopy, fluorescent antibody, immunoperoxidase, reverse transcriptase-polymerase chain reaction (RT-PCR), and nucleic acid probe have become available. The newer methods bring various advantages and disadvantages, but all fall short of the validity of serial propagation of a viral isolate in cell culture as the standard for detecting infection. Without content validity, epidemiologic studies have no value. Therefore it is important with a new virus detection method to determine if it has been validated against viral recovery in cell culture (when possible) and to know its sensitivity and specificity against this standard. Newer methods of viral identification that appear to have greater sensitivity than cell culture are especially suspect until reasonable efforts have been made to assure that findings are valid and do not represent false positives for technical reasons.

Cell Culture

Most of the major respiratory viruses including influenza virus, rhinovirus, respiratory syncytial virus, adenovirus, and the parainfluenza viruses grow well in appropriate cell cultures. An exception is coronavirus, for which sensitive cell cultures have not been developed. Cell culture has the disadvantage, compared to some methods, of the cost of operating a virology laboratory and of the time required for testing. In epidemiologic studies, the time factor is usually not a consideration. Cell culture has the advantage of being the reference standard for most respiratory viruses and of thus producing the highest degree of content validity for an investigation. The various methods of cell culture for respiratory viruses are described in appropriate texts (Lennette 1992).

Serology

Isolation of the respiratory viruses in cell culture provided the viral antigens needed to develop serologic tests for diagnosis of infection. These methods include neutralization, hemagglutination inhibition, complement fixation, and ELISA (Lennette 1992). In some instances, such as with rhinovirus, virus isolation in cell culture is more sensitive than serologic diagnosis. The 100 antigenically distinct rhinovirus serotypes make serologic testing impractical. Serum antibody to respiratory syncytial virus is present in everyone over the age of two years, making detection of antibody rises with this infection not very useful. With other viruses such as influenza, serologic diagnosis may be more sensitive than cell culture in years in which influenza virus strains do not adapt well to cell culture. Newer, rapid serologic tests are commercially available for some of the respiratory viruses. It is important to determine that new serologic tests have acceptable sensitivity and specificity against the performance standard of virus isolation in cell culture before relying on them for diagnosis of infection. Serologic diagnosis, to be most accurate, has the disadvantage of requiring acute and convalescent blood specimens. This adds to the difficulty of specimen collection and delays diagnosis. On the other hand, serologic diagnosis may identify cases that were not detected by virus isolation or other methods and provides useful information on the immunology of the infection under investigation.

Fluorescent Antibody and Immunoperoxidase

Viral antigens in specimens of respiratory secretions or in inoculated cell cultures can be detected by fluorescent antibody (Ahluwalia et al. 1987) and immunoperoxidase techniques (Turner et al. 1982). These methods lack sensitivity under some circumstances and their specificity must be assured if they are to provide valid results.

Reverse Transcriptase-Polymerase Chain Reaction (RT-PCR)

RT-PCR appears to hold promise for diagnosis of infection using samples of respiratory secretions (Hendley 1999). Assays have been developed for rhinovirus and coronavirus (Arruda et al. 1997, Mäkelä et al. 1998) and for simultaneous diagnosis of respiratory syncytial virus, parainfluenza vi-

ruses, and influenza virus (Fan et al. 1998). Because of the low concentrations of virus in respiratory secretions, the amplification obtained by RT-PCR is important for providing the sensitivity needed for accurate diagnosis of infection. With rhinovirus, RT-PCR showed 98%–100% sensitivity compared to testing in two sensitive cell culture lines (Arruda et al. 1997, Mäkelä et al. 1998). Cell cultures showed 76%–82% sensitivity compared to RT-PCR. RT-PCR requires careful attention to detail in performing the test and strict precautions to prevent false positives that result from contamination of specimens with exogenous nucleic acid.

Nucleic Acid Probes

Hybridization with virus nucleic acid in respiratory secretions using labeled synthetic oligonucleotide probes does not have sufficient sensitivity to be practical for use in diagnosis of infection (Hendley 1999). More than 10^2 copies of the viral genome are required for detection with this method. However, nucleic acid probes have been used with in situ hybridization assays to detect virus in respiratory tissue. This technique is useful in studies of viral transmission and pathogenesis where accurate location of viral replication is desired.

SPECIMEN COLLECTION

A variety of specimens has been used for diagnosis of respiratory virus infection using the methods described previously. Nasal and pharyngeal swabs and nasal rinses are generally used for viral isolation. Nasal rinse appears to give better virus recovery on average than the swab method (Cate et al. 1964, Arruda et al. 1996). Conjunctival swabs provide an additional specimen for adenovirus culture. Hand rinses with viral collecting broth have been used to detect rhinovirus on the fingers in transmission studies of rhinovirus colds. Respiratory specimens are usually inoculated into a protein containing viral collecting broth for transportation (and storage) prior to inoculation in cell culture (Lennette 1992). When possible, testing of specimens prior to freezing is desirable. Scrape and punch biopsies of nasal epithelium have been used for viral culture as well as for in situ location of viral nucleic acid using nucleic acid probes (Bardin et al. 1994, Arruda et al. 1995). Sampling of the paranasal sinuses requires sinus aspiration to obtain uncontaminated specimens for culture (Gwaltney 1996). Claims that culture of the middle meatus by endoscopy reflects conditions in the sinus cavity have so far not been adequately substantiated. Specimens of lower respiratory tract secretions collected by bronchoscopy have also been used for viral isolation (Halperin et al. 1983). Bronchoscopic specimens may be contaminated with upper airway virus during collection and thus are difficult to interpret.

Aerosol samples in studies of airborne transmission of infection have been collected by means of air sampling devices such as a large volume air sampler (Artenstein et al. 1968). A simpler method of collecting cough and sneeze specimens has been to have subjects cough or sneeze directly onto petri dishes containing viral collecting broth (Hendley et al. 1973). This method does not distinguish whether the virus is present in a large or small particle aerosol, but by collecting coughs and sneezes separately, sites at which virus-containing aerosols are being generated may be identified.

Biopsies of respiratory epithelium can be obtained by curette and other scraping devices; full thickness specimens of epithelium can be obtained by punch biopsy. Venous blood is processed to provide serum specimens for antibody measurements. Also, nasal washes have been used for measuring antibody produced in the nose. A method to adjust for the dilution of nasal washes has been developed using simultaneous blood and nasal wash urea concentrations (Kaulbach et al. 1993).

EXPERIMENTAL DESIGNS

Virus Challenge Models

Successful experimental virus challenge requires that the subject be susceptible to infection with the challenge virus (Mufson et al. 1963, Hendley et al. 1972). This is ac-

complished by determining that the subject does not have protective levels of antibody to the challenge virus. Most virus challenge studies have been done with rhinovirus and influenza virus. Other respiratory viruses have been used less frequently for the purpose, partially because it is difficult to locate adult subjects without antibody to these viruses.

Challenge models have been used to study transmission (Hendley and Gwaltney 1988), pathogenesis (Naclerio et al. 1988), risk factors (Cohen et al. 1995), vaccines (Murphy et al. 1981), and treatments (Gwaltney and Druce 1997). Experimental infection has a number of advantages over natural infection including control of the time and dose of virus inoculation, predictability of the time of symptom onset, potential for the manipulation of different routes of exposure, close monitoring of clinical parameters, compliance in dosing (in treatment trials), and lower noise to signal ratio (Gwaltney, Buier et al. 1996). Effect sizes are generally larger in treatment trials using the challenge model than in comparable studies of patients with natural colds. Certain aspects of viral transmission and pathogenesis can be studied with more precision in a model than with natural colds and efficacy of treatments more precisely evaluated. On the other hand, experimental infection has the disadvantage of allowing study of only one type of virus at a time and of collecting observations under artificial conditions.

Recruitment and Screening

Most virus challenge studies require subjects to remain in isolation from the general public. Thus subjects are recruited who have periods of five to seven days that can be spared from their regular routines. Since the closing of the Common Cold Research Unit in Salisbury, England (which used vacationers), most subjects have been recruited from college and university populations. The current practice is to measure serum antibody titers of a group of potential subjects against the challenge virus. With rhinovirus challenge, neutralizing antibody titers of 1:2 or less are the cut-off point usually selected for participation.

Virus Challenge

Rhinovirus and influenza virus challenge is usually performed by means of coarse drops delivered into the nose. Other forms of inoculation have included drops onto the conjunctiva (Bynoe et al. 1961, Winther et al. 1986) and aerosols (Couch et al. 1966). Aerosol challenge is not considered safe with viruses such as influenza that have the potential to cause severe and even fatal pneumonia. In studies of transmission routes, rhinovirus has also been introduced into the nose or eye by means of virus-contaminated fingers (Gwaltney et al. 1978). Challenge by means of dropping rhinovirus into the mouth is not efficient (Hendley and Gwaltney 1988) nor is prolonged kissing (D'Alessio et al. 1984). The human infectious dose$_{50}$ for rhinovirus ranges from 0.1 to 5.7 TCID$_{50}$ (Douglas 1970, Hendley et al. 1972). Viral challenge doses in the range of 100 to 1000 are usually given in order to produce consistent infection. With influenza virus, larger challenge doses (~10^5 TCID$_{50}$) are needed to reliably produce infection in susceptible volunteers (Hayden et al. 1996).

Measurement of Illness and Infection

A modification of the previously described Jackson Method of symptom severity scoring and diagnosis of illness is most commonly used in association with measurement of nasal secretion weights. These standard measurements of illness may be supplemented by other methods, depending on the nature of the study. Infection has been detected by isolation of virus from daily cultures of respiratory secretions and measurement of homotypic antibody response. Infection is usually defined as recovery of the challenge virus on one or more days and/or a fourfold rise in serum antibody. Newer methods such as RT-PCR may supplement these techniques in the future.

Sample Size Calculations

Based on calculations using a data set obtained with the rhinovirus challenge model, the relationship between variance, effect size, and probability has been described

(Gwaltney, Buier et al. 1996). The amount of variance in symptom severity in data sets from the rhinovirus challenge model is such that sample sizes of 50 or more subjects per cell are required to detect a "clinically relevant" ($\geq 30\%$) effect size at $p < 0.05$ for cold treatments.

NATURAL INFECTIONS

Recruitment

Colds are frequent during the respiratory disease season (early fall to late spring) and recruiting in suitable populations usually provides subjects for epidemiologic studies.

Surveillance

A major problem with enrolling persons with natural colds is to obtain subjects in the early phase of the illness. The major burden of illness in rhinovirus colds occurs in the first three days of infection (Rao et al. 1995, Gwaltney, Buier et al. 1996). The first three days of infection also is the period of maximum viral shedding (Douglas et al. 1966, Winther et al. 1986) and appears to be the period of maximum contagiousness (D'Alessio et al. 1976). A substantial proportion of subjects with natural colds recruited "off the street" will not be in the first day or two of their illness when they report (Gwaltney, Buier et al. 1966, Gwaltney In press). This problem can be solved to some extent by enrolling a population for prospective surveillance at the beginning of or during the respiratory disease season (late August or early September to early May). These individuals maintain a daily record of the presence or absence of respiratory and general symptoms as described previously and immediately report to the investigative team when any symptoms begin. At this time, they are then enrolled into the phase of the study dealing with its specific investigative goal, such as transmission or treatment.

Sample Size Calculations

Data sets are available for determining variance in symptom severity in patients with natural colds (Turner et al, 1997). As discussed earlier, larger sample sizes are usually required to detect equivalent effect sizes with natural colds than with the challenge model.

Comparison of Natural and Experimental Infection

Natural and experimental rhinovirus colds share a number of features including low viral inoculum to initiate infection (Douglas 1970, Hendley et al. 1972), similar sites of viral shedding (Hendley and Gwaltney 1988), similar symptom profiles and duration of illness (Rao et al. 1995), and similar response or lack of response to specific treatments (Gwaltney In press). Findings in the rhinovirus challenge model have also correlated with the results of natural cold studies in the areas of transmission (Hendley and Gwaltney 1988), and pathogenesis (Naclerio et al. 1988, Proud et al. 1990). Correlations have been observed with experimental and natural influenza infection, but fewer data are available for this virus. Although useful extrapolations can be made from results obtained in challenge model experiments, it is still necessary to confirm important findings obtained with the models by observations from natural infection.

Study of Viral Transmission

To provide valid information, transmission studies must have content validity (accurate identification of illness and infection), sensitive methods of detecting virus in respiratory samples and the environment, and a design that focuses on only one route of transmission at a time. Techniques for the detection and measurement of illness, infection, and viral presence have been discussed. Experimental designs have been developed for focusing on specific routes of viral transmission, especially hand contact and small particle aerosol. In these studies, subjects who are known to be susceptible to the study virus (recipients) are exposed to experimentally infected subjects who are symptomatic (donors). An example of one study design is the hand contamination self-inoculation design. This method of exposure produces high transmission rates and

has been used in a number of studies with rhinovirus (Gwaltney et al. 1978, Gwaltney In press). In another design that focuses on aerosol spread, recipients are placed in elbow restraints that prevent finger-to-nose and finger-to-eye contact (Dick et al. 1987). To produce high transmission rates, this method requires using serial donors with severe cough.

Studies of the hand contact route of transmission have been done under natural conditions in the home setting using a virucidal finger treatment to interrupt cold virus spread (Hendley and Gwaltney 1988). Studies using ultraviolet light to interrupt aerosol spread of natural respiratory infections were performed under natural conditions in the 1940s/50s (Riley 1980). The ultraviolet lights were used primarily in school classrooms. The results of these studies were difficult to interpret because of the inability to apply ultraviolet lighting throughout the environment of the study populations, resulting in exposures in unirradiated atmospheres.

Transmission Postulates

The study of respiratory virus transmission has led to the development of a set of five postulates that address the problem of accurately identifying routes of microbial spread (Table 10–2) (Gwaltney and Hendley 1978). The first four of the postulates are based on inductive inference, while the fifth, and key, postulate, is deductive in nature. The fifth postulate requires (1) that transmission be interrupted by a measure that would only affect the hypothesized route of spread, and (2) that the intervention is effective under natural conditions.

DIRECTIONS FOR FUTURE EPIDEMIOLOGIC RESEARCH

Although progress has been made over the last half century in understanding the natural history and epidemiology of acute respiratory illness, a great deal is still unknown. Important unanswered questions in this field follow.

Table 10–2 Postulates to Address Routes of Microbial Transmission

Postulate	Description
Postulate Number One	Microbial growth occurs at the proposed anatomic site of replication
Postulate Number Two	Microbes are present in secretions or tissues shed from the site of origin
Postulate Number Three	Microbes contaminate and survive in or on postulated environmental substances or objects
Postulate Number Four	Contaminated substances or objects reach a portal of entry of a new host
Postulate Number Five	Interruption of transmission by a hypothesized route reduces the incidence of natural infection

Etiology and Natural History

Despite the discovery of over 200 different respiratory viruses, it has not been possible to assign an etiology to an important proportion of colds, especially during the late fall, winter, and early spring. The reason for this is unknown, with some experts contending that known but underdiagnosed viruses are responsible for the unexplained illness, and others that there are respiratory pathogens that have yet to be discovered. Work on the etiology of acute respiratory illness has virtually ceased because of lack of funding and interest, although new diagnostic methods like RT-PCR detection may help address this question. Without ongoing studies in the field, work on the natural history of acute respiratory illness has also suffered.

Transmission

With rhinovirus, the best studied respiratory virus, an important proportion of infections (40%–60%) appears to result from direct contact spread by hand contamination/self-inoculation. However, the support for this conclusion is, as yet, limited (Hendley and Gwaltney 1988, Corley et al. 1987). Respiratory syncytial virus may also spread by the hand contact route, but data addressing this question are also limited (Hall and Douglas 1981). Measles is generally accepted as spreading in small particle aerosol (airborne route) as the result of clinical observation and epidemiologic investigations of apparent common source outbreaks (Remington et al. 1985). Common source outbreaks of influenza have also been reported, supporting airborne transmission for this

virus (Moser et al. 1979). Also, data have been collected on survival of influenza virus on objects in the environment, supporting the feasibility of hand contact spread. Work on respiratory virus transmission is also progressing poorly because of lack of support and interest.

Interruption of Transmission

The idea of a virucidal hand treatment for interrupting direct contact spread of rhinovirus colds has shown promise (Hendley and Gwaltney 1988), but this approach has not been reduced to practical application. To be most effective, this approach requires compounds that safely provide long-lasting antiviral activity on the skin. Interruption of transmission by the aerosol route presents a difficult problem in practical application. While the technology of air filtration and purification has progressed, its application on a broad enough scale to have practical value in control of airborne infection remains daunting.

Vaccine Development. Control of microbial transmission by creating artificial barriers of immunity with vaccines has been very successful. Work continues on vaccine development for influenza, respiratory syncytial virus, and the parainfluenza viruses. Live influenza vaccines have had successful testing, but their superiority over inactivated vaccines is at best marginal. Live influenza vaccines also present production problems that do not exist with inactivated vaccines. Live adenovirus vaccine has been very successful in controlling acute respiratory disease (ARD) in military recruit populations. It is ironic that the supply of this vaccine is now exhausted, and the military seems unable or unwilling to find a replacement source. Recent experience with military recruits who failed to get the vaccine indicates that adenovirus acute respiratory disease will reemerge as a serious problem unless the vaccination is resumed (Barraza et al. 1999).

Antiviral Development

New antivirals for prophylaxis and treatment of respiratory infections, especially rhinovirus and influenza, are being developed by pharmaceutical companies. Testing of these compounds is in progress in challenge models and in populations with natural infections. Success with rhinovirus treatment has been reported with a combined antiviral-antimediator approach (Gwaltney 1992) and with the use of soluble ICAM receptor to block viral attachment to nasal cells (Turner et al. 1999). Work on antiviral treatment for influenza is also continuing. New compounds that are selective inhibitors of types A and B neuraminidases have shown promise (Hayden et al. 1997). Two neuraminidase inhibitors have been FDA approved for use in the United States.

REFERENCES

Ahluwalia GJ, Embree J, McNicol P, Law B, and Hammond GW. Comparison of nasopharyngeal aspirate and nasopharyngeal swab specimens for respiratory syncytial virus diagnosis by cell culture, indirect immunofluorescence assay, and enzyme-linked immunosorbent assay. J. Clin. Microbiol. 25:763–767, 1987.

Andrewes C. The Common Cold. New York: W.W. Norton, 1965.

Arruda E, Boyle TR, Winther B, et al. Localization of human rhinovirus replication in the upper respiratory tract by *in situ* hybridization. J. Infect. Dis. 171:1329–1333, 1995.

Arruda E, Crump CE, Rollins BS, et al. Comparative susceptibilities of human embryonic fibroblasts and HeLa cells for isolation of human rhinoviruses. J. Clin. Microbiol. 34:1277–1279, 1996.

Arruda E, Pitkäranta A, Witek TJ, Doyle CA, and Hayden FG. Frequency and natural history of rhinovirus infections in adults during autumn. J. Clin. Microbiol. 35:2864–2868, 1997.

Artenstein MS, Miller WS, Lamson TH, and Brandt BL. Large-volume air sampling for meningococci and adenoviruses. Am. J. Epidemiol. 87:567–577, 1968.

Bardin PG, Johnston SL, Sanderson G, et al. Detection of rhinovirus infection of the nasal mucosa by oligonucleotide in situ hybridization. Am. J. Respir. Cell Mol. Biol. 10:207–213, 1994.

Barraza EM, Ludwig SL, Gaydos JC, and Brundage JF. Reemergence of adenovirus type 4 acute respiratory disease in military trainees: Report of an outbreak during a lapse in vaccination. J. Infect. Dis. 179:1531–1533, 1999.

Buchman CA, Doyle WJ, Skoner D, Fireman P, and Gwaltney JM. Otologic manifestations of experimental rhinovirus infection. Laryngoscope. 104:1295–1299, 1994.

Buckland FE, and Tyrrell DAJ. Loss of infectivity on drying various viruses. Nature. 195:1063–1064, 1962.

Bynoe ML, Hobson D, Horner J, et al. Inoculation of human volunteers with a strain of virus from a common cold. Lancet. 1:1194–1196, 1961.

Cate TR, Couch RD, and Johnson KM. Studies with rhinoviruses in volunteers: Production of illness, effect of naturally acquired antibody, and demonstration of a protective effect not associated with serum antibody. J. Clin. Invest. 43:56–67, 1964.

Cohen S, Gwaltney JM Jr, Doyle WJ, et al. State and trait negative affect as predictors of objective and subjective symptoms of a common cold. J. Pers. Soc. Psychol. 68:159–169, 1995.

Connell JT. Rhinometry: Measurement of nasal patency. Ann. Allergy 49:179–185, 1982.

Corley DL, Gevirtz R, Nideffer R, and Cummins L. Prevention of postinfectious asthma in children by reducing self-inoculatory behavior. J. Pediatr. Psychol. 12:519–531, 1987.

Couch RB, Cate TR, Douglas RG Jr, Gerone PJ, and Knight V. Effect of route of inoculation on experimental respiratory viral disease in volunteers and evidence for airborne transmission. Bacteriol. Rev. 30:517–529, 1966.

D'Alessio DJ, Peterson JA, Dick CR, and Dick EC. Transmission of experimental rhinovirus colds in volunteer married couples. J. Infect. Dis. 133:26–36, 1976.

D'Alessio DJ, Meschievitz CK, Peterson JA, Dick CR, and Dick EC. Short-duration exposure and the transmission of rhinoviral colds. J. Infect. Dis. 150:189–194, 1984.

Dick EC, Blumer CR, and Evans AS. Epidemiology of infections with rhinovirus types 43 and 55 in a group of University of Wisconsin student families. Am. J. Epidemiol. 86:386–400, 1967.

Dick EC, Jennings LC, Mink KA, Wartgow CD, and Inhorn SL. Aerosol transmission of rhinovirus colds. J. Infect. Dis. 156:442–448, 1987.

Dingle JH, Badger GF, and Jordan WS Jr. Illness in the Home. A Study of 25,000 Illnesses in a Group of Cleveland Families. Cleveland: The Press of Western Reserve University, 1964: 347.

Douglas RG Jr, Cate TR, Gerone PJ, and Couch RB. Quantitative rhinovirus shedding patterns in volunteers. Am. Rev. Respir. Dis. 94:159–167, 1966.

Douglas RG Jr. Pathogenesis of rhinovirus common colds in human volunteers. Ann. Otol. Rhinol. Laryngol. 79:563–571, 1970.

Elkhatieb A, Hipskind G, Woerner D, and Hayden FG. Middle ear abnormalities during natural rhinovirus colds in adults. J. Infect. Dis. 168:618–621, 1993.

Fan J, Henrickson KJ, and Savatski LL. Rapid simultaneous diagnosis of infections with respiratory syncytial viruses A and B, influenza viruses A and B, and human parainfluenza virus types 1, 2, and 3 by multiplex quantitative reverse transcription-polymerase chain reaction-enzyme hybridization assay (Hexaplex). Clin. Infect. Dis. 26:1397–1402, 1998.

Glezen WP, Fernald GW, and Lohr JA. Acute respiratory diseases of university students with special reference to the etiologic role of Herpes hominis. Am. J. Epidemiol. 101:111–121, 1975.

Gwaltney JM Jr, Hendley JO, Simon G, and Jordan WS Jr. Rhinovirus infections in anindustrial population. I. The occurrence of illness. N. Eng. J. Med. 275:1261–1268, 1966.

Gwaltney JM Jr, Moskalski PB, and Hendley JO. Hand-to-hand transmission of rhinovirus colds. Ann. Intern. Med. 88:463–467, 1978.

Gwaltney JM Jr, and Hendley JO. Rhinovirus transmission: One if by air, two if by hand. Trans. Am. Clin. Climatol. Assoc. 89:194–200, 1978.

Gwaltney JM Jr. The Jeremiah Metzger Lecture. Climatology and the common cold. Trans. Am. Clin. Climatol. Assoc. 96:159–175, 1984.

Gwaltney JM Jr. Combined antiviral and antimediator treatment of rhinovirus colds. J. Infect. Dis. 166:776–782, 1992.

Gwaltney JM Jr. State-of-the-Art. Acute community-acquired sinusitis. Clin. Infect. Dis. 23:1209–1223, 1996.

Gwaltney JM Jr, Buier RM, and Rogers JL. The influence of signal variation, bias, noise, and effect size on statistical significance in treatment studies of the common cold. Antiviral Res. 29:287–295, 1996.

Gwaltney JM Jr, Park J, Paul RA, et al. Randomized controlled trial of clemastine fumarate for treatment of experimental rhinovirus colds. Clin. Infect. Dis. 22:656–662, 1996.

Gwaltney JM Jr, and Druce HM. Efficacy of brompheniramine maleate treatment for rhinovirus colds. Clin. Infect. Dis. 25:1188–1194, 1997.

Gwaltney JM Jr. The use of experimentally infected volunteers in research on the common cold. In: Skoner DP, ed. Asthma and Respiratory Infections. New York: Marcel Dekker, 2000:103–128.

Gwaltney JM Jr, Hendley JO, Phillips CD, et al. Nose blowing propels nasal fluid into the paranasal sinuses. Clinical Infectious Diseases, 30:(2)387–391, Feb. 2000.

Hall CB, Douglas RG Jr, and Geiman JM. Possible transmission by fomites of respiratory syncytial virus. J. Infect. Dis. 141:98–102, 1980.

Hall CB, and Douglas RG Jr. Modes of transmission of respiratory syncytial virus. J. Pediatr. 99:98–103, 1981.

Halperin SA, Eggleston PA, Hendley JO, et al. Pathogenesis of lower respiratory tract symptoms in experimental rhinovirus infection. Am. Rev. Respir. Dis. 128:806–810, 1983.

Hamre D, and Procknow JJ. Viruses isolated from natural common colds among young adult medical students. Am. Rev. Respir. Dis. 88:277–282, 1963.

Hayden FG, Treanor JJ, Betts RF, et al. Safety and efficacy of the neuraminidase inhibitor GG167 in experimental human influenza. JAMA. 275:295–299, 1996.

Hayden FG, Osterhaus ADME, Treanor JJ, et al. Efficacy and safety of the neuraminidase inhibitor zanamivir in the treatment of influenzavirus infections. N. Engl. J. Med. 337:874–880, 1997.

Hendley JO, Gwaltney JM Jr, and Jordan WS Jr. Rhinovirus infections in an industrial population. IV. Infections within families of employees during two fall peaks of respiratory illness. Am. J. Epidemiol. 89:184–196, 1969.

Hendley JO, Edmondson WP Jr, and Gwaltney JM Jr. Relations between naturally acquired immunity and infectivity of two rhinoviruses in volunteers. J. Infect. Dis. 125:243–248, 1972.

Hendley JO, Wenzel RP, and Gwaltney JM Jr. Transmission of rhinovirus colds by self-inoculation. N. Engl. J. Med. 288:1361–1364, 1973.

Hendley JO, and Gwaltney JM Jr. Mechanisms of transmission of rhinovirus infections. Epidemiol. Rev. 10:242–258, 1988.

Hendley JO. Clinical virology of rhinoviruses. Advances in Virus Research, 54:453–466; 1999.

Hilleman MR, Hamparian VV, Ketler A, et al. Acute respiratory illnesses among children and adults. JAMA. 180:445–453, 1962.

Jackson GG, Dowling HF, Spiesman IG, and Boand AV. Transmission of the common cold to volunteers under controlled conditions. I. The common cold as a clinical entity. Arch. Intern. Med. 101:267–278, 1958.

Johnson KM, Bloom HH, Mufson MA, and Chanock RM. Acute respiratory disease associated with Coxsackie A-21 virus infection in military personnel. I. Observations in a recruit population. JAMA. 179:112–119, 1962.

Kaulbach HC, White MV, Igarashi Y, Hahn BK, and Kaliner MA. Estimation of nasal epithelial lining fluid using urea as a marker. J. Allergy Clin. Immunol. 92:457–465, 1993.

Kravetz HM, Knight V, Chanock RM, et al. Production of illness and clinical observations in adult volunteers. JAMA. 657–663, 1961.

Kruse W. Die Erregung von Husten und Schnupfen (The etiology of cough and nasal catarrh) Munch. Med. Wochenschr. 61:1574, 1914.

Kuhn JJ, Hendley JO, Adams KF, Clark JW, and Gwaltney JM Jr. Antitussive effect of guaifenesin in young adults with natural colds. Objective and subjective assessment. Chest. 82:713–718, 1982.

Lennette EH, ed. *Laboratory Diagnosis of Viral Infections*, 2nd ed. New York: Marcel Dekker, Inc. 1992.

Lidwell OM, and Williams REO. The epidemiology of the common cold. J. Hyg. Camb. 59:309–319, 1961.

Mäkelä MJ, Puhakka T, Ruuskanen O, et al. Viruses and bacteria in the etiology of the common cold. J. Clin. Microbiol. 36:539–542, 1998.

McBride TP, Doyle WJ, Hayden FG, and Gwaltney JM Jr. Alterations of eustachian tube, middle ear, and nose in rhinovirus infections. Arch. Otolaryngol. Head Neck Surg. 115:1054–1059, 1989.

Monto AS, Napier JA, and HL Metzner. The Tecumseh study of respiratory illness. I. Plan of study and observations on syndromes of acute respiratory disease. Am. J. Epidemiol. 94:269–279, 1971.

Monto AS. Studies of the community and family:Acute respiratory illness and infection. Epidemiol. Rev. 16:351–373, 1994.

Moser MR, Bender TR, Margolis HS, et al. An outbreak of influenza aboard a commercial airliner. Am. J. Epidemiol. 110:1–6, 1979.

Mufson MA, Ludwig WM, James HD, Gauld LW, Rourke JA, Hopler JC, and Chanock RM. Effect of neutralizing antibody on experimental rhinovirus infection. J. Am. Med. Assoc. 186:578–584, 1963.

Murphy BR, Chanock RM, Douglas RG, et al. Temperature-sensitive mutants of influenza A virus: evaluation of the Alaska/77-*ts*-1 A2 temperature-sensitive recombinant virus in seronegative adult volunteers. Arch. Virol. 65:169–173, 1980.

Murphy BR, Chanock RM, Clements ML, et al. Evaluation A/Alaska/6/77 (H3N2) cold-adapted recombinant viruses derived from A/Ann Arbor/6/60 cold-adapted donor virus in adult seronegative volunteers. Infect. Immun. 32:693–697, 1981.

Naclerio RM, Proud D, Kagey-Sobotka A, et al. Kinins are generated during experimental rhinovirus colds. J. Infect. Dis. 157:133–142, 1988.

Parekh HH, Cragun KT, Hayden FG, Hendley JO, and Gwaltney JM Jr. Nasal mucus weights in experimental rhinovirus infection. Am. J. Rhinol. 6,3:107–110, 1992.

Proud D, Naclerio RM, Gwaltney JM, and Hendley JO. Kinins are generated in nasal secretions during natural rhinovirus colds. J. Infect. Dis. 161:120–123, 1990.

Rao SR, Hendley JO, Hayden FG, and Gwaltney JM Jr. Symptom expression in natural and experimental rhinovirus colds. Am. J. Rhinol. 9:49–52, 1995.

Remington PL, Hall WN, Davis IH, Herald A, and Gunn RA. Airborne transmission of measles in a physician's office. JAMA. 253:1574–1577, 1985.

Riley RL. Historical background. In: RB Kundsin, ed. *Airborne Contagion*, New York: NY Acad Sci, 1980:3–9.

Selwyn BJ on Behalf of the Coordinated Data Group of BOSTID Researchers. The epidemiology of acute respiratory tract infection in young children: Comparison of findings from several developing countries. Rev. Infect. Dis. 12 Suppl 8:S870–S888, 1990.

Sperber SJ, Doyle WJ, McBride TP, et al. Otologic effects of interferon beta serine in experimental rhinovirus colds. Arch. Otolaryngol. Head Neck Surg. 118:933–936, 1992.

Turner RB, Hendley JO, and Gwaltney JM Jr. Shedding of infected ciliated epithelial cells in rhinovirus colds. J. Infect. Dis. 145:849–853, 1982.

Turner RB, Sperber SJ, Sorrentino JV, et al. Effectiveness of clemastine fumarate for treatment of rhinorrhea and sneezing associated with the common cold. Clin. Infect. Dis. 25:824–830, 1997.

Turner RB, Wecker MT, Pohl G, et al. Efficacy of tremacamra, a soluble intercellular adhesion molecule-1 for experimental rhinovirus infection. A randomized clinical trial. JAMA. 281:1797–1804, 1999.

Tyrrell DAJ. Common Colds and Related Diseases. Baltimore: Williams & Wilkins, 1965.

Voors AW, Stewart GT, Gutekunst RR, Moldow CF, and Jenkins CD. Respiratory infection in marine recruits. Influence of personal characteristics. Am. Rev. Respir. Dis. 98:801–809, 1968.

Wells, WF. On airborne infection. Study II. Droplets and droplet nuclei. Am. J. Public Hyg. 20(3):611–618, 1934.

Winther B, Gwaltney JM Jr, Mygind N, Turner RB, and Hendley JO. Sites of rhinovirus recovery after point inoculation of the upper airway. JAMA. 256:1763–1767, 1986.

11

Fecal-Oral Transmission

KARIN E. BYERS, RICHARD L. GUERRANT, and BARRY M. FARR

Infections with organisms transmitted by the fecal-oral route most often manifest in diarrhea. Viruses, bacteria, and protozoa may be responsible for diarrheal illnesses. In recent years, there have been tremendous advances in the understanding of infectious diarrhea and improved sanitation has decreased its occurrence in developed countries. However, gastrointestinal infections remain a major cause of morbidity and mortality worldwide. Diarrhea is still the leading cause of childhood death worldwide with 4.6 to 6 million children dying from diarrheal disease in Asia, Africa, and Latin America every year (Guerrant and Bobak 1991). Even in developed countries, there are frequent outbreaks in child care centers, nursing homes, and hospitals. The fecal-oral pathogens of concern vary geographically and among different age groups. New pathogens are being recognized in patients with immunosuppression due to infection with human immunodeficiency virus (HIV), chemotherapy, and transplantation. Contaminated food and water continue to be common sources of infectious illness due to well-

recognized pathogens (e.g., *E. coli*, *Cryptosporidia*, and *Salmonella*). Risk factors for fecal-oral infections include low socioeconomic status, poor hygiene, malnutrition, not breastfeeding infants, parenthood, work with animals, and time spent in institutional setting, such as day care or nursing homes.

We address in this chapter the biological factors of the host and the pathogens that affect epidemiologic methods, measurement of infection, and study design issues. Other chapters in this book that also touch specifically on research methods for pathogens transmitted by the fecal-oral route are Chapters 14 and 18.

BIOLOGIC FACTORS OF THE HOST

Two general factors that affect the host's risk of infection are the exposure to infectious organisms and the resistance to infection, also known as the host defenses. In this section we describe the aspects of host defenses that are relevant to epidemiologic studies. The types of host defense, their mechanisms of action, and factors that can disrupt them are tabulated in Table 11–1. A more detailed description of general immunology is presented in Chapter 2.

The host defenses are relevant when infection is the outcome (i.e., the dependent variable) of interest, as well as when it is an independent variable, as in a treatment trial. In both instances, variations in immune function between two comparison groups can confound estimates of effect. Therefore it is important to know the variety of host resistance mechanisms and factors affecting host susceptibility.

Host Defenses Against Infection

An individual's host defenses are generally classified as nonspecific or specific, depending on whether they are directed at a specific organism. These are summarized in Table 11–1. The nonspecific host defenses are the first line of defense against the large number of organisms in the intestinal tract. These include natural barriers such as mucous membranes, gastric acidity, gastrointestinal motility, and other physical clearing mechanisms as well as the patient's normal endogenous flora. The specific defenses are an immune response to the agent and depend on the host's nutritional status, age (either very young or old), stress (Shavit 1985, Stein 1985), pregnancy (Weinberg 1984), and underlying diseases such as HIV, renal disease, liver disease, or malignancy (Tramont 1990).

Mucosal integrity prevents direct invasion of pathogens or seeding of the blood stream. When this anatomic barrier is disrupted, such as after chemotherapy, the gut can be an important source of bacteremia. Many pathogens depend on their ability to disrupt this barrier in order to cause disease.

Gastric acidity is important in eliminating organisms before they reach the intestinal tract. The normal pH of gastric juice (<3.0)

Table 11–1 Host Defenses to Infections with Organisms Transmitted by the Fecal-Oral Route

Host Defense	Mechanism of Protection	Method of Disruption
Nonspecific Barrier		
Mucous membranes	Anatomic barrier that prevents direct invasion of pathogens or seeding of blood stream	Chemotherapy
Gastric acidity	Eliminates pathogens prior to their reaching the intestines	Surgery Antiacids H_2 antagonists Proton pump antagonists
Gastrointestinal motility	Prevents bacterial adherence and eliminates pathogens before adherence to the mucosal epithelium	Antimotility drugs Opiates Severe illness
Normal endogenous flora	Competes with pathogens for nutrition; inactivates bacterial toxins; may inhibit bacterial adherence to the intestinal mucosa; stimulates mucosal immune system, which prepares it for exposure to pathogens	Antibiotics Chemotherapy
Specific Immune Response		
IgA	Blocks bacterial adherence to epithelial cells and prevents viral attachment and penetration	IgA deficiency (inherited)
IgE	Protects against parasitic infection	Corticosteroids
IgM, IgG	Activate the classical complement pathway	IgM, IgG deficiency (inherited)
Natural killer (NK) cells	Cytotoxicity to pathogens	Corticosteroids Immunosuppressives
Mucosal macrophages	Phagocytosis of pathogens	Chemotherapy

has bactericidal activity (Sarker and Gyr 1992). When this is altered with H_2 blockers or proton pump inhibitors, there is a consequent increase in intragastric bacterial counts. The condition known as hypochlorhydria has been associated with an increased rate of infection from typhoidal and nontyphoidal strains of *Salmonella* (salmonellosis), bacillary dysentery (shigellosis), *Giardia* (giardiasis), *V. cholerae* (cholera), *Diphyllobothrium latum* (tapeworm), and *Strongyloides* (strongyloidiasis) (Cook 1985, Giannella 1973).

Another important nonspecific defense mechanism is the patient's endogenous flora. The normal flora competes for important nutrients, inactivates bacterial toxins, and may inhibit bacterial adherence to the intestinal mucosa either by competitive inhibition or by secretion of materials that inhibit adherence. These organisms produce bacteriocins and secrete short-chain fatty acids that are directly harmful to some pathogens. Finally, the normal flora stimulates the mucosal immune system that prepares it for exposure to pathogenic organisms (Strober and Brown 1988). When the endogenous flora are altered by antibiotics, for example, the patient becomes susceptible to superinfection with pathogens such as *Clostridium difficile*.

Physical clearing mechanisms prevent bacterial adherence and eliminate pathogens before they can adhere to the mucosal epithelium. Peristalsis is important in preventing bacterial overgrowth as is frequently seen in diabetic patients or patients with blind loop syndrome after surgical resections. Bacterial overgrowth causes malabsorption by altering the intraluminal environment and by direct injury to enterocytes, and can cause diarrhea. Mucus secretions form a thin film that protects the mucosa from pathogen attachment. Mucus blocks toxins and binds and coats pathogens to prevent them from attaching to the mucosa (Strober and Brown 1988).

Other nonspecific factors that are important in creating an unfavorable environment for intestinal pathogens include lactoferrin, IgA antibodies, unconjugated bile salts, lysozyme, and lactoperoxidase. Lactoferrin binds proteins and inhibits the growth of organisms by depriving them of iron. IgA antibodies act through both specific and nonspecific mechanisms by neutralizing virus in infected cells and transporting immune complexes formed in the lamina propria through the adjacent mucosa, preventing absorption into the circulation (Mazanec 1993). Unconjugated bile salts inhibit the growth of anaerobic bacteria primarily in the upper part of the small intestine, and lysozyme lyses organisms. Lactoperoxidase has antimicrobial effects. Various other secreted materials inhibit the attachment of organisms to mucosal surfaces (Strober and Brown 1988).

Specific host defenses generally refer to the humoral arm of the immune system in which specific antibodies are made against the invading organism or other toxins. Each class of immunoglobulin has a specific function. The most important isotypes in gastrointestinal infections are IgA and IgE, while IgM and IgG play a more important role in tissue and systemic infections. IgA acts primarily at mucosal surfaces and is found in human secretions such as saliva, tears, colostrum, milk, and gastrointestinal secretions. It is the predominant class of immunoglobulin in intestinal secretions, where it is most often found in its dimeric form (Kagnoff 1993). Secretory IgA is thought to block bacterial adherence to epithelial cells and to prevent viral attachment and penetration (Strober and Brown 1988, Mazanec 1993). Specific IgA antibody may also be able to neutralize virus intracellularly while it is being transported across the epithelial cell layer (Mazanec 1993). It has been proposed that IgA may function at the level of the lamina propria by binding and then excreting microbial constituents through the mucosal epithelium rather than absorbing them into the circulation (Mazanec 1993). IgE appears to play an important role in protecting against parasitic infections (Butterworth 1977, Densen 1978, Joseph 1983, 1986, Spiegelberg 1983). IgM and IgG are found in the highest concentrations in the serum.

The gastrointestinal tract includes several unique features that are also important in preventing infection. Organized lymphoid aggregates are found throughout the gastrointestinal tract with high concentrations in the tonsils, Peyer's patches, and the appendix. These are morphologically similar to the spleen and lymph nodes. They contain specialized "M cells," also known as follicular-associated epithelium, which have a high degree of affinity for antigenic material. These cells bind microorganisms and present them to the interior of the lymphoid aggregates that contain antigen-responsive B and T cells. At this time it is believed that this function is important in promoting immune protection for the host although it has been proposed that it may give pathogens easy access to the host (Sneller and Strober 1986, Strober and Brown 1988, Strober 1992). These aggregates are able to produce IgA, IgM, and IgG in response to antigenic stimuli (Strober and Brown 1988, Strober 1992).

The gastrointestinal tract also has lymphoid cells that are diffusely distributed along the mucosa. Most of these are plasma cells and the majority of these cells contain IgA. IgM- and IgG-containing cells are also present in smaller numbers (Strober and Brown 1988, Heinzel and Root 1990). Lymphoid cells are distributed differently in two layers, the lamina propria and the intraepithelial layer. In the lamina propria there are more T cells of the helper-inducer type, while in the intraepithelial layer the suppressor-cytotoxic T cells are predominant (Strober and Brown 1988). The intraepithelial layer also contains mast cells that may be distinct from nonmucosal mast cells because they respond to different stimuli and have lesser amounts of histamine (Strober and Brown 1988).

Finally, important cellular mechanisms in the gastrointestinal tract include the natural killer (NK) cells, mast cells, eosinophils, and mucosal macrophages, all of which are important in preventing or limiting infections. These cells act by a number of mechanisms including direct cytotoxicity by NK cells, the production of chemotactic factors and altered vascular permeability mediated by mast cells, phagocytosis by macrophages, and antibody-mediated cell-mediated cytotoxicity by both eosinophils and IgA/IgE (Strober and Brown 1988).

A Compromised Immune System

People with defects in any component of their immune system may be either more susceptible to infection or they may have different manifestations of their infection. For example, in the normal host *Vibrio vulnificus* is most often implicated in soft tissue infections from a contaminated wound. Although in the normal host it rarely causes bacteremia from a gastrointestinal source, it has been strongly linked to primary bacteremia after ingestion of raw oysters in patients with liver disease, illnesses associated with elevated serum iron, or other causes of immunodeficiency (Blake 1979, Klontz 1988, Ah and Raff 1990, Bullen 1991, Koenig 1991). The mortality rate in people with underlying disease is 43%–55% (Blake 1979, Klontz 1988, Levine 1993). *Strongyloides stercoralis* may also cause severe and even fatal infections in patients with impaired cellular immunity or who are on high doses of corticosteroids. This infection is commonly acquired in endemic areas such as the southern United States and tropical regions and is also seen with increased frequency in institutionalized patients. Patients may harbor this infection for many years with minimal symptoms. If they later become immunocompromised they are at risk for life-threatening disseminated disease even years after the initial exposure. This has been seen in patients with lymphomas, leukemias, lepromatous leprosy, and with HIV (Mahmoud 1990).

HIV affects both the cellular and humoral components of the immune system and predisposes patients to a large number of viral, bacterial, fungal, and protozoal infections. Cytomegalovirus (CMV), adenovirus, and herpes simplex virus (HSV) may cause chronic diarrhea in these patients (Smith 1992). CMV and HSV may also cause severe esophagitis. Other novel viruses that have been associated with diarrhea in these patients include astrovirus and picornavirus

(Grohmann 1993). *Salmonella* may also present atypically with a paucity of gastrointestinal symptoms but with recurrent bacteremia in these patients requiring life-long treatment (Celum 1987, Sperber and Schleupner 1987). Fungal infections with *Candida* sp. may cause a severe esophagitis while *Histoplasma capsulatum* has been implicated in colitis. Protozoal infections may also be seen in these patients with *Cryptosporidium, Isospora belli,* or *Enterocytozoon bieneusi* (Microsporidia) (Quinn 1992). Sexual practices of infected homosexual men may put them at risk for proctitis caused by gonorrhea, HSV, syphilis, or chlamydia with symptoms of tenesmus, pain, or diarrhea.

The presence of these or other unusual pathogens or an infection with an atypical and unusually severe presentation may warrant an evaluation for defects in the host defenses. Similarly, patients who are known to be immunocompromised may have unusual pathogens and atypical presentations.

Immunocompromised states also occur among transplant patients; people with severe underlying diseases like liver or renal disease or undergoing chemotherapy for cancer; and people who are malnourished, experiencing high levels of stress, or pregnant.

BIOLOGICAL FACTORS OF THE PATHOGEN

The biological characteristics of pathogens transmitted by the fecal-oral route affect decisions related to epidemiologic study design, such as the timing of data collection measurement. The pathogen-related characteristics we discuss here are the incubation period, the infectious dose, and the particular mechanism of fecal-oral transmission. The most common pathogens and their respective infectious doses and incubation periods are presented in Table 11–2.

Incubation Period

The incubation periods of pathogens causing fecal-oral disease must be taken into consideration when designing questionnaires or surveys. Questions about exposure must include adequate time periods that allow for the pathogen's incubation period. This can be difficult when the pathogen is not known, since incubation periods vary. For example, the incubation period of *Bacillus cereus* can be as short as one hour, while that of *Giardia* can be as long as two weeks. A questionnaire that elicits a retrospective 24-hour food history (or information about exposures in general) would be useful in identifying *Bacillus cereus* as a responsible pathogen (incubation period 1–16 hours) but probably would not be useful in identifying *Campylobacter jejuni* (incubation period 16–72 hours).

If information is sought about possible exposure to pathogens that have long incubation periods, questions may require recall of numerous behaviors (eating, drinking, personal contacts, travel) for several weeks. When information about exposure is retrospective, there is always the potential for inaccurate recall. Knowing the specific mechanism through which fecal-oral transmission occurred can sometimes help in discerning the appropriate time period to investigate, but in many cases, the aim of the study is to determine the mechanism of transmission. In an outbreak investigation (see Chapter 14), the incubation period can be an important clue to the responsible pathogen, but it is often difficult to ascertain unless a number of people who can be associated with each other in some way become infected within a short period of time, or their illnesses, which may be experienced after a longer period of time, can be recognized as a cluster (Goodman and Segreti 1999). In prospective studies of a known pathogen, the follow-up time for persons exposed to the pathogen need to take into consideration the incubation period and allow sufficient time for symptoms to develop.

Infectious Dose

The dose of an organism that is needed to cause infection is highly variable. It is dependent on the specific pathogen, its virulence, and the host susceptibility. To become infected with most enteric pathogens, patients must ingest 10^5 to 10^8 organisms,

Table 11–2   Infecting Dose and Incubation Period of Fecal-Oral Pathogens

Pathogen	Infecting Dose	Incubation Period
Viruses		
Hepatitis A	10–10^2 (U.S. Food and Drug Administration 1992)	60–90 days (45–180 days)
Norwalk virus	Unknown	24–48 hours (10–50 hours)
Rotavirus	Unknown	24–72 hours
Bacteria		
Bacillus cereus	Unknown	1–6 hours emetic syndrome
		8–16 hours diarrheal syndrome
		(Hughes and Tauxe 1990)
Campylobacter jejuni	10^2–10^6 (Guerrant 1990a); $<8\times10^2$ (Black 1988)	16–72 hours (Hughes and Tauxe 1990); 53–68 hours (Black 1988)
Clostridium difficile	Unknown (toxin titers of $\geq10^{-3}$ to 10^{-5}) (Fekety 1990)	4–9 days (Guerrant 1990b), may appear up to 6 weeks after antibiotic exposure (Fekety 1990)
Clostridium perfringens	10^8 (Bartlett 1990)	8–16 hours (Hughes and Tauxe 1990)
Enterohemorrhagic *E. Coli*	Unknown*	3–9 days (Doyle and Padhye 1989)
Enteroinvasive *E. Coli*	10^8 (Doyle and Padhye 1989)	8–24 hours (Doyle and Padhye 1989); 16–48 hours (Hughes and Tauxe 1990)
Enteropathogenic *E. Coli*	2×10^9 (Ferguson 1956)	17–72 hours (Doyle and Padhye 1989)
Enterotoxigenic *E. Coli*	10^8 (Evans 1978, Satterwhite 1978)	16–72 hours (Hughes and Tauxe 1990)
Salmonella sp.	10^{5-8} (Guerrant 1990a)	8–48 hours (Guerrant 1990b)
Shigella	10–10^2 (DuPont and Hornick 1973, Guerrant 1990a)	6 hours–9 days (usually <72 hours) (Guerrant 1990b)
Vibrio parahaemolyticus	Unknown†	9–25 hours (Dadisman 1973, Guerrant 1990b)
Protozoa		
Cryptosporidium	3×10–10^2 cysts (Dupont 1995)	1–12 days (Jokopii and Jokipii 1986)
Giardia lamblia	10–10^2 cysts (Guerrant 1990a)	1–2 weeks ‡ (Hill 1990)

*Estimated to be less than *Salmonella* because implicated meat vehicles are usually only slightly undercooked and subsequently were not held for many hours at warm temperatures that would have permitted bacterial growth (Griffin and Taux 1991).

†1cc of 1/10,000 dilution of broth culture has been reported to cause illness (Takikawa 1958).

‡Symptomatic illness may occur before the cysts can be detected in the stool.

while for more hardy organisms, including *Campylobacter jejuni, Shigella,* and the cysts of *Giardia lamblia* and *Cryptosporidium parvum*, only 10^1 to 10^3 organisms are required to cause disease (Guerrant and Bobak 1991).

Clinical studies in which typhoid fever has been induced by *Salmonella typhi* have used doses ranging from 10^3 to 10^9 organisms. Disease was not seen until doses of 10^5 were ingested. The median incubation period varied inversely with the size of inoculum with a median period of nine days when infected with 10^5 organisms and only five days after ingestion of 10^9 organisms. Once the illness occurred, the clinical courses were similar regardless of the dose used (Hornick 1991). Similar results have been seen with nontyphoidal *Salmonella* infections with most reports indicating that 10^5 organisms are needed to cause infection (DuPont and Hornick 1973, Guerrant 1990a).

Despite these findings, outbreaks have been reported after ingestion of fewer organisms (D'Aoust and Pivnick 1976). In one outbreak attributed to carmine dye contaminated with *Salmonella cubana,* patients became ill after ingestion of as few as 1.5×10^4 organisms. Many of these patients were at increased risk of infection because they were elderly and debilitated or infants with gastrointestinal abnormalities (Lang 1967). As noted earlier, gastric acid is an important host defense. Not surprisingly a higher risk of infection has also been noted when inocula are ingested with acid-neutralizing food or are otherwise protected from the hostile gastric acidity. *Salmonella* is almost always a foodborne or waterborne pathogen, but in certain settings, such as in nursing homes and among hospitalized patients, it may be spread from person to person.

Fewer studies have looked at the inoculum necessary to cause viral gastroenteritis. Studies by Kapikian and colleagues (1983a, b) demonstrated that 5 of 18 volunteers given l mL of a 0.2% stool suspension containing rotavirus had viral shedding and 4 of the 18 volunteers with low titers of antibody developed diarrhea. Twelve of their patients developed serologic evidence of infection. The presence of serum antibody measured by immunofluorescence prior to inoculum or high levels of neutralizing antibody to rotavirus was associated with resistance to diarrheal illness. Two patients who had initially developed diarrhea were rechallenged 19 months later and neither developed diarrhea although one noted constitutional symptoms. The infecting dose for another important pathogen, Norwalk virus, is unknown. For many protozoal diseases (e.g., *Cryptosporidium* and *Giardia*) the inoculating dose is very low (10–30 cysts).

Particularly when an infectious dose is high, a person may come into contact with the organism but not become infected. This can result in misclassification of infection status when exposure to the pathogen is determined by the recall of a study participant or the observation of an investigator but not confirmed by testing biological specimens.

Mechanism of Fecal-Oral Transmission

When seeking the source of an outbreak, it is helpful to know the usual reservoir and mode of transmission for the pathogen in question. Many organisms have been associated with particular food items or environmental exposures. These are summarized in Table 11–3. However, these typical patterns may not always accurately predict the source of an outbreak.

Measurement of environmental exposure to fecal-oral pathogens may require subjective and/or objective techniques, depending on the suspected pathogen and the availability of specimens. Subjective information obtained through questionnaires or interviews usually includes behavioral characteristics of the person, such as hygiene practices, travel or recreational information, eating or drinking patterns, and personal contact. It may also include information about a person's environment, such as source of drinking water, milk supply, agricultural methods used, and swimming pool chlorination (Hertz-Picciotto 1998). Objective information includes field and laboratory data, such as environmental samples (e.g., water, food, or soil) or biologic specimens from humans (e.g., stool samples). If a pathogen is known or suspected, exposure assessment can be limited to specific methods based on the mode of transmission (e.g., food questionnaires for information about exposure to a foodborne pathogen or laboratory analysis of water for the presence of waterborne pathogens). Ideally, exposure assessment should include information about host defense mechanisms, which affect a person's susceptibility to a number of pathogens.

Some measurement issues are specific to the particular mechanism by which fecal-oral transmission occurs. We consider here transmission via food, water, direct contact between people, and contact with environmental sources.

Foodborne transmission

Foodborne pathogens have been identified from unexpected sources including some that were previously thought to inhibit their growth. For example, enterohemorrhagic *E. coli* (EHEC) was initially implicated in outbreaks of diarrheal illness and hemolytic uremic syndrome associated with undercooked beef and was later associated with other meats including pork, poultry, and lamb (Doyle and Padhye 1989). A recent outbreak in New England was not associated with any of these sources and was eventually traced to contaminated apple cider, which had previously been considered to be a "safe" food item because of its acidity. It was later found that E. coli O157:H7 could survive at a pH of 3.6–4.0 and could still be detected after 20 days of refrigeration at 8° (Besser 1993). Fruits whose interior was considered sterile (e.g., cantaloupes) have served as the source of outbreaks when injected with contaminated water to increase their "sale" weight.

Bacillus cereus is another foodborne pathogen of concern because of its ability to form spores and survive high temperatures and then regerminate during cooling. It causes two distinct syndromes. One is an "emetic syndrome" characterized by nausea, vomiting, and malaise that has been attributed to cooked rice from Chinese restaurants or "take-aways" in 95% of cases. The high frequency in this setting has been linked to the common practice of cooking large volumes of rice at one time and then storing it for up to several days without refrigerating it. Any B. cereus present in the raw rice is able to form spores that resist the high temperatures for cooking but which can germinate and grow rapidly at ambient temperatures. The preformed toxins result in illness within several hours of consuming the rice (Kramer and Gilbert 1989).

B. cereus also causes a "diarrheal syndrome" with symptoms of abdominal pain, profuse watery diarrhea, rectal tenesmus, and nausea that do not occur until 10–12 hours after ingestion. This presentation is caused by toxins that are formed in vivo. A number of different food items have been implicated including meat products, soups, vegetables, puddings and sauces. In Hungary, a high incidence of meat-related illness has been attributed not just to meat but also to the use of a large number of spices that contain B. cereus spores (Kramer and Gilbert 1989).

Measurement of pathogens in foodborne illnesses has become challenging in recent years because of the involvement of wide geographic areas, possibly due to food processing, refrigeration, and distribution systems (Goodman and Segreti 1999). Thus contamination of food in one factory with a subsequent regional or national distribution may result in illnesses across the country that are difficult to associate with one another. Furthermore, new food vehicles such as fresh produce, eggs, apple cider, and dishes with combined ingredients have joined traditional food vehicles such as undercooked meat, poultry, seafood, and unpasteurized milk (Tauxe 1997), increasing the risk of exposure as well as the difficulty in measurement. Those experiencing illness may recall consuming foods traditionally associated with foodborne illness but fail to consider other foods now known to also carry the pathogen. In addition, contaminated food often smells and tastes normal (Goodman and Segreti 1999, Tauxe 1997). Waterborne transmission also needs to be considered for some pathogens generally thought of as foodborne.

Waterborne transmission

Giardia lamblia has been reported to be present in up to 20% of people living in the southern United States (Cortner 1959). It is usually acquired after ingestion of fecally contaminated water and was an important cause of diarrhea in travelers to Leningrad in the 1970s. In the United States it was the most common cause of outbreaks of waterborne diarrheal illness between 1965 and 1984. It has been attributed to faulty purification or chlorination systems and untreated water consumed by hikers. It is also spread by person-to-person transmission in child care centers and custodial institutions and among homosexual men (Hill 1990).

Cryptosporidia acquired via waterborne contamination has been involved in several large outbreaks in the United States. The pathogen is relatively resistant to chlorine and hence may survive water purification efforts.

Exposure to waterborne pathogens is difficult to measure for numerous reasons. First, the density of pathogens is variable throughout water. Although current models for quantifying waterborne pathogens as-

Table 11–3 Reservoirs and Modes of Transmission of Selected Fecal-Oral Pathogens

Pathogen	Reservoir	Mode of Transmission	Implicated vehicles	Seasonality
Viruses				
Hepatitis A	Humans	Foodborne, waterborne, contact	Shellfish, personal contact, drinking water	Unknown
Hepatitis E	Humans	Foodborne, waterborne, contact	Drinking water, personal contact	Unknown
Norwalk agent and Norwalk-like viruses	Animals, humans	Foodborne, waterborne, contact	Shellfish, salads, contaminated water, oysters (Hughes and Tauxe 1990, Blacklow and Greenberg 1991)	Winter
Rotavirus*	Animals, humans	Presumed fecal-oral	Personal contact, contaminated food and water	Winter
Bacteria				
Aeromonas sp.	Water, animals	Foodborne, waterborne, contact	Seafood, red meat, poultry, raw milk, water (Stelma 1989)	Summer
Bacillus cereus	Ubiquitous in the environment	Foodborne	Cooked rice, meat products, dairy products, soups, soups, vegetables, puddings, sauces (Kramer and Gilbert 1989, Hughes and Tauxe 1990)	Year round
Campylobacter jejuni	Animals including humans	Foodborne	Unpasteurized milk, poultry, eggs, beef, food handlers, water (Stern 1989, Hughes and Tauxe 1990)	Spring, summer
Clostridium botulinum	Ubiquitous in the environment	Foodborne	Low acid (pH ≥4.4) home canned vegetables and fruit fish, honey (infants)[†] (Hauschild 1989, Hughes and Tauxe 1990)	Summer, fall
Clostridium difficile	Humans	Contact	Person-to-person, fomites (Fekety 1990)[‡]	Year round
Clostridium perfringens	Animals, environment	Foodborne	Beef, poultry, gravy (Hughes and Tauxe 1990)	Fall, winter, spring
Entamoeba histolytica	Animals, environment	Foodborne, waterborne, contact	Personal contact contaminated food and water	Unknown

(continued)

Table 11–3—Continued

Pathogen	Reservoir	Mode of Transmission	Implicated vehicles	Seasonality
Enterohemmorrhagic *E. coli*	Animals, humans	Foodborne, waterborne, contact	Ground beef, poultry, pork, lamb, unpasteurized milk and apple cider, personal contact	Summer, fall
Enteropathogenic *E. coli*	Animals, humans	Foodborne, waterborne, contact	Poor hygiene, coffee substitute, contaminated water (Doyle and Padhye 1989)	Summer
Enteroinvasive *E. coli*	Animals, humans are the major reservoir (Doyle and Padhye 1989)	Foodborne	Cheese (Doyle and Padhye 1989, Hughes and Tauxe 1990), salmon, potato salad, personal contact	Unknown
Enterotoxigenic *E. coli*	Animals, humans are the major reservoir (Doyle and Padhye 1989)	Foodborne, waterborne, contact	Salads, meat, cheese, seafood (Hughes and Tauxe 1990), fomites, contaminated water, personal contact	Summer
Listeria monocytogenes	Ubiquitous in the environment	Foodborne	Raw milk, dairy products, vegetables, processed meats	Unknown
Plesimonas shigelloides	Animals, ubiquitous in the environment	Foodborne	Oysters, salted fish, crab (Lovett 1989)	Unknown
Salmonella sp.	Animals, humans	Foodborne, waterborne, contact	Eggs, poultry, dairy products, beef (Hughes and Tauxe 1990) personal contact with humans and pets (turtles, dogs, parakeets) (D'Aoust 1989)	Summer, fall
Shigella sp.	Animals, humans	Foodborne, waterborne, contact	Egg salad, lettuce (Hughes and Tauxe 1990)	Summer
Staphylococcus aureus	Animals, humans, ubiquitous in the environment	Foodborne, contact	Ham, poultry, egg salad, pastries (Hughes and Tauxe 1990)	Spring, summer, fall
Vibrio cholerae	Animals, humans, ubiquitous in the environment	Foodborne, waterborne, contact	Shellfish, contaminated water (Madden and MacCardell 1989, Hughes and Tauxe 1990)	Variable

(continued)

Table 11–3 Reservoirs and Modes of Transmission of Selected Fecal-Oral Pathogens—Continued

Pathogen	Reservoir	Mode of Transmission	Implicated vehicles	Seasonality
Vibrio parahaemolyticus	Ubiquitous in the environment	Foodborne	Bivalve mollusks, crustaceans (US), saltwater fish (Japan) (Hughes and Tauxe 1990)	Spring, summer, fall
Yersinia enterocolitica	Animals	Foodborne	Pork, milk, tofu (Tauxe 1987, Schiemann 1989, 1989, Pearson and Guerrant 1990)	Winter
Protozoa				
Cryptosporidium parvum	Animals, humans	Waterborne, contact	Drinking water, contact with farm animals and humans	Unknown
Giardia lamblia	Animals, humans, ubiquitous in the environment	Waterborne, contact	Drinking water, personal contact	Unknown

*Most often seen as a cause of infantile diarrhea.

†Preformed toxins are found in these foods. Spores can be isolated from many sites and are insignificant unless they produce toxin or are ingested by an infant. *C. botulinum* spores in honey have been implicated in 20 cases of infant botulism in California.

‡Infection strongly linked to antibiotic use.

sume that the pathogens are dispersed throughout the water, there is some evidence that the pathogens are present in clusters (Gale 1996). The distribution of pathogens affects the exposure to consumers; if pathogens are dispersed, then consumers have low levels of exposure; if pathogens are clustered, then consumers are at risk for high levels of exposure. Models for pathogen density calculate numbers of pathogen per volume of water (e.g., 50 *Cryptosporidium* oocytes in a 100 liter volume of water), which is difficult to translate into exposure for consumers, because people do not consume 100 liters of water daily. Pathogen density models estimate personal consumption at 2 liters per day; in the preceding example, estimates for consumer exposure would be about 1 oocyte per person per day. But if pathogens were clustered, it would be possible for one person to consume 50 oocytes while the remaining 49 people had no exposure (Gale 1996). The difficulty in quantify-ing pathogens in water is complicated even further by seasonal and climatic fluctuations of pathogens and the effects of inadequate treatment techniques.

In assessing exposure to waterborne pathogens, the host defense mechanisms and the biologic properties of the specific organism must be taken into account. In studies assessing the source of exposure to a waterborne pathogen, information should be obtained about source of drinking water, occupational and recreational activities performed in water, and consumption of shellfish or food crops that may have been exposed to contaminated water.

Transmission by direct contact
Person-to-person transmission is common in settings where it is difficult to maintain good hygiene. Children in day care centers are at particular risk because many infants and toddlers are not toilet trained and there is a high risk of fecal soiling among young

children who frequently put their hands and foreign objects in their mouths. In prospective studies of children less than three years old there were 42 cases of gastroenteritis per 100 child-months in day care centers compared with 27 cases per 100 child-months in children at home (Bartlett 1985, Guerrant 1986). The most commonly isolated organisms in this setting include rotavirus, seen predominantly in infants, and *G. lamblia* in toddlers. Other important enteric pathogens include *C. jejuni*, *Shigella*, enteric adenovirus, astrovirus, *Cryptosporidium*, *C. difficile*, and hepatitis A (Pickering 1981, Bartlett 1985, Guerrant 1986, Mitchell 1993). Pathogens with low infectious doses such as *Shigella*, *Giardia*, rotavirus, and possibly *Campylobacter* and *Cryptosporidium* may be spread by direct contact. Asymptomatic carriage of pathogens may be important in the spread of diarrheal disease because caretakers may not be as vigilant about handwashing and other hygienic measures. Secondary attack rates of 12%–79% have been observed in the families of these children: 12%–25% with giardiasis; 26%–46% with shigellosis; and 15%–79% with rotavirus (Guerrant 1986, Guerrant and Bobak 1991). Person-to-person transmission of EHEC has also been well documented in day care settings (Belongia 1993) and in families (Rowe 1994).

Hospitalized patients are also at increased risk. Although only 1.3 cases of nosocomial gastroenteritis per 10,000 hospital discharges were reported to the Centers for Disease Control and Prevention between 1956 and 1979, prospective surveillance studies found rates of 7.7 and 2.3 per 100 admissions to intensive care and pediatric units respectively (Guerrant 1990b). Hospitalized patients usually have impaired resistance to infection because of their underlying illness as well as increased exposure to potential pathogens. Important modes of transmission include direct contact with medical personnel who have not adequately washed their hands and common-vehicle spread. Inadequate sterilization and disinfection of equipment are additional risks.

The most common bacterial pathogens in these settings include cytotoxigenic *C. difficile*, which has been implicated in 45% of cases of nosocomial diarrhea, and *Salmonella*, which has been identified as the cause of 11% of all nosocomial outbreaks (Stamm 1981). McFarland and colleagues (1989) looked at the risk of acquiring *C. difficile* on a general medical ward and found that 21% of patients who initially had negative rectal swab cultures acquired *C. difficile* during their hospitalization. Sixty-three percent of these patients were asymptomatic. Patient-to-patient transmission was evidenced by the earlier acquisition of infection in patients whose roommates had positive cultures with a mean of 3.2 versus 18.9 days to become infected. Fifty-nine percent of health care workers developed positive hand cultures after caring for infected patients and 29% of 216 environmental sites tested were culture positive (McFarland 1989).

Rotavirus is an important cause of diarrhea in the pediatric population and has been associated with outbreaks in nurseries with spread from infant to infant by contact with medical personnel (Chrystie 1975; Bishop 1976, Murphy 1977). Once an outbreak has occurred in a nursery, rotavirus has been detected in 25% of stools described as loose, mucoid, or watery and in 11% of stools described as normal, suggesting that asymptomatic patients may be an important reservoir and their contacts may transmit the infection (Kraus 1981). Other important pathogens that have been reported to cause nosocomial gastroenteritis include *Staphylococcus aureus* and *C. perfringens* with less frequent reports *of Shigella*, *Campylobacter*, *Yersinia enterocolitica*, *E. coli* (enterotoxigenic, enteropathogenic, and enterohemorrhagic), *Aeromonas*, *Plesimonas*, *Giardia*, and *Cryptosporidium* (Jarvis and Hughes 1993).

Humans are important reservoirs for many pathogens, especially if they are asymptomatic carriers. The prevalence of *E. histolytica* is reported to be as high as 50% in underdeveloped countries with poor sanitation and up to 90%–99% of infected individuals are asymptomatic. In the United States the overall prevalence is only about

4% but higher rates are seen in institution-alized patients and male homosexuals with multiple sexual partners. This organism is transmitted through fecally contaminated food or water or through sexual practices with fecal-oral contact (Ravidin and Petri 1990).

Viruses implicated in diarrheal disease in-clude rotaviruses, enteric adenoviruses, and the single stranded RNA viruses that include Norwalk and Norwalk-like viruses, cali-civiruses, astroviruses, enteric coronavirus, and unclassified small round viruses. The group A rotaviruses cause 30%–60% of cases of severe watery diarrhea in infants and young children (Blacklow and Green-berg 1991), while the Norwalk agent and Norwalk-like agents are important patho-gens in older children and adults. These viruses are the cause of 40% of outbreaks of gastroenteritis that occur in recreational camps, on cruise ships, in communities or families, at schools or colleges, in nursing homes and hospital wards, in cafeterias, and on sports teams. Viral gastroenteritis may be spread by close personal contact. In addi-tion, outbreaks may occur due to contami-nated drinking or swimming water, poorly cooked shellfish, oysters from contaminated waters, and contaminated foods (Dolin 1990, Blacklow and Greenberg 1991).

In studies of fecal-oral diseases, measure-ment of exposure is sometimes estimated from a description and quantification of the type of contact between people. For example, in a prospective study of the relationship between child care practices and diarrhea among young children in rural Kenya, phys-ical contact between children and caregivers was observed over a 12-hour period and measured according to predefined protocols (Paolisso 1989). Measurement of physical contact preceded the measurement of out-come (diarrheal illness), strengthening the causal relationship.

Transmission from environmental surfaces
Assessment of exposure to pathogens from contaminated surfaces is more difficult to quantify, as in a day care center where hands may contaminate a surface or pick up con-taminants and transfer them to self or others. Haas and colleagues (1999) describe experi-ments that have attempted to quantify the bacterial transfer rate between hands and surfaces. Methods for detection of patho-gens in the environment often have multiple stages and low sensitivity, or require much time, making it impractical or impossible to measure the pathogens. Furthermore, meth-ods are not available to detect many of the pathogens. For these reasons, measures of pathogens in the environment are probably underestimated.

Spore-forming organisms may be isolated from numerous sources and may be difficult to eradicate because they are resistant to high temperatures. Under appropriate envi-ronmental conditions, they may later reger-minate and lead to infection. For example, *Bacillus cereus* is a ubiquitous organism that has been isolated from soil, dust, and water as well as food sources.

MEASUREMENT OF INFECTION

An important decision by investigators is whether to attempt to ascertain an etiologic diagnosis for an episode of enteritis. We dis-cuss here the use of measures based on lab-oratory tests, clinical observation, and the recall of the study participant.

Laboratory and Clinical Criteria

Obtaining an etiologic diagnosis is both bi-ologically and methodologically difficult. Multiple infectious agents may cause enteric infection and hence one must evaluate the stool for viral, bacterial, and protozoan path-ogens. Detecting toxin-mediated disease and viral pathogens may require sophisticated laboratory support. A single comprehensive microbiologic evaluation of stool may cost hundreds of dollars and require extensive time commitments from trained technicians. Many microbiologic studies performed on stool require a fresh stool sample. Hence, obtaining stool may be difficult. If samples are obtained, there must be a mechanism in place to notify the investigators and a means of transport to the location where the spec-imens will be analyzed. Other methodologic problems include separating colonization from infection, as many potential pathogens may also represent normal stool flora (e.g., *C. difficile, E. coli*) or chronic carriage (e.g., *Salmonella*); determining the etiologic cause of enteritis when multiple pathogens are isolated (common in lesser developed countries); and assessing the relevance of isolating a potential pathogen in an asymptomatic patient. Carriage rates of potential pathogens (e.g., *C. difficile*) may differ by age, geographic location, and immune status.

Parasites can cause infection through several mechanisms, thus raising additional questions about identifying or classifying their infections. They may cause a mechanical barrier to absorption, injure the mucosal lining, produce exotoxins, cause an immune response leading to inflammation, or alter the normal gastrointestinal motility (Cohen 1991). In the case of *Entamoeba histolytica*, the organism is ingested in the cyst form. Encystation or hatching occurs in the lower ileum and the colon. This is followed by invasion of the colonic mucosa and multiplication at which time they establish themselves in mucosal ulcers. Infected patients have colonic lesions that may show frank ulceration and normal or hyperemic mucosa. Polymorphonuclear leukocytes are seen at the edge of the lesions and their destruction may lead to the pathogenesis of the classical "flask-shaped" mucosal ulcers or hepatic abscesses (Guerrant 1981). The amebic destruction of PMNs presumably explains their characteristic absence from stools of patients with amebic dysentery, a factor that has been used to distinguish amebic from "bacillary" dysentery (Anderson 1921, Callendar 1921). Asymptomatic intestinal carriage, which occurs commonly after exposure, affected 5% of the U.S. population during the 1960s (DuPont and Pickering 1980). Recent focus has been on the carrier state, because some patients may have active infection with minimal symptoms or carriers may only have intermittent symptoms, and asymptomatic patients have been noted to have ulceration without clinical evidence of disease (DuPont and Pickering 1980).

Recall by Study Participants

More commonly in epidemiologic studies, the outcome measured is diarrheal disease. Diarrhea is a syndrome without a well-defined operational definition. Most investigators use a combination of stool frequency (e.g., three per day) and stool consistency (e.g., conforming to the shape of a container) to define diarrhea. Commonly, diarrhea among young children in developed countries is defined as three or more loose or watery stools per day. However, it is important to realize that normal stool frequency and consistency vary by age and by diet and thus it is necessary to use a definition that is appropriate to the population being sampled. In addition, the stool habits of all persons are variable and thus many people will have occasional bouts of diarrhea unrelated to infection. The specificity for an infectious etiology can be increased by including in the case definition such symptoms as fever, vomiting, and abdominal pain, and such laboratory findings as an elevated white blood cell count. However, while these findings will improve specificity they will also decrease sensitivity. Dysentery, gastroenteritis due to an invasive pathogen, is associated with the symptom of bloody diarrhea and the laboratory finding of fecal leukocytes.

Seldom is the occurrence of diarrhea directly observed by the researcher. More commonly the researchers rely on a study participant (or a child's caretaker) to recall the occurrence. Recall is subject to memory lapses and discordance over definitions between the investigator and the person recalling the events (Thomas 1989, Boerma 1991). In a study of diarrheal disease in rural Kenya, Thomas and associates measured the misclassification of maternal recall in comparison to the researcher's observation of stool samples obtained from the period to which the recall pertained. They estimated that the maternal recall overestimated the actual occurrence of diarrhea in the study population by nearly twofold (9.5% instead of 4.8%). The resulting misclassification attenuated the "true" odds ratio for one exposure variable (household ownership of a latrine), estimated to be 5.4 (95% confidence interval [CI] = 2.0–14.5), to 2.0 (95% CI = 0.9–4.3). The fact that the 95% confidence interval of the attenuated (observed) odds ratio included 1.0 (i.e., signifying no association) would lead some researchers to disregard this exposure variable when actually its effect on the occurrence of diarrhea may be quite important.

Since some infections can persist for long periods of time and repeat infections are possible, it is also important to determine when one episode has ended and another has begun. Most investigators require a period of "normal" stools between diarrheal episodes. The length of time the individual must be symptom free used in research has ranged from two to 14 days. Baqui (1991) conducted a validation study among Bangladeshi children in which they compared various operational definitions of diarrhea and diarrheal episode and concluded that three or more loose/liquid/watery stools or any number of stools containing blood in a 24-hour period was the best definition for diarrhea, while three prior diarrhea-free days was the best criterion for the beginning of a new diarrheal episode.

The level of respondents' education can affect the accuracy of their recall. Boerma (1991) found that illiterate women reported rates of diarrhea less often than literate women and suggested that the differential reporting was due to misunderstanding by the illiterate women. The higher rate of misclassification of diarrhea episodes in illiterate women could lead to a biased observation that the actual rates of diarrheal episodes between the two groups are different, when in fact only the reported rates are different. Moreover, in cultures where diarrheal illnesses is associated with evil spirits or bad luck, study participants may be reluctant to talk about their bowel habits (Nichter 1991). Despite the problems encountered, the value of recall data should not be underestimated, since individuals (and mothers, in the case of children) are often considered to be the best observers of departures from usual bowel patterns (Baqui 1991).

The use of qualitative data (Kaltenthaler and Drasar 1996), social science research (Nichter 1991), ethnography (Jenkins and Howard 1992), conceptual frameworks (Herman and Bentley 1992), and cultural models (Weiss 1988) to develop culturally sensitive language and methods has improved data collection. Weiss (1988) describes the interaction between ethnographic and epidemiologic methods as synergistic, with ethnography providing culturally informed hypotheses that are appropriate for testing with quantitative epidemiologic methods. Quantitative and qualitative methods can also be mixed effectively in a single study (Paolisso 1989).

STUDY DESIGN

Many of the issues discussed here pertain to epidemiologic studies of fecal-oral pathogens, regardless of the study design. In this section we identify a number of issues related to the use of various study designs for determining risk factors for infection with pathogens transmitted through the fecal-oral route. We discuss risk factor studies, nonindependence of events, and seasonal variation. We focus principally on community-based studies rather than those conducted in an institutional setting, and on the risk of becoming infected rather than the consequences of infection.

Risk Factor Studies

By definition, studies pertaining to risk are concerned with the occurrence of new, or incident infections. Incidence can be described in terms of risk, measured through closed cohort studies, and of rate, measured in dynamic cohorts. In each case, uninfected people are enrolled and followed over time to determine whether they become infected. Most often, only the most severe, life-threatening episodes of diarrhea are brought to the attention of medical caregivers. The detection of these cases can be likened to passive surveillance (types of surveillance are discussed further in Chapter 7). The more common, less severe episodes are usually discovered only by active surveillance conducted by the study investigators. If the follow-up period is long and the disease duration is short (as it can be with diarrhea), the active surveillance will require many visits (e.g., once every one or two weeks for several months). Many younger children are cared for during the day by persons other than their primary caregivers (e.g., day care center staff in developed countries or an older sibling in developing countries) and thus monitoring for illness may involve surveying multiple caregivers. If one adds to this a sizable number of study subjects, such as in a community-based study, it becomes quickly clear that longitudinal studies can be very expensive. Moreover, study participants may not be at home when visited, requiring revisits, or they may tire of multiple visits and withdraw from the study. Studies in institutional settings, such as hospitals or day care centers, are more manageable in this regard.

While case-control study designs are often portrayed as a less expensive alternative to cohort studies, they do not necessarily overcome the need for an expensive surveillance system unless the study is to be limited to severe cases who present themselves to a clinical setting. In this instance, however, the factors that lead a person to become infected often become entangled with the factors that lead the person to obtain care, either at all, or in a particular institution. To identify all new infections, especially if non-life-threatening occurrences are of interest, a surveillance system is still required. The primary advantage to the case-control approach, then, is the time and expense saved by collecting information from only a sample of those who are not infected or diseased. This advantage needs to be weighed against the potential for introducing bias into the study through the method of selecting the sample of controls (as opposed to collecting data from all of the non-cases).

The expense of a surveillance system, and the biases incurred by people dropping out of a study due to fatigue from being visited regularly, are most often circumvented with a cross-sectional study design. This approach, however, has its own inherent limitations. Since information is collected from individuals only at one point in time, prevalent rather than incident diarrhea is identified. Since the likelihood of being found with diarrhea is a function of the duration of the infection, the factors associated with infection can be related to exposure (i.e., acquiring the infection) as well as the disease duration (i.e., keeping the infection). The presence of other infections and the level of competence of the immune system can affect both of these, but their relative contributions to incidence and duration cannot be disentangled in a cross-sectional study.

The relative value and appropriateness of cross-sectional and cohort study designs were compared by Thomas and Neumann (1992) in a study where both designs were employed. They found that the incidence measures (cumulative incidence and incidence density) required significantly more time and resources to obtain and evidenced more underreporting of diarrheal episodes than in the cross-sectional study component. There is no clear study design that is always to be preferred: each has its own assets and liabilities. Determination of the most appropriate study design is a function of the study questions and the resources available.

Non-independence of Events

Risk factor study designs assume that the observations upon which a study is based are independent of each other. In other words, one episode of diarrhea does not make another episode more or less likely to occur. When one episode is closely associated with another, each observation provides less information than if the episodes were unrelated, resulting in the need to adjust the calculation of variance in the estimates of precision (e.g., 95% confidence interval). With organisms transmitted by the fecal-oral route, infections (or episodes of diarrhea) can be associated with each other in two ways: transmission from one person to another, and repeat episodes experienced by one person.

With fecal-oral transmission, one person's infection places those with whom they are in contact at risk of also becoming infected. This is the phenomenon of dependent happenings described in Chapter 5. In community-based studies, the traditional approach to this dependence of events has been to enroll only one person from each family. While this decreases the number of events that are more obviously associated with each other, it fails to account for the fact that essentially every infection is acquired from someone else, whether from within the family or among other contacts. Moreover, different levels of exposure, either by a higher infectious dose from a single source or by contact with multiple sources, can confound measures of association in studies. For example, consider an independent variable such as access to a source of protected water (e.g., a water pump) in an African village. If individuals using the protected water source have greater exposure to infection for some other reason (e.g., they are visited by more friends and relatives than those without such a water source), they may experience more infections in spite of having clean water. It is therefore important in many instances to collect information that will enable one to estimate the degree of exposure and make adjustments for variations in exposure in the data analysis of risk factor studies.

In some instances, it is the dependence of events that is most relevant and interesting. Rather than trying to achieve independence of observations, it may be more fruitful to intentionally design a study that is based on the dependent relationship. For example, a study could focus on the siblings or other contacts of infected persons. Such a study would yield information about the infectivity of the organism in various conditions. With infectivity as the measure of interest, such a study is generally not considered a traditional risk factor study.

In addition to one person infecting another, a particular individual can experience repeat episodes of an infection. A second episode can be due to another pathogen or another exposure to the same pathogen. When the symptoms do not make it clear that another pathogen is involved, laborato-

ry tests to determine the infecting organism will be required if the focus of a study is on one particular pathogen. When it is determined that two infections are with the same pathogen, or when infectious diarrhea, rather than the causative organism, is the outcome of interest, researchers must decide how to handle more than one episode for a given study participant. The two episodes can be related for at least two reasons: the prior infection made the person less resistant to a subsequent exposure; or the factors that led to the first exposure led also to the second exposure. In the former case, it may be important to study second infections separately from first infections in order to identify the factors of the first infection that make a person more likely to experience a second infection. Alternatively, repeat infections can be treated as a "nuisance," in which data collection on a particular study participant would cease once he or she becomes infected the first time.

In studies where communities are the unit of analysis, data on the occurrence of diarrheal disease are typically based on a surveillance system that records all infections during a period of time, including repeat episodes. If researchers are interested rather in the proportion of people experiencing infection, the repeat episodes will have to be identified and excluded from the calculation of a proportion. The use of a rate (i.e., the inclusion of all episodes) may be justified when the overall burden of disease in a community, including repeat episodes, is the outcome of interest.

Seasonal Variation

Exposure to some pathogens can vary with the season. For example, during a dry season in tropical countries, the scarcity of water can result in less hand washing and more transmission of pathogens. This variation in exposure is another instance of the importance of dependent happenings. If a study is focused on a nonseasonal risk factor, the seasonal variations in exposure can confound the observed relation between the risk factor and outcome of interest. This can occur within a particular cohort or in a comparison of two or more populations. In a cohort study that has a phased enrollment or a follow-up time that spans more than one season, some study participants may experience more exposure to a pathogen than do other participants. To control for this it is important to include some measures of season (e.g., calendar months or rainfall) in the analysis.

The same holds true for comparisons between two or more populations. Data collected in the different populations during different seasons can confound some measures of association, as can data collected at the same time but from populations with different climates, due perhaps to differences in altitude.

SUMMARY

As with all infectious diseases, the methods required for an epidemiologic study are determined by the biology of the organism, the study questions, and the resources available. Perhaps more than with pathogens transmitted by other routes, however, studies of fecal-oral infections often rely on non-pathogen-specific symptomatic definitions, such as the number and consistency of stools. Furthermore, researchers must often rely on the study participant (or a care provider) to recall the occurrence of diarrhea. Thus means of improving recall and assuring that the researcher and study participant agree on the outcome of interest are critical.

REFERENCES

Ah MB, and Raff M. Primary *vibrio vulnificus* sepsis in Kentucky. South. Med. J. 83:356–357, 1990.

Anderson JA Dysentery in the field. Lancet 2:998–1002, 1921.

Baqui AH, Black RE, Yunus MD, Hoque AR, Chowdhury HR, and Sack RM. Methodological issues in diarroeal diseases epidemiology: Definition of diarrheal episodes. Int. J. Epidemiol. 20:1057–1063, 1991.

Bartlett AV, Moore M, Gary GW, et al. Diarrheal illness among infants and toddlers in day care centers. II. Comparison with day care homes and households. J. Pediatr. 107:503–509, 1985.

Bartlett J. Gas gangrene (other clostridium-associated diseases). In: Mandell GL, Douglas RG, Bennett JE, eds. Principles and Practice of Infectious Diseases. New York: Churchill Livingstone, 1990:1850–1860.

Belongia EA, Osterholm MT, Sober JT, et al. Transmission of *Escherichia Coli* 0157:H7 infection in Minnesota child day-care facilities. JAMA. 269:883–888, 1993.

Besser RE, Lett SM, Weber TW, et al. An outbreak of diarrhea and hemolytic uremic syndrome from *Escherichia coli* 0157:H7 in fresh-pressed apple cider. JAMA. 269:2217–2220, 1993.

Bishop RF, Hewstone AS, Davidson GP et al. An epidemic of diarrhoea in human neonates involving a retrovirus like agent and "enteropathogenic" serotypes of *Escherichia coli*. J. Clin. Pathol. 29:46–49, 1976.

Black RE, Levine MM, Clements ML, et al. Experimental campylobacter jejuni infection in humans. J. Infect. Dis. 157:472–479, 1988.

Blacklow NR, and Greenberg H. Viral gastroenteritis. N. Engl. J. Med. 325(4):252–264, 1991.

Blake PA, Merson MH, Weaver RE, Hollis DG, and Heublein PC. Disease caused by a marine vibrio. N. Eng. J. Med. 300:1–5, 1979.

Boerma JT, Black RE, Sommerfelt AE, Rutstein SO, Bicego JT. Accuracy and completeness of mother's recall of diarrhoea occurrence in pre-school children in demographic and health surveys. Int. J. Epidemiol. 20:1073–1080, 1991.

Bullen JJ, Spalding PB, Ward CG, and Gutteridge JMC. Hemochromatosis, iron and septicemia caused by *vibrio vulnificus*. Arch. Intern. Med. 151:1606–1609, 1991.

Butler T, Speelman, P, Kabir I, and Banwell J. Colonic dysfunction during shigellosis. J. Infect. Dis. 154:817–823, 1986.

Butterworth AE, David JR, Franks D, et al. Antibody dependent eosinophil mediated damage to 51Cr labeled Schistosomula by *Schistosoma mansoni*: Damage by purified eosinophils. J. Exp. Med. 145:136–150, 1977.

Callendar GR. The differential pathology of dysentery. Am. J. Trop. Med. 14:207–233, 1921.

Cash RA, Music SI, Libonati JP, et al. Response of man to infection with vibrio cholerae. I. Clinical, serologic, and bacteriologic responses to a known inoculum. J. Infect. Dis. 129:45–52, 1974.

Celum CL, Chaisson RE, Rutherford GW, Barnhart JL, and Echenberg DF. Incidence of salmonellosis in patients with AIDS. J. Infect. Dis. 156:998–1002, 1987.

Chrystie IL, Totterdell B, Baker MJ, Scopes JW, and Banatvala JE. Rotavirus infections in a maternity unit. Lancet. 2:79, 1975.

Cohen MB. Etiology and mechanisms of acute infectious diarrhea in infants in the United States. J. Pediatr. 118:S34–S39, 1991.

Cook GC. Infective gastroenteritis and its relationship to reduced gastric acidity. Scand. J. Gastroenterol. (Suppl) 111:17–22, 1985.

Cortner JA. Giardiasis, a cause of celiac syndrome. Am. J. Dis. Child. 98:311–316, 1959.

D'Aoust J-Y, and Pivnick H. Small infectious doses of salmonella (letter). Lancet. 1:866, 1976.

D'Aoust Y-V. (1989). Salmonella. In: Doyle MP, ed. Foodborne Bacterial Pathogens. New York: Marcel Dekker, 1989:327–445.

Dadisman TTA, Nelson R, Molenda JR, and Garver HJ. Vibrio parahaemolyticus gastroenteritis in Maryland. Am. J. Epidemiol. 96:414–426, 1973.

Densen P, Mahmoud AAG, Sullivan J, et al. Demonstration of eosinophil degranulation of the surface of opsonized schistosomules by phase-contrast cinemicrography. Infect. Immun. 22:282–285, 1978.

Dolin R. Norwalk and related agents of gastroenteritis. In: Mandell GL, Douglas RG, Bennett JE, eds. Principles and Practice of Infectious Diseases. New York: Churchill Livingstone, 1990:1415–1419.

Doyle MP, and Padhye VV. Escherichia coli. In: Doyle MP, ed. Foodborne Bacterial Pathogens. New York: Marcel Dekker, 1989:235–281.

DuPont HL, and Hornick RB. Clinical approach to infectious diarrheas. Medicine. 52:265–270, 1973.

DuPont HL, and Pickering LK. Infections of the Gastrointestinal Tract. New York: Plenum Publishing Corporation, 1980.

DuPont HL, Chappell CL, Sterling DR, Okhuysen PC, Rose JB, and Jakubowski W. The infectivity of Cryptosporidium parvum in healthy volunteers. N. Engl. J. Med. 332:855–859, 1995.

Evans DG, Satterwhite TK, Evans DJ, and DuPont HL. Differences in serological responses and excretion patterns of volunteers challenged with enterotoxigenic Escherichia coli with and without the colonization factor antigen. Infect. Immun. 19:883–888, 1978.

Fekety R. Antibiotic-associated colitis. In: Mandell GL, Douglas RG, Bennett JE, eds. Principles and Practice of Infectious Diseases. New York: Churchill Livingstone, 1990:863–869.

Ferguson WW. Experimental diarrheal disease of human volunteers due to Escherichia coli. Ann. NY Acad. Sci. 66:71–77, 1956.

Gale P. Developments in microbial risk assessment models for drinking water—a short review. J. Appl. Bacteriol. 8:403–410, 1996.

Giannella RA, Broitman SA, and Zamcheck N. Influence of gastric acidity on bacterial and parasitic enteric infections. Ann. Intern. Med. 78:271–276, 1973.

Goodman L, and Segreti J. Infectious diarrhea. Disease-A-Month. 45:265–299, 1999.

Griffin PM, and Taux RV. The epidemiology of infections caused by Escherichia coli p157:H7, other enterohemorrhagic E. coli and the associated hemolytic uremic syndrome. Epidemiol. Rev. 13:60–98, 1991.

Grohmann GS, Glass RI, Pereira HG, et al. Enteric viruses and diarrhea in HIV-infected patients. N. Engl. J. Med. 329:14–20, 1993.

Guerrant RL, Brush J, Ravdin JI, Sullivan JA, and Mandell GL. Interaction between Entamoeba histolytica and human polymorphonuclear neutrophils. J. Infect. Dis. 143:83–93, 1981.

Guerrant RL, Lohr JA, and Williams EK. Acute infectious diarrhea. I. Epidemiology, etiology and pathogenesis. Pediatr. Infect. Dis. 5:353–359, 1986.

Guerrant RL. Gastrointestinal infections and food poisoning. In: Mandell GL, Douglas RG, Bennett JE, eds. Principles and Practice of Infectious Diseases. New York: Churchill Livingstone, 1990a:837–847.

Guerrant RL. Inflammatory enteritides. In: Mandell GL, Douglas RG, Bennett JE, eds. Principles and Practice of Infectious Diseases. New York: Churchill Livingstone, 1990b:870–880.

Guerrant RL, and Bobak DA. Bacterial and protozoal gastroenteritis. N. Engl. J. Med. 325:327–340, 1991.

Haas CN, Rose JB, and Gerba CP. Quantitative Microbial Risk Assessment. New York: John Wiley & Sons, 1999.

Hauschild AHW. Clostridium botulinum. In: Doyle MP, ed. Foodborne Bacterial Pathogens. New York: Marcel Dekker, 1989:111–189.

Heinzel FP, and Root RK. Antibodies. In: Mandell GL, Douglas RG, Bennett JE, eds. Principles and Practice of Infectious Diseases. New York: Churchill Livingstone, 1990:41–61.

Herman E, and Bentley ME. Manuals for ethnographic data collection: experience and issues. Soc. Sci. Med. 35:1369–1378, 1992.

Hertz-Picciotto I. Environmental epidemiology. In Rothman KJ, Greenland S, eds. Modern Epidemiology. 2d ed. Philadelphia: Lippincott Williams & Wilkins, 1998.

Hill DR. Giardia lamblia. In: Mandell GL, Douglas RG, Bennett JE, eds. Principles and Practice of Infectious Diseases. New York: Churchill Livingstone, 1990:2110–2115.

Hornick RB, Music SI, Wenzel RP, et al. The Broad Street pump revisited: Response of volunteers to ingested cholera vibrios. Bull. NY Acad. Med. 47:1181–1190, 1971.

Hornick RB, Greisman SE, Woodward TE, et al. Typhoid fever: Pathogenesis and immunologic control. N. Engl. J. Med. 325:327–340, 1991.

Hughes JM, and Tauxe RV. Food-borne disease. In: Mandell GL, Douglas RG, Bennett JE, eds. Principles and Practice of Infectious Diseases. New York: Churchill Livingstone, 1990: 893–905.

Jarvis WR, and H ughes JM. Nosocomial gastrointestinal infections. In: Wenzel RP, ed. Prevention and Control of Nosocomial Infections. Baltimore: Williams & Wilkins, 1993: 708–745.

Jenkins C, and Howard P. The use of ethnography and structured observations in the study of risk factors for the transmission of diarrhea in Highland Papua New Guinea. Med. Anthrop. 15:1–16, 1992.

Jokopii L, and Jokipii AMM. Timing of symptoms and oocyst excretion in human cryptosporidiosis. N. Engl. J. Med. 315(26): 1643–1647, 1986.

Joseph M, Auriault C, Capron A, et al. A new function of platelets: IgE dependent killing of schistosomes. Nature. 303:810–812, 1983.

Joseph M, Capron A, Ameisen JC, et al. The receptor for IgE on blood platelets. Eur. J. Immunol. 16:306–312, 1986.

Kagnoff MG. Immunology of the intestinal tract. Gastroenterology 105:1275–1280, 1993.

Kaltenthaler EC, and Drasar BS. The study of hygiene behaviour in Botswana: A combination of qualitative and quantitative methods. Trop. Med. Int. Health (1):690–698, 1996.

Kapikian AZ, Wyatt RG, Levine MM, et al. Studies in volunteers with human rotaviruses. Dev. Biol. Stand. 53:209–218, 1983a.

Kapikian AZ, Wyatt RG, Levin MM, et al. Oral administration of human rotavirus to volunteers: induction of illness and correlates of resistance. J. Infect. Dis. 147:95–106, 1983b.

Klontz KC, Lieb S, Schreiber M, et al. Syndromes of *vibrio vulnificus* infections. Ann. Intern. Med. 109:318–323, 1988.

Koenig KL, Muller J, and Rose T. *Vibrio vulnificus* hazard on the half shell. West. J. Med. 155:400–403, 1991.

Kramer JM, and Gilbert RJ. *Bacillus cereus* and other *Bacillus* species. In: Doyle MP, ed. Foodborne Bacterial Pathogens. New York: Marcel Dekker, 1989:21–70.

Kraus PJ, Hyams JS, Ballow M, an dKlemas BW. Nosocomial rotavirus in a neonatal intensive care unit. Twenty-first Interscience Conference on Antimicrobial Agents and Chemotherapy. Chicago, abstract 704, 1981.

Lang DJ, Kunz LJ, Martin AT, Schroeder SA, and Thomson LA. Carmine as a source of nosocomial Salmonellosis. N. Engl. J. Med. 276: 829–832, 1967.

Levine WC, Griffin PM, et al. Vibrio infections on the Gulf Coast: results of first year of regional surveillance. J. Infect. Dis. 167:479–483, 1993.

Lovett J. Listeria monocytogenes. In: Doyle MP, ed. Foodborne Bacterial Pathogens. New York: Marcel Dekker, 1989:283–310.

Madden JM, and McCardell BA. Vibrio cholerae. In: Doyle MP, ed. Foodborne Bacterial Pathogens. New York: Marcel Dekker, 1989: 525–542.

Mahmoud AF. Intestinal nematodes (roundworms). In Mandell GL, Douglas RG, Bennett JE, eds. Principles and Practice of Infectious Diseases. New York: Churchill Livingstone, 1990:2139–2140.

Mazanec MB, Nedrud JG, Kaetzel CS, and Lamm ME. A three-tiered view of the role of IgA in mucosal defense. Immunol. Today 14:430–435, 1993.

McFarland LV, Mulligan ME, Kwok RYY, and Stamm WE. Nosocomial acquisition of Clostridium difficile infection. N. Engl. J. Med. 320:204–210, 1989.

Mitchell DK, Van R, Marrow AL, et al. Outbreaks of astrovirus gastroenteritis in day care centers. J. Pediatr. 123:725–732, 1993.

Murphy AM, Aibrey MB, and Crewe EB. Rotavirus infections of neonates. Lancet. 2(Dec 3): 1149–1150, 1977.

Nichter M. Use of social science research to improve epidemiologic studies of and interventions for diarrhea andn dysentery. Rev. Infect. Dis. 13(Suppl 4):5265–5271, 1991.

Paolisso M, Baksh M, and Thomas JC. Women's agricultural work, child care, and infant diarrhea in rural Kenya. In: Leslie J, Paolisso M, eds. Women, Work, and Child Welfare in the Third World. Boulder, CO: Westview Press, 1989.

Pearson RK, and Guerrant RL. Enteric fever and other causes of abdominal symptoms with fever. In: Mandell GL, Douglas RG, Bennett JE, eds. Principles and Practice of Infectious Diseases. New York: Churchill Livingstone, 1990:880–905.

Pickering LK, Evans DG, DuPont HL, Vollet JJ, and Evans DJ. Diarrhea caused by Shigella, rotavirus, and Giardia in day-care centers: Prospective study. J. Pediatr. 99:51–56, 1981.

Quinn TC. Protozoan infections. In: Smith PD, moderator. Gastrointestinal infections in AIDS. Ann. Intern. Med. 116:63–77, 1992.

Ravidin JI, and Petri WA. Entamoeba histolytica (Amebiasis). In: Mandell GL, Douglas RG, Bennett JE, eds. Principles and Practice of Infectious Diseases.New York: Churchill Livingstone, 1990:2036–2049.

Rowe PC, Orrbin EE, Ogborn M, Wells et al. Epidemic *Escherichia coli* 0157:H7 gastroenteritis and helomytic-uremic syndrome in a Canadian Inuit community: Intestinal illness in family members as a risk factor. J. Pediatr. 124:21–26, 1994.

Sarker SA, and Gyr K. Non-immunological defense mechanisms of the gut. Gut. 33:987–993, 1992.

Satterwhite TK, DuPont HL, Evans DG, and Evans DJ. Role of *Escherichia coli* colonization factor antigen in acute diarrhea. Lancet. 22:181–184, 1978.

Schiemann DA. *Yersinia enterocolitica* and *Yersinia pseudotuberculosis*. In: Doyle MP, ed. Foodborne Bacterial Pathogens. New York: Marcel Dekker, 1989:601–672.

Shavit Y, Terman GW, Martin FC, et al. Stress, opiod peptides, the immune system, and cancer. J. Immunol. 135:834s–837s, 1985.

Smith PD. Gastrointestinal infection in AIDS. Ann. Intern. Med. 116:63–77, 1992.

Sneller MC, and Strober W. M cells and host defense. J. Infect. Dis. 154:737–741, 1986.

Sperber SJ, and Schleupner CJ. Salmonellosis during infection with human immunodeficiency virus. Rev. Infect. Dis. 8:925–934, 1987.

Spiegelberg HL, Boltz-Nitulescu G, Plummer JM, et al. Characterization of the IgE Fc receptors on monocytes and macrophages. Fed. Proc. 42:124–128, 1983.

Stamm WE, Weinstein RA, and Dixon RE. Comparison of endemic and epidemic nosocomial infections. Am. J. Med. 70:393–397, 1981.

Stein M, Keller SE, and Schleifer SJ. Stress and immunomodulation: the role of depression and neuroendocrine function. J. Immunol. 135:827s–833s, 1985.

Stelma GN. Aeromonas hydrophila. In: Doyle MP, ed. Foodborne Bacterial Pathogens. New York: Marcel Dekker, 1989:1–19.

Stern NJ. Campylobacter jejuni. In: Doyle MP, ed. Foodborne Bacterial Pathogens. New York: Marcel Dekker, 1989:71–110.

Strober W. Mechanisms of mucosal immunity in relation to AIDS. In: Smith PD, moderator. Gastrointestinal infections in AIDS. Ann. Intern. Med. 116:63–77, 1992.

Strober W, and Brown WR. The mucosal immune system. In: Samter M, ed. Immunological Diseases. Boston: Little, Brown, 1988: 79–55.

Takikawa I. Studies on pathogenic halophilic bacteria. Yokohama Med. Bull. 9(5):313–322, 1958.

Tauxe RV, Vandepitte J, Wauters G et al. Yersinia enterocolitica infections and pork: The missing link. Lancet. I:1129–1132, 1987.

Tauxe RV. Emerging foodborne diseases: An evolving public health challenge. Emerg. Infect. Dis. 3:1–13, 1997.

Thomas JC, Neumann CG, and Frerichs RF. The effect of misclassification of diarrhoea on estimates of its occurrence, the identification of risk factors, and the assessment of prevention efforts. J. Diarrhoeal Dis. Res. 7(3&4):63–69, 1989.

Thomas JC, and Neumann CG. Choosing an appropriate measure of diarrhoea occurrence: Examples from a community-based study in rural Kenya. Int. J. Epidemiol. 21:589–593, 1992.

Tramont EC. General or nonspecific host mechanisms. In: Mandell GL, Douglas RG, Bennett JE, eds. Principles and Practice of Infectious Diseases. New York: Churchill Livingstone, 1990:33–40.

U.S. Food and Drug Administration, Center for Food Safety and Applied Nutrition. (1992). The Bad Bug Book [computer file]: Foodborne Pathogenic Microorganisms and Natural Toxins Handbook. [Online] Available: http://purl.access.gpo.gov/GPO/LPS6 28 [January 1992].

Weinberg ED. Pregnancy–associated depression of cell- mediated immunity. Rev. Infect. Dis. 6:814–831, 1984.

Weiss MG. Cultural models of diarrheal illness: Conceptual framework and review. Soc. Sci. Med. 27:5–16, 1988.

12

Vector-Borne Transmission

FRANK J. SORVILLO, AMY C. MORRISON, and O.G.W. BERLIN

The methodologic issues in epidemiologic studies of infections that are not vector-borne pertain primarily to the sampling and measurement of the people who might experience an infection, including measurement of infection with the organism of interest. When transmission between people involves a vector, another dimension of research is required—one that tracks the biology and behavior of the vector. For this reason, epidemiologic research on vector-borne diseases has traditionally been more biologically oriented, focusing on the factors of vector life cycles that affect transmission. This chapter follows that tradition in that it is structured around considerations of the vector. Methodologic issues are interwoven with the biologic factors.

Over 300 infectious diseases agents encompassing viruses, bacteria, protozoa, and helminths are transmitted by a variety of vectors (Burgdorfer 1981). A list of selected vector-borne diseases by the type of infectious agent is presented in Table 12–1. The characteristics of six vector-borne diseases are presented in Table 12–2. In this chapter

we focus on diseases in which the vector is an arthropod.

Vector-borne diseases exact an enormous toll in terms of human disease and suffering. Malaria alone is estimated to affect 500 million people and cause three million deaths annually, most of them in children (WHO 1997). American trypanosomiasis (Chagas' disease) still devastates large areas of South America and, in its chronic stage, remains incurable (Schofield 1999). Filarial infections continue to be widespread, with onchocerciasis a common and intractable cause of blindness on two continents (Richards 1998). Control of vector-borne diseases is justifiably high among the World Health Organization's (WHO) priorities. The Special Programme for Research and Training in Tropical Diseases cosponsored by the United Nations Development Programme, the World Bank, and WHO has targeted eight priority diseases, six of which are arthropod-borne (malaria, leishmaniasis, Chagas' disease, lymphatic filariasis, African trypanosomiasis, and onchocerciasis) (Godal 1998). As global warming continues, the

Table 12–1   Selected Vector-Borne Diseases and Their Related Agent and Vector

Type of Infectious Agent	Disease	Type of Vector
Viruses	Colorado tick fever	Tick
	Dengue	Mosquito
	Rift valley fever	Mosquito
	St. Louis encephalitis	Mosquito
	Yellow fever	Mosquito
Bacteria	Bartonellosis	Sandfly
	Lyme disease	Tick
	Plague	Flea
	Relapsing fever	Body louse, tick
	Tularemia	Tick, fly, mosquito
Rickettsia	Ehrlichiosis	Tick
	Epidemic typhus	Body louse
	Q fever	Tick
	Rocky Mountin spotted fever	Tick
	Trench fever	Body louse
Protozoa	Babesiosis	Tick
	Chagas' disease	Reduviid (kissing) bug
	Leishmaniasis	Sandfly
	Malaria	Mosquito
	Sleeping sickness	Tsetse fly
Helminths	Dracunculiasis	Copepod (waterflea)
	Filariasis	Mosquito
	Onchocerciasis	Blackfly
	Schistosomiasis	Snail

historical geographic limits of some vector-borne diseases traditionally considered to be "tropical" will expand. Moreover, the last 20 years have seen the emergence of important, newly recognized vector-transmitted infections including such conditions as Lyme disease and ehrlichiosis (Steere 1977, Fritz 1998) and the reemergence of arboviral diseases such as dengue and yellow fever (Holmes 1998). It is not hyperbole to suggest that other vector-borne infections await discovery.

Given the significance of vector-borne diseases, continuing and expanded implementation of sound epidemiologic studies are vital to reducing the effect of these infections. However, numerous unique aspects of vectors, and the agents they transmit, can make such studies difficult. The inclusion of a vector into the ecology of a disease, a third living component beyond the host and agent, considerably increases the complexity of transmission dynamics. In cases of zoonotic vector-borne diseases, where the reservoir of infection is a nonhuman animal, a fourth (or more) living entity is included in the ecology, and the complexity is further heightened. Moreover, the effect of environment is perhaps greater for vector-related infections than for any other type of communicable disease and may have enormous effects on the agent, vector, host, and reservoir. Accordingly, an adequate understanding of the epidemiology of arthropod-borne

Table 12–2 Characteristics of Six Vector-Borne Diseases

Characteristic	Typhus	Yellow Fever	Malaria	Lyme Disease	Onchocerciasis	Schistosomiasis
Infectious agent	Rickettsia: *Rickettsia prowazekii*	Virus: Yellow fever virus	Protozoan: *Plasmodium vivax, P. malariae, P. falciparum, P. ovale*	Bacterium: *Borrelia burgdorferi*	Helminth: *Onchocerca volvulus* (filarial worm)	Helminth: various species of *Schistosoma* genus (blood flukes)
Vector	Body louse: *Pediculus humanus*	Mosquito: various species of *Aedes* genus	Mosquito: female *Anopheles*	Tick: *Ixodes* genera	Blackfly: females of the genus *Simulium*	*Biomphalaria* and *Oncomelania* genera
Reservoir	Humans	Humans (urban areas), monkeys (forests), and mosquitoes	Humans	Ticks (transstadial transmission), transmission to wild rodents and deer	Humans	Humans; other animals depending on parasite species; snails; water
Incubation period (in host)	1–2 weeks	3–6 days	12–30 days, depending on agent	3–32 days (early stages can be asymptomatic)	≥1 year	2–6 weeks
Symptoms	Fever, headache, chills, prostration, macular eruptions	Sudden onset, fever, chills, headache, myalgia, nausea, vomiting. Progresses to further complications	Fever, chills, sweats, headaches. Can progress to further complications	Distinctive skin lesions; systemic symptoms; joint, neurologic, and cardiac involvement	Dermatologic symptoms (altered pigmentation, edema); blindness	Symptoms depend on location of infection; hepatic, intestinal, and urinary symptoms
Laboratory diagnosis	Serologic tests for antigens	Isolation of virus from blood; serologic tests for antigen	Demonstration of parasites in blood films; antigen detection	Serologic tests for antibodies	Demonstration of microfilariae in infected sites	Demonstration of eggs in stool or urine
Treatment	Tetracyclines, chloramphenicol	None	Chloroquine, quinine, and related drugs	Tetracycline, amoxicillin, penicillin, erythromycin, ceftriaxone	Ivermectin	Praziquantel

Based on information in Chin J, ed. *Control of Communicable Diseases Manual* 17th ed. Washington, DC: American Public Health Association, 2000.

infections requires thorough knowledge of arthropod, infectious agent, environment, host, and reservoir(s).

The development of effective antimicrobial drugs and insecticides, as well as the early successes of malaria and *Aedes aegypti* eradication programs, led to the misperception that vector-borne diseases were no longer of primary public health importance. Consequently, there was a reduction in the number of qualified medical entomologists and epidemiologists specializing in vector-borne diseases. Furthermore, many organisms that were once sensitive to antimicrobial drugs have developed resistance to them. Clearly our understanding of vector-borne diseases has not been sufficient for adequate control. Thus there remains a pressing need for epidemiologic research of vector-borne diseases. Research priorities identified by the World Health Organization (WHO 1997) include identification of vectors (Schofield 1999); understanding of vector behavior and interaction with hosts and reservoirs (Richards 1998); identification of reservoirs; and perhaps most important, quantification of the transmission dynamics of these relationships (Godal 1998). Moreover, epidemiologic methods are necessary for the evaluation of interventions to prevent or control vector-borne diseases.

This chapter presents an overview of some of the methodologic considerations in epidemiologic research on vector-borne infections in the context of the biology of disease vectors. Because of the number and variety of vector-borne diseases and the biologic complexity inherent to each of them, in this brief space we can only hope to begin to sensitize readers to the types of methodologic issues that arise from the biologic characteristics of vector-borne transmission. We start with the criteria used for implicating a vector in transmission. Aspects of these criteria are then considered in greater detail in the two main sections that follow pertaining to measurement of infection in humans and biologic aspects of the vector that have implications for epidemiologic research methods.

CRITERIA FOR IMPLICATING VECTOR-BORNE TRANSMISSION

Traditional methods of identifying and incriminating vectors as agents of disease have included the following seven criteria (Harwood 1979):

1. *Demonstration of the spatial co-distribution of the vector and disease.* This spatial association is often not an exact overlap, and vector distribution may exceed that of the disease, or, when transmission occurs by means other than through the vector-borne route, disease distribution can go beyond the range of the suspected arthropod.

The initial hypothesis that Lyme disease might be a vector-borne infection was prompted by patient history, but the overlap of disease in areas populated by *Ixodes* ticks provided early valuable supporting information. However, such ecologic studies must be interpreted cautiously, since they look at "exposure" (in this case, presence of a specific tick species) at the aggregate level (community). Inferences from aggregate-level data to individual risks (e.g., risk of infection with Lyme disease) can be misleading.

2. *Demonstration of temporal association of the vector and disease.* The seasonal activity of the vector should, in most cases, coincide with (and precede) disease occurrence. Clear temporal associations for vector-borne diseases with long incubation periods (e.g. filariasis, Lyme disease, and Chagas' disease) may be more difficult to detect.

3. *Demonstration of association between vectors and humans.* Even if spatial and temporal associations are identified, it must be determined that the arthropod is known to bite or be in close proximity to humans. A vector that interacts only with nonhuman hosts will not be an important threat for transmission of disease to human populations.

It is important to attempt to implicate arthropod exposure as a risk factor for infection in controlled epidemiologic studies. However, several problems can make the assessment of vector exposure difficult and possibly introduce substantial misclassification. These include small vector size (e.g.,

Ixodes ticks, and mites), painless bite (e.g., triatomid bugs), "universal" exposure (e.g. mosquitoes), and, most important, proper species identification of potential vectors. When attempting to evaluate vector contact as a possible risk factor for disease, it is not uncommon for patients to fail to recognize that they have been bitten by an arthropod. For example, a substantial proportion of Lyme disease cases will not report a history of prior tick bite simply because the *Ixodes* tick is very small and the individual in most instances will not recognize an exposure. Exposure to mites, which may not be visible without the aid of a microscope, would be clearly underrecognized by patients. Often arthropods, like triatomid bugs the vectors of Chagas' disease, have a painless bite and typically feed when the human host is asleep. In addition, exposure to some potential vectors such as flies and mosquitoes may be reported by most people and exposure is therefore nearly universal. Moreover, the possible long incubation period of a vector-borne disease, in addition to the difficulty in observing a disease-vector temporal overlap, can create problems of patient recall. Finally, proper species identification is often complicated by the lack of properly trained insect taxonomists and the common occurrence of species complexes, where members can not be distinguished by taxonomic characteristics.

4. *Experimental infection of the vector.* When assessed in the laboratory can the putative vector be infected with the agent under consideration? For this criterion a negative finding is usually more meaningful, since arthropods can often be experimentally infected in the laboratory but may not be important in the transmission of an agent in nature.

5. *Experimental transmission from the vector to a susceptible host.* Supportive evidence of a vector-agent relationship is provided when transmission is observed in the laboratory. However, such transmission under controlled conditions may not be repeated in the field and the results must be interpreted cautiously.

6. *Finding a naturally infected vector.* Recovering the agent from a suspected vector in the field is further important implicating evidence. However, there can be spurious findings. It should be recognized that an agent taken up by an arthropod will live for a short period of time even if there is no multiplication or development within the vector. For example, Western equine encephalitis virus can occasionally be recovered from arthropods such as triatomids that are not vectors of the disease. The positive predictive value of testing when the agent is rare should also be considered. Because of these uncertainties it is important to find repeated natural infections.

7. *Disruption of transmission by control of the vector.* Further supporting evidence implicating an arthropod in disease transmission is provided when disease incidence declines following implementation of vector control measures and reduction of the vector density. However, caution must be exercised, since control measures may affect other factors including other possible vectors.

Several of the above criteria require measurement of infection in humans. We consider the methodologic aspects of these measures next.

MEASUREMENT OF INFECTION IN HUMANS

Techniques to measure the occurrence of infection in humans include clinical examination for manifestations of disease and laboratory tests for infection. Tests in the laboratory are further divided into those that demonstrate the presence of the infecting agent (i.e., antigen) itself and those that measure evidence of infection through an immune response to the agent (i.e., antibody). We discuss the implications of limitations of these methods for epidemiologic research. Malaria, leishmaniasis, and Lyme disease are used as examples.

Clinical Measures

Clinical measures for assessing infectious diseases include history taking, inspection, auscultation, palpation, and percussion. Many diseases have a unique clinical presentation that provides a relatively good proxy measure for infection. However, clinical diagnosis alone generally underestimates actual rates of infection at a population level. For example, with malaria, a relatively rapid and traditional measure of assessing infection prevalence and endemicity has been through the use of surveys for enlarged spleens (Beaver 1984). Malaria infection will typically cause splenomegaly. An enlarged spleen can be readily detected through palpation and the proportion of the population with palpable spleens has been a traditional measure to assess the level of malaria. Four measures of prevalence have been employed based on the following criteria. The term hypoendemic is used when the spleen rate in children (2–9 years) does not exceed 10%; mesoendemic when spleen rate in children is between 11% and 50%; hyperendemic when the spleen rate is high in both children (>50%) and adults (>25%); and holoendemic when the spleen rate in children is over 75% but usually low in adults, who possess partial immunity.

Although the use of spleen surveys is a rapid and traditional method of estimating malaria prevalence, caution must be exercised in the use of this measure. In tropical areas where malaria is endemic, other prevalent diseases, such as leishmaniasis, can cause splenomegaly and will complicate the use of spleen rates as a measure of malaria prevalence (Minodier 1998).

Demonstration of the Infectious Agent

The various clinical laboratory procedures used for diagnosing leishmaniasis have been extensively reviewed (Grimaldi 1993, Manson-Bahr 1987, Palma 1991). They include demonstration of the parasite in tissue or skin lesions, xenodiagnosis, and polymerase chain reaction (PCR) techniques.

Demonstration of the parasite in tissue or skin lesions remains the most definitive diagnostic method available. The limitations of parasitologic diagnosis is that species identification requires isolation and characterization of parasites by isozyme electrophoresis or identification with monoclonal antibodies. This requires either inoculation of hamsters with aspirates of infected tissue, infected sandflies, or in vitro culture of tissue homogenates or aspirates in biphasic media (NNN or Schieders). These procedures are time consuming and the use of in vitro culture under field conditions is often complicated by contamination problems. Furthermore, diagnosis of chronic cutaneous and mucocutaneous leishmaniasis is often made difficult by the paucity of parasites in lesions and visceral leishmaniasis diagnosis requires invasive procedures necessary to obtain bone marrow, lymph node, or splenic aspirates (Grimaldi 1993). The diagnosis of malaria is typically accomplished through microscopic examination of thin and thick blood smears (Ash 1987). This requires sound technique to prevent misdiagnosis and misclassification of disease status in epidemiologic studies. Microscope slides that are not properly cleaned or reagents that are not adequately prepared can lead to errors in diagnosis. Moreover, a trained, skilled microscopist is necessary for accurate identification of malarial parasites. For example, a platelet lying over a red blood cell can be mistaken for a malarial parasite. In conducting prevalence surveys among largely asymptomatic persons the level of parasitemia may be low and false negative findings can occur. When specimens are obtained on clinically ill patients with suspected malaria at the time of paroxysm only small ring stages of the parasite may be present and can be missed, especially by an inexperienced technician.

One of the most sensitive methods of diagnosis of some vector-borne infections is xenodiagnosis (Marsden 1979). In xenodiagnosis infection-free vectors are fed on a host suspected to be infected. The vectors are subsequently dissected and evaluated for presence or absence of infection. This technique can be of value for diseases such as Chagas' disease where parasitemia may be very low. However, one of the problems with this technique is that it requires the ability to maintain sufficient quantities of the arthropod and the assurance of uninfected vectors.

Highly sensitive antigen detection techniques such as the PCR are available for Lyme disease and many other infectious diseases (Goodman 1995). There is an increasing number of specific recombinant probes for numerous *Leishmania* species complexes as well as for probes that may be able to distinguish geographically isolated parasite strains. The PCR technique is a rapid and highly sensitive method for diagnosis of visceral leishmaniasis and is capable of distinguishing between past and current infection (Blackwell 1992). However, while PCR is quite sensitive, genetic heterogeneity of organisms can make development of standardized primers difficult. PCR is also limited to detecting the presence of the agent, which may be present in very low levels, below the threshold of PCR detection. Moreover PCR is not a serologic test and cannot be used to estimate levels of prior infection.

Immunologic Laboratory Tests

A growing number of immunologic and molecular techniques are now becoming available for the diagnosis of leishmaniasis. The most promising for epidemiologic studies are dot blot, dipstick techniques. Several serologic assays are available including ELISA, direct agglutination test, immunoblot, and immunofluorescense to detect anti-*Leishmania* antibodies.

One of the methods most commonly used in prevalence studies has been the leishmanin skin (Montenegro) test, which measures the cutaneous DTH or cellular response to *Leishmania*–derived antigens. The skin test, however, fails to distinguish between current and past leishmanial infections. Furthermore, the Montenegro test is uniformly negative in active visceral leishmaniasis cases, becoming positive between six weeks to one year after recovery.

Patients with Lyme disease often exhibit protean, nonspecific manifestations (Barbour 1993). In addition, *B. burgdorferi* is difficult to isolate from infected patients, in part because of the small numbers of organisms in affected tissues (Berger 1989). As a result, diagnosis is often dependent on serologic testing though it suffers from a number of limitations: a serologic response may be absent in acute Lyme disease, existing serologic tests are not standardized, and considerable interlaboratory variability in results exists (Sherstha 1985, Craft 1984). The problems of case definition and diagnosis of Lyme disease led CDC to attempt to standardize and publish case definition guidelines (Centers for Disease Control and Prevention 1997).

Subsequent to the discovery of the etiologic agent *B. burgdorferi* and development of antibody testing for Lyme disease, there was an explosion of serologic testing for the infection. This was propelled by the protean and nonspecific manifestations of the disease coupled with a plethora of sometimes sensational media stories, including many of dubious accuracy, inundating the public. As a consequence, in the late 1980s thousands of people, many with nonspecific symptoms, were being tested for Lyme disease. Since most of these people were not infected with *B. burgdorferi* the prevalence of infection was often very low among those being tested. In such circumstances even a serologic test of high sensitivity and specificity will produce misleading results (Sorvillo 1990). Specifically, many of those testing positive will be falsely positive and the predictive value of a positive test will be low.

If circumstances permit, the accuracy of testing for Lyme disease and other infections can be improved by testing in series (Dressler 1993). For example, a positive enzyme linked immunosorbent assay (ELISA) or immunofluorescent assay (IFA) can be followed with a Western immunoblot test to improve diagnostic accuracy. Moreover, it is often useful to send duplicate samples to independent laboratories as a means of evaluating and verifying results.

The infectious agent of Lyme disease, *Borrelia burgdorferi*, displays genetic heterogeneity with three genomic groups (*B. burgdorferi* sensu stricto, *Borrelia garinii*, and *Borrelia afzelii*) (Baranton 1992). Strains may vary in infectivity, virulence, incubation period, host and reservoir preferences, tissue tropism, and may significantly affect vector competence. Differences in the strains may be the reason behind different prevalences and clinical characteristics in different regions (e.g., the northeast United States compared to the Pacific coast). Strain differences must be considered in studies evaluating vaccine efficacy and effectiveness and also in assessing the benefits of various therapies when comparisons are made between communities. In addition, strain heterogeneity may lead to suboptimal performance of serologic tests, as has been documented for Lyme disease (Hedberg 1987). This leads, in turn, to inaccurate estimates of disease occurrence and risk through misclassification.

VECTORS AND EXPOSURE OF THE HOST TO INFECTION

For a given host, the probability of infection depends in large part on the prevalence of the vector and the infectious agent, and the effectiveness of the vector in transmitting the infectious agent. We discuss in this section: measuring the presence of the vector, or the "entomologic risk"; ways in which the population biology of the vector affects transmission and exposure; modes of transmission from the vector to the host; transmission of the agent between vectors; and vector feeding behaviors. In estimating associations between exposures and infection it is imperative that a researcher be familiar with these factors affecting the degree of exposure and how they can lead to confounding in a study by varying between comparison groups. A summary of the factors and their implications is presented in Table 12–3.

Entomologic Risk

A measure of exposure to vector-borne infections is the entomologic risk, or the number of a particular vector type actually involved in transmission. To determine the entomologic risk, the vector population must be sampled and the species of the vectors collected must be identified. Measuring the presence of the vector is complicated by the size of the vector, sampling the vector population, and identification of the vector species.

Vector size

It is quite possible that Lyme disease as an entity, and its association with prior tick exposure, would have been discovered much earlier if the *Ixodes* tick was not so small. In implicating a vector, size probably does matter. Larval stages of *Ixodes* are approximately the size of a period on this page, nymphs no larger than a comma (Burgdorfer 1983). Lyme disease exemplifies the problem of assessing vector exposure. Such problems due to size or other factors, including nocturnal activity and painless bite, can lead to misclassification of exposure and the introduction of bias. In such circumstances, surrogates, for example, forest or vegetation contact as a proxy for tick exposure, may be of some value in helping determine possible vector contact. However, care must be exercised in the use of proxy variables as well.

Sampling the vector population

Almost all insect collection methods are biased. For example, in one common collection technique ("human biting counts"), insects are collected and counted as they land on the collector's bare legs. This method selects for blood-seeking females and will not collect other life stages. Most traps similarly attract a biased sample of the vectors.

In studies of leishmaniasis, sampling of the immature sandflies is not practical for monitoring population levels needed for epidemiologic studies. Such efforts have required the removal of large quantities of soil (sometimes in tons) to find larvae (Perfil'ev 1966), or the use of numerous emergence traps monitored over extended time periods to capture recently emerged adult sandflies (Arias 1982). Adult sandflies are not randomly distributed in nature, and there is always sampling bias, regardless of the method used (Young 1991). The spatial distribution of the traps or collections, both horizontal and vertical, will greatly affect estimates of entomologic risk.

The sampling method(s) employed in a study will depend on the study objectives. When there is little knowledge of the existing sandfly fauna in an area or when trying to identify a vector species, surveys should

Table 12–3 Implications of the Biologic Characteristics of Vector-Borne Diseases on Epidemiologic Research

Biologic Characteristic	Implications for Epidemiologic Research
The number and types of the vector present in the environment (entomologic risk)	• A small vector or painless bite can go unnoticed, contributing to misclassification of host exposure. • Contact with forest or other vegetation may be used as a proxy for contact with a tick in some instances. • Techniques for estimating vector population size are often biased. Under- or overestimates of the vector prevalence result in misclassification of exposure in community level studies. Multiple sampling techniques may be needed to more accurately estimate the vector population size. • Variations in vector strains between geographic areas may explain differences in prevalence and incidence of infection. • Strain differences must be considered in assessments of vaccine efficacy/effectiveness.
Vector population biology	• The age distribution of the vectors affects the capacity of the vector population to transmit infection and thus the likelihood of the host to be exposed. Knowledge of the age distribution of the vector population may be important in understanding differences in incidence rates between communities.
Horizontal transmission between hosts and host immune response	• Individual primary and secondary cases can be linked when the extrinsic incubation period is known and infections are not common. • With macroparasites, the parasite load in a host is an important factor in the transmissibility of the infection. • When lifelong immunity is conferred, the incidence of infection can be estimated with serial serosurveys in a population, or pre/post serology in a cohort. • A single serosurvey will provide an estimate of the period prevalence rather than the point prevalence. • The risk of infection cannot be accurately determined when the number of people with immunity (i.e., the number not susceptible to infection) is unknown. • When infection does not result in lifelong immunity, repeat infections are impossible. Depending on the purposes of the study, researchers may need to identify and omit repeat infections from calculations of disease incidence.
Vertical transmission of the agent in vectors	• The propagation of the agent between vectors allows the agent to persist in the environment when vectors are few and infected humans may even be absent. An absence of measured infection may not indicate elimination of an agent from an area or of lasting elimination of infection from a human population.
Vector feeding behavior	• Multiple feeding behaviors of a vector can account for infections among hosts that are temporarily and spatially clustered. • Understanding vector feeding behaviors (e.g., times of day) is important for studies using vector-host proximity as a proxy measure of host exposure to the infectious agent. • Multiple feeding behavior increases host exposure and thus incidence of disease.

employ as many sampling methods as possible. When examining a specific species, the most effective method for capture of both feeding and resting flies should be identified and employed for quantitative studies (Young 1991). Collection methods for adult sandflies have been summarized by Young and Arias (1991). Frequently used methods include direct search and capture with an aspirator, an assortment of traps used to collect flies after disturbing their natural resting sites (Damasceno traps, leaf little traps, funnel traps), sticky paper traps (paper covered with castor oil), human and animal bait collections, light traps (e.g., CDC and Shannon types), and flight trap collection (i.e., Malaise) (Young and Arias 1991).

Vector species identification
A collection of a given vector may need to be further classified into particular species. For example, in many areas where leishmaniasis

is endemic, the sandfly fauna is extremely varied, while only one species is a competent vector. To estimate the entomologic risk, each collected fly must be processed and mounted on a slide to observe internal anatomic structures of females (spermathecae and cibarium) or the genitalia of males under a microscope. The sandflies must be dissected either immediately or after cryopreservation, or macerated for more current PCR assays; each of these procedures precludes species identification from whole specimens. In general, the last abdominal segment and spermethecae of female flies can be mounted for identification after removal of the gut to look for *Leishmania*; in a limited number of cases where local sandfly fauna is well known and homogeneous, flies can be identified by external morphology.

Finally, there are a number of sandfly groups (*Lutzomyia verrucarum*) whose females are morphologically indistinguishable from each other, yet some species are capable of transmitting disease while others are not. If multiple species are present in the same geographic area, the exposure to the vector, or entomologic risk, can be greatly over- or underestimated. Under these circumstances, the proportional distribution of male sandflies, which *can* be distinguished by morphologic characteristics, are used to estimate the numbers of their female counterparts in the collection. However, the behavior of male and female flies is so distinct that the generalization of the male distribution to the female distribution is often erroneous. Species identification methods such as isozyme electrophoresis or PCR assays are more definitive, but are only available for some species complexes (Fryauff 1990, Adamson 1991). However, as mentioned previously, most of these assays require destruction of the adult sample making the determination of *Leishmania* infection rates difficult.

Vector Population Biology

There is a quantitative relationship between vector population levels and pathogen transmission. The nature of this relationship, however, is often poorly understood and is not necessarily linear. Although vector population dynamics can be affected by natural predators and parasites, the physical environment (e.g., rainfall, temperature, and photoperiod) exerts the strongest influence on the capacity of a vector to transmit infection. The daily probability of survival and the frequency of blood-feeding are two important measures of vector transmission capacity (Dye 1992).

Vector survival profoundly affects the size of a vector population that is infective with a pathogen and the duration of its infective life. For example, the extrinsic incubation period for dengue 2 virus in *Aedes aegypti* at 30°C is 12 days (Watts 1987). Considering the earliest age when *Aedes aegypti* ingest their first blood meal (i.e., 2 days post emergence) and the mean temperatures in the tropics (~30°C), females must be 14 days or older to be potentially infective. Even modest variation in daily survival could have a dramatic influence on the number of mosquitoes that become infective and are capable of transmitting virus (Milby 1989, Smith 1975). It has been assumed that the probability of daily survival is constant over time because insect mortality is thought to be caused by predation, weather, and other factors, but not old age. However, a growing body of information suggests that insect mortality is not constant for all age groups and that older arthropods have a lower mortality rate than young ones (Carey 1992, Mueller 1996). This has important epidemiologic implications for disease vectors because it suggests that those arthropods most likely to transmit a pathogen (old ones who have lived long enough to become infectious) have lower rates of mortality and, therefore, greater potential to transmit infection than was previously appreciated.

The age structure of vector populations can be estimated through mark-release-recapture studies (Service 1993). In these studies, the characteristics of a population are estimated through the sampling probabilities of recapturing a proportion of an earlier sample after they have been dispersed.

Transmission from the Agent to the Host (Horizontal Transmission)

Transmission of the agent between hosts, via the vector, is referred to as horizontal transmission. Vertical transmission, discussed in the next section, pertains to transmission of the agent between vectors or different life stages of a vector.

Arthropods may function as vectors between hosts either mechanically or biologically. In mechanical transmission the vector acquires a pathogen from one source and deposits it in other locations, where it may infect a new host. There is no development or multiplication of the pathogen in the vector; that is, there is no incubation period within the arthropod (Burgdorfer 1981). The vector is not infected but rather contaminated for a limited time and transmission typically must occur quickly while the agent is still viable and infectious. For example, *Francisella tularensis*, the causative agent of tularemia, can be transmitted by the bite of a horsefly via contaminated mouthparts.

In contrast to mechanical transmission, biologic transmission requires that the pathogen undergoes an obligatory developmental period within the vector, termed the extrinsic incubation period. The length of the extrinsic incubation period will affect the force of infection (time period between primary and secondary cases of disease) and depending on the survival rate of the arthropod vector will determine the number of potentially infected vectors. To be an efficient vector, a significant number of adults must survive a period greater than the extrinsic incubation period to successfully transmit the disease. Where infections are uncommon, associated cases may be linked if the extrinsic incubation period is known.

Biologic transmission occurs via three forms of multiplication of the agent in the vector: propagative, when the pathogen multiplies within the arthropod to a level necessary for transmission (e.g., yellow fever virus and mosquitoes); cyclopropagative, when the pathogen undergoes both developmental changes and increases in number (e.g., *Plasmodium* sp. and mosquitoes); and cyclodevelopmental, when the pathogen undergoes a series of developmental stages to reach an infectious stage, but without multiplication (e.g., filarial worms and mosquitoes).

Anderson and May (Anderson 1979) divide infectious agents into microparasites and macroparasites. Propagative transmission is most commonly observed in microparasites, smaller organisms (viruses, bacteria, protozoa) that usually have short generation times, often have an acute effect on the host, and generally induce acquired (often lifelong) immunity (Clayton 1997). Thus the spread of these agents through a community will depend directly on the titer or level of the agent within the vector and the contact rate between the vector and host. Furthermore, once infected, a vector can transmit the pathogen for the remainder of its lifetime. Where infection is measured reliably with serologic tests, the incidence of infection can be estimated with a temporally spaced series of serosurveys in a population, or in a cohort with a serologic test at enrollment and at the end of follow up. However, a single serosurvey will provide an estimate of the period prevalence rather than the point prevalence.

Lyme disease, if not treated early, induces a prolonged immunity (Moore 1998). Such lifelong or long-term immunity is common for most viral and bacterial vector-borne diseases. This immunity can complicate determination of populations at risk and subsequent assessment of incidence rates and/or measurement of risk factors for disease. For example, when assessing incidence in a certain health jurisdiction, the annual incidence rate of Lyme disease might be calculated as the number of new cases (numerator) divided by the census population for the jurisdiction (denominator). Yet in a highly endemic area a significant proportion of the population will be immune and should not be considered in the population at risk. Therefore using available population data would inflate the true population at risk.

The incidence rate would consequently (assuming complete identification of cases) be spuriously low because of the inflated denominator. Paradoxically, low incidence may be observed in communities where vector density and vector infection levels are high because of high levels of herd immunity and the availability of relatively few susceptible hosts. In such circumstances using a measure of prevalence may provide a more accurate picture of disease effect.

Multiplication of agents in microparasites can also be cyclopropagative. There are distinct morphologic and biologic differences between the agent within the host and vector (e.g., amastigote versus promastigote stage of *Leishmania*), and these differences have aided the pathogen in combating host immune responses and therefore sterilizing (complete) immunity is not always observed and reinfection can occur. Under these circumstances, calculating attack rates is complicated by the fact that individuals can be infected multiple times.

In contrast, cyclodevelopmental transmission typically occurs in macroparasites, which are usually larger (e.g., helminths) and generally have a progressive (chronic) effect on the host, which is a function of parasite intensity (Clayton 1997). Macroparasites usually show an aggregated frequency distribution among hosts, with most hosts having few or no parasites, and a few hosts having many parasites. Therefore epidemiologic studies of macroparasites often measure load as well as incidence of infection within a community.

Transmission of the Agent Between Vectors (Vertical Transmission)

Vertical transmission refers to the passage of the agent from one life stage to another or directly from parent to progeny. Vertical transmission of infectious agent from the female parent to progeny, termed transovarial transmission, is an important phenomenon in many tick-borne rickettsial diseases (e.g., *Dermacentor andersoni* and *Rickettsia rickettsii,* the causative agent of Rocky Mountain spotted fever) (McDade 1986), and some arboviral diseases (e.g., LaCrosse

virus in *Aedes triseriatus*). Such a mechanism acts to increase the prevalence of an agent in a vector population and can promote pathogen persistence during periods of reduced reservoir abundance or low disease prevalence. Thus an absence of disease among human hosts and of measured infection in vectors may not indicate elimination of the infectious agent from the vector population; resurgence of disease may still be possible.

Transtadial transmission, or retention of infection from stage to stage (i.e., from larva to nymph to adult) is most relevant in tick-borne disease. Without this phenomenon, transmission from host to host would not be possible, since ticks typically feed just once per molt. Moreover, behavioral differences in the larval, nymphal, and adult stages can result in the transmission of a pathogen to different species of hosts.

Vector Feeding Behavior

The transmission of vector-borne diseases is affected by feeding behavior including the place of biting, host preferences, and gonotrophic (ovarian) cycle. Daily activity can be classified as diurnal (active during daylight hours), nocturnal (active at night), and crepuscular (active during twilight hours). Most arthropods have distinct periods of activity when they feed, oviposit, rest, and mate. These patterns are typically species-specific and may often explain transmission patterns of disease. For example, the specific activity patterns of malaria vectors, as well as the human population in a region will determine the effectiveness of a bed net control program. If mosquito activity is highest before 8:00 PM, people become exposed to infective bites before going to bed and bed nets will not afford protection.

Arthropods that rest inside dwellings (endophily) and feed indoors (endophagy) often have a greater probability of host exposure than those vectors that rest outside of dwellings (exophily) and feed outside (exophagy). Host preferences have a strong influence on the capacity to transmit disease. Some arthropods prefer to feed on humans (anthropophilic), others have a preference for nonhuman animals (zoophilic), while some species are considered opportunistic feeders, feeding on whatever species may be available (Gwadz 1996). Vectors are attracted to hosts principally through the detection of warmth, moisture, and carbon dioxide levels (Ribeiro 1996).

Host preference studies are essential to implicate vector-species. Generally, engorged female insects are collected from natural resting sites and the source of the blood meal identified by a variety of serologic methods (Tempelis 1975). Historically, the precipitin method (Tempelis 1963) was the most commonly employed method, but it has been replaced by the ELISA-based method (Chow 1993), and more recently by PCR-based techniques. DNA fingerprinting technology has made it possible to identify specific host characteristics of the same species; that is, identify high risk groups (children versus adults), evaluation of protective measures such as bed nets, and finally to determine the frequency of blood feeding (multiple feeding). These methods are limited to the identification of recent blood meals, generally not much more than 24 hours old, because the digestive processes of the insects degrade the antigens used for blood meal identification. Interpretation of these results depends on the question being asked and the methodology used to collect blood-engorged insects. These types of studies usually require knowledge of the natural resting sites of the vector in question. In addition, some knowledge of the relative availability of blood sources is necessary for proper interpretation of host preference studies. For example, forage ratios can be calculated when an animal census has been carried out. A forage ratio is the ratio of the percentage of vectors feeding on a specific host (calculated from a host preference study) to the percentage of that host species represented in the local animal population. A forage ratio of 1.0 indicates neither preference nor avoidance of the indicated animal host, forage ratios significantly greater than 1.0 indicate selective preferences, and values less than 1.0 indicate avoidance in favor of other hosts. The importance of

using this type of technique is best illustrated by classic studies carried out by Hess and colleagues (1968). These studies demonstrated the strong prference of St. Louis encephalitis (SLE) vectors to feed on birds. Preliminary examination of their results showed only a small percentage of blood meals taken on birds. However, after accounting for the disproportionate number of birds in the sample (using forage ratios) it was apparent that these vectors had an overwhelming preference for bird blood when available, which helped explain the low incidence of human cases.

When studying zoonoses, it is often difficult to test each blood meal against an array of all possible reservoir hosts, where as in the case of anthroponoses, the Blood Index of humans is the only relevant parameter. In the design of host preference studies one must avoid biased sampling. For example, if cattle are a suspected blood source, sampling mosquitoes off cattle shed walls may or may not be informative. If all the samples showed evidence of cattle blood meals the results would not be particularly informative. If, however, some of these mosquitoes at this site had evidence of human blood, one would interpret these results as significant, indicating an important degree of human host preference.

Conventional wisdom has assumed that most insect vectors feed once per gonotrophic cycle. Since a blood meal is necessary for egg production, the gonotrophic (ovarian) cycle of an arthropod will determine when and how frequently a female will feed. Vectors with a short gonadotrophic cycle will feed more frequently. Recently, however, an increasing body of work has challenged the basic assumption that most dipteran vectors are gonotrophically concordant and that many important vector species feed multiple times during a single gonotrophic cycle (gonotrophic discordance). Although this phenomenon is probably more widespread than initially thought, it has been best documented for *Anopheles gambiae* and *Aedes aegypti*, probably the two most important mosquito vectors. In both cases, it appears that the mosquito uses blood to supplement its energy needs as opposed to relying solely on plant sugars as fuel for flight and other daily activities. In the case of *Aedes* aegypti, there appears to be a fitness advantage for mosquitoes that feed exclusively on blood (Scott 1997, Costero 1998, Naksathit 1998, Morrison 1999). Furthermore, characteristics of protein-rich but isoleucine-limited human blood increase mosquitoes' ability to use blood for their energy needs. Therefore these mosquitoes rely more on blood for fuel and have been observed to feed multiple times during a single gonotrophic cycle. This, combined with interrupted feedings, due to host defensive behavior, greatly increases the number of potentially infective contacts of this vector. Multiple feeding behavior can account for observed clusters of arthropod diseases in time and space (Halstead 1968, Christensen 1996). Moreover, the level of host exposure to an infectious agent might be estimated in some studies with a measure of the amount of time the vector and host are in close proximity to each other. To estimate this well, it is important to know the feeding behaviors of the vector.

DIRECTIONS FOR FUTURE EPIDEMIOLOGIC RESEARCH

As we mentioned in the first section of this chapter, the study of vector-borne diseases is not a historical curiosity; it is very much a topic of growing public health importance. To conduct the necessary research, a commitment to improve the epidemiologic capability of personnel in tropical areas is urgently needed. While some quite successful training programs are in operation, additional efforts to enlarge the base of knowledge of epidemiologic methods are necessary.

Those conducting research on the complex biologic systems we have described in this chapter will need to make use of new resources and techniques. We mention two here: geographic information systems and the use of genetically modified vectors in disease control.

Geographic Information Systems

John Snow's classic investigation of cholera represents one of the earliest and well-known successful uses of mapping both disease and factors possibly affecting disease, in this case, source of water. Since then the use of "spot maps" has been a basic and important tool of the field epidemiologist. Geographic information systems (GIS) provide new sophistication to an old concept (Richards 1993, Glass 1995). GIS can be used to map a wide array of variables including location, disease occurrence, and environment, and can provide a valuable analysis tool for epidemiology and public health personnel including those concerned with vector-borne diseases. The availability and relatively low cost of high-speed microcomputers, coupled with improved and easier to use software have combined to make the use of GIS more practical. Performing spatial analyses using GIS to identify clustering patterns can help implicate new vectors, determine environmental factors of importance in the dynamics of arthropod-borne transmission, and aid in predicting possible new areas of disease spread (Kitron 1997). The use of remote sensing data from satellite collection efforts may also provide valuable insight into the epidemiology of arthropod-borne disease (Beck 1997).

To date, the majority of studies utilizing GIS for vector-borne diseases have concentrated on the identification, using remote sensing, of environmental factors that determine the temporal and spatial distribution of both vectors and disease (Beck 1997, Pavolosky 1966) and ultimately to predict areas with highest risk of disease transmission. GIS technology has been successfully applied to the studies of the vectors of numerous water-related diseases, including the mosquito vectors of Rift Valley fever, St. Louis encephalitis, and malaria (Beck 1997, Pavolosky 1966, Wood 1991). In each of these examples, however, the aquatic habitats studied were large, and remotely sensed data were used to identify larval habitats such as temporary or permanent ground pools, marshes, rice fields, rivers, or streams.

GIS has many other advantages for epidemiologic studies. The principal advantage is its spatial analysis capabilities (Clarke 1996). These include data visualization and exploratory data analysis, which allow investigators to interpret spatial data. The graphics and animation features embedded within a GIS are highly effective in demonstrating the spread and dispersal of disease over time. Moreover, spatially referenced data facilitate the use of spatial statistical procedures including geostatistics, spatial autoregressive modeling (Kitron 1997), and pattern analysis (Boots 1988). Spatial statistical methods account for spatial dependence of data (Cressie 1991). In contrast, most ordinary statistics assume that observations are independent. Disease incidence rates commonly exhibit spatial autocorrelation; that is, the tendency for samples collected close to one another to be more similar than samples collected farther away from each other (Boots 1988). For example, pattern analyses consider the distance between each point and all other points to describe and analyze point patterns and characterize disease clustering in time and space (Boots 1988, Marshall 1991). Overall these methods can be applied to identify areas of increased transmission ("hot spots") and dispersal and clustering patterns, and to make spatial comparisons between cases with different demographic characteristics. Recent applications to vector-borne diseases include the demonstration that Lacrosse encephalitis cases in Illinois clustered within three kilometers of the city of Peoria and that transmission was concentrated around specific sites (hardwood ravines and tire piles) (Kitron 1997); and the identification of household clustering of dengue cases in Puerto Rico (Morrison 1998).

GIS is an effective data management system when good maps or baseline information is available. However, caution must be exercised in the interpretation of any mapped information, since within map boundary units such as state, county, or other jurisdiction, there may be great heterogeneity of factors that may not be reflected. Moreover, since many areas lack sufficient geographic and other data, effective mapping may not be possible.

Control Strategies Employing Genetically Modified Vectors

One area of significant interest to vector biologists has been research aimed at developing vectors that are refractory to human pathogens. Considerable research has been directed at identifying genes in insects that make them competent vectors or that afford resistance to infection. Other lines of research have been developing mechanisms to transform mosquitoes using transposable elements and bacterial symbionts (Beard 1998, Jasinskiene 1998). For epidemiologists and ecologists, the most important question related to this issue is how these new refractory traits would be spread in nature and what kind of coverage would be necessary to affect disease. Ongoing research in population genetics and quantitative epidemiology to address these questions is needed.

REFERENCES

Abdel-Wahab MF, Strickland GT, El-Sahly A, et al. Changing pattern of schistosomiasis in Egypt 1935–79. Lancet. 2(8136):242–244, 1979.

Adamson RW, Chance ML, Ward RD, Feliciangeli D, and Maingon RDC. Molecular approaches applied to the analysis of sympatric sand fly populations in endemic areas of western Venezuela. Parasitologia 33:45–53, 1991.

Anderson RM, and May RM. Population biology of infectious diseases: Part I. *Nature* 80:361–367, 1979.

Anderson JF, Johnson RC, Magnarelli LA, Hyde FW, and Myers JE. Prevalence of *Borrelia burgdorferi* and *Babesia mocroti* in mice on islands inhabited by white-tailed deer. Appl. Environ. Microbiol. 53:892–894, 1987.

Arias JR, and de Freitas RA. On the vectors of cutaneous leishmaniasis in the central Amazon of Brazil. 4. Sand fly emergence from a "terra firme" forest floor. Acta Amazonica 12:609–611, 1982.

Ash LR, and Orihel TC. *Parasites: A Guide to Laboratory Procedures and Identification.* Chicago: American Society of Clinical Pathology Press, 1987.

Baranton G, Postic D, Saint-Girons I, et al. Delineation of *Borrelia burgdorferi* sensu stricto, *Borrelia garinii* sp, nov., and Group VS461 associated with Lyme borreliosis. Int. J. Syst. Bacteriol. 42:378–383, 1992.

Barbour AG, and Fish D. The biological and social phenomenon of Lyme disease. Science. 260:1610–1616, 1993.

Beard CB, Durvasula RV, and Richards FF. Bacterial symbiosis in arthropods and the control of disease transmission. Emerg. Infect. Dis. 4:581–591, 1998.

Beaver PC, Jung RC, and Cupp EW. *Clinical Parasitology.* Philadelphia: Lea & Febiger, 1984.

Beck LR, Rodriguez MH, Dister SW, et al. Assessment of a remote sensing-based model for predicting malaria transmission risk in villages of Chiapas, Mexico. Am. J. Trop. Med. Hyg. 56:99–106, 1997.

Berger BW. Dermatologic manifestations of Lyme disease. Rev. Infect. Dis. 11:S1475–1481, 1989.

Blackwell JM. Leishmaniasis epidemiology: all down to the DNA. Parasitology 104(Suppl.): S19–S34, 1992.

Boots BN, and Getis A. Point Pattern Analysis: Newbury Park, UK: Sage, 1988.

Burgdorfer W. The arthropod vector as a selective transport system of animal and human pathogens. In: McKelvey JJ Jr, Eldridge BF, Maramorosch K, eds. *Vectors of Disease Agents: Interactions with Plants, Animals, and Man.* New York: Praeger Publishers, 1981.

Burgdorfer W, and Kierans JE. Ticks and Lyme disease in the United States. Ann. Intern. Med. 99:121, 1983.

Carey JR, Leido P, Orozco D, and Vaupel JW. Slowing of mortality rates at older ages in large medfly cohorts. Science. 258:457–461, 1992.

Centers for Disease Control and Prevention. Case definitions for infectious conditions under public health surveillance. MMWR. 46(RR10);1–55, 1997.

Chin J. *Control of Communicable Diseases Manual* 17th ed. Washington D.C. American Public Health Association, 2000.

Chow E, Wirtz RA, and Scott TW. Identification of bloodmeals in *Aedes aegypti* by antibody sandwich enzyme-linked immunosorbent assay. J. Am. Mosq. Control Assoc. 9:196–205, 1993.

Christensen HA, de Vasquez AM, and Boreham MM. Host-feeding patterns of mosquitoes (*Diptera:* Culicidae) from central Panama. Am. J. Trop. Med. Hyg. 55:202–208, 1996.

Clarke KC, McLafferty SL, and Tempalski BJ. On epidemiology and geographic information systems: a review and discussion of future directions. Emerg. Infect. Dis. 2:85–92, 1996.

Clayton DH, and Moore J. *Host-Parasite Evolution. General Principles and Avian Models.* Oxford: Oxford University Press, 1997:473.

Costero A, Attardo GM, Scott TW, and Edman JD. An experimental study on the detection of fructose in *Aedes aegypti*. J. Am. Mosq. Control Assoc. 14:234–242, 1998.

Craft JE, Grodzicki RL, and Steere AC. Antibody response in Lyme disease: evaluation of diagnostic tests. J. Infect. Dis. 149:789–795, 1984.

Cressie N. Statistics for Spatial Data. Chichester, UK: John Wiley, 1991.

Dressler F, Whalen JA, Reinhardt BN, et al. Western blotting in the serodiagnosis of Lyme disease. J. Infect. Dis. 167:392–396, 1993.

Dye C. The analysis of parasite transmission by bloodsucking insects. Annu. Rev. Entomol. 37:1–19, 1992.

Fritz CL, and Glaser CA . Ehrlichiosis. Infect. Dis. Clin. North Am. 12:123–136, 1998.

Fryauff DT, Kassem HA, Shehata MG, El Awady M, El Said SM. Enzyme electrophoresis as an alternative method for separating the sympatric *Leishmania* vectors *Phlebotomus papatasi* and *Phlebotomus langeroni*. J. Med. Entomol. 27:773–776, 1990.

Glass GE, Schartz BS, Morgan JM III, et al. Environmental risk factors for Lyme disease identified with geographic information systems. Am. J. Public Health. 85:944–948, 1995.

Godal T, Goodman HC, and Lucas A. Research and training in tropical diseases. World Health Forum. 19:377–381, 1998.

Goodman JL, Bradley JF, Ross AE, et al. Bloodstream invasion in early Lyme disease: results from a prospective controlled, blinded sttudy using the polymerase chain reaction. Am. J. Med. 99:6–12, 1995.

Grimaldi G Jr, and nTesh RB. Leishmaniases of the New World: Current concepts and implications for future research. Clin. Microbiol. Rev. 6:230–50, 1993.

Gwadz R, and Collins FH. Anopheline mosquitoes and the agents they transmit. In: Beatty BJ, Marquardt WC, eds. *The Biology of Disease Vectors.* Niwot: University Press of Colorado, 1996.

Halstead SB, Scanlon JE, Umpaivit P,and Udomsakdi S. Dengue and Chickungunya virus infection in man in Thailand, 1962–1964. IV. Epidemiologic studies in the Bangkok metropolitan area. Am. J. Trop. Med. Hyg. 18: 997–1021, 1968.

Harwood RF, and James MT. *Entomology in Human and Animal Health*. New York: Macmillan Publishing Co., 1979.

Hedberg CW, Osterholm MT, MacDonald KL, et al. An interlaboratory study of antibody to *Borrelia burgdorferi*. J. Infect. Dis. 154: 1325–1327, 1987.

Hess AD, Hayes RO, and Tempelis CH. The use of the forage ratio technique in mosquito host preference studies. Mosq. News. 28:386–389, 1968.

Holmes EC, Bartley LM, and Garnett GP. The emergence of dengue: past, present, and future. *In: Emerging Infections*, Richard M. Krause, ed. Academic Press, San Diego, 1998.

Jasinskiene N, Coates CJ, Benedict MQ, et al. Stable transformation of the yellow fever mosquito, *Aedes aegypti*, with the Hermes element from the housefly. Proc. Natl. Acad. Sci. 95:3743–3747, 1998.

Kitron U, and Kazmierczak JJ. Spatial analysis of the distribution of Lyme disease in Wisconsin. Am. J. Epidemiol. 145:558–566, 1997.

Manson-Bahr PEC. Diagnosis. In: Peters W, Killick-Kendric R. (Ed.), *The Leishmaniases in Biology and Medicine*, vol. 2. *Clinical Aspects and Control*. Academic Press: New York, 709–729, 1987.

Marsden PD, Barreto AC, Cuba CC, et al. Improvements in routine xenodiagnosis with first instar *Dipetalogaster maximus* (Uhler 1894) (Triatominae). Am. J. Trop. Med. Hyg. 28:649–652, 1979.

Marshall RJ. A review of methods for the statistical analysis of spatial patterns of disease. J. R. Stat. Soc. v. A154, part 3, 1991.

McDade JE, and Newhouse VF. Natural history of *Rickettsia rickettsii*. Annu. Rev. Microbiol. 40:287–309, 1986.

McDonald G. The analysis of equilibrium in malaria. Trop. Dis. Bull. 49:813–828, 1952.

Milby MM, and Reisen WK.. Estimation of vectorial capacity: vector survivorship. *Bull. Soc. Vector Ecol.* 14:47–54, 1989.

Minodier P, Piarroux R, Garnier JM, Unal D, Perrimond H, and Dumon. Pediatric visceral leishmaniasis in southern France. Pediatr. Infect. Dis. J. 17:701–704, 1998.

Moore KA, Hedberg C, and Osterholm MT. Lyme disease. In: Evans A, Brachman PS, eds. *Bacterial Infections of Humans Epidemiology and Control*. Evans A, and Brachman PS eds,.New York: Plenum Publishing , 1998.

Morrison AC, Getis A, Santiago M, Rigau-Perez JG, and Reiter P. Exploratory space-time analysis of reported dengue cases during an outbreak in Florida, Puerto Rico, 1991–1992. Am. J. Trop. Med. Hyg. 58:287–298, 1998.

Morrison AC,Costero A, Edman JD, Clark GG, and Scott J. Increased fecundity of *Aedes ae-*gypti fed human blood before release in a mark-recapture study in Puerto Rico. Am. Mosq. Control Assoc. 15:98–104, 1999.

Mueller LD, and Rose MR. Evolutionary theory predicts late-life mortality plateaus. Proc. Natl. Acad. Sci. 93:15249–15253, 1996.

Naksathit AT, and Scott TW. Effect of female size on fecundity and survivorship of *Aedes aegypti* fed only human blood versus human blood plus sugar. J. Amer. Mosq. Control Assoc. 14:148–152, 1998.

Palma G, and Gutierrez Y. Laboratory diagnosis of Leishmania. Clin. Lab. Med. 11:909–922, 1991.

Pavolosky EN. The Natural Nidality of Transmissible Disease. Urbana, IL: University of Illinois Press, 1966.

Perfil'ev PP. *Fauna of USSR. Diptera*, vol. 3, no. 2. *Phlebotomidae (Sandflies)*. Academy of Sciences of the USSR. Zoological Institute, Moscow. New series No. 93. 1966. (Translated from Russian by Israel Program for Scientific Translations, Jerusalem, 1968).

Ribeiro JMC. Common problems of arthropod vectors of disease. In: Beatty BJ, Marquardt WC, eds. *The Biology of Disease Vectors*. Niwot: University Press of Colorado, 1996.

Richards FO Jr. Use of geographic information systems in control programs for onchocerciasis in Guatemala. Bull. Pan Am. Health Organ. 27:52–55, 1993.

Richards FO, Miri E, Meredith S, et al. Onchocerciasis. Bull. World Health Organ. 76 (Suppl)2:147–149, 1998.

Schofield CJ, and Dias JC. The Southern Cone Initiative against Chagas disease. Adv. Parasitol. 42:1–27, 1999.

Scott TW, Naksathit A, Day JF, Kittayapong P, and Edman JD. Fitness advantage for *Aedes aegypti* and the viruses it transmits when females feed only on human blood. Am. J. Trop. Med. Hyg. 52:235–239, 1997.

Service MW. *Mosquito Ecology: Field Sampling Techniques. 2nd ed.* London: Elsevier Applied Science, 1993.

Sherstha M, Grdzicki RL, and Steere AC. Diagnosing early Lyme disease. Am. J. Med. 78: 235–241, 1985.

Smith CEG. The significance of mosquito longevity and blood−feeding behaviour in the dynamics of arbovirus infections. Med. Biol. 53: 288–294, 1975.

Sorvillo FJ, and Nahlen B. Lyme disease. N. Engl. J. Med. 322:474–475 (letter), 1990.

Southwood TRE. Ecological Methods. 2n d> ed. London: Chapman and Hall1978.

Spielman A, Levine JF, and Wilson ML. Vectorial capacity of North American Ixodes ticks. Yale Biol. Med. 57:507–513, 1984.

Spielman A. Lyme disease and human babesiosis: evidence incriminating vector and reservoir hosts. In: Englund PT, Sher A, eds. *The Biology of Parasitism*. New York: Alan R. Liss, 1988.

Spielman A, and James AA. Transmission of vector-borne disease. In: Warren KS, Mahmoud AAF, eds. *Tropical and Geographical Medicine*. New York: McGraw-Hill, 1990.

Steere AC, Malwista SE, Newman JH, et al. Lyme arthritis: an epidemic of oligoarticular arthritis in children and adults in three Connecticut communities. Arthritis Rheum. 20:7–17, 1977.

Tempelis CH, and Lofy ML. A modified precipitin method for identification of mosquito blood-meals. Am. J. Trop. Med. Hyg. 12: 825–831, 1963.

Tempelis CH. Host-feeding patterns of mosquitoes: with a review of advances in analysis of blood meals by serology. J. Med. Entomol. 11:635–653, 1975.

Watts DM, Burke DS, Harrison BA, Whitemire R, and Nisalak A. Effect of temperature on the vector efficiency of *Aedes aegypti* for dengue 2 virus. Am. J. Trop. Med. Hyg. 36: 143–152, 1987.

Wood B, Washino R, Beck L, et al. Distinguishing high and low anopheline-producing rice fields using remote sensing and GIS technologies. Prev. Vet. Med. 11:277–288, 1991.

World Health Organization. World malaria situation in 1994. Part I. Population at risk. Wkly. Epidemiol. Rec. 72:269–274, 1997.

13

Sexual Transmission

JAMES C. THOMAS and SARA STRATTON

The number of pathogens known to be transmissible through sexual contact has increased dramatically in the last few decades as new methods of detection have emerged. A list of sexually transmissible pathogens is presented in Table 13–1. The pathogens and the sexually transmitted diseases (STDs) they cause are often grouped by organism taxonomy or symptoms. The organism types, as listed in Table 13–1, include viruses, bacteria, protozoa, and ectoparasites. Clinicians who diagnose STDs are more likely to think in terms of the presenting signs of infection, however. These include urethritis (e.g., chlamydia and gonorrhea); cervicitis and vaginal symptoms (e.g., chlamydia and trichomoniasis, respectively); and skin lesions (e.g., the chancres of syphilis, herpes, and chancroid).

STDs are very common infections. Among developed countries, the rates in the United States are among the highest. An estimated one in four Americans will be infected at one point in their lives (Donovan 1993). Rates of infection are higher in many developing countries in part because treatment for curable infections is less available.

Some of the most commonly studied bacterial STDs are chlamydia, gonorrhea, chancroid, and syphilis. Infections with these organisms are generally curable and acute, but reinfection can occur. Commonly studied viral STDs include hepatitis B and C; herpes simplex, types 1 and 2; human immunodeficiency virus (HIV) infection, which in later stages manifests as acquired immunodeficiency syndrome (AIDS); and genital warts (human papilloma virus). In general, infections with these organisms are incurable and chronic. Some characteristics of these seven STDs are summarized in Table 13–2. As noted in the table, several of the pathogens can also be transmitted nonsexually: "vertically" across the placenta to a fetus (HIV, *T. pallidum*); to a neonate during passage through the birth canal (*N. gonorrhoeae, Chlamydia trachomatis*); and postpartum through breastfeeding (HIV). In this chapter we address only sexual transmission.

Table 13–1   Sexually Transmissible Pathogens and Associated Disease Names

Organism	Disease Name
Viruses	
Cytomegalovirus	CMV infection
Epstein-Barr virus	EBV infection
Hepatitis viruses B, C, and D	Hepatitis
Herpes simplex virus, types 1 and 2	Herpes
Human immunodeficiency virus*	HIV infection and acquired immunodeficiency syndrome (AIDS)
Human papillomavirus*	Genital warts
Molluscum contagiosum virus	Molluscum contagiosum
Bacteria	
Calymmatobacterium granulomatis	Donovanosis; granuloma inguinale
Campylobacter	Campylobacteriosis
Chlamydia trachomatis	Chlamydia; lymphogranuloma venereum[†]
Haemophilus ducreyi	Chancroid
Gardnerella vaginalis	Bacterial vaginitis
Mobiluncus	Bacterial vaginitis
Mycoplasma genitalium	Nongonococcal urethritis
Mycoplasma hominis	Bacterial vaginitis
Neisseria gonorrhoeae	Gonorrhea
Salmonella	Salmonellosis
Shigella	Shigellosis
Streptococcus group B	Streptococcus infection
Treponema pallidum	Syphilis
Ureaplasma urealyticum	Nongonococcal urethritis
Protozoa	
Entamoeba histolytica	Amoebiasis
Giardia lamblia	Giardiasis
Trichomonas vaginalis	Trichomoniasis
Ectoparasites	
Phthirus pubis	Pubic lice
Sarcoptes scabiei	Scabies

*Multiple types.

[†]L serovars of *Chlamydia trachomatis*.

This chapter focuses on epidemiologic methods employed in observational studies of factors contributing to initial infection with an STD. We address research in both clinical and community settings. We do not cover natural history studies of disease progression (e.g., from early HIV infection to the development of AIDS) or treatment trials. Chapter 20 addresses research on HIV and AIDS in further depth. We begin with a description of several fundamental complexities of studying STDs, and then address in turn the measurement of infection, the measurement of sexual behavior, and particular concerns that arise within a variety of study designs.

Table 13–2. Characteristics of Seven Common Sexually Transmitted Diseases

Characteristics	Gonorrhea	Chlamydia	Chancroid	Syphilis	Herpes	Genital Warts	HIV/AIDS
Incubation period	2–10 days	1–3 weeks	2–10 days	2–6 weeks	2–10 days	1–3 months	1–3 months to seroconversion; 10–12 years to AIDS
Symptoms							
Males	Urethral discharge	Urethral discharge; dysuria	Painful chancre	Painless chancre	Chancre, tender, nonindurated	Warts	Initially mononucleosis-like symptoms; lymphadenopathy; opportunistic infections
Females	Endocervical discharge	Endocervical discharge; dysuria	Painful chancre	Painless chancre	Chancre, tender, nonindurated	Warts	Initially mononucleosis-like symptoms; lymphadenopathy; opportunistic infections
Duration	Hours (treated) Months (untreated)	Hours (treated) Months (untreated)	Days (treated) 1 mo–yrs (untreated)	Days (treated) Indefinite (untreated)	Chronic	Chronic	Chronic; length of survival depends on treatment
Sequelae	Disseminated infection; pelvic inflammatory disease; infertility	Salpingitis; ectopic pregnancy; infertility	None significant	Many: tertiary syphilis	Aseptic meningitis; cervical cancer?	Cervical Cancer, penile cancer?	Opportunistic infections
Perinatal transmission	Conjunctivitis	Conjunctivitis; pneumonitis	None known	Congenital syphilis	Meningitis; prematurity; spontaneous abortion	Warts	Opportunistic infections
Treatment	Ceftriaxone; quinalone; spectinomycin; doxycycline	Doxycycline	Erythromycin; ceftriaxone	Penicillin; doxycycline	Antiviral* (to reduce symptoms)	None effective; cryotherapy (cosmetic)	Antiviral† (prolongs survival)

*Acyclovir, famciclovir, and valacyclovir.

†More than 12 agents currently available.

FUNDAMENTAL COMPLEXITIES IN STUDYING STDS

There are several difficulties inherent to epidemiologic research on STDs. They can be grouped roughly into factors that are based on the biology of the organisms, human biology and psychology, and the environment in which the organism and host both exist.

Biology of the Organisms

Organisms that in general are transmitted predominantly by sexual contact do not survive well outside the human host and require intimate contact for transmission to occur. Infections that become systemic, such as syphilis, hepatitis B and C, and HIV, can also be transmitted nonsexually through exchanges of blood or blood products. However, most STDs do not become systemic and their transmission is limited to sexual contact. Also, humans are generally the only animals for which these infections are pathogenic. The fragility of these organisms and the lack of simple animal models make them difficult to study outside of the human host. For these reasons much of the pathogenesis of STDs remains a mystery.

Many STDs are difficult to detect because often they produce no overt symptoms, especially in women. While men are usually infected in the urethra and external surface of the penis and genitalia, women are most often infected in the cervix and inner walls of the vagina. Infections of women in these sites are hidden from view and may result in less pain than would occur with infection of the urethra. Thus infections are asymptomatic more often among women than among men. Asymptomatic infection is important for epidemiologic studies, but it is also an important factor in transmission, since in the absence of symptoms there are no cues to the infected person to avoid sexual contact and transmission can still occur.

Human Biology and Psychology

Aspects of human biology and psychology strongly influence factors of exposure to STDs. Some of these are involuntary, while others involve an element of volition. Many reproductive behaviors are based on human instincts that are to some degree hormonally stimulated. In conjunction with other factors determining human need, they rank among those that the psychologist, Abraham Maslow stated to be the most basic: physiologic need, and the need for love and belonging. Such drives often function independently of reason and can confound some reasoned searches for means to decrease exposures. Even conscious decisions to engage in sex are often made with the knowledge that the other person may be infected. Such decisions may involve taking a calculated risk in which the immediate benefits are perceived to outweigh the likelihood of eventual adverse consequences.

Environment

Factors of one's environment, such as early family life, have a profound influence on subconscious motivations for sex as an adult. For example, people who were sexually abused as children have been found to have a greater number of sexual partners than those who were not abused (Luster 1997) and female prostitutes have been found to be more likely than other women to have been abused as children (Widom 1996). Human culture is another element of the environment that influences sexual behavior. One's beliefs about the age to begin having sex, the desired duration and quality of relationships, and behaviors associated with sex are all influenced by the attitudes and practices of one's peers as well as images portrayed in the media. Essentially all human cultures have deemed a wide variety of sexual behaviors to be taboo, and in many cultures, discussion of any sexual activity is also avoided. Thus, sexual behaviors are performed in private and cannot be objectively observed. Therefore, researchers often have to rely on study participants to report their sexual behaviors; these reports can vary widely in quality.

Factors of the social environment that lead to or perpetuate poverty influence both the actual and observed occurrence of STDs. The unavailability or inaccessibility of health care for curable infections may result in infections of longer duration, increasing the opportunity for continued transmission and thereby contributing to a higher incidence. The observed patterns of infection are influenced by the predominance of cases among low income people being diagnosed and reported in public health clinics. Private physicians often fail to report to the health department the STDs they diagnose even though reporting is legally mandated (Rothenberg 1980, Lansky 1992, Smucker 1995). Thus, the infections of wealthier people who can afford care by a private physician, and those of people who pay for private care with Medicaid, are underrepresented in aggregated STD data.

These characteristics of the infecting organisms, the host, and the environment present formidable challenges for epidemiologic researchers of STDs. In the following sections we discuss approaches to measurement of infection and sexual activity, study design, and data analysis that attempt to address these complex issues.

MEASUREMENT OF INFECTION

Current infection

Sexually transmitted diseases, particularly those that are commonly asymptomatic, are not reliably identified by a clinical examination alone. Diagnosis usually requires the aid of laboratory tests or microscopy. Estimates of the sensitivity and specificity of commonly used tests for seven STDs are presented in Table 13–3 (see the Appendix for the references and methods used to construct Table 13–3). Theoretically, the sensitivity and specificity of a diagnostic test are not affected by the prevalence of disease (only the predictive values are affected). However, the sensitivity and specificity for some STD diagnostic tests are commonly reported according to the prevalence of disease in a population. These measures can vary with the prevalence because they are affected by the stage of disease and the distribution of various stages may vary with disease prevalence (e.g., a larger proportion of infections may be more advanced when social conditions result in widespread infection).

All tests are dependent upon the appropriate selection of anatomic sites for specimen collection. Clinicians not suspecting anal intercourse or oral sex are unlikely to collect specimens from these sites and thus may miss some infections. However, collecting specimens indiscriminately from all sites is not cost-effective. The substantial marginal cost added by analyzing extra specimens on all patients may result in a negligible yield of additional infections identified. In screening for gonococcal infection, one group found 2% of women and 31% of men reporting homosexual activity were infected only in the anal canal (Hook 1990). Others infected in the anal canal were also infected in the urethra and cervix, sites from which specimens are usually first taken. Key to a cost-effective diagnostic protocol is an environment in which the patient trusts the clinician enough to accurately report behaviors such as receptive anal intercourse. Clinicians not trained in such questioning, or who are embarrassed by these questions, are likely to miss infections where this is the only infected site.

In some studies, laboratory tests for infection (e.g., urine tests for gonorrhea and chlamydia) are used as a means of verification of some sexual behaviors. A respondent's report of not having sex in the last month, or of consistent condom use, will be called into question by a prevalent gonorrhea infection. But the absence of infection says very little about the reliability of a respondent's reports of sexual behavior.

If an infection is diagnosed in a person who has been infected with the same organism before, there are some additional questions to resolve. The diagnosed infection may be a newly acquired infection following the cure of a prior infection. Alternatively, it may reflect an incomplete cure of the index infection. Ideally, the latter possibility is ruled out through a "test of cure," in which a person gets tested again for infection immediately following completion of the prescribed course of treatment, with a negative test confirming that the person was cured. However, many people do not return for a test of cure. In the absence of such a negative

Table 13–3 Sensitivity and Specificity of Selected Diagnostic Tests for Sexually Transmitted Infections

Organism	Test	Specimen Source	% Sensitivity	%Specificity	Reference Standard	Reference*
N. Gonorrhoeae	Culture[a]	Male urethra (symptomatic)	NA	NA	NA	NA
		Male urethra (asymptomatic)	NA	NA	NA	NA
		Endocervix	81–96	NA	Contact[p]	Caldwell et al. 1971
	Gram stain	Male urethra (symptomatic)	90–95	95–100	Culture	Hook and Handsfield 1990
		Male urethra (asymptomatic)	50–70	95–100	Culture	Hook and Handsfield 1990
		Endocervix	50–70	95–100	Culture	Hook and Handsfield 1990
	Pace2[b]	Male urethra	92–100	96–99[o]	Culture	Koumans et al. 1998
		Endocervix	85–100	94–100[n]	Culture	Koumans et al. 1998
	LCR[c]	Male urethra	98–100	98–99[n]	Culture	Koumans et al. 1998
		Endocervix	91–100	97–98[n]	Culture	Koumans et al. 1998
		Urine (women)	94–100	98–99[n]	Culture	Koumans et al. 1998
		Urine (men)	98–100	100[o]	DA	Koumans et al. 1998
	PCR[d]	Urethral and cervical swabs	100	89	Culture	Ho et al. 1992
C. trachomatis	Culture	Urethra (men)	61–83[o]	100[o]	DA	Shafer et al. 1993; Chomvarin et al. 1997
		Endocervix	70–96	100	Culture	Chomvarin et al. 1997; Barnes 1989
	DFA[e]	Urethra (men)	49–100	72–99	Culture	Barnes 1989; Stamm and Mardh 1990
		Endocervix	56–100	89–99	Culture	Barnes 1989; Stamm and Mardh 1990
	EIA[f]	Urethra (men)	67–92	90–100	Culture	Barnes 1989; Stamm and Mardh 1990
		Endocervix	78–100	86–98	Culture	Barnes 1989; Stamm and Mardh 1990
	Pace[b]	Urethra (men)	92	100	DA	Chomvarin et al. 1997
		Endocervix	78–96	100	DA	Pasternack et al. 1996; Chomvarin et al. 1997
	LCR[c]	Urethra (men)	100[o]	100[o]	DA	Pasternack et al. 1998
		Urine (men)	94[o]	100[o]	DA	Puolakkainen et al. 1998
		Endocervix	82[o]	100[o]	DA	Puolakkaine n et al. 1998
		Urine (women)	93[o]	100[o]	DA	Puolakkaine n et al. 1998

Organism	Test	Specimen	Sensitivity (%)	Specificity (%)	Method	Reference
C. trachomatis (*continued*)	PCR[d]	Urethra (men)	51[o]	100[o]	DA	Quinn et al. 1996
		Urine (men)	88[o]	97[o]	DA	Quinn et al. 1996
		Endocervix	82–86[o]	99–100[o]	DA	Quinn et al. 1996; Pasternack et al. 1996
		Urine (women)	82–93[o]	98–100[o]	DA	Quinn et al. 1996; Pasternack et al. 1996
H. ducreyi	Culture	Genital lesion	60–80	100	DA	Jessamine and Ronald 1990; Orle et al. 1996
	Immunofluorescence	Genital lesion	89–93	50–63	Culture	Karim et al. 1989; Jessamine and Ronald 1990
	EIAfIgG	Serum	94–100	84	C&C[r]	Desjardinis et al. 1992
	EIAfIgM	Serum	92–74	64	C&C	Desjardinis et al. 1992
	PCR[d]	Genital lesion(men)	98–100[o]	86–100[o]	DA	Orle et al. 1996; Johnson et al. 1995
T. pallidum	Dark field microscopy	Serum	NA	NA	NA	NA
	VDRL[g]	Serum (primary)	74–87	96–99	NS	Larsen et al. 1995
		Serum (secondary)	100	96–99	NS	Larsen et al. 1995
		Serum (latent)	88–100	96–99	NS	Larsen et al. 1995
		Serum (late)	37–94	96–99	NS	Larsen et al. 1995
	RPR[h]	Serum (primary)	77–100	93–99	NS	Larsen et al. 1995
		Serum (secondary)	100	93–99	NS	Larsen et al. 1995
		Serum (latent)	95–100	93–99	NS	Larsen et al. 1995
		Serum (late)	73	93–99	NS	Larsen et al. 1995
	FTA-Abs[i]	Serum (primary)	70–100	94–100	NS	Larsen et al. 1995
		Serum (secondary)	100	94–100	NS	Larsen et al. 1995
		Serum (latent)	100	94–100	NS	Larsen et al. 1995
		Serum (late)	96	94–100	NS	Larsen et al. 1995
	MHA-TP[i]	Serum (primary)	69–90	98–100	NS	Larsen et al. 1995
		Serum (secondary)	100	98–100	NS	Larsen et al. 1995
		Serum (latent)	97–100	98–100	NS	Larsen et al. 1995
		Serum (late)	94	98–100	NS	Larsen et al. 1995
	PCR[d]	Serum	91	99	DA	Orle et al. 1996

(*continued*)

Table 13–3   Sensitivity and Specificity of Selected Diagnostic Tests for Sexually Transmitted Infections—Continued

Organism	Test	Specimen Source	% Sensitivity	%Specificity	Reference Standard	Reference*
HSV[k]	Culture	Ulcerative lesion of primary HSV	70–80	100	DA	Orle et al. 1996; Van Dyck et al. 1999
		Vesicles	90	100	NS	Van Dyck et al. 1999
		Ulcerative lesion from recurrent infection	50	100	NS	Van Dyck et al. 1999
		Crusted lesions	25	100	NS	Van Dyck et al. 1999
	Immunofluorescence	Genital lesion	84	NA	Culture	Pouletty 1987
	EIA[f]	Genital lesion	95	91	NS	Neurkar 1984
	PCR[d]	Genital lesion	100	100	DA	Orle et al. 1996
HPV[l]	PCR[d]	Cervical lesion	100	61	NS	Zazove et al. 1998
HIV[m]	EIA[f]	Serum	>99	90–100	NS	Van Dyck et al. 1999; Adimora et al. 1994
	Western blot	Serum	>99	>99	NS	Adimora et al. 1994
	PCR[d]	MNC[q]	10–100	40–100	Concordant pairs	Owens et al. 1996

*See Appendix to this chapter.

[a] Modified Thayer-Martin medium.   [b] Pace2 = Gen-Probe, nonamplified DNA probe test.   [c] LCR = Ligase chain reaction.   [d] PCR = Polymerase chain reaction.   [e] DFA = Direct fluorescent antibody.   [f] EIA = Enzyme immunoassay.   [g] VDRL = Venereal Disease Research laboratory test.   [h] RPR = Rapid plasma regain test.   [i] FTA-Abs = Fluorescent treponemal antibody absorption test.   [j] Microhaemagglutination assays for antibodies.   [k] HSV = Herpes simplex virus.   [l] HPV = Human papillomavirus.   [m] HIV = Human immunodeficiency virus.   [n] Estimates before discrepant analysis.s   [n] Estimates before discrepant analysis.   [o] Estimates after discrepant analysis.   [p] Reference standard: Sexual contact history. Women who were the only sexual co ntact of man with culture confirmed gonorrhea infection within a period of time longer than the incubation period of the disease.   [q] A734 Peripheral blood mononuclear cells,   [r] C&C = Combination of clinical diagnosis and cuture.   NA = Not available.   DA = Discrepant analysis.   NS = Not specified.

confirmatory test, researchers commonly assume that an infection is new if it follows the prior treated infection by two weeks or more.

Viral infections, for the most part, are not curable and thus, by definition, cannot be reacquired (with the exception of "superinfection" with multiple strains of some organisms, such as HIV). However, they can alternate through periods of overt clinical symptoms and latency. Most people with HSV develop recurrent symptoms but over time recurrences tend to decrease in severity and frequency. HIV infection is accompanied by symptoms early and late in the course of infection, typically with several years of latency in between. Syphilis is a bacterial infection with a complex natural history. When left untreated, it progresses through several stages, each with different symptoms, alternating with periods of latency. Distinguishing between the different stages requires a combination of serologic tests and clinical examinations. With many chronic infections, however, it is often difficult to determine when the initial infection occurred. The inability to determine when an infection occurred can seriously limit an investigator's ability to study risk factors for infection, which logically must precede the infection.

Populations of organisms such as gonorrhea and HPV consist of many different strains. In the case of HPV, strain typing is critical, since only a few strains are associated with the development of cervical cancer. Typing of gonococcal strains can also enhance one's understanding of the epidemiology of the organism. By determining the particular strain of each gonococcal infection in Durham County, North Carolina, investigators were able to reveal the pattern of spread of a newly identified antibiotic-resistant strain of gonococcus (Faruki 1985). Fox and colleagues used typing methods to demonstrate the absence of strain-specific immunity to gonorrhea among people repeatedly infected (Fox, 1999).

Past infection

In some cases, a researcher may want to know whether a person has experienced a prior STD. The recall of prior infections is generally unreliable (Kleyn 1993). The respondent will often not know or not accurately recall the name of any symptomatic infections, however, and of course cannot recall any infections that did not manifest in symptoms.

Because several STDs are reportable, more historical information is available on them than for nonreportable STDs. (STDs of public health importance that are reportable in the United States include syphilis, gonorrhea, chlamydia, chancroid, and AIDS.) However, as noted previously, private physicians typically have a low level of suspicion for STDs and a poor record for reporting diagnosed infections. Local health departments follow standards of record keeping set by the Centers for Disease Control and Prevention (CDC) or their respective state health department. Local records typically include the patient's complaint, clinical impressions, laboratory test results, and limited information on sexual behavior, such as number of sexual partners since they noticed symptoms. Less information is included in STD reports from private clinicians to health departments, and often even less in reports from the local health departments sent to the state office and CDC (these reports may be limited to a count of the number of infections occurring during some period of time).

Because of the sensitive nature of STDs, medical records including this information may be relatively inaccessible, particularly in private physicians' offices. Excluding patient identifiers from the data abstracted reduces the sensitivity of a researcher's data and, of course, records that already lack identifiers will be more accessible.

MEASUREMENT OF SEXUAL BEHAVIOR

Since it is known that STDs are transmitted through sex, what reasons are there to study sexual behaviors? One might wish to know whether a particular type of sex favors transmission more than another (e.g., anal versus vaginal intercourse), or whether behaviors accompanying sex affect transmission (e.g., the use of barrier contraceptives). To study variables such as these it is often important to also know about other parameters such as the frequency of sex and the genders of the respective people having sex. Moreover, when it is well established that transmission is likely to occur in certain circumstances (e.g., when a pathogen is present and a barrier is not), epidemiologic studies of factors associated with particular behaviors rather than with infection are often appropriate (e.g., factors associated with condom use).

Sexual behaviors that are commonly measured in studies of STDs include the number of sexual partners; variation in behaviors with different partner types (e.g., main versus casual partners); the degree to which partners are alike in terms of the number of partners they each have (referred to as concordance/discordance or assortive/dissortive mixing [Anderson 1991, Aral 1999]); whether a person with multiple partners during a particular period had sexual relationships that were concurrent or if one relationship ended before the other started (Morris 1997); the rate of changing partners; the frequency and types of sex; and barrier methods used during sex.

Because information on sexual behaviors is sensitive, researchers are rightly concerned about the quality of data on reports of sexual behaviors. In comparing the independent responses of couples, Padian (1990) found high consistency of reports of sexual practices among HIV discordant couples (e.g., the correlation (r) for the number of vaginal intercourse contacts was 0.84); Similarly, Seage and colleagues (1992) found a high level of agreement on sexual histories among homosexual couples. Reliability has also been assessed by asking the same person the same question, but at different times (typically at least several days apart). Rohan and associates (1994) observed a high degree of reliability of information on age at first coitus and lifetime number of sexual partners among women attending a clinic (intraclass correlation coefficients ≥ 0.94). Saltzman and coworkers (1987) interviewed

homosexual men at two times, an average of six weeks apart. They report kappa statistics for the degree of agreement. The respective kappa statistics for reports of income, diet habits, and number of sexual partners in the last six months were 0.87, 0.63, and 0.56, respectively. They suggest that the agreement for information on income was "almost perfect," and for the other two variables was "moderate."

The reliability of any question will depend a great deal on the context in which it is asked and the question wording. We provide next an overview of survey instrument types and the wording of questions. Further details on these and other methodologic issues related to gathering data on sexual behaviors can be found in Ostrow and Kessler's *Methodological Issues in AIDS Behavioral Research* (1993).

Instrument Type

Researchers commonly rely on participants to report their own sexual activity through a structured instrument that is either self-administered or conducted through a face-to-face interview. Because self-administered questionnaires do not involve an interviewer, they are less expensive to administer than face-to-face interviews, and enhance the privacy of responses under certain conditions. Computer-assisted self-interviewing (CASI) is more expensive than paper-based interviews, but it can use pictures instead of words or letters for responses or can present the questions through earphones or a speaker. The privacy afforded by self-administered questionnaires is thought by some to facilitate honest reporting of sensitive information (Catania 1986, Kissinger 1999). The underlying assumption is that higher reported frequencies of behaviors are more valid. Under some situations, however, respondents may exaggerate their behaviors or not understand the question. Thus greater frequency cannot always be equated with validity.

A self-administered questionnaire must use simple, clear language and avoid skip patterns (where a respondent is instructed to skip some questions and proceed to another portion of the questionnaire based on his or her answer to a particular question) unless a computer-guided system is being used to make skips automatically. The length must be carefully pretested to avoid respondent fatigue.

Studies requiring long, detailed accounts of behavior have typically relied on face-to-face interviews because of the decreased likelihood of respondent fatigue (Committee on AIDS Research and the Behavioral, Social, and Statistical Sciences 1990). With this format, interviewers can use visual aids (e.g., a calendar, sketches of behaviors), provide and interpret verbal and nonverbal cues, probe responses, and explain questions. Face-to-face interviews enable the interviewer to establish rapport with the respondent; many assume that the rapport enhances reporting and results in more valid responses. However, one cannot assume that validity is related to rapport; the presence of an interviewer and the rapport established may also make respondents more inclined to seek to please the interviewer by providing the responses the respondent thinks the interviewer is seeking (Catania 1990). Also, a poorly trained interviewer can introduce serious biases into the data. Another limitation of face-to-face interviewers is the expense of training interviewers and conducting the interviews.

Interviews conducted over the telephone combine some of the advantages of self-administered questionnaires and face-to-face interviews. One group of researchers found that, compared to face-to-face interviews, telephone interviews yielded more reliable information on sensitive behaviors (ASCF 1992). Yet telephone interviewing in a low income population where a significant number of potential respondents do not have a telephone can introduce a participation bias into the study.

Question Wording

The text edited by Davis and colleagues (1998) provides a compendium of sets of questions for a wide variety of sexuality-related topics. Three aspects of asking questions we address here are terminology, question timeframe, and means of aiding recall.

Careful thought must be given to the varieties of ways in which respondents will interpret basic terms such as "sex" and "partner." Some respondents may think sex does not include intercourse with a condom, oral sex, or anal intercourse. For some, a person with whom they have had a "one night stand" or other "casual" sex may not qualify as a true "partner." The term "prostitute" has lost some meaning with increased awareness of the many ways in which people can barter for sex. Even the more recent generic term "commercial sex worker" (which is unlikely to be understood in a questionnaire) does not encompass those who exchange sex for drugs or other favors. To elicit such information, it is often more effective to avoid labels and refer only to specific behaviors, such as accepting or giving money or other goods in return for sex.

Although study participants often may not be familiar with clinical terms, such as "intercourse," caution must be exercised in resorting to the use of slang terms. Slang terminology for sexual and drug-related behaviors vary from one group to another and are subject to frequent change. Some slang may also be seen as crass coming from an interviewer or written in a questionnaire and thus offend some respondents. It is imperative that question wordings be pretested among the target population.

The time period for which behaviors are recalled depends largely on the study question and organism of interest. If risk factors for infection are of interest, then a person diagnosed with AIDS will have to recall a period of time more distant than will a person recently diagnosed with gonorrhea, because of the different incubation periods of the two organisms. Apart from such considerations, questions commonly pertain to the respondent's lifetime, the last year, or the last few months (typically one or three months). Recall is better for shorter and more recent periods (Kauth 1991). For longer recall periods it is more likely that respondents must rely on estimates of behaviors. The accuracy of the estimate depends on the regularity of the event and the strategy used to arrive at a response. But this "guesstimation" may result in over- or underreporting of sexual behaviors. The frequency of behaviors of interest, however, declines with shorter time periods, thereby decreasing statistical power.

To help respondents recall events, some researchers have asked study participants to maintain a diary, or coital log, in which they record information daily or weekly. Coital logs have been found to elicit higher levels of reporting, possibly because they may be completed prospectively and thus facilitate memory, and they are completed in the privacy of one's home. Coital logs have been used successfully among populations with low literacy levels with the aid of pictograms and positive reinforcement for the participants (Zekeng 1993). Coital logs record data prospectively, however, and cannot be used when there is only one research encounter with the respondent (e.g., a cross-sectional study).

USES OF QUALITATIVE DATA

Structured instruments facilitate quantification of comparisons between individuals or groups, but they are limited in the types of information they can capture. To obtain the full range and depth of information needed to understand and prevent disease transmission, other research techniques must be brought to bear. The methods of anthropology have been shown to complement well those of epidemiology (Janes 1986). Anthropological techniques not only can expose deeply held beliefs but can provide an explanation of why events occur or beliefs are held. Allowing people to speak freely, rather than restricting their answers to strict categories, provides an insight into the insider's perspective as well as a cultural and historical context for understanding sexual behaviors (Committee on AIDS Research and the Behavioral, Social, and Statistical Sciences 1990, Thomas 1999, McDonald in press).

Qualitative methods often prove to be an invaluable complement to epidemiologic studies. Information obtained by these means can generate hypotheses for epidemiologic studies (Thomas 1999); provide insights to appropriate terminology to use in a questionnaire; provide guidance in the design of interventions (McDonald in press); and help in the interpretation of study results (Thomas 1999).

In general, anthropologists search for rich descriptions about phenomena by observing and participating in activities, interviewing key people, taking life histories, conducting case studies, and examining existing documents (Steckler 1992). In research on STDs and illicit drug use these approaches have been modified somewhat to address concerns about the safety of the researcher and problems associated with observing illegal or very private behavior. Thus an STD researcher will more often be a listener and less often an observer or a participant, and may rely on intermediaries such as indigenous outreach workers for descriptions of behaviors and terminology (Committee on AIDS Research and the Behavioral, Social, and Statistical Sciences 1990).

Ethnographic interviews typically treat the respondent as a "collaborator" rather than as a "participant." To get the full benefit of ethnographic methods, the researcher needs to appreciate that the respondent has information and perceptions that the researcher does not even know to ask about. Thus within a given area of interest, the respondent is allowed to set the agenda of a conversation with the researcher. Topics thus arise and information surfaces that would not have if the researcher had guided the conversation. This procedure is referred to as unstructured data collection. In some situations, a researcher may approach a population with a narrow agenda. He or she may only wish to know, for example, men's attitudes and beliefs about women's roles in sexual relationships. In a semistructured ethnographic approach a researcher in this situation might interview a number of men and women of each race of interest, but guide discussions through a standard set of issues. This approach elicits some information on a specific topic that would not be obtainable through a standardized questionnaire.

The sampling goals for ethnographies differ from those of epidemiologic studies. The purpose of an ethnography is to learn about the range of activities or beliefs, rather than to determine measures of central tendency that can be generalized to a larger population. Thus the aim in selecting respondents for an ethnography is to find people who are observant, knowledgeable, reliable, and lucid, rather than those who are "representative" of some group. The number of people interviewed is related to the breadth and depth of information sought. One often looks to hear similar information from several respondents (termed "saturation") before determining that an adequate number of people have been interviewed.

Focus group discussions, with their origin in marketing rather than anthropology, are another form of data collection that is increasingly common in STD research. They typically consist of a facilitated discussion of about one hour in length between six to ten people. Through these discussions a researcher can hear the participants build on each other's ideas, challenge each other's comments, and at times reach a consensus. The composition of the group depends on the information sought. It is often of value to make the group homogeneous according to gender, race, age, and potentially other factors. In all cases, the facilitator must be well trained and highly skilled; a focus group is not simply a discussion.

STUDY DESIGN

Sampling and Enrollment

The types of people to be included in a study depend on the study question. The appropriate source of study participants may be a general population (e.g., a telephone survey or household interview); a particular group at high risk of infection (e.g., commercial sex workers); or people attending an STD clinic. In each case there are factors that affect whether a potential study participant actually participates in the study, each factor potentially introducing bias into the data. For example, one study found that nonparticipants were likely to be at lower risk of HIV infection than participants (Copas 1997).

Many studies are conducted in STD clinics, more because of the high probability of finding infected people than because a clinic population is appropriate for the study question. Where risk factors for infection are of interest in a clinical setting, these must be distinguished from factors that determined whether and why the person came to the clinic (i.e., care-seeking behaviors). Factors that determine if and where a person seeks care for an STD include a person's financial resources; the options for care in a particular community; the cultural sensitivity of the various sources of care (Schuster 1995); patterns of referral from other clinics in the community; practices of self-treatment among those who are infected (Irwin 1997); and partner notification practices (i.e., the effort expended to identify the sexual partners of an infected person and bring them into a clinic for treatment). The comparisons made in clinic-based samples will be confounded to the degree that any of these factors is associated with the probability of the outcome and risk factors under consideration. Researchers can explore for evidence of confounding if they collect data on the reasons a person attended the clinic, such as whether they experienced symptoms, were referred by someone else, or if they have attended other clinics in the past.

Individual-Level Measures of the Occurrence of the Outcome

Conventional epidemiologic study designs focus on the occurrence of some event in a previously susceptible individual and are based on the assumption that the occurrence of the outcome in one person has no bearing on whether any other person experiences the outcome (i.e., statistical independence). As explained in Chapter 5, however, infectious diseases violate this assumption, since each person's risk of infection is dependent in part upon the occurrence of infection among other people, or rather different levels of exposure. Thus, in an extreme example, a lower number of sexual contacts will appear as a risk for infection if all of the contacts among those with the low number of partners are infected, and none of the contacts of those with the high number of partners are infected. Differences in exposure between two groups represent a type of confounding.

In calculating prevalence or incidence the denominator should include only those who can experience the outcome of interest. While a person can be infected with an STD at any age, infection before puberty is uncommon and reflects circumstances that are different from those affecting transmission among adolescents and adults. Thus the inclusion of infants, for example, in the calculation of rates among adults results in an underestimate of the actual rate. The magnitude of inaccuracy will vary with the age distribution of a population. The sexually active population is estimated more accurately by excluding those under 10 years of age. An upper age range for sexual activity is harder to estimate (Marx 1989).

Measures other than prevalence and incidence that have been devised for studying the epidemiology of STDs include the probability of transmission, the infector number, and the force of infectivity. The probability of transmission is estimated in studies where exposure to infection is known. In STD research, studies of partners in which one is infected and the other is not are often used to obtain such estimates (see the section in this chapter on partner studies).

The infector number is the number of susceptible people to whom infection is transmitted from a given infected person during the infectious period of a single infection. This empirically measured value is analogous to the reproductive number (R_0) estimated in models and described in Chapter 4. The public health importance of a particular group of people in spreading infection can thus be highlighted by comparing their average infector number with that of other groups of people.

The force of infectivity relates to delays in treatment of people who are contacts of STD cases. The "contact treatment delay" is the number of days between the date of the last reported sexual encounter between a case and a contact and the date of treatment of the contact. The sum of the contact treatment delays for all of the contacts of a case is referred to as the "force of infectivity" for that case (Rothenberg 1988). As with the infector number, the public health importance of a particular group of people can be shown by comparing their force of infectivity with that of other groups. However, calculation of this measure depends on the ability to identify contacts and measure their time to treatment. The interplay between illicit drugs and sex, for example, has made the identification of contacts difficult (Andrus 1990).

Population-Level Measures

Studies of population-level factors consist of comparisons of groups of people, such as counties or states, not of individuals. In such studies, aggregate measures of infection among people in the group are the outcome of interest. Examples for rates of syphilis and gonorrhea in counties include the 10-year average rate of infection (Kilmarx 1997), overall decline or increase over a 10-year period (Gaffield 1999), and year-to-year fluctuations (Cook 1999).

Population measures of infection are typically based on reported diseases, thus they are often limited to studies of reportable diseases. Disease reporting reflects practices in disease detection as well as reporting detected infections. Disease detection is a function of the presence of symptoms, care-seeking behaviors, and physician practices (e.g., treatment without a laboratory confirmation of infection). The reporting of detected infections is usually most thorough when handled by someone other than the diagnosing physician, such as clinic office staff and laboratory technicians (Smucker 1995). Thus reporting of an infection such as syphilis is relatively thorough because clinicians seldom treat it without a laboratory test and laboratories are required to report any positive tests.

The thoroughness of reporting, and thus the potential for misclassification, varies by disease and geographic reporting area. Smucker and colleagues (1995) found reporting for syphilis to be nearly complete in one rural North Carolina county, followed in thoroughness by gonorrhea and then chlamydia. Gaffield and Thomas (1999) found that adjustment for potential underreporting of gonorrhea in urban counties and counties that did not have a health department did not markedly affect the associations identified between county gonorrhea rates and county characteristics.

Reports of HIV infection are notoriously poor, in large part because the infection is asymptomatic for long periods of time and some of those who suspect they are infected do not get tested because they do not want to know they are infected, or they do not want others to know. Thus rates of HIV infection based on passive surveillance do not lend themselves well to comparisons of populations defined by geographic or political boundaries. Reporting of AIDS is marginally better, but because of the long incubation period between HIV infection and AIDS, it is difficult to draw implications about population-level factors affecting initial infection from AIDS trends. Even if one accounts for the incubation period by using data on independent variables that reflect a period 10 years before the AIDS data, this analysis does not account for the immigration and emigration of people with HIV and AIDS that has occurred during the incubation period (Rumley 1991). Moreover, the official definition of AIDS has changed on a couple of occasions, a factor that has independently affected reported rates (Selik 1990).

Studies of population-level factors yield information that inform population-level interventions (see Chapter 16). It is inappropriate (i.e., the "ecological fallacy") to use population-level data to make inferences about the risks to individuals or to inform individual-level interventions. Some studies gain extra analytic leverage by combining population- and individual-level data (Grady 1993, Guttmacher 1997).

Cross-Sectional Studies

The term "cross-sectional" usually implies collecting data from people at only one point in time. In contrast to follow-up studies where new infection is identified in a person who was first determined not to be infected with the organism of interest (i.e., infection incidence), in cross-sectional studies a researcher can often only establish

whether someone is currently infected (i.e., infection prevalence). The ability to estimate when an infection began varies by organism. Some bacterial infections have a short incubation period and are brief in duration. Thus when infection with one of these organisms is detected, the infection probably began within the previous few days or weeks and thus more closely resembles an incident infection. But this level of certainty is not possible with many viral infections. This distinction is important in the identification of factors that facilitated infection. For example, for an infection detected one year after it began, behaviors during the three months prior to detection (ascertained through a questionnaire) may not reflect those prior to the infection. This misclassification of exposure will obscure the true risk factors.

When not followed by additional measurements at a later date, the identity of the study participant is not needed for the purpose of linking information with follow-up data. Thus any interview or questionnaire can be conducted anonymously (i.e., without a means of linking data with a particular person) rather than confidentially (i.e., having identifying information on the respondent but not disclosing it to others). A respondent's sense of anonymity can result in more candid responses to some sensitive questions. Reinfection with bacterial STDs is common, however, and data may have to be collected confidentially to avoid including individuals more than once in a sample when collecting data over an extended period of time. In one study an estimated 4 out of 10 patients with gonorrhea or chlamydia experienced another gonococcal or chlamydia infection within 16 months of their index infection (Thomas 2000).

Cohort Studies

In follow-up or longitudinal studies, people are assessed for infection at one or more times following initial enrollment. If study participants are to be contacted and/or identified again at a later date, they cannot be studied anonymously at the time of enrollment in the study. When participants are asked for their name or address they may report false information in the desire to remain anonymous. In addition, study participants may move during the study and be lost to follow up even if they remain in the same neighborhood if notice of their move is not obtained.

Identifying infection during a follow-up period is complicated by asymptomatic infections. Some people will present themselves for follow up simply by revisiting a clinic with a newly suspected infection (though some may take their new infection to a clinic other than where they enrolled in the study). But to detect the occurrence of asymptomatic infections clinical specimens must be collected from study participants who ordinarily would not be presenting themselves for these tests. Thus complete follow up for infection cannot be achieved with phone calls. In many situations follow up also is not feasible with household visits. We have observed that some clientele of one health department STD clinic move frequently or maintain residences in several locations simultaneously in the same community. Paying study participants to return to the clinic for a follow-up visit has met with mixed success (Thomas JC, unpublished data). But if not done frequently, even follow up of this type will fail to detect asymptomatic infections that resolve spontaneously and have no measurable immune response, as with gonorrhea.

When an infection is curable and does not confer lifelong immunity, and is thus repeatable, researchers must decide whether they wish to include repeat infections in their analysis. If the outcome of interest is the burden of disease in a population, repeat infections may be relevant. In such cases, the rate of infection (i.e., the number of infections divided by the population time at risk) is an appropriate measure. Where the study question pertains to the probability of infection in an individual, the outcome of interest is typically one or more infections; that is, the person is counted as a case after the first infection and subsequent infections are not counted. Here the measure is a proportion rather than a rate.

Ratios of two incidences are used to identify factors that increase the risk or rate of infection. But in some situations the data accompanying the disease occurrence are only superficial, as with infections reported to the health department. Associations with infection are often limited to routinely collected data, and race or ethnicity is one of the factors most commonly identified. But other factors associated with race, such as behaviors and access to health care, are more directly responsible for disease transmission. These factors are thus the "real" risk factors, while their association with race makes race only a marker for their occurrence. Thus race and other factors acting similarly should not be presented as risk factors (Osborne 1992). The predictive value of race as a marker will vary between different groups within a given race.

Since aspects of the anatomy and physiology of women and men differ, as well as the social factors affecting them, the effects of various factors on infection should often be expected to differ for the two genders. Therefore gender often needs to be treated as an effect modifier or interaction term, limiting analyses to same gender comparisons. Researchers will need to adjust sample size calculations to accommodate gender-specific analyses.

Case-Control Studies

In case-control studies a sample of noncases is selected for comparison with a group of cases. This presents the issue of which of the noncases to select for comparison. The most important factor determining appropriate control selection is the study question, or the comparison of interest. For example, in studying factors associated with infection with human papillomavirus (HPV), one can compare cases with those uninfected with any STD or with those infected with another STD. The former comparison can provide information about avoiding infection altogether, while the latter comparison highlights differences between infection with HPV versus other STDs.

The source of the cases is another factor that guides the selection of controls. Ideally, controls are people who, if they were to become a case, would have the same probability of being included in the study as the other cases. Therefore controls for cases identified in an STD clinic should represent those who would present to that clinic if they were infected, and should not represent all noncases in the community. However, even controls selected from those in the STD clinic who are not infected may not meet this criterion. People are usually in the clinic because they believe they are experiencing symptoms, they have been told they were exposed, or they suspect they were exposed. People who have been exposed but do not suspect it, and who would go to the STD clinic if they did suspect exposure, are underrepresented. If reasons for suspecting exposure and going to the clinic are associated with sexual behaviors, then noncases selected from the clients in the clinic are more likely to practice behaviors similar to the cases than are the noncases who are not in the clinic. This can be considered "overmatching" and it introduces biases into the data.

To more closely approximate the potential clientele of the STD clinic, one might select controls from sexually active individuals who came to the clinic for reasons other than a suspected STD, say for an immunization or prenatal checkup. For some STDs, these people would need to agree to a genital exam. Alternatively, controls could be selected from those not in the clinic. They might be selected from the list of people who have an active patient file in the clinic, or from among the neighbors of a case. If the absence of infection is to be determined clinically, they might need to come to the clinic for an exam. With neighborhood controls there may be some difficulty maintaining the confidentiality of the case and there is no assurance that, if infected, the neighbor would go to the same clinic the case went to.

Partner Studies

Different levels of exposure between comparison groups introduce bias into a conventional epidemiologic study. One way around this is to eliminate some of the unknowns about exposure by linking each susceptible person with one (and ideally only one) infected person. The probability that the susceptible person's contact (i.e., partner) is infected is thus one (1.0). Ideally, the number of times the partners have sexual contact with each other can be counted and the probability of transmission per contact can then be calculated (i.e., the inverse of the number of sexual encounters between the two partners between the time of infection of the index case and the time of infection of the partner). Partner studies have been used most for the study of HIV transmission (Padian 1987, 1991, Seidlin 1993).

The accuracy of the estimate of the probability of transmission depends on the accuracy of the dates of infection of the index cases, the dates of infection of susceptibles and the number of sexual contacts between the partners between the two dates. Factors modifying the transmission probability must also be monitored, such as the type of sex (vaginal, anal, or oral), use of contraceptives, and any sex the uninfected partner has with others. Separate analyses are performed according to the genders of the infected and uninfected partners.

Some partner studies have been retrospective in that some of the once susceptible partners were already infected at the time of data collection. The date of infection of the index case often may not be known unless infection occurred through a means that can be dated (e.g., blood transfusion). Likewise, the information available on the partner of the index case may be only the infection status at the time of data collection, and not the date of infection. There may even be some uncertainty about which of the two partners was infected first. More accurate data on the date of infection of the nonindex case may be obtained through prospective follow up of couples where one is known to be infected at the time of enrollment and the other known not to be infected (i.e., "discordant" couples). The precision of this date will depend on the frequency of tests for infection.

Network Studies

When all of the infected contacts of an index case are identified, and in turn their infected contacts are identified, and so on, a "network" of infected contacts is established. Thus network samples represent a "snowball" sampling technique in which each person studied leads to the next people sought for enrollment. The source population for the interconnected cases is not easily determined, however, thus a population-based denominator is seldom inferred. With high rates of partner change among some members of a network and with infections that are often asymptomatic, it becomes difficult to know who infected whom during a given sexual encounter, or even if transmission occurred during that particular encounter. This limits the usefulness of network samples for estimating the probability of transmission. The primary utility of the network studies is in understanding the spread of organisms in a community (Faruki 1985).

FUTURE DIRECTIONS

While advances have been made in the last few decades in the study of behaviors putting individuals at risk of infection, population-level factors affecting the patterns of disease in communities are relatively neglected. The units of analysis (both exposure and outcomes) for studies of these factors include counties, census tracts, and towns. To advance this area of research new measures of various characteristics of populations are needed. Some of these measures will emerge from studies of social capital (often in the literature on cardiovascular diseases) (Lochner 1999).

New and improved techniques of molecular typing of organisms are being developed at a rapid pace. With these techniques researchers can identify subepidemics within the overall rate of infection in a community and identify sexual networks. When combined with geocoding, these subepidemics can be analyzed geographically (Pierce 1999). These typing techniques will enable researchers to refine models of transmission and estimate transmissibility more specifically for individual strains of an organism.

As interventions to prevent STDs are developed, they will need to be systematically evaluated for their effectiveness in preventing disease, as well as their relative cost-effectiveness. Anticipated vaccines to prevent infections with agents such as HIV, HSV, and HPV are examples of interventions to be evaluated. These vaccines may not confer complete or lifelong immunity because of the variety of strains or the ability of a particular strain to change over time. To the degree the vaccine is not completely efficacious yet incurs a sense of safety, vaccination may be associated with a decrease in the use of barrier contraceptives and/or an increase in sexual partners, and thus an increased risk of transmission that contravenes against the protection afforded by the vaccine. Thus the development of vaccines will raise a great number of questions to be addressed with epidemiologic study methods.

The authors thank Olga Sarmiento, M.D., M.P.H., for assistance in the construction of Table 13–3.

REFERENCES

Anderson RM. The transmission dynamics of sexually transmitted diseases: the behavioral component. In: Wasserheit JN, Aral SO, Holmes KK, Hitchcock PJ, eds. Research Issues in Human Behavior and Sexually Transmitted Diseases in the AIDS Era. Washington, DC: American Society for Microbiology, 1991.

Andrus JK, Fleming DW, Harger DR, et al. Partner notification: can it control epidemic syphilis? Ann. Intern. Med. 112:539–543, 1990.

Aral SO, Hughes JP, Stoner B, et al. Sexual mixing patterns in the spread of gonococcal and chlamydial infections. Am. J. Public Health. 89:825–833, 1999.

ASCF Principal Investigators and their associates. Analysis of sexual behaviour in France (ASCF). A comparison between two modes of investigation: telephone survey and face-to-face survey. AIDS. 6:315–323, 1992.

Catania JA, McDermott L, and Pollack L. Questionnaire response bias and face-to-face interview sample bias in sexuality research. J. Sex. Res. 22:52–72, 1986.

Catania JA, Gibson DR, Chitwood DD, and Coates TJ. Methodological problems in AIDS behavioral research: influences on measurement error and participation bias in studies of sexual behavior. Psych. Bull. 108:339–362, 1990.

Committee on AIDS Research and the Behavioral, Social, and Statistical Sciences. Methodological issues in AIDS surveys. In: Miller HG, Turner CF, Moses LE, eds. AIDS: The Second Decade. Washington, DC: National Academy Press, 1990.

Cook RL, Royce RA, Thomas JC, and Hanusa BH. What's driving an epidemic? The spread of syphilis in rural North Carolina along an interstate highway. Am. J. Public Health. 89:369–373, 1999.

Copas AJ, Johnson AM, and Wadsworth J. Assessing participation bias in a sexual behaviour survey: implications for measuring HIV risk. AIDS. 11:783–790, 1997.

Davis CM, Yarber WL, Bauserman R, Schreer G, and Davis SL, eds. Handbook of Sexuality-Related Measures. Thousand Oaks, CA: Sage Publications, 1998.

Donovan P. Testing Positive: Sexually Transmitted Disease and the Public Health Response. Washington, DC: The Alan Guttmacher Institute, 1993.

Faruki H, Kohmescher RN, McKinney WP, and Sparling PF. A community-based outbreak of infection with penicillin-resistant Neisseria gonorrhoeae not producing penicillinase (chromosomally mediated resistance). N. Engl. J. Med. 313:607–611, 1985.

Fox KK, Thomas JC, Weiner DH, Davis DH, et al. Longitudinal evaluation of serovar-specific immunity to Neisseria gonorrhoeae. Am. J. Epidemiol. 149:353–358, 1999.

Gaffield ME, and Thomas JC. An ecologic analysis of gonorrhea endemicity in the south. International Society of Sexually Transmitted Disease Research, Denver, CO: October, 1999.

Grady WR, Klepinger DH, and Billy JO. The influence of community characteristics on the practice of effective contraception. Fam. Plann. Perspect. 25:4–11, 1993.

Guttmacher S, Lieberman L, Ward D, et al. Condom availability in New York City public high schools: relationships to condom use and sexual behavior. Am. J. Public Health. 87:1427–1433, 1997.

Hook EW, and Handsfield HH. Gonococcal infections in the adult. In: Holmes KK, Per-Anders M, Sparling PF, et al. eds. Sexually Transmitted Diseases. 2nd ed. New York: McGraw-Hill, 1990.

Irwin DE, Thomas JC, Spitters CE, et al. Self-treatment patterns among clients attending sexually transmitted disease (STD) clinics and the effect of self-treatment on STD symptom duration. Sex. Transm. Dis. 24:372–377, 1997.

Janes C, Stall R, and Gifford SM, eds. Anthropology and Epidemiology. Boston: D. Reidel Publishing Company, 1986.

Kauth AU, St. Lawrence JS, and Kelly JA. Reliability of retrospective assessments of sexual HIV risk behavior: a comparison of biweekly, three-month, and twelve-month self-reports. AIDS Educ. Prev. 3:207–214, 1991.

Kilmarx PH, Zaidi AA, Thomas JC, et al. Ecologic analysis of socio-demographic factors and the variation in syphilis rates among counties in the United States, 1984–93. Am. J. Public Health. 87:1937–1943, 1997.

Kissinger P, Rice J, Farley T, et al. Application of computer-assisted interviews to sexual behavior research. Am. J. Epidemiol. 149:950–954, 1999.

Kleyn J, Schwebke J, and Holmes KK. The validity of injecting drug users' self-reports about sexually transmitted diseases: a comparison of survey and serological data. Addiction. 88:673–680, 1993.

Lansky A, Thomas JC, and Earp JA. Visits to private physicians in urban North Carolina for sexually transmitted diseases. N.C. Med. J. 427–430, 1992.

Lochner K, Kawachi I, and Kennedy BP. Social capital: a guide to its measurement. Health Place. 5:259–270, 1999.

Luster T, and Small SA. Sexual abuse history and number of sex partners among female adolescents. Fam. Plann. Perspect. 29:204–211, 1997.

McDonald MA, Thomas JC, and Eng E. When is sex safe?: Insiders' views on sexually transmitted disease prevention and treatment. Health Educ. & Behav. (in press).

Marx R, and Aral SO. Gonorrhea rates: what denominator is most appropriate? Am. J. Public Health. 79:1057–1058, 1989.

Morris M, and Kretzschmar M. Concurrent partnerships and the spread of HIV. AIDS. 11:641–648, 1997.

Osborne NG, and Feit MD. The use of race in medical research. JAMA. 267:275–279, 1992.

Ostrow DG, and Kessler RC. Methodological Issues in AIDS Behavioral Research. New York: Plenum, 1993.

Padian N, Parquis L, Francis DP, et al. Male-to-female transmission of human immunodeficiency virus. JAMA. 258:788–790, 1987.

Padian NS. Sexual histories of heterosexual couples with one HIV-infected partner. Am. J. Public Health. 80:990–991, 1990.

Padian NS, Shiboski SC, and Jewell NP. Female-to-male transmission of human immunodeficiency virus. JAMA. 266:1664–1667, 1991.

Pierce RL, Thomas JC, Sparling PF, et al. An epidemiologic evaluation of the use of microbiologic tools for identifying gonorrhea infection networks. Int. J. STD AIDS. 10:316–323, 1999.

Rohan TE, McLaughlin JR, and Harnish DG. Repeatability of interview-derived information on sexual history: a study in women. Epidemiology. 5:360–363, 1994.

Rothenberg R, Bross DC, and Vernon TM. Reporting of gonorrhea by private physicians: a behavioral study. Am. J. Public Health. 70:983–986, 1980.

Rothenberg RB, and Potterat JJ. Temporal and social aspects of gonorrhea transmission: the force of infectivity. Sex. Transm. Dis. 15:88–92, 1988.

Rumley RL, Shappley NC, Waivers LE, and Esinhart JD. AIDS in rural eastern NC—patient migration: a rural AIDS burden. AIDS. 5:1373–1378, 1991.

Saltzman SP, Stoddard AM, McCusker J, Moon MW, and Mayer KH. Reliability of self-reported sexual behavior risk factors for HIV infection in homosexual men. Public Health Rep. 102:692–697, 1987.

Schuster J, Thomas JC, and Eng E. Bridging the culture gap in sexually transmitted disease clinics. NC Med. J. 56:256–269, 1995.

Seage GR, Mayer KH, Horsburgh R, Cai B, and Lamb GA. Corroboration of sexual histories among male homosexual couples. Am. J. Epidemiol. 135:79–84, 1992.

Seidlin M, Vogler M, Lee YS, and Dubin N. Heterosexual transmission of HIV in a cohort of couples in New York City. AIDS. 7:1247–1254, 1993.

Selik RM, Buehler JW, Karon JM, Chamberland ME, and Berkelman RL. Impact of the 1987 revision of the case definition of Acquired Immune Deficiency Syndrome in the United States. J. Acq. Immun. Defic. Syndromes. 3(1):73–82, 1990.

Smucker D, and Thomas JC. Evidence of thorough reporting of sexually transmitted diseases in a Southern rural county. Sex. Transm. Dis. 22:149–154, 1995.

Steckler A, McLeroy KR, Goodman RM, Bird ST, and McCormick L. Toward integrating qualitative and quantitative methods: an introduction. Health Educ. Q. 19(1):1–8, 1992 Spring.

Thomas JC, Clark M, Robinson J, et al. The social ecology of syphilis. Soc. Sci. Med. 48:1081–1094, 1999.

Thomas JC, and Thomas K. Things ain't what they ought to be: social forces underlying high rates of sexually transmitted diseases in a rural North Carolina county. Soc. Sci. Med. 49:1075–1084, 1999a.

Thomas JC, Weiner DH, Earp JA, and Schoenbach VJ. Frequent reinfection in a community with hyperendemic gonorrhea and chlamydia: appropriate clinical actions. Int. J. STD AIDS. 11:46–47, 2000.

Widom CS, and Kuhns JB. Childhood victimization and subsequent risk for promiscuity, prostitution, and teenage pregnancy: a prospective study. Am. J. Public Health. 86(11):1607–1612, 1996.

Zekeng L, Feldblum PJ, Oliver RM, and Kaptue L. Barrier contraceptive use and HIV infection among high-risk women in Cameroon. AIDS. 7:725–731, 1993.

APPENDIX

Table 13–3 shows the estimates of sensitivity and specificity for selected diagnostic tests for sexually transmitted diseases and the corresponding reference standards (also referred to as "gold standards") used to calculate these values. These estimates should be interpreted with some caution because of limitations of the reference standards and the adjustment methods (e.g., discrepant analysis) used to obtain the estimates.

Discrepant analysis was used in a number of the estimates to combine the results of two different tests, such as those of a new molecular technique and the conventional reference standard. In this procedure, if the results of the new test agree with those of the current gold standard, these two tests are considered equivalent. If the results of the two tests disagree, then the discordant results (i.e., false positives and false negatives, or only the false positives) are retested. This retesting, however, violates the assumption of independence that the new test and the reference should meet, and on average tends to overestimate the sensitivity and specificity (Hadgu 1997).

REFERENCES FOR TABLE 13–3

Adimora A, Hamilton H, Holmes K, and Sparling P. Sexually transmitted diseases: companion handbook. New York: McGraw-Hill, 1994.

Barnes CR. Laboratory diagnosis of human chlamydial infetions. Clin. Microbiol. Rev. 2:119–136, 1989.

Caldwell JG, Price EV, Pazin GJ, and Cornelius CE III. Sensitivity and reproducibility of Thayer Martin culture medium in diagnosing gonorrhea in women. Am. J. Obstet. Gynecol. 109:463–468, 1971.

Chomvarin C, Chantarsuk Y, Thongkrajai P, Waropastrkul N, and Tesana N. An assessment and evaluation of methods for diagnosis of chlamydial and gonococcal infections. Southeast Asian J. Trop. Med. Public Health. 28:791–800, 1997.

Desjardins M, Thomspson CE, Filion LG, et al. Standardization of an enzyme immunoassay for human antibody to *Haemophilus ducreyi*. Clin. Microbiol 1992;30:2019–2024, 1992.

Hale YM, Melton ME, Lewis JS, and Willis DE. Evaluation of the PACE 2 *Neisseria gonorrhoeae* assay by three public health laboratories. J. Clin. Microbiol. 31(2):451–453, 1993.

Ho BSW, Feng WG, Wong BKC, and Egglestone SI. Polymerase chain reaction for the detection of *Neisseria gonorrhoeae* in clinical samples. J. Clin. Pathol. 45:439–442, 1992.

Hook EW, and Handsfield HH. Gonococcal infections in the adult. In: Holmes K, Mardh P, Sparling PF, Wiesner PJ, eds. Sexually Transmitted Diseases. New York: McGraw-Hill, 1990:149–165.

Jessamine PG, and Ronald AR. Chancroid and the role of genital ulcer disease in the spread of human retroviruses. Med. Clin. North Am. 74(6):1417–1431, 1990.

Johnson SR, Martin DH, Cammarata C, and Morse SA. Alterations in sample preparation increase sensitivity of PCR assay for diagnosis of chancroid. J. Clin. Microbiol. 33:1036–1038, 1995.

Karim QN, Finn GY, Easmon CSF, et al. Rapid detection of *Haemophilus ducreyi* in clinical and experimental infections using monoclonal antibody: a preliminary evaluation. Genitourin. Med. 65:361–365, 1989.

Koumans EH, Johnson RE, Knapp JS, and Sta Louis ME. Laboratory testing for *Neisseria gonorrhoeae* by recently introduced nonculture tests: a performance review with clinical and public health considerations. Clin. Infect. Dis. 27:1171–1180, 1998.

Larsen SA, Steiner BM, and Rudolph AH. Laboratory diagnosis and interpretation of tests for syphilis. Clin. Microbiol. Rev. 8:1–21, 1995.

Nerurkar LS, Namba M, Brashears G, et al. Rapid detection of herpes simplex virus in clinical specimens by use of a capture biotin-streptavidin enzyme-linked immunoabsorbent assay. J. Clin. Microbiol. 20:109–114, 1984.

Orle KA, Gates CA, Martin DH, Body BA, and Weiss JB. Simultaneous PCR detection of *Haemophilus ducreyi, Treponema pallidum*, and herpex simplex virus types I and 2 from genital ulcers. J. Clin. Microbiol. 34:49–54, 1996.

Owens DK, Holodniy M, Garber AM, et al. Polymerase chain reaction for the diagnosis of HIV infections in adults. A meta-analysis with recommendations for clincal practice and study design. Ann. Intern. Med. 124:803–815, 1996.

Pasternack R, Vuorinen P, Kuukankorpi A, Pitkajarvi T, and Miettnen A. Detection of *Chlamydia trachomatis* infections in women by amplicor PCR: comparison of diagnostic performance with urine and cervical specimens. J. Clin. Microbiol. 34:995–998, 1996.

Pouletty P, Chomel JJ, Thouvenot D, et al. Detection of herpes simplex virus in direct specimens by immunofluorescence assay using monoclonal antibody. J. Clin. Microbiol. 25:958–959, 1987.

Puolakkainen M, Hiltunen-Back E, Reunala T, et al. Comparison of performance of two commercially available tests, a PCR assay and a ligase chain reaction test, in detection of urogenital *Chlamydia trachomatis* infection. J. Clin. Microbiol. 36:1489–1493, 1998.

Quinn TC, Welsh L, Lentz A, et al. Diagnosis by AMPLICOR PCR of *Chlamydia trachomatis* infection in urine samples from women and men attending sexually transmitted disease clinics. J. Clin. Microbiol. 34:1401–1406, 1996.

Shafer MA, Schachter J, Moncada J,et al. Evaluation of urine -base screening strategies to detect *Chlamydia trachomatis* among sexually active asymptomatic young males. JAMA. 270:2065–2070, 1993.

Stamm W, and Mardh P. In: Holmes K, Mardh P, Sparling PF, Wiesner PJ, eds. Sexually Transmitted Diseases Second Edition. New York : McGraw-Hill, 1990:917–925.

Van Dyck E, Meheus AZ, Piot P, eds. Laboratory Diagnosis of Sexuallly Transmitted Diseases. World Health Organization, 1999.

Zazove P, Reed BD, Gregoire L, et al. Low false negative rate of PCR analysis for detecting human papillomavirus related cervical lesions. J. Clin. Microbiol. 36:2708–2713, 1998.

Part IV

OUTBREAK INVESTIGATION

AND EVALUATION RESEARCH

14

Investigation of Outbreaks

DAVID J. WEBER, L. BERNARDO MENAJOVSKY,
and RICHARD WENZEL

The historical foundations of infectious disease epidemiology are surveillance and outbreak investigations. Surveillance traces its heritage to William Farr, who in his 42 years (1838–1880) as statistician to the General Register Office in London developed and implemented such epidemiologic techniques as the standardized collection of morbidity and mortality data, the assessment of the determinants of the public health, and the application of these data to the prevention and control of disease (Susser 1975, Langmuir 1976). Modern outbreak investigative techniques date to John Snow, who investigated an outbreak of cholera in London in 1854, linked acquisition of cholera to use of water from the Broad Street pump, and terminated the epidemic by removing the pump handle (Winkelstein 1995, Brody 1999).

UTILITY OF OUTBREAK INVESTIGATIONS

Outbreak investigations have played a critical role in understanding and controlling infectious diseases in at least the five following ways. First, outbreak investigations have the immediate goal of discerning the cause of an outbreak, eliminating the source of infection or interrupting transmission, and providing postexposure prophylaxis to exposed persons. Postexposure prophylaxis is available for many communicable diseases including hepatitis A, hepatitis B, meningococcal infections, measles, pertussis, rabies, and varicella (Lutwick 1996, Peter 1997, Chin 2000).

Second, outbreak investigations continue to uncover new infectious agents and diseases (Butler 1996). In recent years, outbreak investigations have led to the discovery of *Legionella* spp. (McDade 1977) and the description of legionnellosis (Fraser 1977), *Sin nombre* virus (Nichol 1993) and its disease Hanta-virus pulmonary syndrome (Durchin 1994), toxic shock syndrome due to toxogenic strains of *Staphylococcus aureus* (Todd 1978) and its association with tampon use (Davis 1980, Shands 1980), and Ebola virus and its disease viral hemorrhagic fever (WHO 1978a,b).

Third, spread of a known virus to a new geographic area may be uncovered such as the recent description of West Nile-like viral encephalitis in New York (CDC 1999). Infectious agents may be the cause of outbreaks in new geographic areas via immigrants (Cote 1995), returning tourists (Narain 1985, Moore 1989), infected imported animals (CDC 1990a,b), or contaminated food (Herwaldt 1997, 1999). The West Nile-like viral encephalitis outbreak in New York (CDC 1999) and a recent outbreak of human psittacosis (Moroney 1998) were uncovered by investigations of disease clusters in animals. These outbreaks highlight the importance of veterinary epidemiology, since more than 200 diseases, known as zoonoses, can be transmitted from animals to man (Weber 1997, Weber 1999).

Fourth, outbreak investigations have improved our understanding of infectious disease epidemiology by uncovering new means of disease transmission. For example, although *E. coli* O157:H7 infections are most associated with eating undercooked hamburger meat (Slutsker 1998), outbreak investigations have documented transmission of *E. coli* O157:H7 via swimming in pools (Brewster 1994, Friedman 1999) and lakes (Keene 1994, Ackman 1997); ingestion of lettuce (Ackers 1998, Hilborn 1999), alfalfa sprouts (CDC 1997), municipal water (Dev 1991, Swerdlow 1992), and unpasteurized milk (Martin 1986), commercial apple juice (CDC 1996) and fresh pressed apple cider (Besser 1993); and person-to-person transmission (Spika 1986, Pavia 1990, Belongia 1993).

Finally, outbreak investigations have led to public health regulations and recommendations designed to prevent future disease outbreaks. Examples of public health recommendations based on outbreak investigations include thoroughly cooking ground hamburger to prevent *E. coli* O157:H7 infections (CDC 1993), recalling intrinsically contaminated medications (Matsaniotis 1984, CDC 1998, Wang 2000), recommending rubella immunity for women of childbearing age (especially pregnant women) traveling on cruise ships (CDC 1998), and placing hospitalized patients with active tuberculosis in specially engineered rooms (≥6 air-exchanges per hour, negative pressure, air exhausted directly to the outside) to prevent nosocomial transmission of tuberculosis (CDC 1994). Finally, outbreaks have aided in the assessment of public health guidelines. For example, measles outbreaks in highly immunized populations validated recommendations for a two-dose measles immunization strategy (CDC 1999). Outbreak investigations during the 1980s and 1990s documented the association of *Salmonella enteritidis* infection with the ingestion of raw or undercooked shell eggs (Angulo 1998) and led to introduction of control measures. Additional outbreak investigations have documented the success of these control measures and suggested additional control measures (CDC 2000).

In contrast to the above points, Rothman (1989) has argued that cluster studies yield little, if any, scientific information for the following reasons. First, individual clusters of disease are usually too small to constitute a useful epidemiologic study, with adequate control of confounding variables. Second, reported clusters often have vague definitions of disease, with cases that may be too heterogeneous for useful study. Third, the exposure or exposures that fall under investigation are also very often poorly chacterized, heterogeneous, and low in concentration. Finally, the cluster often generates a torrent of publicity, making the unbiased collection of data difficult or impossible, especially by interview or questionnaire. Rothman's view is supported by the low success rate in discovering the etiology of non-infectious disease clusters. For example, in 61 investigations of reported cancer clusters, only 16 confirmed that an excess of cases actually occurred (Schulte 1987). Rothman noted that of these 16 actual clusters little or no etiologic insight emerged. Similarly, the CDC noted that although investigations of disease "outbreaks" or "clusters" are common, true clusters (i.e., common etiology or cause) explain fewer than 5% of all clusters (CDC 1990). However, evaluation of infectious disease clusters is likely to be more successful. For example, between 1980 and 1990 the Centers for Disease Control and Prevention performed 125 on-site epidemiologic investigations of hospital outbreaks with none being reported as due to an unknown etiology (Jarvis 1991).

Although outbreak investigations are an important activity of local, state, and federal agencies responsible for public health, the number of total outbreak investigations conducted each year by public health authorities is unknown. However, it is clear that outbreak investigations are frequently performed by public health departments. For example, local and state public health departments investigated 2423 foodborne outbreaks involving 77,373 persons between 1988 and 1992 (Bean 1996), and 59 waterborne outbreaks involving 11,016 persons between 1995 and 1996 (Levy 1998). Nosocomial (i.e., hospital acquired) outbreaks were reported to occur with a frequency of 1 for every 10,000 to 12,000 discharges (Wenzel 1983, Haley 1985) with 3.7% of all patients developing a nosocomial infection being associated with an outbreak (Wenzel 1983).

DEFINITION OF AN OUTBREAK

An "epidemic" [from the Greek *epi* (upon) and, *demos* (people)] has been defined as the occurrence in a community or region of cases of an illness, specific health-related behavior, or other health-related events clearly in excess of the normal expectancy (Last 1995). The area (community or region) and the time frame in which the cases occur are precisely specified. An epidemic is thus relative to the usual frequency of the disease in the same area, among the specified population, at the same season of the year. A single case of a communicable disease long absent from a population (e.g., human rabies in the United States) or first invasion by a disease not previously recognized (e.g., West Nile-like virus in New York) may constitute an epidemic. Conversely, multiple cases of some communicable diseases (e.g., viral influenza) may represent only the endemic level.

Surveillance is critically important in outbreak evaluations both because it provides a measure of the endemic rate, which is a necessary component of the definition of an epi-

demic, and it may provide early warning that an epidemic is underway (see Capter 7). Although one can "eyeball" surveillance rates to detect an epidemic, more precise methods have been developed to aid in deciding whether the number of recently reported disease cases constitutes more than statistical fluctuation. Statistical process control (SPC) was developed in the first half of the twentieth century by Walter Shewart. Subsequently W. Edwards Demming promoted the use of statistical process control to guide management decisions in industry. In recent years, control charts have been adapted for use in health care to improve quality (Finison 1993), and are now being used by hospital epidemiologists to detect increases (i.e., epidemics) in the rate of nosocomial infections (Sellick 1993, Benneyan 1998a,b,c, Humble 1998). A control chart contains data points that graphically represent the performance of a process (e.g., infection rate in a population), measured against statistically determined limits (Finison 1993). As summarized by Benneyan (1998a), process data are collected at certain intervals over time and formed into rational time-ordered subgroups (such as by day or week). Some value of interest is calculated from each subgroup soon after being collected, plotted in chronologic sequence on the chart, and then evaluated for typical versus statistically irregular behavior. At least 25 subgroups are recommended to start a control chart. Along with these subgroup values, three horizontal lines are also calculated and plotted on the chart: the centerline, the upper control limit, and the lower control limit. Generally the centerline is set equal to the arithmetic mean and the control limits are set at plus and minus three standard deviations of the plotted values (Fig. 14–1). The control chart allows one to separate expected statistical variation ("common cause variation") from unexpected variation ("special cause variation"). When infection or disease rates are plotted by time, significantly elevated levels may represent an "epidemic." Rules have been developed to aid in assessing whether the variation is statistically significant enough to warrant in-

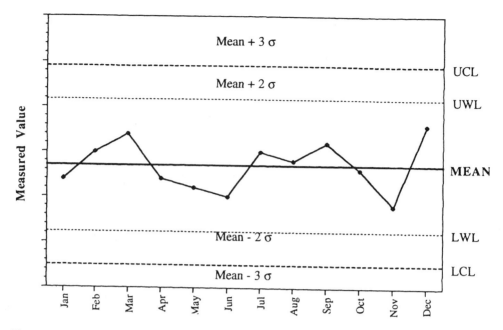

Figure 14–1. Sample statistical process chart, p chart, of surgical site infection rate. *Source*: Adapted from Sellick 1993.

vestigation (Sellick 1993, Benneyan 1998b). The selection of an appropriate control chart for any given situation, is based on identifying the type of process data to be investigated (Table 14–1). In brief, either an *np* or *p* control chart should be used when analyzing discrete data from binomial distributions, either a *c* or *u* chart should be used for categorical data generated by Poisson distributions, both an *X* or an *S* chart should be used together for normally distributed continuous data, and either a *g* or *h* chart should be used for categorical data generated by geometric distributions. The methods to construct control charts and further discussion of limitations are available in published reviews (Benneyan 1998a,b,c, Humble 1998).

Although most epidemics are time limited, they may be very prolonged (e.g., HIV). "Outbreaks" or "clusters" are often used synonymously with the term "epidemic" but probably should be defined as an unusual aggregation, real or perceived, of health events that are grouped together in a short time period and limited geographic area (CDC 1990). The Centers for Disease Control and Prevention (CDC) has summarized

the standard statistical and epidemiologic techniques for assessing excess risk that are often used to evaluate reported clusters (CDC 1990). Tabulating frequencies of the illness event, and examining related descriptive statistics is a useful first step in the evaluation. Mapping the data is also helpful. If the number of cases is sufficient and population data are available, examination of rates (ideally age-, race-, gender-adjusted) and standardized mortality and morbidity ratios may determine whether there is an excess number of events. If the number of events is too small to show meaningful rates, statistical approaches include chi-square tests of observed versus expected frequencies (based on the Poisson distribution for low frequency data) and Poisson regression (used for comparison of rates). Whether the rate for a geographic area or time period is excessive may be determined by comparing it with rates of other areas or times. If a spatial cluster is being assessed, the occurrence in the geographic area can be compared with that in adjacent areas, with other areas of similar size, or with that for a larger area (e.g., rate for a city with rate for the sur-

Table 14–1 Features of Different Types of Control Charts Based on the Type of Data to Be Analyzed

	Categorical (In SPC: "attributes")	Ordinal	Continuous (In SPC: "variables")
Also known as	Nominal, discrete, binary (0/1)	Ordinal category	Measurement, interval
Examples	Infection count	Number of intravenous catheters that result in infection	Timing of preoperative relative to surgical wound infections
Usually reported as	% in each category	% in each category	Mean, median
Usual statistical test of differences between groups	Chi-square	Chi-square for trend unless dichotomized	t tests
Control chart*	p if rate >0.01 u if $0.01 >$ rate ≥ 0.001 c if rate <0.001	Depends on scale, data distribution, and whether regrouped	X and S Median and range Individuals chart

*Most commonly used types; lists not exhaustive.

Source: Adapted from Humble 1998.

rounding county). If a temporal cluster is being assessed, the occurrence in the time period can be evaluated in the context of previous or subsequent periods. When such comparisons are being made, the referent population must be chosen carefully to ensure its appropriateness. If standard approaches cannot be used in an investigation of clusters because the number of cases is too small, data on the population at risk are unavailable, or space-time clustering is suspected, numerous statistical tests are available for use in detecting spatial, temporal, and space-time clustering (CDC 1990, Mantel 1967, Wartenberg 1993, Jacquez 1993, 1996a,b). Because a detailed epidemiologic investigation can be expensive and time consuming, the CDC recommends testing for clusters of cases using available data based on disease cluster statistics as an initial response (Fig. 14–2) (Jacquez 1996a). Only if a cluster is confirmed should additional resources be allocated to an in-depth investigation.

The issue of defining a cluster and detecting an outbreak have been discussed. It is obvious that failure to detect a cluster precludes an outbreak investigation. Equally important to stress is that overly sensitive definitions of clusters may lead to exhaustion of human and financial resources investigating "clusters" that only represent statistical variation of endemic rates.

METHODOLOGIC CHALLENGES IN OUTBREAK INVESTIGATIONS

Several methodologic issues may complicate outbreak investigations (Table 14–2). Outbreaks are unplanned events and as such must be studied retrospectively. Classically, retrospective cohort studies and case-control studies have been used to assess the risk factors for infection. Problems with the retrospective nature of these investigations include locating cases and controls, discerning the initial time of illness to construct an epidemic curve, obtaining appropriate clinical specimens, locating potential sources (e.g., food) prior to disposal, and recall bias among cases and controls when assessing risk factors.

Although outbreaks may involve thousands of people, many outbreaks are small, which may severely limit the power to assess risk factors. Unlike standard cohort or intervention trials where the sample size may be chosen by the investigator, the number of cases in an outbreak is beyond the control of the investigators. However, it is critical that cases be ascertained by active rather than passive surveillance (see Chapter 7). The precison of case-control studies can be improved by increasing the number of controls. However, since the additional precision achieved by increasing the number of controls rapidly diminishes, it is rarely use-

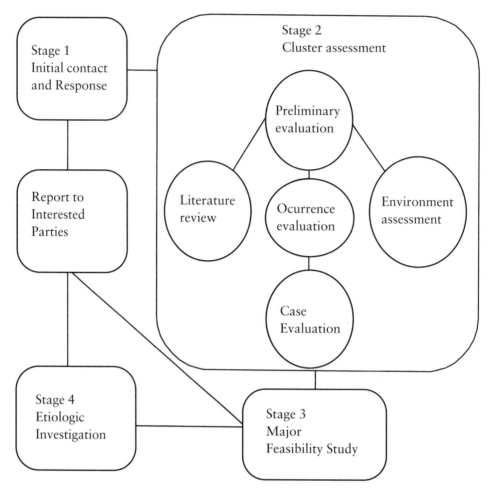

Figure 14–2. Flowchart of the multistep approach for investing disease clusters. *Source*: Adapted from Jacques 1996a.

ful to obtain more than two or three controls per case.

Many outbreaks occur in a limited locale (e.g., hospital, school) but some outbreaks may involve multiple states. Clusters involving large geographic areas may present problems with recognition of the outbreak and with evaluating cases. Failure to evaluate either all cases or a random selection of cases may lead to a failure to appreciate the magnitude of the outbreak, a biased assessment of risk factors, and failure to identify the source of the outbreak.

Point source outbreaks (outbreaks in which transmission occurs at a single point in time) may be caused by multiple pathogens acquired simultaneously (Keene 1994, CDC 1998, 1999, Feikin 1999). Multiple pathogens complicate the outbreak investigation, since the outbreak curve represents the superimposition of two curves reflecting the epidemiology of each pathogen (i.e., incubation period, duration of infectivity, infectiousness). In addition, the two pathogens may produce different symptoms, which may misdirect the investigators from obtaining the correct microbiologic studies to identify all causative agents.

In some outbreaks, the etiologic agent may be transmitted by more than one mode.

Table 14–2 Methodologic Issues Potentially Complicating Outbreak Investigations

Determining a cluster (outbreak) exists

Evaluation of risk factors must be retrospective

Small numbers of cases may limit statistical power to evaluate risk factors

Statistical analysis must take into account multiple comparisons

Cases may occur over a large geographic area

Cases may be scattered over an extended period of time

Novel pathogens may be responsible

Novel routes of transmission may be responsible

Novel sources or reservoirs may exist

The outbreak may be due to multiple pathogens

The etiologic agent may be transmitted by multiple routes

Disease may be limited to susceptible hosts

For example, a gastrointestinal pathogen could be spread to numerous people through contaminated food and then be transmitted to additional persons by person-to-person spread (Gordon 1990).

Finally, outbreaks may be caused by novel pathogens or represent infection due to novel mechanisms of transmission or sources. Outbreak investigations may be unable to isolate the causative pathogen. It is unclear to what extent these failures represent as yet undiscovered pathogens, inappropriate laboratory techniques, or late acquisition of specimen samples.

GOALS OF AN OUTBREAK INVESTIGATION

The primary goals of an outbreak investigation are to rapidly identify the source and reservoir of the outbreak, to implement interventions to control and eliminate the outbreak, and to develop policies to prevent future outbreaks.

The basic principles of outbreak investigations remain the same regardless of the epidemic or setting (Gregg 1996a, Wendt 1997, Checko 1996). First, although the investigative process is usually diagrammed as a linear process, the process is dynamic and multiple activities are conducted simultane-

ously. At every stage of the investigation, the investigators should constantly be refining their hypothesis, study design, and control measures. Second, it is critical to maintain communication between the investigators, public health officials, stakeholders, and often, the general public. Third, epidemiologic and statistical principles regarding study design and analysis must be appropriately applied (Philips 2000). Fourth, investigators must meticulously record all steps taken in the investigation and all information gathered. Fifth, a careful and critical review should be undertaken of the pertinent medical literature (Dash 2000). Such a review may suggest potential reservoirs and sources of the outbreak pathogens, modes of transmission, and control measures. Finally, investigators must maintain an open mind regarding the source of the outbreak as new pathogens and/or means of transmission may be uncovered.

The importance of maintaining an open but critical mind in determining the source of an outbreak must be stressed. Outbreaks due to natural biologic toxins, heavy metals, and chemical poisoning may mimic those due to infectious agents in regard to signs and symptoms of illness (e.g., gastroenteritis), epidemic curve, and means of transmission (e.g., contaminated food or water). Of outbreaks in the United States with a proven etiology, 14.3% with foodborne (1988–1992) and 31.8% with waterborne transmission (1995–1996) resulted from chemical agents including heavy metals, mushroom poisoning, ciguatoxin, scombotoxin, chlorine, liquid soap, sodium hydroxide, and nitrite (Bean 1996, Levy 1998). Outbreaks have resulted from unintended illegal activities or purposeful contamination (biologic terrorism). An outbreak of *Pseudomonas pickettii* sepsis among hospitalized patients apparently resulted when an employee replaced a narcotic with contaminated water (Maki 1991). The practice by growers of injecting water into watermelons to increase weight and sale price has led to outbreaks of shigellosis (Fredlund 1987). Failure to acknowledge participation in an illegal "floating" card game led to failure to ascertain persons exposed to a source case with tuberculosis (Bock 1998). Biologic terrorism has resulted in at least two outbreaks in the United States: a large community outbreak of salmonellosis resulted from the intentional contamination of restaurant salad bars (Torok 1997) and an outbreak of *Shigella dysenteriae* type 2 occurred among laboratory workers due to intentional food contamination (Kolavic 1997). Laboratory error (misdiagnosis) or contamination of a specimen may lead to so-called pseudoinfection or pseudooutbreaks. Finally, mass hysteria may simulate an infectious disease outbreak (Boss 1997).

Rare and exotic diseases may also be imported via travelers or immigrants (Roden 1968). In the United States a significant proportion of measles (CDC 1999) and tuberculosis (CDC 1998) occurs in immigrants. Infected travelers or immigrants have led to transmission in the United States of such tropical diseases as malaria (Zucker 1996).

PREPARING FOR A FIELD INVESTIGATION

An epidemiologic field investigation entails considerably more effort than simply following the recommended steps outlined in this section (Goodman 1996). In addition to the collection, tabulation, and analysis of data, many operational issues must be addressed. The initial preparation for a field investigation has been reviewed (CDC 1990, Goodman 1996). Goodman and colleagues (1996) have summarized the key issues to be considered; what resources (including personnel) will be available locally? what resources will be provided by the visiting team? who will direct the day-to-day investigation? who will provide overall supervision and ultimately be responsible for the investigation? how will the data be shared and who will be responsible for the analysis? and if a report of the findings will be written, who will write it, to whom will it go, and who will be the senior author of a scientific paper should one be written?

Most field investigations of presumed infectious diseases will require a team of people with skills in epidemiology, questionnaire design, interview techniques, biostatistics, data management, and microbiology. It is critical to have access to a microbiology laboratory skilled in handling large numbers of samples, isolation of fastidious pathogens from human and environmental sources, and ability to characterize pathogens using molecular techniques (Gregg 1996b). Prior to initiating an investigation, all personnel should be assembled and technical items (e.g., culture media) be obtained. Legal jurisdictions and local interests must be informed and respected.

Once on site, Goodman and colleagues (1996) suggest the following steps. First, review and update the status of the problem. Second, identify and review primary contacts. Third, identify the principal collaborator who can serve as the local contact. Fourth, identify local resources (e.g., office space, clerical support). Fifth, create a method and schedule for providing updates to local authorities. Finally, review sensitivities likely to be encountered during the investigation, including potential problems with institutions and individuals. Key to conducting a large investigation are recording all decisions, accuracy in recording data, maintaining communication internally with the investigative team and externally with stakeholders, simplifying the problem, storing all data in a retrievable form, and maintaining collaboration with local personnel.

Outbreaks often generate intense public interest and hence investigators must understand the factors that influence the various media in their selection and presentation of stories (e.g., the desire for a pictorial/visual component, the presence of conflict or controversy, the presence of strong emotive content, and the availability of targets to blame) (Greenberg 1990). Investigators should be prepared to stress key points; provide the background necessary for understanding the cause, evaluation, and control of the outbreak; and be straightforward regarding what is fact, what is speculation, and what is not known (CDC 1990). Most important, investigators must remain cooperative and responsive to the media. Investigators also need to be aware of the legal considerations in conducting field investigations including the legal basis for public health investigations, ethical and legal guidelines for research involving human subjects, privacy laws, and compulsory isolation and quarantine (Neslund 1996). Investigative reports are likely to be used in litigation (CDC 1990) and for that reason investigators should be aware of the basic concepts of tort law including negligence (breach of duty that caused or substantially contributed to harm or damage), breach of warranty (understanding that an action or situation is safe), strict liability (focuses on product rather than conduct), and failure to warn (Black 1990).

OUTBREAK INVESTIGATION

The components of an outbreak investigation are listed in Table 14–3. They are listed roughly in the order that they occur logically, but in reality there is no strict order.

Confirming the Diagnosis and Developing a Case Definition

Prior to launching a major investigation, the infectious disease epidemiologist should confirm that an outbreak exists. The first step in this process is to develop a case definition and identify persons who meet the case definition. A preliminary case definition can be based on the signs and symptoms of infection, the etiologic agent, or both (Wendt 1997). The definition should include the

period under investigation and the geographic area or population in which the problem occurred. If the agent presumed to be causing the outbreak is known, it can be included in the case definition. The case definitions used by the CDC for surveillance can be used as an aid in formulating an initial case definition (CDC 1997). As the investigation proceeds, the case definition may be refined to increase its specificity. Often "cases" are divided into subgroups based on the strength of etiologic diagnosis into "definite" (e.g., laboratory confirmed), "probable" (e.g., cases with objective signs and symptoms consistent with the case definition), and "possible" (e.g., cases with subjective signs and symptoms consistent with the case definition).

If an etiologic cause has been putatively identified, the investigators should review the basis for the microbiologic diagnosis. Laboratory error (misdiagnosis) can lead to pseudoepidemics. For example, more than 150 people received postexposure prophylaxis after contact with a bear cub initially diagnosed with rabies; subsequent analysis failed to confirm infection (CDC 1999). Pseudoinfection, defined as the presence of microorganisms by stain/culture of a body fluid/tissue that does not correlate clinically with signs or symptoms of infection characteristics of microorganisms, may also lead to outbreak investigations. Cunha (1999) in a review of nosocomial pseudoinfections and pseudooutbreaks listed more than 100 published reports. Epidemiologic causes of pseudooutbreaks include incorrect diagnosis of the clinical entity, failure to separate colonization from infection, increased surveillance efficiency, and chance clustering. Laboratory causes of pseudooutbreaks include contamination during specimen collection, transport, or processing (due to contaminated media, solutions, or equipment), and inadequate laboratory methods or techniques (McGowan 1996).

Ascertainment of Cases

Following development of a case definition, the investigators should rapidly move to active surveillance to ascertain any additional cases. In closed populations (e.g., hospitals,

Table 14–3 Steps in the Investigation of an Outbreak (multiple steps should be undertaken simultaneously)

Confirm the diagnosis	Contact cases and obtain the following information using a written protocol: demographics (age, gender, occupation), date of onset of illness, clinical symptoms and signs, potential risk factors for infection
Develop a case definition	
Document and organize findings at each step in the investigation	
Ascertain all cases via active surveillance: obtain information regarding person, place, and time	Formulate a hypothesis about the source and reservoir for infection and likely mode of transmission
Plot the epidemic curve and geographic area involved	Institute preliminary control measures
Demonstrate that an epidemic exists by showing the epidemic rate is higher than the baseline rate	Confirm the hypothesis by performing a case-control study or retrospective cohort study
Communicate with public health department	Document the source, reservoir, and mode of transmission microbiologically
Perform a literature review	
Notify all persons who need to be informed	Demonstrate the biologic plausibility of the suspected source and reservoir and mode of transmission; confirm using molecular epidemiology
Request that personnel save all isolates from patients and suspected sources or vehicles	
Assemble a team of investigators	Update control measures
Appoint a spokesperson to ensure that consistent information is disseminated; be prepared to answer questions and address the concerns of the community	Revise policies to preclude further outbreaks
	Document efficacy of control measures by continued surveillance
Record all actions taken by the team	Write a report and publish report of investigation and control measures

extended care facilities, day care centers, military) it may be possible to identify and interview all persons potentially exposed during the outbreak period. In more dynamic situations (e.g., restaurants) one may need to canvass local physicians, emergency rooms, and other sources to find additional cases. Prudent use of the communication media may aid in identifying additional people meeting the case definition. As cases are identified, investigators should collect general information including age, gender, underlying diseases, race, and means to contact the person. Relevant information regarding risk factors should also be collected. Failure to collect pertinent risk factor information will likely lead to an inability to determine the exact source of the outbreak.

In investigating cases, the investigator should characterize the person, place, and time of illness. Person includes age, gender, and underlying diseases. Place may include specific locations within a closed environment (e.g., school), sites of routine activities (e.g., restaurants, use of pools), and location where the person lives. Assessment of time

should include exact timing of symptoms, activities during potential exposure period, and date(s) of medical evaluations (if any).

Construction of an Epidemic Curve

An epidemic curve is a graph in which the cases of a disease that occurred during an epidemic period (outbreak) are plotted according to the time of onset of illness in the cases (Fig. 14–3). An epidemic curve often provides information on the probable time of exposure of the cases to the source(s) of infection; the probable incubation period; whether the outbreak was due to a common point source (e.g., contaminated food), propagated (i.e., person-to-person spread), or both; and whether the outbreak was time limited or ongoing. Checko (1996) provides an excellent discussion of the uses and attributes of an epidemic curve. An epidemic curve is a histogram. Cases are plotted on the Y-axis by date of onset of illness. The time intervals (X-axis) must be based on the incubation period or latency period of the disease and the time period over which cases are distributed. The time interval should be

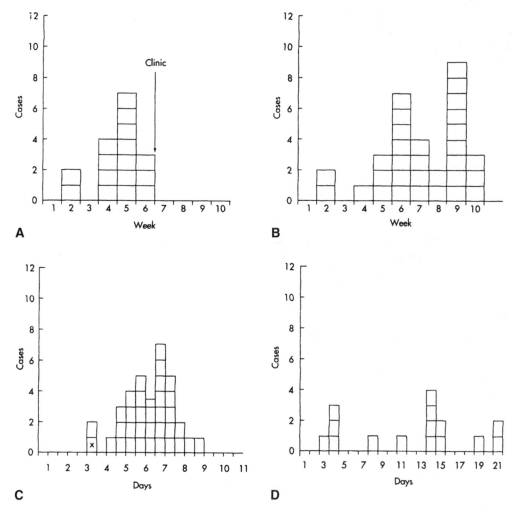

Figure 14–3. Epidemic curves; common versus propagated source outbreak. In practice, other information gathered in the course of investigation is also used to interpret epidemic curves. **A,** Propagated source: single exposure, no secondary cases (e.g., measles). **B,** Propagated source: secondary and tertiary cases (e.g., hepatitis A). **C,** Common source: point exposure (e.g., salmonellosis following a company picnic) (food handler = x). **D,** Common source: intermittent exposure (e.g., bacteremmia associated with contaminated blood product).
Source: Adapted from Checko 1996.

chosen based on the etiologic agent and the length of time the outbreak persists. For example, the time intervals for a short incubation disease such as *Staphylococcus aureus* food poisoning should be hours. The time intervals for a long incubation disease such as hepatitis B or tuberculosis should be days or weeks. Failure to use an appropriate time interval may obscure the temporal distribution.

An epidemic curve may be useful in distinguishing a common source from a propagated (continuing) outbreak. A common-

source outbreak is defined as an outbreak due to transmission from a single environmental or human source. Propagated infections are transmitted from person to person. Outbreaks may begin as a common-source outbreak that is followed by person-to-person spread. For example, an outbreak of viral gastroenteritis in an extended care facility was initiated by ingestion of contaminated shrimp (common source) and was followed by person-to-person spread of disease (propagated source) (Gordon 1990). This is

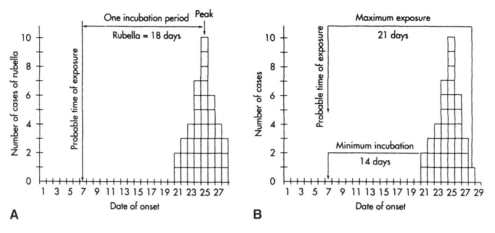

Figure 14–4. Determining the probable period of exposure in common-source outbreaks using mean or median incubation period (*A*) or minimum and maximum incubation period (*B*). *Source*: Adapted from Checko 1996.

most common with food- or waterborne outbreaks of gastrointestinal pathogens. An epidemic curve due to common-source outbreak approximates a normal distribution if there are a sufficient number of cases and if cases are limited to a short exposure with a maximum incubation of a few days or less (point source). Exposure may be continuous or intermittent; intermittent exposure to a common source produces a curve with irregularly spaced peaks. When an outbreak is due to a propagated source, cases occur over a longer time period than in outbreaks due to a common source. Person-to-person transmission may lead to multiple waves of infection (e.g., varicella); if secondary and tertiary cases occur, the intervals between peaks usually approximate the incubation period. As successive waves occur, the histogram usually demonstrates lower peaks due to exhaustion of susceptibles and each wave covers a longer time period owing to variation in the incubation period.

Formulating a Hypothesis

The goal of an outbreak investigation is not only to identify the causative agent (toxin, pathogen) but also to determine the source of the outbreak and to institute proper control methods. Knowledge of the causative agent or potentially likely agents allows one to formulate an initial hypothesis regarding

the source of the outbreak and means of disease acquisition.

A review of signs and symptoms of disease exhibited by the cases often allows one to narrow the spectrum of possible disease entities. For example, gastrointestinal symptoms (i.e., nausea, vomiting, diarrhea) suggest an ingested toxin or pathogen. Pulmonary symptoms (i.e., cough, radiographic evidence of pneumonia) suggest an inhaled toxin or pathogen. Evaluation of the epidemic curve may allow one to calculate the probable incubation period, which would further narrow the spectrum of potentially causative agents. Isolation of a pathogen from the cases allows development of an even more specific hypothesis regarding potential source of the outbreak.

Based on the actual agent or potential agent, one may develop the list of potential risk factors associated with infection. These risk factors should be formally assessed using an appropriate study. A detailed and comprehensive review of the literature should be undertaken prior to testing the hypothesis. Failure to assess all potential risk factors may lead to missing the crucial risk factor for the outbreak.

Assessment of Risk Factors

If the initial evaluation supports the existence of an outbreak a formal study to assess the risk factors for infection and to identify a tentative source is warranted. In a closed environment (e.g., hospital, school, day care center, military) a retrospective cohort study may be used. More common, a case-control study design is used because the population at risk cannot be unequivocally defined and/or fully enumerated. Case-control studies are especially suited to investigating outbreaks, because they are structured so that multiple etiologic hypotheses can be tested concurrently, they are unbiased by the absence of full enumeration at the time of interim analyses, and they are an efficient use of time and resources (Dwyer 1994). Examples of outbreak investigations using retrospective cohort studies and/or case-control studies are provided in Table 14–4.

Retrospective cohort studies compare attack rates among exposed and unexposed individuals in a cohort and usually measure their association by means of the risk ratio or relative risk (i.e., the attack rate in the exposed divided by the attack rate in the unexposed) (Dwyer 1994). When the outbreak involves only a small cohort, one should attempt to identify and interview all individuals. In large identifiable cohorts, it is often desirable to sample only a fraction of eligible individuals; however, the entire cohort must be identifiable in order to select a random sample. Enumeration of a known sampling fraction of cases and unaffected individuals must be achieved if accurate attack rates and relative risks are to be calculated as unbiased measures of association. Even if a retrospective cohort study can be conducted, it may be more efficient to avoid enumerating the whole cohort and use a case-control study to test hypotheses (Dwyer 1994). In poorly defined cohorts, use of case-control methods is essential to identify risk factors.

Case-control studies, unlike retrospective cohort studies, do not require enumeration of the whole cohort; rather, an unknown fraction of cases and unaffected persons (i.e., controls) are compared. However, it is assumed that the cases are representative of all cases and that the controls are representative of all persons capable of being a case

if they had become infected in order for the comparison to be an unbiased measure of association between disease and exposure. Case-control studies may be the most appropriate method of formal testing hypotheses in an outbreak investigation in three instances (Dwyer 1994). First, when the cohort could be fully enumerated but it is desirable to sample only a fraction of persons (e.g., very large outbreak). Second, where the population at risk cannot be adequately defined to determine a discrete cohort or cannot be fully enumerated. Finally, nested case-control studies that select a subset of cases and control may be used to test specific hypotheses. Nested case-control studies may include only persons who definitively meet the case definition.

The proper choice of controls is crucial to any successful case-control study. When an outbreak occurs in a closed population (e.g., hospital), controls are generally sampled from persons potentially exposed during the outbreak period but without disease. Depending on the suspected source of exposure, controls may also be selected by telephone survey, from friends of cases, or from the same neighborhood as cases. Multiple control groups may be obtained to reduce the risk of selection bias in the choice of controls. Multiple case-control studies using different controls may be conducted as the investigators refine their hypotheses (Maki 1991).

Regardless of the study design, it is important for investigators to attempt to minimize likely sources of bias. Selection bias may be an important problem, especially if cases are ascertained only through passive surveillance. Recall bias is especially likely if the outbreak investigation is conducted after a prolonged period of time. Decker (1986) and colleagues videotaped a potluck luncheon and collected food histories from participants 50 to 69 hours after the luncheon; less than 15% of the persons correctly identified all the food items they ingested. Misclassification of people as cases and controls may occur for a variety of reasons including failure to test all persons for asymptomatic infection; failure to obtain an etiologic diagnosis and thereby include cases with multiple

Table 14–4 Selected Outbreak Investigations

Reference	Setting	Cases	Pathogen(s)	Evaluation of Risk Factors	Source	Demonstration of Linkage
Kehrberg, 1981	State, UT	52	Staphylococcus aureus (toxin producing)	Case-control study	Tampon*	—
Seals, 1981	Denver, CO	7	Clostridium botulinum	Case-control study	Potatoes	Culture
Taylor, 1982	Multiple states, US	62	Salmonella muenchen	Case-control studies	Marijuana	Molecular analysis (plasmid analysis)
Langley, 1988	House, poker game, Canada	12	Coxiella burnetti	Case evaluation	Parturient cat	Culture, serology
Linnan, 1988	Community, CA	93	Listeria monocytogenes	Case-control study	Mexican cheese	Serotyping, phage typing
Gordon, 1990	Retirement facility, CA	183	Snow Mountain agent	Case-control study	Shrimp meals then person-to-person	Immune electron microscopy
Ostroff, 1990	Restaurant, WA	37	E. Coli O157:H7	Case–control study	Ground beef	Molecular analysis (plasmid profile)
Maki, 1991	Hospital, WI	9	Pseudomonas pickettii	Case-control studies	Tampered narcotic	Culture
Thomas, 1991	Jail, CA	21	Neisseria meningitidis	Case– control study	Person-to-person	Molecular analysis (isoenzyme typing)
Mahoney, 1992	Grocery store, LA	33	Legionella pneumophila	Case-control study	Mist machine	Monoclonal antibody subtyping
Edlin, 1992	Hospital, US	18	Multidrug resistant Mycobacterium tuberculosis	Case– control study	Person-to-person	Molecular analysis (RFLP)
Keller, 1996	Community, MA	11	Legionella pneumophila	Case-control study	Cooling towers	Molecular analysis (MAS, PCR, PFGE)
Beller, 1997	Fairbanks, AL	>20	Norwalk-like viruses	Case-control study	Contaminated well	Molecular analysis (PCR)
Kenyon, 1996	Airplane, US	6	Mycobacterium tuberculosis	Retrospective cohort	Person-to- person	Tuberculin skin test
Nuorti, 1998	Nursing home, OK	11	Streptococcus pneumoniae	Retrospective cohort study	Person-to- person	Molecular analysis (PFGE)
CDC, 1999	Restaurants, US	>200	Shigella sonnei	Retrospective cohort and case-control studies	Uncooked parsley	Molecular analysis (PFGE)
CDC, 1999	County fair, NY	15,921	E. Coli O157:H7, C. jejuni	Case control study	Well water	Molecular analysis (PCR)
Hutin, 1999	Schools, MI & ME	236	Hepatitis A	Case– control studies	Frozen strawberries	Molecular analysis (PCR)
Holmes, 1999	Hospital, MS	268	Burholderia cepacia	Retrospective cohort and case-control studies	Person-to-person	Molecular analysis (ribotype RFLP)
Hoffmann, 2000	Ambulatory surgery clinic, NC	5	Pseudomonas aeruginosa	Retrospective cohort study	Phacoemulsifer	Molecular analysis (PFGE)
Brennen, 2000	High School, MA	54	Bordetella pertussis	Retrospective cohort study	Person- to-person	Molecular analysis (PFGE)

*Infection from patient's own flora; tampons major risk factor.

Abbreviations: MAS = monoclonal antibody subtyping; PCR = polymerase chain reaction; PFGE = pulse-field gel electrophoresis; RFLP = restriction fragment length polymorphism.

pathogens causing a similar symptom complex (e.g., gastroenteritis); and failure to exclude endemic infection (i.e., infection nonoutbreak strain of pathogen) among cases by using appropriate molecular methods.

The odds ratio is a measure of association obtained in case-control studies. When the outcome is rare, the odds ratio approximates the relative risk in a population. Although, the disease being studied in an outbreak may be rare in the general population, during an outbreak the disease may not be rare in the cohort under study or among those exposed to the risk factor. Under these circumstances the odds ratio will not accurately estimate the increased risk (i.e., relative risk or risk ratio) related to exposure. Nevertheless, the odds ratio for the various suspected causes will allow the investigators to rank the potential causes and identify the ones exerting the most influence (Dwyer 1994).

Laboratory Investigation

Laboratory investigation is crucial to the successful evaluation of infectious disease outbreaks for three reasons (McGowan 1996). First, laboratory investigation of the cases is required to isolate or otherwise identify the specific toxin or pathogen. Second, laboratory investigation of the environment may be indicated when an environmental source is possible. Finally, molecular analysis of isolates from cases and, if available, from the environment may conclusively demonstrate the presence of an outbreak and linkage to an environmental source.

Every attempt should be made to isolate the causative pathogen from the cases. Isolation of a specific pathogen allows one to narrow the possible initiating sources for outbreak, and to link cases with molecular epidemiology. It also aids in planning control measures. Standard culture methods should be used in isolating pathogens (Murray 1999). All isolates should be saved for potential molecular analyses. Care must be taken to avoid contamination of specimens leading to pseudoepidemics. When cultures are obtained from nonsterile sites (e.g., skin) one must consider whether the isolated organisms represent colonization or infection. Appropriate safety precautions must be used when culturing microorganisms to minimize risks of infection to laboratory personnel (CDC 1999). Additional methods of determining the causative pathogen may be required in many circumstances, including circumstances where techniques to culture the pathogen do not exist (e.g., hepatitis C), culture is technically difficult or not available (e.g., arboviruses causing encephalitis), culture is not sufficiently sensitive (e.g., *Bordetella pertussis*), and where cases were ascertained after the infectious period. In these instances one most often relies on measurement of antibodies to the infectious agent. Generally acute infection may be demonstrated by either a diagnostic level of IgM or a fourfold increase of IgG (see Chapter 2).

Environmental cultures should be obtained only when epidemiologic or microbiologic evidence suggests an environmental source. Environmental cultures are often difficult to interpret, especially if the etiologic agent commonly contaminates the environment or if the affected patients contaminate the environment secondarily. Validated and sensitive methods for isolating pathogens from environmental sources (e.g., potable water, foods) may not exist.

Molecular typing of microorganisms has become a valuable epidemiologic tool (Maslow 1996, Pfaller 1997, Weber 1997, Tenover 1997). For example, molecular typing was used by the CDC in 79% of its investigations of nosocomial outbreaks in which a pathogen had been isolated between 1991 and 1994 (Jarvis 1994). Molecular methods (see Chapter 8) allow one to demonstrate that microorganisms are clonal, thereby demonstrating a common-source outbreak. Just as important, molecular analysis may demonstrate that although statistical clustering occurred, the isolated pathogens were not linked (Benaouddia 1997, CDC 1999). Molecular analysis may also link human cases to an environmental source (Table 14–4). While typing methods are useful tools they cannot replace good epidemiology and they have important limitations (Wendt 1997). For example, typing methods can determine only that two isolates give the same results to a specific test; they cannot establish causality or the direction of spread.

Control Measures

At every step of an outbreak investigation, the epidemiologists should be prepared to recommend preliminary control measures. Initial control measures often focus on interrupting transmission from the suspected reservoirs. However, care should be taken to preserve all suspect reservoirs until all needed laboratory specimens are obtained. For example, if specific food items are considered a possible source, cultures should be obtained prior to the destruction of the food item.

When multiple control measures are possible, the criteria for selection of the most appropriate one should be based on effectiveness for interrupting the epidemic, ease of implementation, expense, and safety. Engineering changes (e.g., disinfection of contaminated equipment, recall of contaminated food) are generally easier than interventions that require behavioral change (e.g., substituting pasteurized egg products in recipes that call for raw eggs).

Additional follow-up studies should be undertaken to assess the effectiveness of the control measures. Failure to reduce the incidence of illness may be attributed to inappropriate control measures; an etiologic agent with more than one reservoir or spread by more than one mode; and people who do not comply with recommendations made to eliminate the outbreak.

Preparing a Report

Careful and detailed notes should be maintained of all outbreak investigations. After instituting control measures and assessing their effectiveness, the team should write a report that describes the extent of the outbreak, results of the investigation, control measures that were implemented, and effectiveness of the measures (Wendt 1997). Appropriate public health institutions to inform include the state health department, Food and Drug Administration (for medications, foods, medical devices), and Centers for Disease Control and Prevention. The investigators should consider publishing their report, especially if the outbreak had unusual features. Published reports are extremely useful because they aid other public health epidemiologists in preventing or investigating similar outbreaks.

CONCLUSIONS

Outbreak investigations have proven to be a valuable tool in identifying and controlling infectious disease outbreaks. Knowledge and skills in a variety of disciplines are critical to designing and implementing a successful outbreak investigation.

REFERENCES

Ackers M, Mahon BE, Leahy E, et al. An outbreak of *Escherichia coli* O157:H7 infections associated with leaf lettuce consumption. J. Infect. Dis. 177:1588–1593, 1998.

Ackman D, Marks S, Mack P, et al. Swimming-associated haemorrhagic colitis due to *Escherichia coli* O157:H7 infection: evidence of prolonged contamination of a fresh water lake. Epidemiol. Infect. 119:1–8, 1997.

Angulo FJ, and Swerdlow DL. *Salmonella enteritidis* infections in the United States. JAMA. 213(12):1729–1731, 1998.

Bean NH, Goulding JS, and Lao C. Surveillance for foodborne-disease outbreaks—United States, 1988–1992. MMWR 45(SS–5):1–55, 1996.

Belongia EA, Osterholm MT, Soler JT, et al. Transmission of *Escherichia coli* O157:H7 infection in Minnesota child day-care facilities. JAMA. 269(7):883–888, 1993.

Benaoudia F, and Bingen E. Evidence for the genetic unrelatedness of nosocomial *Alcaligenes xylosoxidans* strains in a pediatric hospital. Infect. Control Hosp. Epidemiol. 18:132–134, 1997.

Benneyan JC. Statistical quality control methods in infection control and hospital epidemiology. Part I. Introduction and basic theory. Infect. Control Hosp. Epidemiol. 19(3):194–214, 1998a.

Benneyan JC. Statistical quality control methods in infection control and hospital epidemiology. Part II. Chart use, statistical properties, and research issues. Infect. Control Hosp. Epidemiol. 19(4):265–283, 1998b.

Benneyan JC. Use and interpretation of statistical quality control charts. Int. J. Qual. Health Care. 10(1):69–73, 1998c.

Besser RE, Lett SM, Weber JT, et al. An outbreak of diarrhea and hemolytic uremic syndrome from *Escherichia coli* O157:H7 in fresh-pressed apple cider. JAMA. 269(17):2217–2220, 1993.

Black B. Matching evidence about clustered health events with tort law requirements. Am. J. Epidemiol. 132:S79–S86, 1990.

Bock NN, Mallory JP, Mobley N, DeVoe B, and Taylor BB. Outbreak of tuberculosis associated with a floating card game in the rural south: lessons for tuberculosis contact investigations. Clin. Infect. Dis. 27:1221–1226, 1998.

Boss LP. 1997. Epidemic hysteria: a review of the published literature. Epidemiol. Rev. 19(2): 233–243, 1997.

Brewster DH, Brown MI, Robertson D, et al. An outbreak of *Escherichia coli* O157 associated with a children's paddling pool. Epidemiol. Infect. 112:441–447, 1994.

Brody H, Vinten-Johansen P, Paneth N, and Rip M. John Snow revisited: getting a handle on the Broad Street pump. The Pharos, 1999.

Butler JC, Kilmarx PH, Jernigan DB, and Ostroff SM. Perspectives in fatal epidemics. Infect. Dis. Clinics North Am. 10(4):917–937, 1996.

Centers for Disease Control and Prevention and National Institutes of Health. Biosafety in Microbiological and Biomedical Laboratories. 4th ed. Washington: US Government Printing Office, 1999.

Centers for Disease Control and Prevention. Guidelines for preventing the transmission of *Mycobacterium tuberculosis* in health-care facilities, 1994. Federal Register. 59(208): 54242–54303, 1994.

Centers for Disease Control and Prevention. Surveillance for foodborne-disease outbreaks—United States, 1988–1992. MMWR. 45(SS-5):1–65, 1996.

Centers for Disease Control and Prevention. Surveillance for waterborne-disease outbreaks—United States, 1995–1996. MMWR. 47(SS-5):1–29, 1998.

Centers for Disease Control and Prevention. Reported tuberculosis in the United States, 1997. July 1998.

Centers for Disease Control. Guidelines for investigating clusters of health events. MMWR. 39(RR-11):1–23, 1990.

Centers for Disease Control. Update: Filovirus infection in animal handlers. MMWR. 39(13):221, 1990.

Centers for Disease Control. Update: Filovirus infections among persons with occupational exposure to nonhuman primates. MMWR. 39(16):266–267, 1990.

Centers for Disease Control. 1993. Update: Multistate outbreak of *Escherichia coli* O157:H7 infections from hamburgers—Western United States, 1992–1993. MMWR. 42(14):258–263, 1993.

Centers for Disease Control. Outbreak of *Escherichia coli* O157:H7 infections associated with drinking unpasteurized commercial apple juice—British Columbia, California, Colorado, and Washington, October 1996. MMWR. 45(44):975, 1996.

Centers for Disease Control. Case definitions for infectious conditions under public health surveillance. MMWR. 46(RR-10):1–55, 1997.

Centers for Disease Control. Outbreaks of *Escherichia coli* O157:H7 infection associated with eating alfalfa sprouts—Michigan and Virginia, June–July 1997. MMWR. 46(32): 741–744, 1997.

Centers for Disease Control. Nosocomial *Ralstonia pickettii* colonization associated with intrinsically contaminated saline solution—Los Angeles, California, 1998. MMWR. 47(14):285–286, 1998.

Centers for Disease Control. *Plesiomonas shigelloides,* and *Salmonella* serotype Hartford infections associated with a contaminated water supply—Livingston County, New York, 1996. MMWR. 47(19):394–396, 1998.

Centers for Disease Control. Rubella among crew members of commercial cruise ships—Florida, 1997. MMWR. 46(52 & 53):1247–1250, 1998.

Centers for Disease Control. Epidemiology of measles—United States, 1998. MMWR. 48 (34):749–753, 1999.

Centers for Disease Control. Outbreak of *Escherichia coli* O157:H7 and *Campylobacter* among attendees of the Washington County Fair—New York, 1999. MMWR. 48(36): 803–804, 1999.

Centers for Disease Control. Outbreak of West Nile-like viral encephalitis—New York, 1999. MMWR. 48(38):845–849, 1999.

Centers for Disease Control. Outbreaks of *Shigella sonnei* infection associated with eating fresh parsley—United States and Canada, July–August 1998. MMWR. 48(14):285–289, 1999.

Centers for Disease Control. Public health response to a potentially rabid bear cub—Iowa, 1999. MMWR. 48(42):971–973, 1999.

Centers for Disease Control. Transmission of measles among a highly vaccinated school population—Anchorage, Alaska, 1998. MMWR. 47(51 & 52):1109–1111, 1999.

Centers for Disease Control. Use of pulsed-field gel electrophoresis for investigation of a cluster of invasive group A streptococcal illness—Spokane, Washington, 1999. MMWR. 48 (31):681–683, 1999.

Centers for Disease Control. Outbreaks of *Salmonella* serotype enteritidis infection associated with eating raw or undercooked shell eggs—United States, 1996–1998. MMWR. 49(4):73–79, 2000.

Checko PJ. Outbreak investigation. In: Bowlus B, ed. Infection Control and Applied Epidemiology. Mosby-Year Book, St. Louis, Missouri. 1996.

Chin J, ed. Control of Communicable Diseases Manual. 17th ed. American Public Health Association, 2000.

Cote TR, Convery H, Robinson D, et al. Typhoid fever in the park: epidemiology of an outbreak at a cultural interface. J. Community Health. 20(6):451–458, 1995.

Cunha BA. Pseudoinfections and pseudo-outbreaks. In: Mayhall CG, ed. Hosp. Epidemiol. And Infection Control. Philadelphia: Lippincott Williams & Wilkins, 1999.

Dash GP. Conducting a Literature Search. In: Quick Reference to Outbreak Investigation and Control in Health Care Facilities. Maryland: Aspen Publishers, 2000.

Davis JP, Chesney PJ, Wand PJ, et al. Toxic-shock syndrome: epidemiologic features, recurrence, risk factors, and prevention. N. Engl. J. Med. 303(25):1429–1435, 1980.

Decker MD, Booth AL, Dewey MJ, et al. Validity of food consumption histories in a foodborne outbreak investigation. Am. J. Epidemiol. 124(5):859–863, 1986.

Dev VJ, Main M, and Gould I. Waterborne outbreak of Escherichia coli O157. Lancet. 337:1412, 1991.

Duchin JS, Koster FT, Peters CJ, et al. Hantavirus pulmonary syndrome: a clinical description of 17 patients with a newly recognized disease. N. Engl. J. Med. 330(14):949–955, 1994.

Dwyer DM, Strickler H, Goodman RA, and Armenian HK. Use of case-control studies in outbreak investigations. Epidemiol. Rev. 16 (1):109–123, 1994.

Edlin BR, Tokars JI, Grieco MH, et al. An outbreak of multidrug-resistant tuberculosis among hospitalized patients with the acquired immunodeficiency syndrome. N. Engl. J. Med. 326:1514–1521, 1992.

Feikin DR, Moroney JF, Talkington DF, et al. An outbreak of acute respiratory disease caused by Mycoplasma pneumoniae and adenovirus at a federal service training academy: new implications from an old scenario. Clin. Infect. Dis. 29:1545–1550, 1999.

Finison L, Finison K, and Bliersbach CM. The use of control charts to improve healthcare quality. JHQ. 15(1):9–23, 1993.

Fraser DW, Tsai TR, Orenstein W, et al. Description of an epidemic of pneumonia. N. Engl. J. Med. 297(22):1189–1197, 1977.

Fredlund H, Back E, Sjoberg L, and Tornquist E. Water-melon as a vehicle of transmission of shigellosis. Scand. J. Infect. Dis. 19:219–221, 1987.

Friedman MS, Roels T, Koehler JE, et al. Escherichia coli O157:H7 outbreak associated with an improperly chlorinated swimming pool. Clin. Infect. Dis. 29:298–303, 1999.

Goodman RA, Gregg MB, Gunn RA, and Sacks JJ. Operational Aspects of Epidemiologic Investigations. In: Gregg MB, ed. Field Epidemiology. New York: Oxford University Press, 1996.

Gordon SM, Oshiro LS, Jarvis WR, et al. Foodborne Snow Mountain agent gastroenteritis with secondary person-to-person spread in a retirement community. Am. J. Epidemiol. 131:702–710, 1990.

Greenberg M, and Wartenberg D. Risk perception: understanding mass media coverage of disease clusters. Am. J. Epidemiol. 132(1): S192–195, 1990.

Gregg MB, ed. Conducting a Field Investigation. In: Field Epidemiology. New York: Oxford University Press, 1996a.

Gregg MB, ed. Laboratory Support for the Epidemiologist in the Field. In: Field Epidemiology. New York: Oxford University Press, 1996b.

Haley RW, Tenney JH, Lindsey JO, Garner JS, and Bennett JV. How frequent are outbreaks of nosocomial infection in community hospitals? Infect. Control. 6(6):233–236, 1985.

Herwaldt BL, and Ackers M. An outbreak in 1996 of cyclosporiasis associated with imported raspberries. N. Engl. J. Med. 336(22): 1548–1556, 1997.

Herwaldt BL, and Beach MJ. The return of cyclospora in 1997: another outbreak of cyclosporiasis in North America associated with imported raspberries. Ann. Intern. Med. 130(3):210–220, 1999.

Hilborn ED, Mermin JH, Mshar PA, et al. A multistate outbreak of Escherichia coli O157:H7 infections associated with consumption of mesclun lettuce. Arch. Intern. Med. 159(15): 1758–1764, 1999.

Jacquez GM, ed. Papers from the Workshop on Statistics and Computing in Disease Clustering. Stat. Med. 12(19/20):1751–1967, 1993.

Jacquez GM, Waller LA, Grimson R, and Wartenberg D. The analysis of disease clusters. Part I. State of the art. Infect. Control Hosp. Epidemiol. 17(5):319–327, 1996a.

Jacquez GM, Grimson R, Waller LA, et al. The analysis of disease clusters, Part II: Introduction to techniques. Infect. Control Hosp. Epidemiol. 17(6):385–397, 1996b.

Jarvis WR. Usefulness of molecular epidemiology for outbreak investigations. Infect. Control Hosp. Epidemiol. 15:500–503, 1994.

Jarvis WR, and the Epidemiology Branch. Nosocomial outbreaks: the Centers for Disease Control's Hospital Infections Program experience, 1980–1990. Am. J. Med. 91 (suppl 3B):101S–106S, 1991.

Keene WE, McAnulty JM, Hoesly FC, et al. A swimming-associated outbreak of hemorrhagic colitis caused by *Escherichia coli* O157:H7 and *Shigella sonnei*. N. Engl. J. Med. 331(9):579–584, 1994.

Kehrberg MW, Latham RH, Haslam BT, et al. Risk factors for staphylococcal toxic-shock syndrome. Am. J. Epidemiol. 114:873–879, 1981.

Kolavic SA, Kimura A, Simons SL, et al. An outbreak of *Shigella dysenteriae* type 2 among laboratory workers due to intentional food contamination. JAMA. 278(5):396–398, 1997.

Langley JM, Marrie TJ, Covert A, Waag DM, and Williams JC. An urban outbreak of Q fever following exposure to a parturient cat. N. Engl. J. Med. 319(5):354–356, 1988.

Langmuir AD. William Farr: founder of modern concepts of surveillance. Int. J. Epidemiol. 5(1):13–18, 1976.

Last JM, ed. A Dictionary of Epidemiology. 3rd ed. New York: Oxford University Press, 1995.

Levy DA, Bens MS, Craun GF, et al. Surveillance for waterborne-disease outbreaks—United States, 1995–1996. MMWR 47(5):1–34, 1998.

Linnan MJ, Mascola L, Lou XD, et al. Epidemic listeriosis associated with Mexican-style cheese. N. Engl. J. Med. 319(13):823–828, 1988.

Lutwick L. 1996. Postexposure prophylaxis. Infect. Dis. Clin. North Am. 10(4):899–915, 1996.

Maki DG, Klein BS, McCormick RD, et al. Nosocomial *Pseudomonas pickettii* bacteremias traced to narcotic tampering. JAMA. 265(8):981–986, 1991.

Mantel N. The detection of disease clustering and a generalized regression approach. Cancer Res. 27(2):209–220, 1967.

Martin ML, Shipman LD, Potter ME, et al. Isolation of *Escherichia coli* O157:H7 from dairy cattle associated with two cases of haemolytic uraemic syndrome. Lancet. 2(8514):1043, 1986.

Maslow J, and Mulligan ME. Epidemiologic typing systems. Infect. Control Hosp. Epidemiol. 17:595–604, 1996.

Matsaniotis NS, Syriopoulou VP, Theodoridou MC, et al. Enterobacter sepsis in infants and children due to contaminated intravenous fluids. Infect. Control. 5(10):471–477, 1984.

McDade JE, Shepard CC, Fraser DW, et al. Isolation of a bacterium and demonstration of its role in other respiratory disease. N. Engl. J. Med. 297(22):1197–1203, 1977.

McGowan JE, and Metchock BG. Basic microbiologic support for hospital epidemiology. Infect. Control Hosp. Epidemiol. 17:298–303, 1996.

Moore PS, Schwartz B, Reeves MW, Gellin BG, and Broome CV. Intercontinental spread of an epidemic group A *Neisseria meningitidis* strain. Lancet. 2:260–262, 1989.

Moroney JF, Guevara R, Iverson C, et al. Detection of chlamydiosis in a shipment of pet birds, leading to recognition of an outbreak of clinically mild psittacosis in humans. Clin. Infect. Dis. 26:1425–1429, 1998.

Murray PR, ed. Manual of Clinical Microbiology, 7th ed. Washington, DC: American Society for Microbiology, 1999.

Narain JP, Farrell JB, Lofgren JP, and Gunn A. Imported measles outbreak in a university. AJPH. 75(4):397–398, 1985.

Neslund VJ. Legal Considerations in a Field Investigation. In: Gregg MB, ed. Field Epidemiology. New York: Oxford University Press, 1996.

Nichol ST, Spiropoulou CF, Morzunov S, et al. Genetic identification of a hantavirus associated with an outbreak of acute respiratory illness. Science. 262(5):914–917, 1993.

Ostroff SM, Griffin PM, Tauxe RV, et al. A statewide outbreak of *Escherichia coli* O157:H7 infections in Washington State. Am. J. Epidemiol. 132(2):239–247, 1990.

Pavia AT, Nichols CR, Green DP, et al. Hemolytic-uremic syndrome during an outbreak of *Escherichia coli* O157:H7 infections in institutions for mentally retarded persons: clinical and epidemiologic observations. J. Pediatr. 116:544–551, 1990.

Peter G, ed. Red Book: Report of the Committee on Infectious Diseases. 24th ed. American Academy of Pediatrics 1997.

Pfaller MA, and Herwaldt LA. The clinical microbiology laboratory and infection control: emerging pathogens, antimicrobial resistance, and new technology. Clin. Infect. Dis. 25:858–870, 1997.

Phillips DY, and Arias KM. Statistical methods used in outbreak investigation. In: Quick Reference to Outbreak Investigation and Control in Health Care Facilities. Rockville, Maryland: Aspen Publishers, 2000.

Roden AT. Imported disease as a public health problem. J. R. Coll. General Practitioners. 2(19):19–31, 1968.

Rothman KJ. A sobering start for the Cluster Busters' conference. Am. J. Epidemiol. 132 (1):S6–S13, 1989.

Schulte PA, Ehrenberg RL, and Singal M. Investigation of occupational cancer clusters: theory and practice. AJPH. 77(1):52–56, 1987.

Seals JE, Snyder JD, Edell TA, et al. Restaurant-associated type A botulism: transmission by potato salad. Am. J. Epidemiol. 113:436–444, 1981.

Sellick JA. The use of statistical process control charts in hospital epidemiology. Infect. Control Hosp. Epidemiol. 14(11):649–656, 1993.

Shands KN, Schmid GP, Dan BB, et al. Toxic-shock syndrome in menstruating women: association with tampon use and *Staphylococcus aureus* and clinical features in 52 cases. N. Engl. J. Med. 303:1436–1442, 1980.

Slutsker L, Ries AA, Maloney K, et al. A nationwide case-control study of *Escherichia coli* O157:H7 infection in the United States. J. Infect. Dis. 177:962–966, 1998.

Spika JS, Parsons JE, Nordenberg D, et al. Hemolytic uremic syndrome and diarrhea associated with *Escherichia coli* O157:H7 in a day care center. J. Pediatr. 109(2):287–291, 1986.

Susser M, and Adelstein A. An introduction to the work of William Farr. Am. J. Epidemiol. 101(6), 469–476, 1975.

Swerdlow DL, Woodruff BA, Brady RC, et al. A waterborne outbreak in Missouri of *Escherichia coli* O157:H7 associated with bloody diarrhea and death. Ann. Intern. Med. 117 (10):812–819, 1992.

Taylor DN, Wachsmuth IK, Shangkuan Y, et al. Salmonellosis associated with marijuana: a multistate outbreak traced by plasmid fingerprinting. N. Engl. J. Med. 306(21):1249–1253, 1982.

Tenover FC, Arbeit RD, Goering RV, and the Molecular Typing Working Group of the Society for Healthcare Epidemiology of America. How to select and interpret molecular strain typing methods for epidemiological studies of bacterial infections: a review for healthcare epidemiologists. Infect. Control. Hosp. Epidemiol. 18:426–439, 1997.

Thomas JC, Bendana NS, Waterman SH, et al. Risk factors for carriage of meningococcus in the Los Angeles County men's jail system. Am. J. Epidemiol. 133:286–295, 1991.

Todd J, Fishaut M, Kapral F, and Welch T. Toxic-shock syndrome associated with phage-group-I staphylococci. Lancet. 2:1116–1118, 1978.

Torok TJ, Tauxe RV, Wise RP, et al. A large community outbreak of salmonellosis caused by intentional contamination of restaurant salad bars. JAMA. 278(5):389–395, 1997.

Wang SA, Tokars JI, Bianchine PJ, et al. *Enterobacter cloacae* bloodstream infections traced to contaminated human albumin. Clin. Infect. Dis. 30:35–40, 2000.

Wartenberg D, and Greenberg M. Solving the cluster puzzle: clues to follow and pitfalls to avoid. Stat. Med. 12:1763–1770, 1993.

Weber DJ, Rutala WA. Zoonotic infections. Occupational Medicine 14(2):247–284, 1999.

Weber S, Pfaller MA, and Herwaldt LA. Role of molecular epidemiology in infection control. Infect. Dis. Clin. North Am. 11(2):257–278, 1997.

Wendt C, and Herwaldt LA. Epidemics: Identification and Management. In: Wenzel RP, ed. Prevention and Control of Nosocomial Infections, 3rd ed. Baltimore: Williams & Wilkins, 1997.

Wenzel RP, Thompson RL, Landry SM, et al. Hospital-acquired infections in intensive care unit patients: an overview with emphasis on epidemics. Infect. Control. 4(5):371–375, 1983.

WHO/International Commission. Ebola haemorrhagic fever in Zaire, 1976. Bull. World Health Organ. 56(2):271–293, 1978a.

WHO/International Study Team. Ebola haemorrhagic fever in Sudan, 1976. Bull. World Health Organiz. 56(2):247–270, 1978b.

Winkelstein W. A new perspective on John Snow's communicable disease theory. Am. J. Epidemiol. 142(9):S3–S9, 1995.

Zucker JR. Changing patterns of autochthonous malaria transmission in the United States: a review of recent outbreaks. Emerg. Infect. Dis. 2(1):37–43, 1996.

15

Clinical Trials

HARRY A. GUESS and GARY B. CALANDRA

This chapter outlines aspects of clinical trial methodology that are particularly relevant to evaluating the safety and efficacy of new antibiotics and vaccines. The focus is on the sequence of clinical trials needed either to support initial licensing approval of a new investigation antibiotic or vaccine or to provide the safety and efficacy data needed for regulatory approval of a new indication for an existing antibiotic or vaccine. We do not discuss special considerations applicable to trials of HIV vaccines or of therapies for HIV infections. For further information on the design, conduct, and analysis of clinical trials in general, the reader should consult one of the many excellent textbooks (Friedman et al. 1998, Hulley and Cummings 1988) on clinical trial methodology. Also of interest are recent articles providing criteria for judging the validity of clinical trials (Guyatt et al. 1993), guidelines for what information should be provided in papers reporting results of clinical trials (Begg et al. 1996), guidelines for the design and analysis of trials to demonstrate therapeutic equiva-

lence of two treatments (Jones et al. 1996), and regulatory standards for clinical trials (Food and Drug Administration 1998a).

GENERAL PRINCIPLES APPLICABLE TO ALL DRUG AND VACCINE TRIALS

Conceptual Planning

All clinical trials, whether controlled or not, are conducted to answer specific questions. It is essential that the primary questions to be answered be stated clearly before starting the trial. For investigational drugs, antibiotics, and vaccines, the questions that must be answered include those necessary to meet specific regulatory requirements, to address competitive issues, and to provide appropriate guidance to physicians and patients who will use the product after license approval. Plans to provide pharmacoeconomic data to support use of the new product should, also, be considered. The initial step is to outline what one wants to be able to say in the recommendations for use by physicians and then to make sure that the clinical trial program includes studies to support all of the points. In particular, the desired indications for usage will dictate the objectives of the main efficacy trials. Once the study objectives have been developed, a conceptual outline of the whole clinical trial program should be prepared, along with a brief outline of objectives and plan for each proposed clinical trial.

Another way in which review of the proposed prescribing information can be helpful is to focus attention on what is the intended *target population* for each specific indication for the product. Knowing the intended target population provides guidance on how the *study populations* for the trials should be selected and defined in terms of inclusion and exclusion criteria. While the study population for the main efficacy trials may be considerably more homogeneous than the intended target population, it will probably be necessary to conduct additional studies in a broader range of patients. Such studies are generally needed to provide data on use in male and female patients in different age ranges and racial groups, to determine whether special dosing regimens or precautions are needed in patients with impaired drug metabolism or organ insufficiency, and to investigate possible drug or vaccine interactions. One of the most common deficiencies in the body of investigational data supporting a new drug or antibiotic is in the definition of dosing regimens, especially for patients with impaired drug metabolism. Selection of the right dose is often a time consuming and difficult task.

Once the study questions have been formulated, it is useful to restate them in the form of *study objectives*, to develop operational definitions of terms, and finally to restate the objectives as the *hypotheses* to be tested statistically. The process of formulating operational definitions requires that the methods of measurement be specified and that evidence of their reliability, validity, clinical relevance, and responsiveness to known interventions be documented. For laboratory assays such processes are well accepted; however, some clinical measurements often come into wide use and gain acceptance by clinicians without ever having been standardized for clinical trial use. In particular, symptom scales and quality of life questionnaires require considerable testing and validation work before they can be accepted as valid, reproducible measures. Careful attention to the study questions and their operational measurement in the clinical trial has to be made at a very early stage of clinical trial planning so that any studies necessary to standardize or validate measurements may be undertaken.

For each clinical trial the specific hypothesis tests, case definitions, response criteria, statistical methodology, and methods of analysis need to be defined in advance and included in the protocol. Ideally, the level of detail should be such that a knowledgeable statistician could reproduce the analyses, given the data and the protocol.

The clinical relevance of any proposed endpoints and response criteria needs to be established. If it is desired to base efficacy analysis on a surrogate endpoint (e.g., serologic response to a vaccine) rather than a clinical endpoint (e.g., development of the study disease), then it is essential that the validity of the surrogate endpoint as a substitute for a clinical endpoint be well documented and accepted by the regulatory agencies for purposes of supporting license approval.

In addition to the methodologic aspects of study design and analysis, it is necessary to outline the logistic, administrative, and operational aspects in considerable detail so that resource implications and overall feasibility within available time constraints can be determined and potential problems can be identified and solved before they occur. The need to define study procedures carefully is one reason why a clinical trial needs not only a protocol but also a *manual of operations*.

The study investigator, oversight groups such as ethical review boards, and regulatory agencies need the medical background of illnesses being prevented or treated and all the previous data on the compound or vaccine being studied. These are provided in an investigators' brochure, which presents all the data about the preclinical investigations, previous clinical trials, and other information pertinent to the benefit-to-risk use of the investigative product.

The prior discussion is intended to serve only as a brief introduction to the subject of designing and conducting clinical trials of investigational antibiotics and vaccines. Before undertaking such a trial an investigator should have a full understanding of clinical trial design, study protocols, and operations manuals for related trials, and consult with investigators having experience in the design, conduct, and analysis of clinical trials similar to the one being planned.

Phases of Clinical Investigations

Clinical trials required for approval of drugs and biologics, including vaccines, are conducted in accordance with regulations of the Food and Drug Administration (FDA) or other national authority and are subject to auditing by FDA inspectors, with both civil and criminal penalties for noncompliance. These regulations include requirements for monitoring, recording, and reporting adverse events occurring during the course of clinical trials.

All human clinical studies must be reviewed by an Institutional Review Board (IRB) to assure protection of human subjects and to ensure compliance with standards for informed consent. Subjects may not be forced to waive any legal rights or to release the investigator or sponsor from legal liability for negligence. The elements of informed consent include a description of the research purposes, study duration and procedures, foreseeable risks and discomforts, anticipated potential benefits, compensation and medical treatment available in case of injury, whom to contact for further information in case of injury, and a statement that discontinuation is permitted at any time, and that refusal to participate or discontinuation of participation will not involve any penalties.

As outlined in the Code of Federal Regulations (CFR), the clinical investigation of a drug or antibiotic that has not been previously tested in humans is generally divided into three phases, which are typically conducted in sequence after in vitro tests and preliminary animal toxicity tests have been completed (21 CFR § 312.21).

Phase I refers to the initial human studies that are designed to determine the absorption, distribution, metabolism, elimination ("ADME"), and pharmacologic actions of the drug, any acute toxicity or side effects associated with increasing doses, and, if possible, some early evidence of effectiveness. Phase I studies may also be conducted to explore drug mechanisms of action, structure-activity relationships, and dose tolerability. The testing in Phase I is less well defined for vaccines and primarily consists of safety and dose ranging to test immune response. However, there are a number of circumstances that could lead to extensive preclinical testing for a new vaccine candidate. The vaccine could contain material that could theoretically generate cross-reacting antibodies to host tissue. Use of novel adjuvants could require extensive preclinical evaluation in animals. New modes of delivery such as polynucleotide ("naked DNA") vaccines have led to extensive preclinical testing, which is beyond the scope of this chapter. In summary, preclinical testing requirements for vaccines may require careful attention in response to new technologies and evolving regulatory standards. For potentially toxic drugs, Phase I studies are conducted in patients for whom there are no effective therapies. For drugs in which serious toxicity is not expected, Phase I studies are typically conducted in normal volunteers. Initial Phase I studies are typically closely monitored, beginning with single dose studies and proceeding to multiple dose studies, ultimately involving about 20 to 80 total subjects. During Phase I, sufficient information about acute dose-related toxicity, pharmacokinetics, and pharmacologic effects should be obtained to permit the design of well-controlled, scientifically valid Phase II studies.

Phase II studies include controlled clinical studies conducted to evaluate effectiveness of the drug for a particular indication in patients with the disease under study and to determine any common short-term side effects and risks associated with the drug. (In clinical epidemiology the term "effectiveness" commonly refers to how well the treatment performs when used in everyday clinical practice, and "efficacy" refers to how well the intervention works in randomized controlled trials. However, the Code of Federal Regulations does not make this distinction and uses both terms to refer to clinical trial conditions.) Early Phase II studies are often conducted as dose-ranging studies, while late Phase II studies may include randomized, double-blind, controlled trials to provide efficacy data needed for drug approval.

Phase III studies include both randomized, double-blind, controlled studies to assess efficacy and uncontrolled studies to assess safety in a broader range of patients than those studied in Phase II. Phase III studies typically include from several hundred to several thousand patients and are intended to provide additional information on both safety and efficacy in support of the prescribing information for physicians.

Adequate and Well-Controlled Studies

Approval of claims of effectiveness of a drug, antibiotic, or vaccine must be supported by "substantial evidence" from "adequate and well-controlled studies" (21 CFR § 314.126). An adequate and well-controlled study has the following characteristics:

1. a study protocol that provides a clear statement of the objectives of the investigation and a summary of the methods of analysis.
2. a design that permits a valid comparison with a control group to provide a quantitative assessment of drug effect,
3. a method of selecting subjects that provides adequate assurance that they have the disease being studied or evidence of susceptibility and exposure to the condition against which prophylaxis is directed,
4. a method of assigning patients to treatment and control groups that minimizes bias and is intended to assure comparability of the groups with respect to perti-

nent variables, such as age, sex, severity of disease, duration of disease, and use of therapy other than the study agent,
5. adequate measures to minimize bias on the part of the subjects, observers, and analysts of the data,
6. methods and criteria used to assess response that are well defined, reliable, and adequately described in the study protocol,
7. methods of analysis, including statistical methods, that are adequate to assess effects of the study agent and are described in the study report. The analysis should assess comparability of the test and control groups with respect to pertinent variables and should assess how any interim analyses performed are taken into account in the final analysis.

Internal and External Validity of Studies Needed for Approval

The regulatory standards for "adequate and well-controlled" studies are intended to provide assurance that effects of the study agent can be distinguished from other influences, such as spontaneous changes in the course of the disease, placebo effect, or biased observations. In the language of clinical epidemiology this refers to the *internal validity* of the study, that is, the extent to which the drug effects can be separated from other effects within the study itself (Hulley and Cummings 1988). One article on the interpretation of clinical trial results (Guyatt et al. 1993) emphasized two other aspects of clinical trial design needed for internal validity. The first requirement is that the analysis address all patients randomized and that all patients be analyzed in the groups to which they were originally randomized, even if they never received the study agent. This method of analysis is known as an "intention-to-treat analysis." The second, closely related requirement is that the outcome of all patients randomized be ascertained as of the completion date of the trial. This requires follow up of all trial dropouts through either their date of death or the completion date of the trial, whichever is earlier. Since the latter requirement may not be met in some trials it is necessary to determine if the number of patients in each group whose status with respect to the clinical trial endpoints were not known as of the completion date of the trial is sufficient to compromise validity of study conclusions. It is worth noting that in clinical trials designed to demonstrate therapeutic equivalence of two or more active treatments (e.g., typical antibiotic clinical trials), the intention-to-treat analysis may not be the most conservative, and per-protocol analyses also need to be conducted (Jones et al. 1996).

Establishing valid case definitions is essential for the internal validity of both antibiotic and vaccine clinical trials. Estimates of efficacy can be highly sensitive to the choice of case definition (Salmaso et al. 1997). Incomplete ascertainment of mild cases of disease in a vaccine trial may result in an overestimate of vaccine efficacy (Cherry et al. 1998).

Another point of concern is the *external validity*, which refers to the degree to which conclusions in the study can be generalized to the target populations of patients who will be treated with the study agent in clinical practice. The very carefully controlled conditions needed to assure internal validity may not be representative of how drugs, antibiotics, and vaccines are used in clinical practice. Such differences may involve characteristics such as compliance, disease severity, comorbidity, and organ system impairment. A number of authors have noted that preapproval clinical trials required to demonstrate efficacy under controlled conditions do not provide as much information as might be desired about the effectiveness of the agent as used in clinical practice (Epstein 1990) or about how the agent compares with existing agents under conditions typical of clinical practice (Ray et al. 1993). Requirements for preapproval clinical trials tend to maximize internal validity at the possible expense of external validity. Hence preapproval studies should be viewed as testing a therapeutic principle under carefully controlled conditions rather than as providing valid estimates of the magnitude of the effect under clinical conditions.

CLINICAL EVALUATION
OF VACCINES

Consideration of Some Issues about the Vaccine to Be Tested

A major difference between vaccines and drugs is that drugs can often be characterized from a composition and structural standpoint. Vaccines are usually made from a biologic system rather than chemical synthesis. The first vaccine candidate is often changed from the one for licensure because of attempts to make it more immunogenic or to change the biologic production system to enhance factors such as productivity. Even small changes in production could lead to a different trial vaccine even if unintended. To have the final vaccine to use for all clinical trials would be best. Unfortunately, it is more likely that changes will be introduced to the vaccine during clinical trials. It is critical that investigators start with a well-characterized vaccine candidate. Any and all changes for the production must be recorded and reported to the regulatory authorities. If a change is deemed significant, then the prior studies must be linked to present and future studies. There must be a validated test, referred to as a release test, which provides the potency of the vaccine so as to be able to link all the studies. The researcher or investigator must be able to show that the progression of tests and outcomes is valid from Phase I to licensure. The release test can be an in vitro test and/or an in vivo test. It also may be tentative at the start of clinical trials until verified by clinical results.

Considerations Applicable to Combination Vaccines

Combination vaccines, which provide protection against two or more diseases or against multiple serotypes of a single disease, are increasingly used to help reduce the number of injections required for childhood immunizations (Guess 1999). Such vaccines offer the potential for increasing compliance with existing regimens and for facilitating the addition of new vaccines into routine use. Regulatory guidance on production, testing, and clinical trials of combination vaccines has recently been provided by the FDA (Food and Drug Administration 1998b). This topic is beyond the scope of this chapter and is mentioned here only to call attention to the fact that there are special regulatory requirements and scientific considerations involving all aspects of preclinical and clinical development and evaluation of combination vaccines.

Initial Safety Studies

As with drugs, suitable animal toxicity tests for vaccines are required by many countries to begin any human clinical trials. There generally are no well-defined tests required for toxicity for vaccines as for drugs, although some countries or groups of countries do require some preclinical testing. There are now major ongoing discussions to define which tests should be done and to harmonize the testing among the major regulatory groups in the world. In the initial human studies of investigational new vaccines, single doses of the vaccine are administered to small numbers of healthy adult volunteers to evaluate safety. If practical, the subjects should be seronegative for the disease under study, although for certain childhood diseases seronegative healthy normal adults may be impossible to find. The initial human studies of a new vaccine are typically conducted without use of either a placebo or an active control vaccine. However, some initial studies could include an equal in size group of adults receiving placebo to detect any background conditions in study population. While there is little to no power to compare the two groups, the investigator is alerted if both groups have symptoms such as diarrhea or upper respiratory tract infections that there are important background conditions to consider for the analysis of the vaccines. Prevaccination serology is drawn, the vaccine is administered, and the vaccinees are observed in-clinic for up to an hour with checks of vital signs and monitoring for immediate allergic reactions, vasovagal reactions, or other acute responses. The vaccinees are then followed by telephone or diary cards as outpatients for several weeks with daily temperature checks for at least the first several days and inquiries about any local reactions (e.g., erythema, swelling, induration, pain) or systemic adverse events. Precise rules for collecting solicited events from the diary cards and nonsolicited events (potential adverse events) must be prospectively defined. Monitoring to ensure compliance with the protocol both by the subjects and the investigator must also be conducted. One or more postvaccination serologies are subsequently drawn beginning at around the time of expected peak serologic response, which is often four to six weeks after vaccination. Follow up for safety to a defined time (usually 30–42 days postvaccination) must be done. Further safety studies in lower age groups may be done in a step-down by age manner.

Studies to Evaluate Immunogenicity as a Surrogate Marker of Efficacy

Once initial safety has been established, dose-ranging studies are conducted to establish immunogenicity and provide further evidence of safety in larger number of vaccines. These studies, analogous to Phase II drug studies, are sometimes conducted without a control group. However, the use of control groups as soon as possible is beneficial to establish the safety and tolerability profile of the vaccine and to decrease the potential bias in assessment of adverse event causality. It is customary to enroll seronegative subjects of both sexes and of different ethnic backgrounds in a number of different age ranges and body weights to choose an optimum dose. The ultimate aim of the program of immunogenicity trials is to select a vaccine composition and dose that will provide a sufficiently immunogenic response in initially seronegative vaccinees representative of the target populations. Phase II studies are often restricted to subjects with no medical illness. It is, therefore, necessary to conduct studies on specific populations to determine whether the vaccine is useful for all people regardless of background medical conditions.

To interpret an immunogenicity trial it is necessary to have some information about what level of antibody is associated with protection in a population similar to the population under study. Such information is often obtained from epidemiologic studies or clinical trials in which antibody levels in persons who developed disease can be studied (Kayhty et al. 1983). If a protective level is known, the immunogenicity trial may be analyzed in terms of the percentage of vaccinees achieving protective levels of antibody. When the protective level of antibody is unknown, the answers may only be derived from efficacy trials.

Information collected on each vaccinee in an immunogenicity trial should include major factors likely to affect immune response. These include age, sex, smoking (Shaw et al. 1989, Wood et al. 1993) body weight, recent exposure to immunosuppressive drugs, and diseases affecting immunity (e.g., chronic renal failure on dialysis). Buttock injections have been shown to yield lower immune response than deltoid injections for hepatitis B (Shaw et al. 1989). With buttock injections immune response is affected by both needle length and skin fold thickness. Hence, injection site and a measure of obesity should be recorded on all subjects in an immunogenicity trial. The preferred injection site for adults and older children is the deltoid and for young children is the anterolateral thigh.

Immunogenicity trials are conceptually similar to dose-ranging studies of drugs but are much more complex because the dose is not the only vaccine-related factor being tested. Differences in antigens, adjuvant material, manufacturing parameters, stability characteristics, and other factors are also being evaluated. The process of making minor adjustments in vaccine composition and testing these in small groups of human vaccinees in an ongoing series of small immunogenicity studies does not parallel the clinical trials of drugs or antibiotics, where the chemical composition of the product is typically well defined before the start of human trials.

Immunogenicity trials, as well as safety ones, require careful attention to well-established statistical principles of experimental design so that the effects of different factors can be separated from each other and tested in the most efficient manner. Statisticians must be involved in the design of the immunogenicity testing program from the very beginning and must approach the design of the entire program of immunogenicity studies in a unified way with full attention to all of the factors that will have to be tested. Failure to do this can yield highly imbalanced data sets where certain important effects cannot be separately tested. For example, without careful attention to experimental design one type of manufacturing process could be tested in many adults and few children while another type of manufacturing process is tested in many children and few adults, yielding insufficient statistical power to separate manufacturing effects from age effects.

Once the vaccine composition and dosing regimen have been established, expanded trials, similar to Phase III drug trials, are conducted to provide further safety, immunogenicity, and persistence of antibody data on the final composition in larger numbers of initially seronegative subjects. Trials must also be done to prove no clinically relevant interference with concomitantly administered vaccines. The manufacturer must demonstrate that the vaccine can consistently be made immunogenic, effective, and safe. The composition of the lots used in these trials is defined by the regulatory agencies. All these studies serve to meet a regulatory requirement that the final vaccine manufacturing process used to produce the vaccine intended for marketing show an acceptable level of consistency in human serologic response and tolerability in large numbers of vaccinees.

During the course of vaccine development, problems are sometimes identified in manufacturing processes. Such problems can include an unacceptably high lot-to-lot variability in vaccine potency, inefficient processes that have to be changed in order to be economically viable, or problems with vaccine composition. Sometimes the manufacturing problems are identified by results from the clinical trials. Once the manufacturing processes have been changed, it is often necessary to repeat much of the animal and human safety and immunogenicity testing. Unless appropriate bridging studies can be done, it may also be necessary to repeat lot consistency trials. Thus the process of vaccine development can be an iterative one, where trials can lead to changes in manufacturing processes, which necessitate new trials, which may lead to further manufacturing changes and more trials.

Licensing approval of new versions of existing vaccines may sometimes be given on the basis of safety and immunogenicity data, without an added requirement of a clinical efficacy trial. For example, a *Haemophilus influenzae* type b conjugate vaccine manufactured by Pasteur Mérieux and distributed by SmithKline Beecham [Haemophilus b Conjugate Vaccine (Tetanus Toxoid Conjugate)] was approved on the basis of immunogenicity testing (Decker et al. 1992, Granoff et al. 1992) without the requirement of a clinical efficacy trial to demonstrate that the incidence of *Haemophilus influenzae* type b infections is lowered. This is discussed in the manufacturer's prescribing information supplied with the vaccine. The waiver of a requirement for a clinical efficacy trial in this case can be justified because: (1) a placebo-controlled trial would be unethical, since there are existing vaccines of known efficacy recommended for universal use in the age group of interest, (2) a trial to confirm clinical equivalence with a vaccine of known efficacy would have been prohibitively large, and (3) the relationship between antibody levels and clinical protection has been well established with existing vaccines.

Clinical Efficacy Trials

Approval for licensure of vaccines to prevent diseases for which there is no approved vaccine requires not only evidence of safety and immunogenicity but also evidence of clinical efficacy in "adequate and well-controlled" studies. An example of a nonblinded efficacy trial meeting regulatory requirements for U.S. license approval was a design used in Finland (Makela et al. 1977), where all eligible children in the country received either a *Haemophilus influenzae* vaccine or a *Neisseria meningitidis* vaccine, with the choice of vaccine depending on whether the child's birthday fell on an odd or even numbered day of the year. In such a design every child has a potential benefit and each vaccine serves as an inactive control against the other. Such designs are quite unusual, however. In nearly all instances the clinical trials used to provide demonstration of clinical efficacy for purposes of license approval have been double-blind and randomized, with either placebo control or an active control. Examples of such trials include the randomized, double-blind, placebo controlled clinical efficacy trials for vaccines against hepatitis B (Szmuness et al. 1980), chickenpox (Weibel et al. 1984), *Haemophilus influenzae* type b (Santosham et al. 1991), rotavirus (Rennels et al. 1997), and Lyme disease (Steere et al. 1998, Sigal et al. 1998).

When planning clinical efficacy trials it is especially important to select a population in which the incidence of the disease is sufficiently high. Proper choice of a study population can result in substantial reductions in study size, cost, and duration relative to what would be required with a lower risk population (Werzberger et al. 1992, Santosham et al. 1991).

Postmarketing Studies of Vaccine Effectiveness in Clinical Use

Although it is customary to think of effectiveness under conditions of ordinary clinical use as being lower than would be expected on the basis of efficacy data from preapproval clinical trials, it is possible that effectiveness may actually be higher than efficacy. An example of this is the decline in the incidence of *Haemophilus influenzae* type b disease beyond that which could be directly attributed to vaccine use (Murphy et al. 1993), combined with evidence that vaccine recipients had decreased nasopharyngeal carriage of the organism (Murphy et al. 1993). It appears that widespread vaccine use decreased the transmission of the disease to nonvaccinees, thereby causing a decreased likelihood of disease among both vaccinees and nonvaccinees. Studies of vaccine effectiveness under conditions of ordinary clinical use are typically conducted as observational studies (e.g., case-control studies) rather than as randomized clinical trials. Methodologic aspects of such studies have been discussed by a number of authors (Orenstein et al. 1988, Halloran et al. 1992, Halloran and Struchiner 1991) but are beyond the scope of this chapter.

CLINICAL EVALUATION OF ANTIINFECTIVE DRUGS

International Guidelines

Guidelines for the clinical evaluation of antiinfective drugs have been developed and published in a joint effort between the U.S. Food and Drug Administration (FDA) and the Infectious Diseases Society of America (IDSA). In addition to guidelines covering aspects common to all antiinfective clinical trials (Beam et al. 1992) were guidelines in the same journal (Beam et al. 1992) pertaining to clinical bacteriology and to specific types of infections including intraabdominal and pelvic infections; respiratory tract infections; infective endocarditis; sexually transmitted diseases other than HIV infections; skin, skin structure, bone, and joint infections; central nervous system infections; febrile episodes in neutropenic patients; urinary tract infections; gastrointestinal infections; systemic fungal infections; systemic mycobacterial infections; and prophylaxis of surgical infections. Related guidelines for clinical evaluation of antiinfective drugs have been published by the British Society for Antimicrobial Chemotherapy (Finch 1990, British Society 1989, Lunde 1990). In addition, the U.S. guidelines were modified for European use by a European Working Party and published (Beam et al. 1993). Guidelines for AIDS clinical trials also have been published (Cotton et al. 1993, Norrby and Withney 1993). In addition, in 1998 the FDA published a draft guidance for industry for the clinical evaluation of antimicrobials (Food and Drug Administration 1998b). The discussion in this chapter provides an introductory overview of these guidelines, which should be studied in detail prior to planning any clinical evaluation of such drugs.

Clinical trials evaluating antibiotics have almost exclusively been sponsored by pharmaceutical companies. The studies have been done for the registration of the antibiotic or after the antibiotic has been approved (often called postlicensure or postmarketing studies). Many of the patients in the trials used for licensure of an antibiotic have not been studied in a comparative randomized design because of the need to obtain a defined number of infections by pathogen and by body system to get a claim for a single indication. Almost all of the pre- and postlicensure studies that have been randomized and comparative have not been blinded. While comparative studies may have had statistically significant outcomes, the power has been relatively low. Many of these problems have been discussed previously (Polk and Hepler 1986).

A large number of noncomparative clinical efficacy trials have been done with historical controls. This is most appropriate for diseases such as endocarditis or meningitis where an unfavorable outcome for untreated patients is the rule. For other infections such as certain skin and soft tissue infections this may be less appropriate.

Preclinical Studies

Prior to studies in animals or humans, in vitro studies and animal in vivo studies are required to provide preliminary evidence of antiinfective activity against specific microorganisms. In addition, toxicology studies such as genotoxicity, bone marrow toxicity, interference with coagulation mechanisms, and induction of certain enzymes that could affect metabolism of other drugs can be done prior to animal testing. In vitro studies are also needed to establish mechanisms of antiinfective action and development of resistance, to identify interactions with other antiinfective drugs, and to develop appropriate culture systems. Animal studies of antiinfective drugs required prior to human studies include acute and chronic toxicity measurements in several animal species over prolonged time. As a rule, the primary toxicities of a drug need to be defined before proceeding to humans. In particular, when use in pregnancy is anticipated, suitable animal studies should be conducted to evaluate any fetal toxicity, congenital malformations, premature labor, or postnatal effects of fetal exposure. Suitable animal models of fetal toxicity typically include rabbits and often primates. A detailed discussion of requirements for animal studies is given in the U.S. Code of Federal Regulations (21 CFR 58). Since other countries may have different regulations, the reader should consult regulations of specific countries of interest.

Phase I Studies

All Phase I studies of antiinfective drugs are closely monitored and involve both frequent recording of clinical observations and laboratory tests including serum and urine drug levels, biochemistry, hematology, coagulation, hepatic function, and renal function. The first studies administer single doses with timed collection of blood and urine specimens to establish single-dose pharmacokinetics and set dosing intervals for the multiple-dose Phase I studies that follow. For most antiinfective drugs the Phase I studies are undertaken in healthy volunteers; however, potentially toxic drugs intended for treatment of life-threatening infections may be initially evaluated in patients. For example, Phase I studies of drugs to treat patients with HIV may be conducted in HIV-infected patients (Cotton et al. 1993).

Phase II Studies

The definition of Phases II and III differ somewhat by various groups. Phase II is usually the first time patients with infections are treated. However, in pediatrics, Phase I studies are often done in children with resolving infections. Since the dose for adults without renal or hepatic insufficiency can be predicted reasonably well from the antibiotic in vitro studies, animal models, and pharmacokinetics, Phase II can be done with fixed dose regimens. Data from Phase II may require dose-ranging studies to be done. Most of the early data are from well-defined

infections treated from 3 to 14 days. The Phase II studies should be done with a double-blind comparative design against the best available antibiotic or antibiotics with comparable in vitro profile and pharmacokinetics. Phase II studies escalate from the least severe to more severe infections. Once the dose is confirmed (or in some cases determined) in Phase II, Phase III studies are conducted to evaluate the effectiveness and safety in a large number of patients.

Extensive patient information is typically collected in such trials in order to document safety and efficacy to the standards needed for regulatory approval. In the United States it is customary to review the clinical program with FDA periodically to ensure that there is agreement on adequacy of the design of the overall program in general and of the double-blind, randomized, controlled clinical efficacy trials in particular. As a part of this process an "End of Phase II Meeting" is commonly held to review results to date and outline plans for Phase III. Randomized, double-blind, controlled trials from Phase II may also serve as "adequate and well-controlled" trials required to establish efficacy for particular indications.

Phase III Studies

Phase III studies include both randomized, double-blind, controlled efficacy trials and expanded uncontrolled trials of several hundred to several thousand patients with a variety of clinical conditions. The uncontrolled studies are conducted once preliminary evidence of efficacy has been obtained and are intended to provide further evidence of safety and efficacy in patients typical of those encountered in clinical practice. Patients in Phase III trials typically include those with concomitant illnesses and impaired organ function that may affect drug absorption, distribution, metabolism, and excretion. Special patient populations such as adolescents, children, infants, neonates, pregnant women, and the elderly (65 years of age and older) may be included in Phase III, if the drug is intended for use in such populations. Such studies may suggest the need for further dose adjustment in special patient populations. An example where this occurred was in studies of the antibiotic imipenem/cilastatin in patients with renal impairment (Calandra et al. 1988). These studies led to changes in the manufacturer's recommended doses for such patients.

The entire program of in vitro and animal studies and Phases I through III program should provide the adequate evidence of safety and efficacy necessary to secure regulatory approval of the drug for marketing. The initial set of approved indications can be expanded based on later efficacy studies, conducted according to the standards discussed previously.

Phase IV Studies

Phase IV studies are those undertaken after regulatory approval. Such studies include those undertaken to provide further evidence concerning particular safety questions as well as studies to obtain new indications and to give investigators experience with new uses. As an example, while some experience is gained early in the treatment of immunocompromised patients, large-scale trials in this group of patients are often conducted in Phase IV. Often, specific Phase IV studies will be suggested by an FDA Advisory Committee or may be requested by the FDA at the time of regulatory approval.

Requirements for Study Design and Analysis

There will have been a number of events leading up to raising the question to be addressed. For example, the spectrum of an antibiotic may suggest that as monotherapy it could be as effective as combination antibiotic therapy for intraabdominal infections. Testing in animal models could be done to see if results are consistent with this. Nonrandomized probe studies in patients with intraabdominal infections would be done to ensure that such patients can be treated. Thereafter, the hypothesis would be defined that the antibiotic in question is as good as or better than combination antibiotic therapy in all or a defined group of patients.

Protocol preparation

Clinical study protocols should provide all information needed for the design, conduct, and analysis of the study. This includes a clear statement of the objectives of the proposed study; the specific study hypotheses; study design and randomization requirements; study size and duration; inclusion and exclusion criteria; dosage and dosing intervals, information to be collected, the timing of data collection; adverse experience monitoring and reporting procedures, and statistical considerations. Copies of case report forms showing all information to be collected on each patient are included as a part of each protocol.

The final design of an antibiotic clinical trial is the result of the cooperative interaction of a number of groups. For industry sponsored trials the question must be medically relevant and economically realistic. The input for the question may come from a basic science group (Is a compound useful for an infection?), from a clinical group, or others such as marketing (Is an antibiotic used in a certain way more cost-effective than other forms of therapy?). Early statistical input is needed in determining how large a trial may be needed. For an investigational drug, groups from process research, formulation research, and toxicology must all be involved. Because of the high cost of answering important clinical questions, the question should be one that results in novel information.

Study size and power to detect clinically meaningful differences

The statistical analysis section of the protocol should specify the hypotheses to be tested, planned analyses, analytic methods to be used, and statistical criteria for declaring differences to be statistically significant. In the usual case where more than one hypothesis is to be tested the criteria for statistical significance must address the effect of multiplicity on the Type I error. Clinical efficacy trials of antiinfective drugs in which an active control drug is used are typically designed to show that the efficacy of the new drug is not worse than that of the active control drug. Such trials intended to show therapeutic equivalence must be sufficiently large to provide adequate power (typically at least 80% power) to detect a predetermined clinically meaningful difference in treatment outcomes. These considerations need to be discussed in the protocol as part of the discussion justifying the choice of study size, duration, and power. A justification of what constitutes a clinically meaningful difference should also be given or referenced.

Interim analyses and stopping rules

For trials in which interim analyses are planned, the specific analyses to be performed must be specified in the protocol along with the timing of the analyses and the criteria for stopping the study. The p-values must be adjusted for the effects of the interim analyses, so as to preserve the overall Type I error rate at its nominal level (usually 0.05), taking into account the interim analyses. A number of statistical techniques for these purposes are in common use. The choice depends in part on the planned purposes of the interim analyses. For further discussion the reader should consult a textbook of clinical trial design (Friedman et al. 1998).

Exclusions of randomized patients

In clinical efficacy trials of antiinfective drugs, patient eligibility typically requires a positive culture from the infection site. Since it may take several days for the culture results to become available and since antiinfective treatment is required in the interim, it is often necessary to randomize patients before one can confirm that they are eligible. If the rate of negative cultures is high and turns out, by chance, not to be distributed equally between treatment groups, the resulting imbalance in numbers of patients who are evaluable for efficacy can compromise the results of the randomization process. As a general rule, any exclusion of a randomized patient requires justification (Guyatt et al. 1993). The FDA guidelines (Beam et al. 1992) suggest comparing ex-

clusion rates by center and examining efficacy in those centers with low exclusion rates. It is important also to ensure that the blinding is working and that investigators are not excluding randomized patients on the basis of knowing the treatment group to which the patients were randomized. If investigators keep a list of all patients who might have entered the trial but did not, and keep a record of why patients were not entered, bias in this aspect of the trial can be decreased. The FDA guidelines also suggest doing an intention-to-treat (ITT) analysis, in which all randomized patients are counted and followed for clinical outcomes, regardless of whether they met eligibility criteria (Beam et al. 1992). If the overall conclusions of the study differ depending on the method of analysis, then the validity of the study conclusions regarding comparative efficacy would come into question. For purposes of safety analyses, including evaluation of rates of adverse drug reactions, it is customary to include all patients who received at least one dose of the study drug, regardless of whether they had positive cultures (Beam et al. 1992).

Patients to be studied

The populations to be studied should be relatively obvious, but sometimes difficult to obtain. For example, to answer the initial question about whether an antibiotic is generally safe and effective in Phase II studies, patients with serious infections of mild to moderate severity are treated. For a parenteral antibiotic, there is a problem of acquiring infections mild enough to not put the patient in jeopardy but yet to require hospitalization long enough to test the antibiotic. Specific inclusion criteria (e.g., well-defined infections with high probability of defining the pathogen) and exclusion criteria (e.g., no renal or hepatic insufficiency prior to definition of the pharmacokinetics of the antibiotic in these states) must be provided.

Care must be taken for overt and covert exclusions to a study. For example, for a new antimicrobial agent, certain concomitant drugs may be excluded for part of the trial. This could bias a safety analysis. Additionally, certain suspected infections could be excluded by the investigators if they had concerns about the in vitro evidence of effectiveness. This could bias comparisons among sites if there were different patterns of patient entry.

The infections to be studied must be well defined. For example, pneumonia as a category must be defined by apparent etiology, symptoms, signs, radiologic findings, or other clinical criteria to avoid ambiguities when the data are analyzed. For example, it is inappropriate to include community acquired pneumonia that has a high probability of *Mycoplasma* in a trial of a cephalosporin with no anti-*Mycoplasma* activity. Also, the claim for use of an antibiotic for pneumonia due to *Pseudomonas aeruginosa* should be based upon true pneumonia and not exacerbation of chronic bronchitis.

Eligibility criteria for inclusion of previously treated patients

Patients enrolled in a clinical efficacy trial of an antiinfective drug should normally not have received previous treatment for the current infection. However, there are circumstances, defined in FDA guidelines (Beam et al. 1992) in which patients who have received inadequate treatments may be eligible for enrollment. For example, an otherwise eligible patient infected with an organism resistant in vitro to the initial antiinfective drug may be enrolled in a clinical efficacy trial of a new antiinfective drug provided that there is a positive culture of the organism from the infection site obtained within 48 hours prior to enrollment.

Types of controls

Most clinical efficacy trials of antiinfective drugs use an active control drug that is approved for the indication studied and that represents an accepted standard treatment. Use of an active control agent that is not approved for the indication may be acceptable under appropriate circumstances; the FDA guidelines recommend prior consultation (Beam et al. 1992). This problem sometimes arises in international clinical trials when an active control that is standard approved therapy in another country is not yet approved in the United States. Placebo controls are generally used only when no agent is known to be effective or when the infection is benign and self-limited. Historical controls would only be appropriate for infections in which there is no known effective therapy and the infection has been well documented to be fatal.

Randomization and blinding

Random assignment should be used in all controlled clinical efficacy trials. For multicenter trials block randomization within each center is used to ensure an adequate balance of patients in both arms of the trial within each center. Stratification is used to decrease the chances of an imbalance in important prognostic factors. Since such imbalances can be addressed at the analysis stage by multivariate analysis, it is generally not advisable to stratify so finely that there are too few patients (e.g., <5) in any one stratum.

Clinical efficacy trials are conducted with both patients, investigators, and evaluators blinded as to therapy. This is often difficult to achieve in practice and yet if auditing reveals inadequate blinding, the trial results may be judged unacceptable for purposes of meeting regulatory requirements for drug approval. Comparative antibiotic studies should be done with agents of similar pharmacokinetics and antimicrobial spectrum. When the dose, dosing interval, mode of administration, or physical characteristics of the comparison agent differs from that of the study drug it is necessary to employ a double-blind, double-dummy technique to maintain blinding. An example of this is the study by Solomkin and colleagues (1990), who compared one antibiotic (imipenem/cilastatin) to two (tobramycin and clindamycin) for serious intraabdominal infections. The patients were stratified for severity of illness by an Apache II score or grading system.

Failure to appropriately blind the patients to treatment group can lead to several areas of bias. For example if patients feel that one treatment arm is more effective and they are on the other one, they might try to get into the other arm. Also, if they feel that one drug more likely has a side effect than another, they might be quicker to report a similar effect if they think they are on the suspect drug. If the investigators know which drug the patient is taking, they could be biased for both efficacy and safety. For example, investigators may be more willing to declare a failure on one drug than another if there was a perceived difference in potency. Also, investigators may be more likely to call an adverse event drug related if they think the patient was on a drug with a known side effect.

Definition of clinical response

Explicit criteria for the expected response to treatment or prophylaxis must be clearly defined in the protocol. Response is usually classified as a cure, failure, or intermediate outcome (Beam et al. 1992) based on clinical and microbiologic criteria. Clinical outcome has to be based upon measurable criteria such as change in sputum, improved PO_2, and/or improved X-ray in pneumonia. Microbiologic outcome criteria have been well defined for urinary tract infections. For other body sites the definitions must be quite clear. When material for culture is available and the patient is not put at risk by the sampling technique, a posttreatment culture should be done. For patients with infections of chronic lesions such as decubiti, the definition of what the reculture results mean is very important. The outcome of patients treated with parenteral antibiotics may be more difficult to decide if they are switched to oral therapy. Therefore, treatment outcome definitions need to take this into consideration. The FDA guidelines applicable to specific infections should be consulted for what would be considered acceptable response criteria. Case report forms should maintain appropriately timed records of clinical observations, white blood cell counts and differentials, radiographs, and cultures. Standards for microbiologic outcome should use the terminology specified in FDA guidelines (Beam et al. 1992).

In antibiotic trials, predictive markers and sampling of outcome markers are usually not difficult issues. In other antimicrobial trials such as for AIDS anti-HIV therapy one must define any surrogate markers being used (Lagakos 1993). The timing of measurement of these markers may be important if there are transient effects to be measured.

Also in antibiotic trials there are usually no problems with the validity and reliability of measures, except perhaps in the area of health economics. However, in other areas such as anti-HIV therapy, use of plasma free viral titers, viral RNA copy number, or other measures require confirmation of their validity and reliability.

Preparation of clinical study reports

The clinical information included in the clinical and statistical sections of new drug applications must meet FDA requirements applicable to all drugs (Food and Drug Administration 1988). Narrative clinical discussions of study results must be accompanied by statistical summaries, analyses, and conclusions. The FDA guideline (Beam et al. 1992) notes that, as a minimum, the following tables are needed: (1) a listing of all randomized subjects, by center and indication, with date of randomization, final disposition, and all data; (2) all subjects who dropped out after randomization, together with the reason for drop-out and the date of dropout; (3) all adverse drug experience (AE) reports listing the type of AE, investigator rating of causality, seriousness (according to the FDA definition), the treatment group, and the outcome; (4) all pathogens by center, indication, treatment, and outcome; (5) intermediate summary tables summarizing efficacy, safety, and AEs.

Other Antimicrobial Trials

There are a number of antimicrobial clinical trials that may differ from the general example given for antibiotics and some are presented hereafter for reference for the readers. Many of the examples are in the area of treatment or prophylaxis for HIV infections or opportunistic infections in AIDS patients. There is also an exceptional series of trials for aminoglycosides.

Most of the antibiotic trials for licensure have contained enough dose-ranging data so that only changes in dose for organ dysfunction have been done postlicensure. An exception is the studies to evaluate once-daily dosing of aminoglycosides (Prins et al. 1993). While no large study was done to support the claim for efficacy, on the basis of all the studies done, the Food and Drug Administration has approved this claim for aminoglycosides.

An example of a prophylaxis study was one done by the Canadian HIV Clinical Trials Network against *Mycobacterium avium* complex (Nightingale et al. 1993). The studies were randomized, double blind, and large enough to detect significant differences in the development of *Mycobacterium avium* complex bacteremias between rifabutin and placebo.

Hughes and associates (1993) is an example of a treatment study for *Pneumocystis carinii* pneumonia. This study was randomized, double blind, and controlled.

Large clinical trials testing antifungal drugs have been done for a number of pathogens. For example, White and colleagues (1998) compared amphotericin B colloidal dispersion versus amphotericin B.

The U.S. AIDS Clinical Trials Group has studied antiviral agents for infections other than HIV. A small study compared vidarabine to foscarnet for acyclovir-resistant mucocutaneous herpes simplex and showed very early a lack of effect of vidarabine and toxicity due to that drug (Saffrin et al. 1991).

The first pivotal trial of an anti-HIV drug was the double-blind, randomized test for licensure of zidovudine (Fischl et al. 1987). This trial (results published in 1987) set a standard by which other nucleoside analogues might be given accelerated approval on the basis of surrogate markers. However, controversy remained over the use of surrogate markers (Volberding et al. 1990, Hamilton et al. 1992, Seligman et al. 1994). The choice of surrogate markers rapidly evolved to markers specific to patient status (CD4+ cells) plus measurements of viral burden (measurements of HIV RNA) and to trials that involved combination therapy (Eron et al. 1995, Gulick et al. 1997). Testing of new classes of anti-HIV therapy such as a protease inhibitor has led to new studies of measurement of patient benefit (Hammer et al. 1997). As newer agents and new classes of drugs are developed, the design of clinical trials for anti-HIV drugs becomes more complex and difficult. New designs to study patients with HIV infection have been proposed (Gilbert et al. 1998) and will have to evolve as the pathogenesis of HIV infections is further unraveled.

CONCLUSIONS

The range of clinical trials that can be conducted in infectious disease is extremely broad. This chapter has given only a few examples and has emphasized vaccine and antibiotic trials designed to obtain government approval for registration. However, the principles of trial design presented should be valid for almost all proposed studies. The keys are to define the question, set forth the hypothesis, define the appropriate size and characteristics of the population to be tested, define the appropriate endpoint(s), and set forth the appropriate statistical analysis to demonstrate the validity of the outcome. When done with forethought and ingenuity, infectious disease study trials can provide useful and rewarding results.

REFERENCES

Beam TR, Gilbert DN, and Kunin CM. Guidelines for the evaluation of antiinfective drug products. Clin. Infect. Dis. 15 (Suppl 1):S1–S346, 1992.

Beam TR, Gilbert DN, and Kunin CM. General guidelines for the clinical evaluation of anti-infective drug products. Clin. Infect. Dis. 15 (Suppl 1):S5–S32, 1992.

Beam TR, Gilbert DN, and Kunin CM, with modifications by a European working party. European guidelines for the clinical evaluation of anti-infective drug products. Eur. Soc. Clin. Microbiol. Infect. Dis. 1–354, 1993.

Begg C, Cho M, Eastwood S, et al. Improving the quality of reporting of randomized controlled trials. JAMA. 276(8):637–639, 1996.

British Society of Antimicrobial Chemotherapy. The clinical evaluation of antibacterial drugs. J. Antimicrob. Chemother. 23(B):1–42, 1989.

Calandra G, Lydick E, Carrigan J, Weiss L, and Guess H. Factors predisposing to seizures in seriously ill infected patients receiving antibiotics: experience with imipenem/cilastatin. Am. J. Med. 84:911–918, 1988.

Cherry JD, Heininger U, Stehr K, and Christenson P. The effect of investigator compliance (observer bias) on calculated efficacy in a pertussis vaccine trial. Pediatrics. 102(4 Pt 1): 909–912, 1998.

Cotton DJ, Powderly WG, Feinburg J, et al. Guidelines for the design and conduct of AIDS clinical trials. Clin. Infect. Dis. 16:816–822, 1993.

Decker MD, et al. Comparative trial in infants of four conjugate Haemophilus influenzae type b vaccines. J. Pediatr. 120:184–189, 1992.

Epstein AM. The outcomes movement: will it get us where we want to go? NEJM. 323:266–269, 1990.

Eron JJ, Benoit SL, Jemsek J, et al. Treatment with lamivudine, zidovudine, or both in HIV-positive patients with 200 to 500 CD4+ cells per cubic millimeter. N. Engl. J. Med. 333: 1662–1669, 1995.

Finch RG. The clinical evaluation of antibacterial drugs: guidelines of the British Society for Antimicrobial Chemotherapy. Eur. J. Microbiol. Infect. Dis. 9:542–547, 1990.

Fisch MA, Richman DD, Grieco MH, et al. The efficacy of azidothymidine (AZT) in the treatment of patients with AIDS and AIDS-related complex: a double-blind placebo-controlled trial. N. Engl. J. Med. 317:185–191, 1987.

Food and Drug Administration. Center for Drug Evaluation and Review. Guideline for the format and content of the clinical and statistical sections of new drug applications. Rockville, MD: Department of Health and Human Services, 1988.

Food and Drug Administration. Developing antimicrobial drugs—general considerations for clinical trials. (Draft FDA Guidance Document Issued for Comment July 1998). Available at: http://www.fda.gov/cder/guidance/index.htm. Accessed November 21, 1998a.

Food and Drug Administration. Guidance for industry for the evaluation of combination vaccines for preventable diseases: production, testing and clinical studies, April 1997. Available at: http://www.fda.gov/cber/gdlns/combvacc.txt. Accessed December 15, 1998b.

Friedman LM, Furberg CD, and DeMets DL. Fundamentals of Clinical Trials. 4th ed. Berlin/Heidelberg: Springer-Verlag, 1998.

Gilbert P, DeGruttola V, and Hammer S. Efficient trial designs for studying combination antiretroviral treatments in patients with various resistance profiles. J. Infect. Dis. 178:340–348, 1998.

Granoff DM, et al. Differences in the immunogenicity of three Haemophilus influenzae type b conjugate vaccines in infants. J. Pediatr. 121: 187–194, 1992.

Guess HA. Combination vaccines: issues in evaluation of effectiveness and safety. Epidemiol Rev. 21(1):89–95, 1999.

Gulick RM, Mellors JW, Havlir D, et al. Treatment with indinavir, zidovudine, and lamivudine in adults with human immunodeficiency virus infection and prior antiretroviral therapy. N. Engl. J. Med. 337:734–739, 1997.

Guyatt GH, Sackett DL, and Cook DJ. The medical literature: users' guides to the medical literature. II. How to use an article about therapy or prevention: A. Are the results of the study valid? JAMA. 270:2598–2601, 1993.

Halloran ME, Haber M. and Longini IM Jr. Interpretation and estimation of vaccine efficacy under heterogeneity. Am. J. Epidemiol. 136:328–343, 1992.

Halloran ME, and Struchiner CJ. Study designs for dependent happenings. Epidemiology. 2: 331–338, 1991.

Hamilton JD, Hartigan PM, Simberkoff MS, et al. A controlled trial of early versus late treatment with zidovudine in symptomatic human immunodeficiency virus infection. Results of the Veterans Affairs Cooperative Study. N. Engl. J. Med. 362:437–443, 1992.

Hammer SM, Squires K, Hughes MD, et al. A controlled trial of two nucleoside analogues plus indinavir in persons with human immunodeficiency virus infection and CD4 cell counts of 200 per cubic millimeter or less. N. Engl. J. Med. 337:725–733, 1997.

Hughes N, Leoung G, Kramer F, et al. Comparison of atovaquone (566C80) with trimethoprim-sulfamethaxazole to treat Pneumocystis carinii pneumonia in patients with AIDS. N. Engl. J. Med. 328:1521–1527, 1993.

Hulley SB, and Cummings SR. Designing Clinical Research: An Epidemiologic Approach. Baltimore: Williams & Wilkins, 1988:5.

Jones B, Jarvis P, Lewis JA, and Ebbutt AF. Trials to assess equivalence: the importance of rigorous methods. Br. Med. J. 313:36–39, 1996.

Kayhty H, Peltola H, Karanko V, and Makela PH. The protective level of serum antibodies to the capsular polysaccharide of Haemophilus influenzae type B. J. Infect. Dis. 147:1100, 1983.

Lagakos SW. Surrogate markers in AIDS clinical trials: conceptual basis, validation, and uncertainties. Clin. Infect. Dis. 16(Suppl 1): S22–S25, 1993.

Lunde I. Guidelines of the World Health Organization for clinical trials with antimicrobial agents. Eur. J. Microbiol. Infect. Dis. 9:548–551, 1990.

Makela PH, Peltola H, Kayhty H, et al. Polysaccharide vaccines of group A Neisseria meningtitidis and Haemophilus influenzae type b: a field trial in Finland. J. Infect. Dis. 136 (Suppl):S43–50, 1977.

Murphy TV, Pastor P, Medley F, Osterholm MT, and Granoff DM. Decreased Haemophilus colonization in children vaccinated with Haemophilus influenzae type B conjugate vaccine. J. Pediatr. 122:517–523, 1993.

Murphy TV, White KE, Pastor P, et al. Declining incidence of Haemophilus influenzae type b disease since introduction of vaccination. JAMA. 269:246–248, 1993.

Nightingale SD, Cameron DW, Gordin FM, et al. Two controlled trials of rifabutin prophylaxis against Mycobacterium avium complex infection in AIDS. N. Engl. J. Med. 329:828–833, 1993.

Norrby SR, Whitley RJ, and the European Working Party of the European Society of Clinical Microbiology and Infectious Diseases. Evaluation of new anti-infective drugs for the treatment of infection with human immunodeficiency virus. Clin. Infect. Dis. 17:794–801, 1993.

Orenstein WA, Bernier RH, and Hinman AR. Assessing vaccine efficacy in the field. Further observations. Epidemiol. Rev. 10:212–241, 1988.

Polk RE, and Hepler CD. Controversies in antimicrobial therapy: critical analyses of clinical trials. Am. J. Hosp. Pharm. 43:630–640, 1986.

Prins JM, Büller HR, Kuijper EJ, Tange RA, and Speelman P. Once versus thrice dailiy gentamicen in patients with serious infections. Lancet 341:335–339, 1993.

Ray WA, Griffin MR, and Avorn J. Evaluating drugs after their approval for clinical use. Sounding Board. NEJM. 329:2029–2032, 1993.

Rennels MB, Glass RI, Dennehy PH, et al. Safety and efficacy of high-dose rhesus-human reassortant rotavirus vaccines—report of the multinational trial. Pediatrics. 97:7–13, 1997.

Safrin S, Crumpacker C, Chatis P, et al. A controlled trial comparing foscarnet with vidarabine for acyclovir-resistant mucocutaneous herpes simplex in the acquired immunodeficiency syndrome. N. Engl. J. Med. 325:551–555, 1991.

Salmaso S, Moiraghi A, Barale A, et al. Case definitions. Dev. Biol. Stand. 89:135–142, 1997.

Santosham M, Wolff M, Reid R, et al. The efficacy in Navajo infants of a conjugate vaccine consisting of Haemophilus influenzae type b polysaccharide and Neisseria meningitidis outer-membrane protein complex. N. Engl. J. Med. 324:1767–1772, 1991.

Seligmann M, Warrell DA, and the Concorde Coordinating Committee. Concorde: MRC/ANRS randomized double-blind controlled trial of immediate and deferred zidovudine in symptom-free HIV infection. Lancet. 343:871–881, 1994.

Shaw FE Jr, Guess HA, Roets JM, et al. Effect of anatomic injection site, age and smoking on the immune response to hepatitis B vaccination. Vaccine. 7:425–430, 1989.

Sigal LH, Zahradnik JM, Lavin P, et al. A vaccine consisting of recombinant Borrelia burgdorferi outer-surface protein A to prevent Lyme disease. N. Engl. J. Med. 339:216–222, 1998.

Solomkin JS, Dellinger EP, Christou NV, and Busuttil RW. Results of a Steere multicenter trial comparing impenem/cilastatin to tobramycin/clindamycin for intra-abdominal infections. Ann. Surg. 212:581–591, 1990.

Steere AC, Sikand VK, Meurice F, et al. Vaccination against Lyme disease with recombinant Borrelia burgdorferi outer-surface lipoprotein A with adjuvant. N. Engl. J. Med. 339(4):263–264, 1998.

Szmuness W, Stevens CE, Harley EJ, et al. Hepatitis B vaccine: demonstration of efficacy in a controlled clinical trial in a high risk population in the United States. NEJM. 303:833–841, 1980.

Volberding PA, Lagakos SW, Koch MA, et al. Zidovudine in asymptomatic human immunodeficiency virus infection. A controlled trial in persons with fewer than 500 CD4-positive cells per cubic millimeter. N. Engl. J. Med. 322:941–949, 1990.

Weibel RE, Neff BJ, Kuter BJ, et al. Live attenuated varicella virus vaccine. Efficacy trial in healthy children. NEJM. 310:1409–1415, 1984.

Werzberger A, Mensch B, Kuter B, et al. A controlled trial of a formalin-inactivated hepatitis A vaccine in healthy children. NEJM. 327:453–457, 1992.

White MH, Bowder RA, Sandler ES, et al. Randomized, double-blind clinical trial of amphotericin B colloidal dispersion vs. Amphotericin B in the empirical treatment of fever and neutropenia. Clin. Infect. Dis. 27:296–302, 1998.

Wood RC, MacDonald KL, White KE, Hedberg CW, Hanson M, and Osterholm MT. Risk factors for lack of detectable antibody following hepatitis B vaccination of Minnesota health care workers. JAMA. 270:2935–2939, 1993.

16

Community Intervention Studies

JAMES C. THOMAS

Most of the chapters in this book describe methods for observational research on infectious diseases, research in which the investigators do not manipulate any of the variables. This chapter and the chapter on clinical trials focus primarily on methodologic issues in studies where a factor affecting an infection is altered in the hope of decreasing the risk or duration of the infection. The two most common rubrics for intervention research in epidemiology are clinical trials and community trials. Typically, a clinical trial is a study of a clinical intervention among individuals, while community trials are characterized by an emphasis on whole communities as the unit of analysis. However, the distinction between clinical and community trials can be blurred, as when the evaluation of a clinical intervention, such as a new vaccine, entails implementation in a community or comparison between different communities. While recognizing the absence of a clear distinction, this chapter focuses predominantly on study methods in those situations where evaluation of an in-

tervention entails the prevalence or incidence of disease in a community.

The term "community" is used so indiscriminantly in contemporary parlance that its use in this context deserves some definition. In their seminal work, *Habits of the Heart*, Bellah and colleagues (1985) distinguish between a "community of interest" and a "community of memory." These categories are not mutually exclusive, but they bring to light some important distinctions. A community of interest is constituted of people who share an interest but may not live in the same neighborhood or city. For example, people who are infected with HIV are sometimes referred to as the "HIV-infected community" even though they are scattered throughout a region. In contrast, a community of memory consists of people of diverse interests who share in the history of a particular place and thus are physically proximate to each other. Physical proximity and personal interactions that enable transmission are key for most infections. It is this concept of community that is most relevant to this chapter. We present in these pages an overview of evaluation theory as it applies to infectious disease interventions in communities commonly described as counties, cities, neighborhoods, and villages. We discuss types of interventions, types of evaluation, study designs, measurement, and practical considerations.

TYPES OF INTERVENTION

The essence of community is interactions and interdependencies between people. Such human relationships underscore the improbability of independence or strict autonomy of individuals and the enduring importance of relationships in the face of an increasingly technological world. They also bring into question the relationships between the people conducting a study and the people studied. We address the methodologic implications of each of these points.

Unit of Intervention

The object intervened upon in a community intervention is not necessarily the community. For example, health education can be delivered in a community to one person at a time as through a door-to-door campaign, or to the population as a whole through mass media. Lomas (1998) thus draws a distinction between population-*based* and population-*level* interventions. In a population-based intervention the term "community" typically connotes that it does not transpire in a clinical setting. In other words, it is used from the perspective of someone working in a clinic to describe what happens "out there" when people are not in the clinic. Such community-based interventions are typically delivered to individuals but outside of the clinical setting. An example of this might be a needle exchange outreach on "street corners" to drug users to prevent transmission of HIV and hepatitis viruses. In contrast, a population-level intervention is one that aims to influence the dynamics or social environment of an entire population. An example of this would be a program to improve the skills of community members to work together in identifying a shared problem and rallying resources to address the problem. Such communal skills, referred to as community competence, community efficacy, and social capital, benefit the entire community. For example, in a study of an intervention to decrease rates of sexually transmitted diseases (STDs), African-American women living in the highest STD incidence neighborhoods of one town were trained to interact with each other and local institutions to represent the interests of their peers in STD prevention (Thomas 1998). The women active in this intervention were not necessarily those who experienced STDs, but their coordinated efforts brought new skills to the community in furthering an agenda that would benefit the entire community.

McLeroy and colleagues (1988) describe not just two but six categories in their model of social ecology: intrapersonal (e.g., beliefs and attitudes); interpersonal (e.g., peer norms); network (e.g., dissemination of information and skills); institutional (e.g., the accessibility of services); community (e.g., community competence, as described previously); and policy (e.g., a state-level policy on anonymous testing for HIV). This model describes the social ecology of humans. A broader ecologic perspective for infectious diseases would also include the ecology of the infecting organism. Interventions aiming to simultaneously affect more than one level of the social ecology are referred to as multilevel interventions. Awareness of the level(s) or unit(s) of intervention is critical for identifying the necessary components of the intervention, the appropriate study design, and the data collection instruments.

Levels of Dependence on Technology

The stereotypical infectious disease intervention in the current era is a vaccine or an antibiotic. The eradication of smallpox with a vaccine is one shining example. Historically, however, infectious diseases have had a mixed relationship with technological innovations. The advent of the hospital, for example, led to new transmission opportunities and even a new branch of infectious diseases research: nosocomial epidemiology. In some instances, the means of stemming an epidemic has been the reversal of earlier technological advances. Such was the case with the encouragement of breastfeeding over bottle feeding and of oral rehydration therapy in lowering the incidence and case fatality of childhood diarrhea. In some instances, an intervention may aim to affect behaviors related to the use of an existing technology. One of the preeminent theories of health behavior, the Health Belief Model, was developed to explain and counteract low participation rates in tuberculosis screening programs (Strecher 1997). Finally, some interventions can be virtually nontechnological. Such would be the case in a program to decrease transmission of STDs by enhancing the social status of women and providing them with education and employment opportunities, thereby decreasing the number who engage in commercial sex (Gupta 1993). Similarly, the Grameen Bank in Bangladesh has provided small loans to rural women to enable them to develop self-employment activities. The program has been found to result in empowerment of women to control personal decisions and an associated increase in contraceptive use (Schuler 1994).

Active versus Passive Participation

Some interventions require the beneficiaries to make a conscious decision to actively participate; e.g., to attend a clinic or follow the advice of a health educator. Other interventions may require the volition of an institution, such as a national or local government, but not of the individual beneficiaries. The chlorination and fluoridation of public drinking water would be one example of such a "passive" intervention. Interventions based on diffusion theory have both active and passive components. Key individuals in a community are trained to actively share information, skills, or attitudes within their network of friends and relatives (for example, see Kelly 1997). The information that is shared can eventually become a social norm that is unconsciously adopted or followed by community members who do not

interact directly with the people who were initially trained. Many infectious disease interventions have a passive effect on some members of the community. As the intervention decreases the prevalence of infection, the average rate of exposure to the pathogen declines. Halloran et al. (1991) refer to this as an indirect benefit to those who did not directly (i.e., actively) participate in the intervention.

Another measure of activity is the degree to which the members of the community participate in the research component of the intervention apart from cooperating with the data collectors. In some instances, the community has no voice in the conduct of the research, while in others the researchers may form a research advisory board consisting of community members (Thomas 1998). In some types of participatory action research (PAR) community members collect data about themselves. PAR is based in part on the assumption that the act of gathering information leads to discovery and new realizations that can, themselves, be considered an intervention. By engaging the community in a study of themselves, community members achieve new insights and adopt new behaviors or solutions. In the modernist tradition of research (in contrast to some postmodern philosophies), where observation means not affecting the study subjects, the Hawthorne effect is a term used to describe the unintended influence that research can have on the study participants (Last 1988). For example, administering a questionnaire can put new ideas into the minds of the respondents. In PAR, however, the influence of the research process on the people being studied is embraced and even encouraged. For more information on PAR, we refer the reader to the text by Whyte (1991).

TYPES OF EVALUATION

Interventions are evaluated on the basis of their ability to work under ideal conditions (efficacy), their ability to yield measurable benefits in 'real life' conditions (effectiveness), and how they compare with alternative interventions (efficiency).

Efficacy

The aim of efficacy research is to establish the "proof of concept," that is, whether a given intervention *can* have the anticipated effect. The distinctions between efficacy and effectiveness derive from the development of individual-level interventions. For example, the efficacy of an antibiotic is measured in a highly controlled experiment of human volunteers who have the relevant infection. The effectiveness is then a measure of how the antibiotic works to contain the infection in a community setting. An antibiotic is an individual-level intervention for which a highly controlled setting can be arranged. Moreover, with individuals as the unit of analysis a community of people can provide a sizable sample of individuals for the purposes of statistical testing. But for community-level interventions there is no "ideal" setting other than a real community, and a single community represents a sample of one. Thus the terms efficacy and effectiveness lose some of their original meaning when applied to community-level interventions.

For the purpose of drawing a distinction between levels of evaluation in community-level interventions, we can consider the application of the intervention in a single community to be a measure of the efficacy, that is, an assessment of whether the intervention *can* work with the maximum number of resources brought to bear (Table 16–1). Such a study is often referred to as a demonstration project. A demonstration project has the additional aim of refining the intervention and evaluation methods in anticipation of a multisite trial. A multisite trial might then be considered the best assessment of the community-level intervention's effectiveness, or its ability to work in a variety of settings.

The ideal conditions of a community-based efficacy study generally involve the maximum achievable or optimal application of the intervention with intensive monitoring of all aspects of the application and outcomes. An intervention that does not yield the desired outcome under optimal trial conditions is unlikely to be useful in the far more variable and less-than-ideal conditions to be found in other communities where the intervention may be replicated. A nonefficacious intervention also will not merit the tremendous expense of a multisite study. Alternatively, an intervention shown to be efficacious under ideal conditions may not be feasible, replicable, or sustainable when applied in other communities under suboptimal conditions. Thus demonstrated efficaciousness is not the final word; there remains the need for effectiveness studies.

Effectiveness

An assessment of effectiveness includes a wider variety of conditions that an intervention is likely to encounter when broadly implemented. For an individual-level intervention this entails a variety of individuals. For example, will latex condoms (with known efficacy in blocking HIV transmission) reduce HIV transmission in a given population after factoring in the vicissitudes of

Table 16–1 The Number and Type of Study Units for Evaluating the Efficacy and Effectiveness of Interventions

Unit of Intervention	Individual (e.g., pharmaceutical)	Community (e.g., mosquito abatement)
Efficacy: Can the intervention work in isolated cases?	One or more persons	One community
Effectiveness: Does the intervention work in a variety of "real world" situations?	A population of people or a community	Multiple communities

product distribution, resistance to the adoption of new behaviors, and improper use? For a community-level intervention, the effectiveness is measured in a variety of communities. For example, will a program to lower STD infection rates by enhancing social capital (demonstrated as efficacious in one community) have a similar effect when applied in a variety of other communities?

If an intervention is shown to be ineffective, new questions arise. Might the intervention have worked if its implementation had been different; if it had been monitored more carefully; if it had been conducted in a different setting, under a different schedule, with different workers; or if any of a dozen other factors had been different? Unfortunately, researchers and health professionals generally do not have the luxury to conduct multiple effectiveness trials in various contexts. Thus an intervention that might be effective under other conditions is at risk of being discarded on the basis of a single study. The collection of copious information on the intervention application, or "process data," can mitigate against such an overly conservative conclusion. Process data help researchers understand why an intervention was ineffective or why it was effective. Because of the inherent difficulties of community trials, some have even argued that, following a demonstration of the efficacy of an intervention, research should turn to process evaluation in different settings with less emphasis on expensive outcome evaluation and the associated risk of rejecting an intervention on the basis of a single community trial (Fortmann et al. 1995).

Efficiency

The question of which of two or more effective interventions works best is a concern about efficiency. Which program works best in which conditions? Which program provides the optimal balance between cost and benefit? For example, how does clinic-based screening for sexually transmitted diseases (STDs) compare to using community groups to screen outside of the clinic setting in terms of cost and effect on the incidence of STDs in the community? Studies to answer ques-

tions of efficiency deal with concepts such as cost-benefit and cost-effectiveness. We do not describe these approaches in this chapter but we refer the reader to the text by P. Rossi and H. Freeman (1999) (Chapter 11: Measuring Efficiency) for an overview of these concepts.

STUDY DESIGNS

The aspects of study design we discuss in this section are the types of comparisons made to assess the relative effect of an intervention; the level of exposure to the intervention; sampling; approaches to dealing with confounding; approaches to minimizing information biases; and multilevel interventions and analyses.

Types of Comparisons

The types of comparisons made for assessing an infectious disease intervention depend principally on the unit of the intervention and the effects of interest. In Chapter 5, Study Design, Halloran identifies and diagrams four types of effect: direct, indirect, total, and overall. When an intervention is received by individuals in a community, as with a vaccine, the vaccinated people benefit directly from the vaccine, while the unvaccinated people benefit indirectly because of a decrease in the number of potentially infectious individuals as a result of the vaccination program. To isolate the direct effect of such a program, the incidence of infection among those receiving the intervention is compared with those in the same community not receiving the intervention. An estimate of the indirect effect is obtained by comparing the incidences of infection between those not receiving the intervention in the intervention community and those in another community that did not receive the intervention. The combined direct and indirect effects are estimated by comparing the incidence of infection among those receiving the intervention in the intervention community with the incidence among those in another community not receiving the intervention.

A comparison of the combined incidence of infection in the intervention community (i.e., a weighted average of those who received the intervention and those who did not) with the incidence in a community without the intervention yields an estimate of the overall effect of the intervention. This is simply a comparison of the incidences of two communities. Where the unit of intervention is at the community level, as with a mosquito abatement program, the only suitable comparison is between communities (i.e., overall effects).

In some instances the communities compared may actually be the same community at different points in time, once before the intervention and again sometime after initiation of the program. For example, trends in diarrhea rates after the installation of protected water sources for a village can be compared to rates in previous years, assuming that background effects are constant. An example of an individual-level intervention assessed in a community is the occurrence of infant illnesses before and after a program to increase breastfeeding (Wright 1998). Such data can be persuasive if consistent trends are seen over a prolonged time. If the outcome of interest is a disease that is reported through standard surveillance, then comparisons can be made with the rates in other communities to estimate whether any noted changes in the intervention community might be attributed to secular trends in the society at large.

As already noted, however, a study of a community-level intervention in a single community is equivalent to a measure of efficacy. An assessment of effectiveness, as we are using the term here, would require intervention implementation in several communities. In a multisite study, several communities receive the intervention and another several do not. The comparison communities may receive nothing more than they usually have, a placebo, or an alternative intervention. Measurements of the outcome are made before and after the intervention and the average change in the outcome among the intervention communities is compared to the average change among the other communities. Two programs aiming to lower the incidence of HIV and STD by lowering the community prevalence of STDs were conducted in eastern Africa. Each studied several communities and included several nonintervention communities (Mayaud 1997, Wawer 1999).

Individual-level interventions are sometimes conducted with a cross-over design, in which one group of participants receives the intervention while a second set receives another. At a predetermined midpoint, the interventions are switched between the two groups. Rates of infection are assessed in both groups before, at the midpoint, and at project end. A cross-over design provides reasonable guarding against the effects of secular change. This design may be difficult to implement for community-level interventions, however. Logistically, it would be complex to switch interventions. Politically, if one intervention were to appear to be more effective, acceptable, or popular, it would be difficult to replace it with another. There may also be a lag in time between an intervention and its effects. Such a lag in effect could be erroneously attributed to the intervention implemented after a cross-over.

Exposure

The risk of a new infection depends in large part upon the prevalence of infection in the community and thus the likelihood of exposure. The application of an efficacious intervention may be greater in one community compared to another, but if the prevalence of infection (i.e., the level of exposure) is markedly higher in the intervention community, the number of new infections will be elevated relative to what it would be if the infection prevalence were the same as in the nonintervention community, possibly leading to the false impression that the intervention is ineffective.

Exposure to the intervention can also vary in critical ways. By the time some interventions have progressed through stages of development and evaluation to where their efficacy is known, the general public is also aware of them and may have begun adopting them spontaneously. This is particularly true for interventions at the individual level that are readily accessible. The use of condoms for the prevention of STDs would be one example. Condoms were originally designed as a contraceptive and were widely available as such before they were promoted for disease prevention. Before studies were conducted to evaluate the effectiveness of condom campaigns to limit STD transmission, condoms were being promoted on the basis of their physical properties as a barrier to STDs (i.e., their efficacy in vitro). As more people adopted the use of condoms, intervention studies bore the onus of showing an advantage not only to a condom campaign over the absence of condoms in another community but of a campaign over and above the natural (and increasing) occurrence of "spontaneous" condom use.

Such spontaneous adoption of a behavior, referred to as a secular trend, has plagued even the best-funded and most well executed community trials of interventions against noninfectious diseases. In the Stanford Five-City Project to lower cardiovascular disease risk, changes in social norms toward low fat diets, exercise, and nonsmoking in many instances obviated the researchers' ability to demonstrate the effectiveness of the intervention components with statistical significance (Green 1995). Such trends are less of a problem where the intervention is not generally available, as with a new antibiotic or vaccine.

Sampling

In some instances, the outcome of interest is a disease that is reported as part of standard surveillance. In many developed countries, syphilis is one such disease. Theoretically, all diagnosed cases of the disease are reported. Thus the reported incidence represents the entire population of interest rather than a sample of the population. Where there is no sampling involved, it can be argued that it is inappropriate to assess the precision of the rate or the statistical significance of differences between two rates: the observed rate simply *is* the rate, and the observed difference simply *is* the difference. However, measures of precision, such as confidence intervals, apply when the researchers are making inferences beyond the populations from which data were collected, inferring the likely generalizability of findings to other communities not included in the study or to other times in the same community.

In reality, however, some diagnosed infections are not reported. Thus the data available do not accurately represent the occurrence of diagnosed infection in the entire population. Unreported cases are unlikely to occur randomly. More likely, they result from a particular clinician who regularly fails to report cases, or from many clinicians who choose not to report in certain instances. Underreporting is thus a systematic rather than a random error. It is inappropriate to assess the degree of systematic errors with statistical measures based on random errors, such as confidence intervals.

Reported cases of infection also do not account for undiagnosed or asymptomatic infections. Thus comparisons based on surveillance data must be interpreted strictly as differences in reported infections. Reported cases can provide a reasonable proxy for infections in some instances where the reporting is relatively thorough and resources for empirically measuring infection status are unavailable. Empirical measurement is made more feasible when it is conducted on only a sample of the population. Once sampling is applied, then estimates of precision (e.g., confidence intervals) are appropriate.

Changes in the occurrence of infection in a sample of the community can be assessed by testing the same people repeatedly (i.e., a cohort) or by testing a new sample each time (i.e., a series of cross-sectional samples). If the intervention is at the individual level, and the level of exposure each individual experiences can be assessed, then a cohort can provide the strongest evidence of a relation between the intervention and the outcome, provided there are not large discrepancies in the loss to follow up between the intervention and nonintervention groups. If a community-level intervention affects all members of the community to a fairly uniform degree, as would, say, a new protected source of water, then a series of cross sections may adequately reflect the experience of the community. Other factors also come into consideration when choosing between a cohort or serial cross sections. In some instances the need for anonymous rather than confidential data will obviate the ability to identify a cohort, and where a population is highly mobile, significant loss to follow up can occur in a cohort.

Confounding

Comparisons can be complicated by confounding of the effects of the intervention between the intervention and nonintervention communities. In essence, confounding is a type of bias where there is a systematic difference between the intervention and control communities in variables related to both the intervention and the measured outcome. Confounding can be reduced through restriction and adjustment, and in theory through randomization. Each approach has advantages and disadvantages.

With restriction, the observations are limited to those participants (or communities) who share a particular level of a confounding variable. For example, if community size is a confounder, the analysis may be restricted to communities within a particular population range. (For an example of this, see Kilmarx 1997). This restriction can be implemented during study enrollment if the confounder is known in advance. This approach eliminates the ability to evaluate the intervention in the communities excluded from the study. However, in some instances, the effect in the other communities may be of less interest or relevance, in which case the restricted enrollment is an appropriate cost-saving measure. If the confounding influence is determined after the data are collected, the restriction can be implemented by selecting particular participants out of the data set. If not anticipated with a large sample, this restriction can severely reduce the sample size and thus the ability to estimate intervention effects with precision.

When confounding is identified after the data are collected, it is more common to adjust for the confounder through stratified analysis or statistical modeling and thereby minimize the amount of discarded data. However, a small number of observations within one of the levels of the confounder can limit the statistical power of this approach. If the need to adjust is anticipated, the study enrollment can be manipulated to include the needed numbers of participants with particular characteristics. This is commonly known as matching. For example, in a community-level study, for each intervention community of a particular population size a control community of similar size can be enrolled. In a matched study, the effect of the matching variable on the study outcome cannot be estimated. In addition, overly restrictive matching criteria can make it very difficult to find and enroll participants with the desired criteria.

Regardless of efforts to adjust for identified confounders, variables that were not measured may also confound the data. Random assignment of the intervention to various communities is an approach that aims to overcome the influence of unforeseen and unmeasured confounders. The basic assumption is that the randomness of the assignment will lessen any systematic differences between the intervention and nonintervention groups. This would be true on average over many replications of identical community trials, but in the instance of a single community trial, randomization can fail. That is, the intervention and nonintervention groups can still differ from each other on some variables. Thus adjustment for confounding can still be necessary, though it is less likely than in a nonrandomized study.

Problems Resulting from Population Dynamics

Communities are constantly changing in their constituents. Babies are born into the community, some people die, others migrate in or out. The prevailing norms in attitudes and behaviors can change solely on the basis of changes in the people who make up the community. Where such changes are not balanced across the study communities, these dynamics can confound the effects of interventions. Moreover, infections can be brought into or taken out of a community as people enter and leave. For example, one town clamping down on prostitution may cause commercial sex workers to leave that town and move to another for business. The rate of an infectious disease in one community may be affected in part by the rate in neighboring communities because of the interactions among people between the communities. Analytic methods that take into account "autocorrelation" can control for the lack of independence between contiguous communities. Alternatively, communities can be selected for study that are not contiguous with each other. Although they will still be affected by the communities that surround them, they will be less affected by, and thus more statistically independent of, other communities in the study.

Information Bias

Systematic bias in the measurement of variables can occur for a multitude of reasons. Two means of minimizing information bias that are of particular relevance to intervention studies of infectious disease are *masking* and *placebos*.

If the researchers know which group is receiving the intervention, they may systematically look more carefully in the intervention communities for evidence of a positive effect. To preserve objectivity in a study where individuals are the unit of analysis, the researcher may therefore give to someone else the task of assigning participants to the intervention and nonintervention groups, and ask not to be informed (i.e., to be masked to) who is in which group. Masking is often associated with randomization, but randomization can be done without masking and masked assignment can be nonrandom if done by someone other than the researcher. Keeping the researcher masked is less feasible when communities are the unit of analysis. The effort required to elicit a measurable effect on a community is often substantial and difficult to conceal.

If study participants know whether they are receiving an intervention, they may alter their responses in an evaluation either in favor of or against the intervention. Masking study participants from knowledge of who is receiving the intervention is typically done by giving a placebo to the nonintervention group. To be effective, a placebo must be indistinguishable from the actual intervention. Where the intervention is a pill or a shot, this may be feasible. But where it is a community-level program, it is essentially impossible to provide a placebo program. Where masking is not feasible for either the participants or the researcher, the printouts of data analyses can be masked to reduce the possibility of subtle differences in data interpretation.

Multilevel Interventions and Analyses

We have presented here relatively straightforward interventions occurring either at the individual or community level. Some interventions work at multiple levels and thus require analyses that simultaneously account for the different units of analysis. For example, an intervention to prevent diarrheal disease may provide protected water supplies to a village (a group-level variable) and aim to influence villagers' attitudes and behaviors related to water use (individual-level variables). Multilevel modeling can accommodate both individual- and group-level variables simultaneously. We refer the reader to the text by Bryk and Raudenbush (1992) for more information on this technique.

An analysis of group- or community-level interventions can also be based on data collected from individuals in the group (see the description of contextual variables in the section on measurement). An example of this would be when bed nets are distributed to an entire village and data are collected from individuals regarding their actual use of the nets (or the actual condition of the nets) and their infections with malaria. However, the exposures and outcomes of individuals in a cluster (or "class") reflect some degree of interaction between the individuals. Thus the data do not represent fully independent observations. Corrections for "intraclass correlation" are available in some data analysis software programs such as SUDAAN and Stata.

MEASUREMENT

To evaluate *whether* an intervention has had its intended effect, researchers collect data on the occurrence of the outcome of interest. To understand *how* an intervention worked, data are collected on the process of intervention implementation. We describe here the measurement issues for both outcomes and processes in infectious disease community interventions.

Variables that measure some aspect of an entire community are of two general types, labeled by Susser (1994) as integral and contextual. An *integral variable* is one that affects essentially all members of the community, such as latitude, degree of rurality, and location on a highway (see, for example, Cook 1999). A *contextual variable* is one that is an aggregate of the values for individuals in the community. It might be the mean income of the residents, the ratio of males to females, or the occurrence of disease in the community. Outcome and process data can consist of both integral and contextual variables.

Infection Outcomes

Several stages in the natural history of infection can serve as outcomes that an intervention aims to affect, including infection incidence, duration of infection, disease, disability, and case fatality. The measurement of particular infections is addressed in Chapters 10–13. When an intervention is at the individual level, then the epidemiologic parameter of interest may be the difference in or ratio between the incidences or prevalences of infection in those receiving the intervention compared to those not receiving it. For an individual-level intervention the incidence is a summary measure of individual experiences. When the intervention is at the community level, the incidence reflects the experience of a single community. A community trial would then compare differences in a summary measure of the incidences (e.g., the mean incidence) between the intervention and the nonintervention communities.

When interpreted as the experience of a community, the incidence of infection is a relatively crude measure. The distribution of infection across other parameters of interest provides additional information. For example, individual infections can be mapped geographically according to the residence of the infected person or the location of exposure to provide information about the distribution of disease in the community (see, for example, Pierce, 1999). Factors affecting the geographic distribution can then be compared across communities. Similarly, comparisons of the distribution of infection across age groups, ethnicity, class, and gender can be informative. As this chapter was being written, there were at least two requests for research proposals from federal institutions for interventions to decrease the racial disparity of rates of disease (e.g., "Understanding and Eliminating Minority Health Disparities," RFA # HS-00-003, released October 1999 from the Agency for Health Care Policy and Research). In the instance of disparities, the difference in disease rates between various races in a given community would be the outcome of interest.

Intermediate Outcomes

The absence of an observed effect on infection is inconclusive evidence of the ineffectiveness of an intervention. An inadequately administered intervention will not be effective, and other factors acting differentially in the intervention and nonintervention communities (i.e., confounders) can cause the effectiveness to be underestimated or overestimated. The influences of these two contingencies are often monitored through process data, which are discussed in the next section.

An effective intervention may also be judged to be ineffective if evaluated prematurely. Interventions that require change on the part of individuals or communities obviously need to allow time for the natural processes of change. The transtheoretical model of behavior change holds that individuals progress through five stages: precontemplation (i.e., never thought of the change); contemplation (i.e., have considered the change); preparation (i.e., taking concrete steps to begin change); action (i.e., adopting the new behavior); and maintenance (i.e., incorporating the change into one's life style) (Prochaska 1997). Relapse to prior stages is also part of the normal process in this model. The time to progress through these stages will vary with the type of change and the culture in which it occurs. For example, in most cultures, adopting the use of a bed net for protection against mosquitoes will be more readily adopted than the use of condoms to prevent STDs, assuming there are no barriers to the availability of either. Cultural factors, such as an association between low social status and bed nets could greatly slow the adoption of bed nets. There is very little information about the amount of time for various behaviors to be adopted. Moreover, there is little information on stages of adoption of community-level changes.

An intervention may be quite effective in moving individuals or communities through stages of change. But an effect on infection rates may not be observable until there is a critical number of people or communities who proceed to the action and maintain stages. A measure of infection prior to this point would conclude inappropriately that the intervention is ineffective. For this reason it is important to collect information on behaviors and attitudes (e.g., contemplation) when an intervention entails individual change.

When a particular behavior has a known effect on transmission, as with compliance to a schedule of childhood vaccines, research may focus on the behavioral outcome alone, e.g., immunization coverage instead of infection rates. Often, though, both biologic and behavioral data are needed for a complete evaluation of an intervention. Some behavioral researchers have felt that biologic specimen collection is obtrusive and will decrease participation in research, while some clinical researchers have felt that behavioral information is superfluous, or that asking questions will also decrease study participation. However, recent research on such socially sensitive infections as HIV and STDs has demonstrated the feasibility of collecting both detailed behavioral data and biologic specimens. The feasibility of specimen collection has been enhanced by the development of home-based and self-administered procedures, such as urine-based tests for STDs. The combination of biologic and behavioral data maximizes the opportunities for explanatory analyses.

Intervention Processes

Process evaluation pertains to the implementation of the intervention and monitoring of potential confounders. The components of intervention implementation that are commonly measured include the quantity and quality of the intervention (referred to as output), the intervention acceptability, and implementation barriers. (For example, see Kroeger 1997.) The data for both process and outcome evaluation that were gathered for a community-level intervention based on dissemination and empowerment principles are listed in Table 16–2.

Output evaluation refers to the quantification of program activities. Outputs can include numbers of service providers trained, clients served, treatments or immunizations delivered, and preventive health brochures produced and distributed, to give but a few examples. Output evaluation assesses whether an intervention program is functioning at the intended level and thus whether the study can be regarded as an evaluation of the intervention efficacy or effectiveness.

The quality of an intervention may be reflected in such factors as the nature of a training program for people administering the intervention, the degree to which people understand a message in a mass media campaign, the actual use rates of condoms that have been distributed, and the reliability with which vaccines that require refrigeration are kept refrigerated.

Information on factors that can affect the outcome differentially in the intervention and nonintervention communities is also critical. If these are anticipated during the study design, then collection of data on these factors may be incorporated into the study schedule. However, unforeseen fac-

Table 16–2 Types of Outcome and Process Data Collected for the Evaluation of the Efficacy of a Community-Level Intervention* to Lower the Rate of Sexually Transmitted Diseases

Data Type	Information Collected
Outcomes	
Behaviors	• Household survey of the reported occurrence of the targeted behaviors, both before the survey and after 18 months of the intervention.
Disease	• Occurrence of cases of reportable STDs (syphilis, gonorrhea, chlamydia) during the six months prior to the intervention and six months following the intervention.
Institutional characteristics	• The competence of local institutions to deliver services in a culturally sensitive manner to the populations most affected by STDs. An institutional assessment instrument, consisting of interviews and observations, was developed and administered in four institutions both before and after the intervention.
Processes	
Attitudes	• Items in the household survey pertaining to attitudes about the targeted behaviors, such as intentions to engage in them in the future. Data on trends in attitudes allow researchers to monitor the progress through stages of change.
Behaviors	• The number and proportion of people seeking care for an STD in the county STD clinic within three days of symptoms. • The number and proportion of people seeking care for a potential STD in the county STD clinic following suspected exposure. • The number and proportion of people seeking care in the county STD clinic who reported using a condom during the last episode of sex.
Intervention activity (output)	• Qualitative interviews with the program staff (not LHAs) about the degree to which the selected LHAs have proven to match the desired criteria for LHAs. This information also enables the refinement of the selection process for any future LHA programs. • Evaluation of the training program for the LHAs. • Items in the household survey about interactions with LHAs and exposure to any other HIV or STD interventions during the six months prior to the intervention, and during the intervention. • Recall among the LHAs of the number and type of interactions they had with people about STD prevention. The data were collected through telephone conversations every four months with each LHA. • Field notes kept by the intervention coordinator about her own activities, conversations with the LHAs, the monthly meetings with the LHAs, meetings of the community advisory group, group activities conducted by the LHAs, and other miscellaneous meetings and events.
Intervention confounders and barriers	• Items in the household survey about exposure to any other HIV or STD interventions during the six months prior to the intervention, and during the intervention. • Clippings from the local newspaper reporting on the activities of local groups and institutions that might affect the targeted behaviors.
Empowerment among the lay health advisors	• Field notes reporting on the interactions of the LHAs with local institutions

*The intervention is a lay health advisor (LHA) program to disseminate skills, information, and attitudes about three behaviors, and to enhance social capital through the empowerment of the lay health advisors. The targeted behaviors were: (1) seeking care for a symptomatic sexually transmitted disease (STD) within three days of the symptoms; (2) seeking testing for a potential infection following suspected exposure to an STD, and (3) condom use with one's main sexual partner (Thomas 1998).

tors can also exert an influence. Some factors may be readily recognized as they occur and may even lend themselves to objective measurement. For example, researchers may be aiming to reduce the incidence of HIV through a program enhancing social cohesion. After initiating the intervention the researchers may observe that, apart from their program, neighborhood crime causes neighbors to join efforts to combat the crime (an expression of social cohesion). A crime wave that differentially affects nonintervention communities would thus dilute the observed effect of the program. However, the researchers could obtain crime statistics to document the influence of this factor on the study.

Other factors may not be immediately evident or measurable. The influence of such factors can sometimes be captured in field notes. These are notes that researchers and staff keep to document their own activities, observations, and thoughts during the course of the study. Upon reviewing these or sharing them with other researchers, the investigators can gain new insights. In one of my studies (Thomas, unpublished data), we subscribe to the local newspaper of the respective towns in our study. The project field director reads the papers and clips articles about events that may have an effect on the delivery of our intervention (a lay health advisor program) or the occurrence of the outcome (STD infection) in either the intervention or nonintervention community. Through this process we have learned about some STD prevention programs conducted by community-based organizations that we had not heard about through our other connections in the towns.

PRACTICAL CONSIDERATIONS

A population-based study can consist of a random sample of individuals scattered throughout a region. These individuals may never meet each other or know who else is in the study: they are largely independent of each other. In a study of a "community of memory" (i.e., geographically defined) the individuals who make up the community are interdependent; they talk to each other, help each other, and form political alliances. Gaining and maintaining the trust and cooperation of community members and leaders cannot be done with efficiency or expediency. There is no substitute for meeting with people in person, and relations are best maintained through frequent communications and meetings.

Enrolling a community in a study of an intervention that entails personal or community compliance is like entering into a committed relationship that requires frequent attention. One should not enter such a relationship lightly. Prior to enrolling a community in a study it is critical to gather some preliminary information, including the rates of the target condition or behavior to guide sample size determination, the likelihood of the community to accept and comply with the intervention, and the occurrence of other factors that may affect study implementation. A community with a very low rate of HIV incidence, for example, would not be suitable for assessing intervention effects on HIV acquisition, because any decrease in the incidence would nonetheless be a small change. A community embroiled in turf battles between health care providers may not be a good place to conduct an efficacy study of an intervention that depends on coordination between the providers. The barriers to intervention implementation in this instance would interfere with the assessment of whether the intervention *can* have the intended effect.

In a multisite study there are few efficiencies of scale when it comes to the required human interactions between researchers and the community. Thus in addition to the concerns of careful implementation of the intervention, and thorough and accurate evaluation, multisite intervention studies are enormously complex and very expensive. Furthermore, because multisite studies are conducted in what are ultimately selected populations that meet the requirements for compliance and follow up, and because their conduct is highly monitored, results may not be generalizable to other populations. These complexities and costs have led to cautious attitudes toward large outcome studies and a new appreciation for process evaluation of replications of efficacious interventions (Fortmann 1995, Koepsell 1995).

Since effectiveness studies of community-level interventions entail data collection in several communities, empirical data collection requires resources and organizational structures in excess of those for a standard individual-level, population-based study. Research components that need to be adapted from population-based designs include community-level information and outreach to prepare the target population; development of outreach and contact (it may be unrealistic to expect community participants to come to clinics or other central sites for follow up); logistic support for any worker or client travel and for transport of samples; and development of analyses appropriate to community and cluster designs.

Ethics

Ethical considerations pervade research. We mention here three issues of particular relevance to infectious disease community intervention studies: the testing of expensive interventions in poor communities; informed consent at the community level; and the provision of services in nonintervention communities.

Often, poor communities offer favorable conditions for research because they have a high incidence of the disease in question. Moreover, if the intervention is effective, the intervention communities reap the benefit of preventing or curing at least some infections, more than they would have prevented or cured without the intervention. But when the study is over, sustaining the intervention is likely to require resources that the community does not have. Critics of such studies argue that wealthy communities take unfair advantage of poor communities because the wealthy can afford the intervention but they do not have to take the risks involved in testing it. Regardless of the degree of wealth or power that a particular community selected for a study may have, the community must be informed of the potential benefits and risks of participation in the study. In studies where the intervention is at the individual level, informed consent is obtained from the persons who are study candidates. In the case of a community-level intervention, however, it is not clear who should be informed and from whom consent should be obtained. The community leaders may not represent the interests of some segments of the community. Researchers, and the institutional review boards that consider the ethics of their studies, must give considerable attention to the identification of and interaction with those segments of a community that will be most affected by an intervention. Several theoretical and practical aspects of ethical research in communities are addressed in a book edited by King, Henderson, and Stein (1999).

Whether those not receiving an intervention receive a placebo or another intervention for which the effect is known, they must be provided with at least the prevailing standard of care. There is currently debate about whether the standard should reflect what is locally available or what could be available under ideal conditions. This is an issue of particular pertinence in developing country settings. This question, which has arisen most notably with respect to provision of intensive AZT therapy for the prevention of mother-to-child HIV transmission, is very complex and has not been fully resolved. Detailed ethical review and comment by both in-country and donor human subjects committees are critical in the design of an international trial.

Some researchers question whether it is ethical to have a control community at all if the effects of the intervention being tested can be plausibly assumed to be good. (This ethical conundrum is portrayed in Sinclair Lewis's *Arrowsmith [1925]*). This view must be weighed against other ethical considerations such as the expenditure of valuable resources to implement a program that is not known to be effective. To mitigate against the former error, researchers can conduct interim analyses of the intervention effectiveness. If the intervention is found to be significantly more effective than the placebo or a competing strategy, the trial can be halted and the more effective measure provided to the nonintervention group.

SUMMARY

The most important distinction between a clinical trial conducted in a community and a community trial is the ability of the latter to study population-level factors through the comparison of communities. Population-level factors have been largely neglected in the study and control of infectious diseases in both observational and intervention

research. Thus they constitute an important
and exciting line of inquiry for future research. These studies will necessarily entail
the development of new measures that reflect groups rather than individuals and
analyses that do not assume independence
among individuals. The methodologic complexity and the sheer size of studies of multiple communities make them complex,
time-consuming, and expensive. The promise of developing and demonstrating the effectiveness of interventions working at new
levels depends, then, on the careful and
thorough implementation of preliminary
steps leading up to a full-scale trial comparing multiple communities.

Acknowledgment: The author thanks Maria J. Wawer,
MD for her input to this chapter.

REFERENCES

Bellah RN, Madsen R, Sullivan WM, Swidler A,
and Tipton SM. Habits of the Heart: Individ-
ualism and Commitment in American Life.
New York: Harper and Row, 1985.

Bryk AS, and Raudenbush SW. Hierarchical Linear Models: Applications and Data Analysis
Methods. Thousand Oaks, CA: Sage, 1992.

Cook RL, Royce RA, Thomas JC, Hanusa BH.
What's driving an epidemic? The spread of
syphilis in rural North Carolina along an interstate highway. Am. J. Public Health 89:
369–373, 1999.

Fortmann SP, Flora JA, Winkelby MA, et al.
Community intervention trials: reflections on
the Stanford Five-City Project experience.
Am. J. Epidemiol. 142:576–586, 1995.

Green SB, Corle DK, Gail MH, et al. Interplay between design and analysis for behavioral intervention trials with community as the unit
of randomization. Am. J. Epidemiol. 142:
587–593, 1995.

Gupta GR, and Weiss E. Women's lives and sex:
implications for AIDS prevention. Cult. Med.
Psychiatry. 17:399–412, 1993.

Halloran ME, and Stuchiner CJ. Study designs
for dependent happenings. Epidemiology.
2:331–338, 1991.

Kelly JA, Murphy DA, Sikkema KJ, et al. Randomised, controlled, community-level HIV-
prevention intervention for sexual-risk behaviour among homosexual men in US cities.

Community HIV Prevention Research Collaborative. Lancet. 350:1500–1505, 1997.

Kilmarx PH, Zaidi AA, Thomas JC, et al. Ecologic analysis of socio-demographic factors
and the variation in syphilis rates among
counties in the United States, 1984–93. Am.
J. Public Health. 87:1937–1943, 1997.

King NMP, Henderson GE, and Stein J. Beyond
Regulations: Ethics in Human Subjects Research. Chapel Hill: University of North Carolina Press, 1999.

Koepsell TD, Diehr PH, Cheadle A, and Kristal
A. Invited commentary: symposium on community intervention trials. Am. J. Epidemiol.
142:594–599, 1995.

Kroeger A, Meyer R, Mancheno M, Gonzalez M,
and Pesse K. Operational aspects of bednet
impregnation for community-based malaria
control in Nicaragua, Ecuador, Peru, and
Colombia. Trop. Med. Int. Health. 2:589–
602, 1997.

Last JM. A Dictionary of Epidemiology. 2nd ed.
New York: Oxford University Press, 1988.

Lewis S. Arrowsmith. New York: Harcourt,
Brace, and World, 1925.

Lomas J. Social capital and health: implications
for public health and epidemiology. Soc. Sci.
Med. 47:1181–1188, 1998.

Mayaud P, Mosha F, Todd J, et al. Improved
treatment services significantly reduce the
prevalence of sexually transmitted diseases in
rural Tanzania: results of a randomized controlled trial. AIDS. 11:1873–1880, 1997.

McLeroy KR, Bibeau D, Steckler A, and Glanz K.
An ecological perspective on health promotion programs. Health Educ. Q. 15:351–377,
1988.

Pierce RL, Thomas JC, Sparling PF, et al. An epidemiologic evaluation of the use of microbiologic tools for identifying gonorrhea infection
networks. Int. J. STD AIDS. 10:316–323,
1999.

Prochaska JO, Redding CA, and Evers KE. The
transtheoretical model and stages of change.
In: Glanz K, Lewis FM, Rimer BK, eds.
Health Behavior and Health Education. San
Francisco: Jossey-Bass Publishers, 1997.

Rossi PH, and Freeman HE. Evaluation: A Systematic Approach. 6th ed. Thousand Oaks,
CA: Sage, 1999.

Schuler SR, and Hashemi SM. Credit programs,
women's empowerment and contraceptive
use in rural Bangladesh. Stud. Fam. Plann.
25:65–76, 1994.

Strecher FJ, and Rosenstock IM. The Health Belief Model. In: Glanz K, Lewis FM, Rimer BK,
eds. Health Behavior and Health Education.
San Francisco: Jossey-Bass Publishers, 1997.

Susser M. The logic in ecological. I. The logic of
analysis. Am. J. Public Health. 84:825–829,
1994.

Thomas JC, Eng E, Clark M, Robinson J, and Blumenthal C. Lay health advisors: sexually transmitted disease prevention through community involvement. Am. J. Public Health. 88:1252–1253, 1998.

Wawer MJ, Sewankambo NK, Serwadda D, et al. Control of sexually transmitted diseases for AIDS prevention in Uganda: a randomised community trial. Rakai Project Study Group. Lancet. 353:1522–1523, 1999.

Whyte WF. Participatory Action Research. Newbury Park, CA: Sage, 1991.

Wright AL, Bauer M, Naylor A, Sutcliffe E, and Clark L. Increasing breastfeeding rates to reduce infant illness at the community level. Pediatrics. 101:837–844, 1998.

17

Evaluation of Immunization Programs

ROBERT T. CHEN and WALTER A. ORENSTEIN

Immunizations are among the most successful and cost-effective disease prevention interventions available (World Bank 1993). In the United States, the introduction of routine immunizations has greatly reduced the incidence of several vaccine preventable diseases (Table 17–1). Similar success in disease reduction has been demonstrated by immunization programs in many other countries (Acres 1985, Feery 1981). The World Health Organization's Expanded Programme on Immunizations (EPI), with assistance from the United Nation's Children's Fund (UNICEF) and other donors, has made great strides in extending these benefits to developing countries (WHO 1999). Immunizations permitted the global eradication of smallpox (Fenner 1988) and may do the same for poliomyelitis (Satcher 1999) and some other diseases. Interest in immunization programs continues to grow as countries attempt to improve the rational allocation of their scarce health resources. Developments in biotechnology and immunology offer the promise of new vaccines against many diseases old and new,

ranging from malaria to acquired immunodeficiency syndrome (AIDS) (Johnson 1999), including some noninfectious diseases like cancer (Greten 1999). In sum, immunization programs represent an impressive attempt by the human species, via science and social organization, to purposefully alter the ecology of certain infectious diseases in its favor. While some people may view this as hubris against nature (Illich 1976), most of us willingly accept that less disease is better.

Epidemiologic studies and principles, experimental and observational, play a critical role in guiding almost all steps of a successful immunization program (Begg 1990). Before licensure, a vaccine must demonstrate its safety and efficacy in phased clinical trials. After licensure, continued close monitoring of the vaccine's safety and effectiveness is needed, especially early on. But equally important to a vaccine's ultimate success is the close monitoring of the immunization program itself.

Surveillance for measurable indicators like vaccine coverage, disease incidence, and ad-

Table 17–1   Comparison of Maximum and Current Reported Morbidity Vaccine Preventable Diseases and Vaccine Adverse Events, United States, 1995

Disease	20th Century Annual Morbidity	1999*	Percentage Change
Diphtheria	175,885	1	−100
Measles	503,282	100	−100
Mumps	152,209	391	−99.7
Pertussis	147,271	7,298	−95.0
Polio (wild) (paralytic)	16,316	0	−100
Rubella	47,745	267	−99.4
Cong. rubella synd.	823	6	−99.3
Tetanus	1,314	42	−96.8
Invasive Hib disease	20,000[†]	254	−98.7
Vaccine adverse events	0[†]	11,827	

*Final totals of reported cases to the Centers for Disease Control.

[†]Estimated because no national reporting existed in the prevaccine era.

equacy of the cold chain provide the benchmarks for an immunization program to judge its progress. Rigor in design, conduct, and analyses of epidemiologic studies to understand the corresponding risk factors for nonvaccination, vaccine failure, and cold chain failure permits development of accurate and timely adjustments to immunization programs and policies to ensure their ultimate success. This review discusses the epidemiologic methods used in the various phases of an immunization program drawing largely, though not exclusively, on the experience in the United States.

PRELICENSURE

Clinical Trials

The goals of the prelicensure studies are to (1) identify a candidate vaccine, (2) show that the vaccine is safely tolerated in terms of local and systemic reactions ("safety"), and (3) demonstrate that the vaccine confers protection against the target disease ("efficacy"), either directly in terms of disease reduction, or indirectly, in terms of elicitation of protective antibodies. Prelicensure studies are carefully phased in design and conduct. Impressive progress in biotechnology during recent decades has revolutionized not only the capability to rapidly identify the causative organisms for new illnesses

(Barre-Sinoussi 1983) but also to engineer and produce vaccines that are potentially safer, more effective, easier to produce, and less costly (Woodrow 1997). This biotechnology revolution poses a tremendous challenge to the traditional "vaccine development system" to provide adequate and timely assessments so that maximum benefits might be reaped from these advances (Mahoney 1999).

After isolation and characterization of the causative organism for a disease, inactivation or attenuation permits the development of candidate vaccines (Levine 1997). Such candidate vaccines are tested in animals (Lee 1995) before advancing to phased human clinical trials. Phase I trials usually enroll 10–100 adult volunteers to assess initial safety tolerance and acceptable vaccine dosage in humans. Phase II trials seek to expand knowledge about the safety, optimal dose, route of administration, and schedule (primary series, and if needed, boosters) of the candidate vaccine. Sample sizes usually range from 25–1000 persons.

Phase III clinical trials aim to show that the candidate vaccine is efficacious in conferring protection on a targeted, at-risk population under controlled conditions (Halloran 1999). Safety issues are also examined to the extent the sample size (calculated primarily on efficacy considerations) and study duration permit. As with any clinical trial, issues such as case definition, case finding, trial design, and sample size must be considered carefully (Tackett 1997). Classically, a prospective, double-blind, randomized, controlled design in a closed cohort is used (Takala 1998, Steere 1998, Monto 1999). Occasionally, studies with an open cohort (Eskola 1987), historic controls (Fritzell 1992), or using a household secondary attack rate (Mortimer 1990) are used.

Based on a comparison of the disease incidence rate of vaccinated to unvaccinated individuals, the percentage reduction in disease as a result of the vaccination, or vaccine efficacy, is calculated (see the section on vaccine efficacy and vaccine effectiveness studies) (Greenwood 1915, Halloran 1999). Comparison of adverse event rates between the two groups is also made. The accurate ascertainment of cases and, therefore, the accuracy of the vaccine efficacy calculation depend greatly on which endpoint is selected for the trial.

The endpoint "case definition" may be a laboratory result, a clinical finding, or a combination of both. The goal of the immunization may be to prevent infection [e.g., by human immunodeficiency virus (HIV)], to prevent the final disease (e.g., AIDS), or prevent severe disease (e.g., pertussis). Whatever the endpoint chosen, the specificity of the diagnosis is more critical to the accuracy of the vaccine efficacy estimate than the sensitivity of diagnosis (Orenstein 1988). Clear thinking about these and other questions of interest in such trials will assist in appropriate study design on factors ranging from unit of observation, comparison groups, and level of information required (Halloran 1999). Many lessons can be learned from analyzing the similarities and differences in study design among recent acellular pertussis vaccine trials (Fine 1997). Another key goal of Phase III trials is to establish a laboratory correlate of human protection if possible (Siber 1997). This permits a potency test to be developed and standardized for use in prerelease testing as well as a surrogate endpoint in future trials.

Program Goals and Strategies

After a vaccine completes the clinical trials and licensure is imminent, several decisions must be made prior to its introduction into a vaccine program. The goals of the program and the appropriate strategies to reach them need to be defined. This in turn determines how widely the vaccine can be used, which target populations should receive it, and how rapidly use of the vaccine must be implemented. The disease control strategy is dictated to a large degree by (1) the *epidemiologic features of the disease* (Fine 1993), (2) the *adequacy of the health infrastructure*, and (3) the *resources available* (Mahoney 1999, Wenger 1999). Vaccination strategies in developing countries may confront difficult choices (Cutts 1999), especially in terms of the balance between a "vertical" (immunization is directed from the national level as a separate program) versus an "integrated" (where it is part of a comprehensive primary care effort) immunization program (Taylor 1997).

After considerable experience in disease control through immunization, elimination or eradication of the vaccine preventable disease (the absence of disease with, and without, a continuing threat of reintroduction, respectively) is usually considered. Special strategies like "ring immunization" for smallpox (Foege 1971) or "national immunization days" for poliomyelitis (Hull 1994) are usually required to move from simple disease control to eradication.

Disease surveillance data on age groups, special populations at risk, and illness complications are important in evaluating the cost and benefits of vaccination. Measles was a disease that affected many young children prior to school entry, while rubella was uncommon before school age (Langmuir 1962, Witte 1969). For example, surveillance data were useful in designing strategies for vaccination against measles and rubella. Thus measles immunization programs needed to target both children at one year of age and those in elementary school. In contrast, vaccination efforts against rubella could either be narrowly targeted at prepubertal females (Dudgeon 1985) or be used universally among all children of both sexes (Bart 1985). The latter strategy has been shown to be more successful as vaccine coverage is higher and provides greater herd immunity by reducing rubella transmission but at a higher cost (Gudnadottir 1985). When adequate surveillance data are available, different options for control strategies can be modeled mathematically to obtain quantitative insights in lieu of mere intuition (Anderson 1991).

Once a vaccine has shown good results in an *efficacy* study, an *effectiveness* study may be needed to determine if the use of the vaccine in routine public health practice is indicated. The initial evaluation of the Ty21a oral typhoid vaccine was done with a liquid formulation that was efficacious but was not suitable for mass production. Subsequent trials compared more convenient capsule and enteric-coated tablets against the liquid formulation (Clemens 1996). New health programs today frequently also need to demonstrate *cost-effectiveness*, as was done prior to licensure of the *Haemophilus influenzae* type b (Hib) polysaccharide (Cochi 1985), varicella (Lieu 1994, Scuffham 1999), and rotavirus (Tucker 1998) vaccines.

By necessity, Phase III trials must evaluate the efficacy of the candidate vaccine when used alone. With the increasing number of antigens routinely recommended in infants and children, simultaneous or combined administration of multiple antigens becomes increasingly attractive to minimize the costs and the number of health care visits and injections needed to complete the immunization series (King 1994). The safety and immunogenicity of simultaneous or combined vaccinations require careful evaluation to ensure there is no interference in immunogenicity or enhancement of adverse reactions (Williams 1995, Guess 1999). Such "Phase IIIb" trials are practical only if a serologic correlate of efficacy is established during the "Phase IIIa" trials (Cherry 1998), as was done for the licensure of combined DTP-Hib vaccines (CDC 1993). Should the goal of a trial be improving the efficacy of an existing moderately efficacious vaccine, large simple randomized clinical trials may be needed (Guess 1999).

POSTLICENSURE

Once a vaccine has been shown to be efficacious, it would be unethical to deliberately withhold it from certain populations in further studies to provide a comparison group. Therefore in contrast to prelicensure studies, which have the relative "simplicity" of experimental designs, most postlicensure studies are observational and epidemiologic in nature. Issues of confounding and bias, which were minimized by random allocation of vaccinated and unvaccinated persons in prelicensure studies, must now be either rigorously controlled for in study design and analyses, or taken into account during the interpretation of the data.

Because of the limits in size, duration, and population heterogeneity of preclinical trials, usually much remains to be learned about the characteristics of a vaccine and its optimal use after licensure. Rarer adverse events, such as vaccine-associated paralytic poliomyelitis (Henderson 1964), mumps vaccine–associated aseptic meningtitis (McDonald 1989), or rotavirus vaccine–associated intussusception (CDC 1999) may not have been detected earlier. Certain batches of vaccine may turn out to be unsafe or inefficacious, leading to improvements in manufacturing and quality control (Nathanson 1963). Some issues, such as duration of vaccine-induced immunity, may require decades to assess (Christenson 1994).

Surveillance on several aspects of an immunization program are needed to assure its optimal performance. This may include collection of data on vaccine distribution (Santoli 1999), adequacy of the cold chain (Gold 1999), adequacy of sterilization (Hutin 1999), the cost of the vaccine, public attitudes toward the importance of immunizations (Freeman 1999), barriers to immunizations and missed opportunities (Santoli 1998), characteristics of populations who have not been vaccinated (Reichler 1998), characteristics of remaining cases of disease (Jafari 1999), characteristics of persons experiencing adverse reactions (Stetler 1985), and even the number of lawsuits filed against vaccine manufacturers (Orenstein 1990). Special studies (e.g., epidemiologic, laboratory, combination or others) may be needed to better understand and solve potential problems identified by these immunization program surveillance/information systems. Health services research may be needed to identify the most effective way of improving immunization coverage rates (Shefer 1999).

As immunizations change the epidemiology of vaccine preventable diseases, the immunization schedule may require fine tuning based on risk data from outbreak investigations. This was the basis for changing the age for measles vaccination in the United States from 9 months upon initial licensure to 12 months, to 15 months (Orenstein 1986), then two doses (Markowitz 1989). A large outbreak in Greece showed the hazards of immunizing against rubella without a clear planned strategy (Panagiotopoulos 1999). Modeling studies may then be used to better analyze strategy options (Rohani 1999). Ad-

ditional cost-effectiveness studies may be needed to garner continued program support (Margolis 1995). Serosurveys may be used to assess any major gaps in immunity that could result in future outbreaks (Evans 1980).

A sophisticated surveillance system is also needed because of the dynamic nature of the relationship between (1) disease incidence, (2) vaccine coverage, and (3) vaccine adverse events as an immunization program progresses from preimplementation to final disease elimination/eradication (Fig. 17–1). Information about at least these three variables is needed by health authorities with responsibilities for weighing the costs, risks, and benefits of an immunization program and recommendations for the use or discontinuation of a vaccine. After sustained control, the cumulative burden of the vaccine-induced illnesses may exceed that from the wild disease itself. The United States Advisory Committee on Immunization Practices (ACIP) recommended that routine smallpox vaccination (CDC 1971) and use of oral polio vaccine (CDC 1999) be discontinued prior to global eradication of their target diseases. To assure the correct decisions are made, the information system needed will

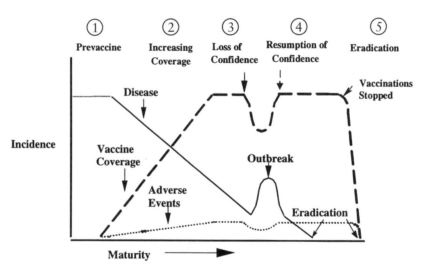

Figure 17–1. Evolution of immunization program and prominence of vaccine safety. Source: Chen 1994b.

have to be tailored to each phase. At all times, both surveillance and special studies are needed. However, the level of sophistication required of both types of information generally increases with each phase.

SURVEILLANCE OF VACCINE PREVENTABLE DISEASES

General Issues

Surveillance systems differ from special studies in that they are usually designed to monitor trends, detect and describe problems, and establish hypotheses to be tested in more refined research designs (Thacker 1988). Surveillance systems are ongoing, limited data are collected on each case, and data analysis is traditionally straightforward. In contrast, special studies are usually designed to test specific hypotheses and are usually time limited, data collection can be complex, and analyses are often sophisticated.

All passive surveillance systems tend to generate incomplete data. Cases of disease reported to surveillance systems are likely to reflect a subset of all cases, and they may not provide an unbiased representation of the total. For example, reports of pertussis cases tend to include persons with the most severe disease. About 40% of the pertussis cases reported to the Centers for Disease Control and Prevention (CDC) were hospitalized (CDC 1995), compared with less than 10% in community-based studies (Royal 1981). Despite underreporting and other potential biases, surveillance data have been remarkably useful in serving the needs of public health programs (Teutsch 1994).

Analysis of age-group-specific measles surveillance data during the 1989–1990 measles outbreak pointed to the importance of unimmunized preschool children as the main risk group (Gindler 1992). A gradual increase in pertussis incidence after a long historic decline may reflect waning immunity in adolescents and adults due to decreased circulation of pertussis mostly from a successful vaccination program (Guris 1999). Analysis of surveillance data may point out

areas for special vaccination campaigns. Examination of the U.S. measles surveillance data from 1980 to 1989 showed that measles was endemic in only 0.5% of the nation's 3137 counties (Hersh 1992). Measles cases from these counties were probably responsible for much of the measles transmission during these years. These data added impetus to programs targeted at age-appropriate immunization of children by age two in the United States (NVAC 1991).

Innovative analysis of surveillance data may provide insight into the pathogenesis of vaccine preventable diseases. The lack of expected increase in the interepidemic period with increasing pertussis vaccination levels led Fine and Clarkson (Fine 1982) to hypothesize that pertussis vaccine was more effective in protecting against disease than against infection. This hypothesis has since been supported by other studies (Blackwelder 1991). The rapid disappearance of diphtheria (Chen 1985) and Hib (Adams 1993) relative to population vaccination levels suggests that, in addition to individual protection, immunization may play a role in reducing carriage of pathogenic organisms. Comparison of measles immunization rates, obtained via retrospective school surveys with measles attack rates among census tracts in Milwaukee, Wisconsin, provided insight on the level of herd immunity necessary to halt transmission (Schlenker 1992).

Sources of Data

Most surveillance systems generally rely upon case reports by physicians, other health care workers, or laboratories. This is particularly true for diseases like measles and mumps with characteristic clinical symptoms and signs and for which few cases are hospitalized and few attempts are made to confirm cases through the laboratory. School-based surveillance, usually based on the school nurse, needs to identify reasons for absenteeism. Frequently such reports are delayed because ill students may otherwise escape detection until their return to school. This can impede control efforts if vaccinations need to be started at the time of the first case.

For surveillance of diseases like invasive *Haemophilus influenzae* type b disease, laboratories and hospitals can be more useful because most cases of invasive illness are both hospitalized and confirmed via the laboratory (Jafari 1999). Laboratory surveillance is also important for pertussis, rubella, and hepatitis B, because of the difficulties in making the clinical diagnosis. Mortality records are used for evaluating health impact and the characteristics of persons who die with a given disease. A special surveillance system including deaths registered in 121 U.S. cities each week is used to determine the existence of an epidemic of influenza by comparing the reported proportion of total deaths due to pneumonia and influenza with expected proportions based on nonepidemic years (Choi 1981).

In the United States, the Council of State and Territorial Epidemiologists (CSTE), in collaboration with the CDC, develops the list of diseases recommended to be reported by states to the CDC (Roush 1999). Canada and most other countries have a similar process (Advisory Comm 1991). Among the vaccine preventable diseases, cases of diphtheria, tetanus, pertussis, polio, Hib (invasive disease), measles, mumps, rubella, congenital rubella syndrome, hepatitis A, and hepatitis B are currently officially reportable via health departments of the states and the District of Columbia on a weekly basis to the CDC. For selected diseases like measles, pertussis, tetanus, polio, additional details on each case are gathered via a supplementary surveillance form by county and state health staff. In addition, there are special surveillance systems for Hib and hepatitis B disease. As diseases like varicella become newly vaccine preventable (CDC 1999), new surveillance systems will be needed to better monitor the impact of immunizations, or lack thereof.

Case Definitions

Case definitions vary with the goals of the surveillance system. For example, prior to beginning a vaccination program or during its early phases, all physician reports are usually accepted (i.e., the case definition is a physician diagnosis). However, as disease incidence decreases and a greater degree of disease control is achieved, individual cases are investigated by health department personnel, and case definitions tend to become more precise. For example, the case definition for measles can also require laboratory confirmation or epidemiologic linkage to another case meeting the same clinical criteria. Clinical information from reported suspected cases of poliomyelitis is now reviewed by a panel of three experts before being accepted as a case (Strebel 1992). These stricter definitions increase the predictive value positive of reported cases. The predictive value positive would normally fall as disease incidence decreases unless stricter definitions are used.

The current case definitions used by the CDC for notifiable vaccine preventable diseases have been published (CDC 1990). Similar definitions have been elaborated by Canada (Advisory Comm 1991). Most of these definitions are based on clinical and epidemiologic experience; some have been evaluated for sensitivity and specificity during special investigations. For example, outbreak investigations in Wisconsin, Delaware, and Missouri revealed that a case definition for pertussis of cough for 14 or more days duration was 81% to 92% sensitive and 58% to 90% specific in the outbreak setting (Patriarca 1988b, Strebel 1993). The ideal sensitivity and specificity of case definitions depend upon the outcomes desired from surveillance. For controlling outbreaks, particularly during disease elimination and eradication, high sensitivity with rapid reporting becomes important for early action. For studies, such as vaccine efficacy evaluation, specificity assumes greater importance (Orenstein 1988).

Disease Registries, Sentinel and Universal Surveillance

Because of the expense and other difficulties of conducting large-scale active surveillance on an entire population, some programs target sentinel sites for special emphasis. For example, the CDC has conducted intensive surveillance and investigations of hepatitis in at least four sentinel counties (Alter 1987). This surveillance suggested that hepatitis B disease was underreported by 50%. In addition, the comprehensive nature of the surveillance allowed greater confidence to be placed in the data that showed decreasing prominence of persons citing homosexual behavior as a risk factor and increasing prominence of intravenous drug abusers and persons engaging in heterosexual activity (CDC 1988).

Well-developed sentinel surveillance systems are used by some European countries to provide information on disease occurrence (Chauvin 1998), though Europe-wide harmonization is still distant (Salisbury 1999). The World Health Organization's Expanded Programme on Immunization (EPI) has encouraged many developing countries to adopt sentinel systems in which reports are accepted from selected providers within a community, generally the large hospitals (Cutts 1993). Such sentinel systems, while generally inexpensive, may give biased information depending upon how representative the sites are of the general community. For example, hospital-based systems are more likely to report sicker children who tend to be younger and unvaccinated than cases occurring in the community at large. Nevertheless, even these surveillance data are useful for evaluating trends and estimating the initial impact of the vaccination program (Chen 1994c). Such systems may become less useful as wide vaccine use reduces disease incidence.

Special registries may be maintained for rare diseases of special interest. The CDC maintained a registry that compiled data on women vaccinated with rubella vaccines within three months of conception (CDC 1989). The women were followed prospectively to determine whether vaccination was associated with adverse pregnancy outcomes. In 1989, the registry was discontinued when adequate data had been accumulated to indicate that the risk of congenital rubella syndrome (CRS) following vaccination, if any, was less than 1.2%. A similar registry has been started to follow pregnan-

cy outcomes after varicella vaccination (CDC 1996). A subacute sclerosing panencephalitis (SSPE) registry was created to determine both whether vaccination against measles prevented the disease or whether it could be caused by vaccination (Modlin 1977). These data showed that SSPE had virtually disappeared from the United States (Bloch 1985).

Evaluation

Guidelines for evaluation of public health surveillance systems have been developed (Klaucke 1994). Such evaluations consist of determining usefulness, simplicity, flexibility, acceptability, sensitivity in detecting the true number of cases or epidemics, positive predictive value of reported cases (i.e., the proportion of cases reported that are true cases), representativeness of reported cases, timeliness of reporting, and cost-effectiveness. With regard to immunization, major questions have revolved around sensitivity and predictive value positive.

Estimates of underreporting are possible for diseases like measles that are essentially universal childhood infections. Prior to the licensure of measles vaccines in 1963, approximately 400,000 to 500,000 cases were reported annually at a time when roughly four million children were born each year (Langmuir 1962). Thus the 400,000 to 500,000 cases reported represented approximately 10% of the total cases occurring in the United States. Surveillance data were supplemented by special population-based studies which corroborated the validity of the surveillance information (Witte 1969).

Once the disease burden decreases as a result of vaccination, however, the total remaining burden is difficult to estimate. Particular use has been made of the Chandrasekar and Deming method of estimating the reporting efficiency for various vaccine preventable diseases in the United States (Sutter 1990, 1992, Prevots 1994, Cochi 1989). This method requires two independent surveillance systems detecting the same illness and measures the degree of overlap to estimate the total burden. It is similar to capture-recapture systems used to estimate animal populations. The efficiency of measles no-tification in England and Wales has been estimated to be 40%–60%, while that of pertussis is 5%–25% (Clarkson 1985). Ef-ficiency of vaccine adverse events reporting can be evaluated if population-based esti-mates based on prior studies are available (Rosenthal 1995, Verstraeten 2000). Predic-tive values positive studies use gold stan-dards such as laboratory confirmation to evaluate the proportion of cases, given a particular case definition, that are laborato-ry confirmed (Patriarca 1988b).

SEROLOGICAL SURVEILLANCE

Immunization programs aim to substitute vaccine-induced immunity for immunity in-duced by disease. Neither history of disease or vaccination may be an accurate marker of true immunity. Therefore, if a serologic correlate of protective immunity against a vaccine preventable disease exists, periodic serologic surveys are useful in (1) evaluating the success of an immunization program, and (2) identifying groups with low immu-nity that might require changes in vaccina-tion strategy (Evans 1980, Bottiger 1998).

The United Kingdom switched from a se-lective to a universal rubella immunization policy after results of routine antenatal test-ing showed an unacceptably high rate of sus-ceptibility (Miller 1991). Several countries have conducted special measles vaccination campaigns based on results of serosurveys (Agocs 1992), especially when combined with mathematical modeling (Babad 1995). Serosurveys in recruits have been used to refine immunization policy in the military (Kelley 1991). Serosurveys in all countries with longstanding childhood vaccination programs against diphtheria have shown a high proportion of adults to be susceptible (Chen 1985). Not surprisingly, adolescents and adults constitute a high proportion of diphtheria cases in the recent resurgence in Russia and Ukraine (Hardy 1996). A Euro-pean Sero-Epidemiological Network has been established to coordinate data collec-tion on immunity to vaccine preventable diseases (Osborne 1997).

As with all surveys, representativeness of the sample, participation rate, and definition of "protective titers" (Chen 1990) are criti-cal to interpreting the results. More impor-tant, requirements for obtaining, shipping, and laboratory assay of serologic specimens make serosurveys relatively expensive. These factors plus the relative slow change in pop-ulation immunity profiles suggest that sero-surveys need not be conducted frequently [e.g., decennial National Health and Nutri-tion Examination (NHANES) in the United States (McQuillan 1990) versus annual].

Occasionally, in addition to serosurveys, specially designed immunogenicity trials are critical to assessing immunization strategy. An increasing proportion of children in the United States, for example, responded to the measles vaccine at younger ages because of lower levels of passively acquired maternal measles antibodies (Markowitz 1996). This is because more and more mothers derive their immunity from vaccine rather than wild measles. This resulted in lowering the age of first measles vaccination from 15 to 12 months. A trial of diphtheria toxoid boost-ers in Ukrainian adults revealed that many persons 30–49 years of age missed both their primary vaccinations and exposure to natural diphtheria, and therefore needed a complete primary series, not just a booster dose to protect them during the recent diph-theria resurgence (Hardy 1996).

VACCINATION COVERAGE

Because no vaccine is perfectly efficacious, vaccination levels are not the same as im-munity levels. Once rates of primary and secondary vaccine failure are known from special studies, an estimate of immunity levels is possible in conjunction with knowl-edge of the vaccination levels. In practice, because primary and secondary vaccine fail-ure rates are fairly low for most routinely recommended vaccines, vaccination levels provide a reasonable measure of the prog-ress of a vaccination program. Vaccination coverage can be monitored via direct meas-urement of vaccination levels, or estimated indirectly by several ways including (1) surveys, (2) reports of doses of vaccine administered, and (3) reports of doses of vaccine distributed. As vaccine coverage reaches high levels, indirect measurements may not provide the accuracy and precision needed to improve the marginal coverage. Accurate ascertainment of vaccination history is also critical to any epidemiologic study of vaccines, as this represents the "exposure." The ability to ascertain accurate vaccination history in U.S. children is increasingly threatened owing to an increasingly complex immunization schedule, diversity of combination vaccines used, and high turnover among health plans (Weniger 1998), and calls for innovative solutions like barcodes, standard peel-off labels (Schwartz 1998), and computerized immunization registries (Wood 1999).

Direct Measurement (Vaccination Registry, School Entry Census)

Since 1978, national immunization levels in the United States have been assessed at school entry. Each state Health Department reports the results of its assessment to the CDC where a national estimate is calculated. School enterer levels are not measured by sample survey but represent a census of the immunization status of *all* enterers. Each school must review the immunization status of each new enterer because of laws requiring specified immunizations prior to admission to school. Data from each school are usually compiled by school nurses or other school officials from immunization records on file for each student. State immunization program personnel perform sample validation surveys to confirm the school reports (Eddins 1993).

The major advantage of this approach is that coverage levels are based on records rather than parental recall. Since many parents do not have immunization records of their children at home, persons doing telephone surveys, or even home visits, would have to list persons without records as unknown or rely on parental recall. Another advantage of the school enterer assessment is that to the degree it achieves a complete census, there is no potential bias from sampling.

The major disadvantage is that immunization levels are measured several years after vaccination should have been administered. A second problem relates to validity of the records. Most states require physician confirmation of immunization status. However, if physicians rely on parental recall rather than records to certify immunization, falsely high immunization levels may be reported. Finally, assessment of newly recommended infant vaccinations like Hib and hepatitis B on a timely basis are not possible from examining school enterer vaccination data.

In the United States, requirements for recording of vaccinations by providers was legislated in the late 1980s. These requirements plus the increasing automation of health care practice have led several health maintenance organizations (HMOs) to fully computerize their vaccination records (Chen 1997). This permits easy, timely assessment of vaccination levels by physician, by clinic, for the health maintenance organization, as well as for recall (Payne 1993). Several regional computerized immunization registries are under development in the United States (Wood 1999). In England and Wales, computerized preschool child registers combined with vaccination histories have permitted more rapid, frequent, and accurate assessment of vaccine coverage in almost all districts (Begg 1989). This system recently detected a drop in measles vaccination uptake after new safety allegations (CDSC 1998).

Indirect Measurement—EPI 30 Cluster Survey

Surveys are commonly used to provide a more efficient estimate of vaccination levels. Perhaps the best known is the 30 cluster two stage stratified random survey initially developed for use during the smallpox eradication program (Henderson 1973). This method has since been used widely in World Health Organization's EPI as a "gold standard" (with validity generally ±10% of the actual levels) to validate administrative estimates of vaccine coverage (Henderson 1982). It has also been adapted to examine rates of neonatal tetanus deaths and polio lameness (Cutts 1988). Coverage Survey Analysis System (COSAS), a software to rapidly analyze the results of EPI 30 cluster surveys, has been developed (Desve 1994).

The EPI survey has been criticized because the sampling frame is not based on households but a convenience sample of the target population living in close proximity to the selected starting point (Brogan 1994). Evaluation of the 30 cluster method, however, has shown it to be generally accurate within the desired 10% of the true levels, though it is particularly insensitive to pockets of unvaccinated persons (Lemeshow 1985). This can be ameliorated by expanding the number of clusters to what the resources permit (Turner 1996). The advantage of the 30 cluster method includes its relative ease of use with moderate training. Its standard methodology permits aggregation of results from smaller geographic areas.

A big disadvantage of the EPI survey is that the method requires a sampling frame for the population of interest. Any census data available may be woefully out-of-date, especially in rapidly growing urban areas in developing countries (Ferrinho 1992). Home vaccination records may be limited or lost. Substantial logistical resources may also be needed for the survey team to travel to remote locations selected for study. The EPI survey can be particularly difficult to interpret if a substantial proportion of respondents lack accurate vaccination records. This problem is likely to worsen as EPI adds more vaccines, requiring greater recall by parents. The utility of the EPI survey is also reduced at higher coverages since its low precision cannot detect smaller increases in coverage. Techniques for improving the accuracy and precision of the cluster survey method have been proposed (Brogan 1994, Turner 1996).

Indirect Measurement—Other Surveys

The United States has tried a variety of approaches to estimating vaccination levels among preschool children, none of which are entirely satisfactory. From 1959 to 1985, an annual survey of households to determine immunization levels for all key age groups (United States Immunization Survey, USIS) was performed (published and unpublished data. US Immunization Survey Reports, Division of Immunization, CDC, Atlanta, Georgia, 1959–1985). Beginning in 1972, the data were collected principally by telephone interview. Most of the answers were based on parental recall and the results were generally substantially lower than the results of the school enterer assessments. In 1979, a question on whether parents were reading from records was added. Vaccination levels based upon the approximately one-third of respondents with records more closely approximated results from the school enterer assessments (Eddins 1982). Because of concerns about the accuracy and cost of the USIS, it was abandoned after 1985.

The continuing need for timely data on national vaccination levels by age two, however, led to resumption of such surveys in 1991 via the National Health Interview Survey (NHIS), using household interview of parents (CDC 1994). The most difficult problem for the NHIS was the lack of validity of parental history. In general, parents tended to underestimate the number of doses of multidose vaccine their child received and overestimate single dose vaccines (e.g., measles). When asked whether their child is up-to-date, however, parents tend to overestimate coverage (Goldstein 1993). To compensate for these problems, beginning in 1992, a spontaneous response of "my child is up-to-date" was accepted and children with unknown history were excluded. These changes caused estimates to correlate better with other survey results. Beginning in 1994, parental responses are verified with providers. Preliminary data for the first two quarters of 1994 suggest such verification will generally raise coverage by about 5% (CDC 1995).

In 1994, the National Immunization Survey was also initiated in the United States. Using random digit dialing technology to locate eligible children, this survey collects data quarterly to estimate immunization coverage in 19–35-month-old children in all 50 states and 28 large urban areas (CDC 1995, 1999). Consent is obtained from the interviewee to validate the vaccination history with the provider. Data are adjusted for children from households without telephones based on NHIS data (CDC 1996). This survey has become the standard means for measuring coverage in the United States (Orenstein 1999).

Other approaches to measuring preschool levels have included statewide follow up of a sample of children at two years of age who were selected from state birth certificates (Hutcheson 1974). This technique also was abandoned in most states because response rates were frequently low, often less than 50%, casting concerns on the validity of the results. More recently, most states began measuring immunization levels retrospectively using data obtained at school entry. Using date specific information, immunization personnel calculate immunization levels for these enterers as of the date of their second birthday (CDC 1992).

Guidelines and software for assessing vaccination levels of the two-year-old population in clinic settings have also been developed (NIP 1994). Standards for definition of a two-year-old, active versus inactive files, age markers for assessing vaccination levels, definition of "up-to-date" and complete vaccination levels, and sampling of clinic charts may permit comparisons of clinics within and between states. Such routine assessment and feedback of vaccination rates (CDC 1996) combined with reducing "missed opportunities" for vaccinations (Szilagyi 1996) have been shown to be highly effective in raising and sustaining high vaccination rates. Because the increasingly complicated childhood vaccination schedule (CDC 2000) will increase the difficulty of accurately ascertaining vaccination history via interview, computerized immunization registries are increasingly looked to as the answer for timely and accurate assessment of vaccine coverage (Wood 1999).

Indirect Measurement—Administrative Estimate, Biologics Surveillance, and Other Approaches

If the number of doses of vaccine administered and the number of children in the target age group (e.g., number of surviving infants) are known, an inexpensive "administrative" estimate of vaccine coverage can be calculated. Again, if the same method is used everywhere, then aggregation of data is possible. This is the method used routinely by World Health Organization's EPI to estimate vaccine coverage (Cutts 1999). This method is most useful when the great majority of vaccinations are performed in government-financed clinics (e.g., most developing countries) and accurate denominator data on the population at risk are known. Commonly, however, these results are higher than actual coverage, as the census data used to estimate denominators tend to be low.

Since 1962, the CDC has received data from vaccine manufacturers concerning the number of doses of vaccines they distributed minus the number of doses returned (published and unpublished data, US Biologics Surveillance, National Immunization Program, CDC, Atlanta, Georgia, 1962–1996). Data on the "net doses" of vaccines distributed have been helpful in tracking use of various types of measles vaccines. Biologics data have also been useful in tracking DTP and DTaP use and confirming the greater safety profile of DtaP postlicensure (Rosenthal 1996). The advantage of the biologics surveillance system is that data become available relatively rapidly. If school entry data were required, it would have taken about five years to obtain any information on infants born and immunized following the onset of the adverse publicity.

In the United States, about 60% of the childhood vaccines are purchased by the government via annual negotiated contracts with the vaccine manufacturers (Orenstein 1999). A database recording purchases from this contract also provides an alternative source of denominators. The major uses of these data have been in monitoring the proportion of the population served by the public sector and in calculating rates of adverse events reported following vaccination in the public sector.

DISEASE SURVEILLANCE

The ultimate purpose of immunization is to prevent disease and complications of disease. Surveillance data on reported cases are critical to determine whether the program is having an impact, to assess why disease is still occurring, to evaluate whether new strategies are necessary, and to detect problem areas and populations that require more intensive program input.

Disease surveillance systems initially need to be simple. Physician diagnosis is usually the case definition, and reported information may include date of onset or report, age, and place of residence. Such limited data have been useful to demonstrate the marked impact of vaccination on disease incidence and for analyzing how best to reduce remaining morbidity. For example, surveillance data were used to develop policies to enhance rubella vaccination of postpubertal populations in the United States (Cochi 1989).

Surveillance data were instrumental in the spread of regulations to require vaccination for schoolchildren in the United States. Beginning in the mid 1970s, surveillance data clearly showed that states without laws requiring vaccination at school entry had 1.7- to 2.0-fold higher incidence rates of reported measles than states with laws (Orenstein 1978). This information was extremely useful in the universal adoption of school enterer requirements by showing legislators that laws could lead to significant impact. By the late 1970s, the epidemiology of measles had changed. Cases were more prominent in junior high and high school students (CDC 1982). These students were not covered by the recently enacted school enterer laws, since they had already been enrolled when such regulations went into effect. This led to adoption of comprehensive laws covering all students, kindergarten through 12th grade.

Surveillance data showed such states had lower incidence rates for measles than other states and led to adoption of comprehensive laws by most states (Robbins 1981).

An analysis of reported mumps cases by age and by state demonstrated that the marked increases in incidence were due to failure to vaccinate large numbers of older children and adolescents rather than to vaccine failure (Cochi 1988). The highest incidence rates were in states without comprehensive school laws requiring mumps immunization. If vaccine failure were the predominant concern, increased incidence should have occurred in all states. Thus evaluation of the role of vaccine failure was possible without any data on vaccination status of cases. More recently, an analysis of measles surveillance data and religious and philosophical exemption status of the cases showed that such exempters were at 35-fold increased risk of measles compared to nonexempters (Salmon 1999).

Case Investigations

As programs mature and cases become more uncommon, surveillance tends to move from simply the passive collection of limited data on cases to more sophisticated individual case investigations by health department personnel. During these investigations, staff generally collect relevant clinical and laboratory data as well as information on disease complications, hospitalizations, vaccination status, and other desired information such as potential sources and contacts of the case. Health Department personnel may assist in collecting critical laboratory specimens such as acute and convalescent phase sera or providing transport media for bacterial and/or viral cultures. In the United States, special case investigation forms were used historically for congenital rubella syndrome, diphtheria, tetanus, pertussis, and hepatitis B. Detailed information is collected on individual measles and polio cases. More recently, electronic systems to compile this information directly have been developed. These data are used to analyze cases in greater depth particularly with regard to health impact and problems with vaccination. The advent of molecular epidemiologic techniques has added new insights into geographic spread of vaccine preventable diseases (Rico-Hesse 1987).

A major question in control of vaccine preventable diseases is whether a given case represents a failure of implementation of the vaccine strategy (a preventable case), or failure of the strategy (a nonpreventable case). For example, a preventable case of measles is disease in someone who was eligible for vaccine but was unvaccinated.

In the past, such persons must have been born after 1956, be at least 16 months of age, be a U.S. citizen, have no medical contraindications against measles vaccination, have no religious or philosophical exemptions to vaccination under state law, and have no evidence of measles immunity (CDC 1983). Measles immunity was defined as documented evidence of prior physician-diagnosed disease, receipt of live vaccine on or after the first birthday, or laboratory evidence of immunity. Analyses of cases by preventability status played a major role in new policy recommendations for more aggressive revaccination efforts. In the mid-late 1980s, only a minority of cases were preventable, and especially among school-age children, vaccine failure was the predominant reason for nonpreventability (Markowitz 1989). Analyses of large school-age outbreaks in 1985 and 1986 (≥ 100 cases) reported through the measles surveillance system demonstrated as many as 69% of cases in such outbreaks were appropriately vaccinated with one dose of measles-containing vaccine. Of the school-age cases in these outbreaks, a median of 71% were vaccinated, ranging up to 90%. Case reports, many of them initiated by physicians, played a crucial role in recommendations for a routine two-dose schedule for measles and for more aggressive outbreak revaccination efforts (CDC 1989). In contrast, the oubreaks during the 1989–91 resurgence occurred largely among preschool unvaccinated black and Hispanic children residents of large inner cities (Gindler 1992). This resulted in a successful special initiative to raise vaccine coverage in preschool children (National Vaccine Advisory Comm 1991, Orenstein 1999).

Outbreak Investigation

Disease outbreaks in a vaccinated population can raise doubts as to the efficacy of the vaccine and the vaccination program (Cutts 1990, Agocs 1992, Chen 1994, 2000, Hennessey 1999). Such outbreaks may result from accumulation of susceptible persons from (1) lack of vaccination, (2) primary vaccine failures (persons vaccinated but not immunized), and/or (3) secondary vaccine failures (persons successfully immunized initially but whose immunity subsequently wanes) (Hinman 1992). Special studies to determine which of these factor(s) caused the outbreak are needed to prevent recurrence and maintain public confidence in the vaccination program.

Special studies may be laboratory and/or epidemiologic in design. Testing of residual vaccine used in outbreak areas may indicate poor potency, suggesting problems in production (Hlady, 1992), formulation (Patriarca 1988a), or refrigeration during shipping (Hayden 1979). Careful analysis of descriptive epidemiologic data from surveillance or outbreak investigations may offer insights and hypotheses on possible causes worth testing via a controlled epidemiologic study. Case-control studies were used in two measles outbreaks to show that lack of provider verification of a school record of measles vaccination and vaccination at less than 12 months of age were independent risk factors for measles disease (Wassilak 1985, Chen 1989). When the outbreak persisted despite a mass immunization campaign, a case-control study showed that cases occurring after the campaign had all received vaccine from one jet injector team, possibly due to poor administration technique (Wassilak 1985). The same studies showed that children who had been vaccinated in earlier years were no more likely to be at risk for measles than recent vaccinees, suggesting waning immunity did not play a role. During the early stages of the resurgence of diphtheria in the former Soviet Union in the 1990s, multiple etiologies ranging from new mutant strains to poor host immunogenicity due to Chernobyl were hypothesized, a case-control study showing excellent vaccine efficacy helped to rule out most of these hypotheses (Chen 2000).

Unusual circumstances during outbreaks or trials may permit the design of studies to answer longstanding questions. A blood drive serendipitously scheduled before a measles outbreak on a college campus permitted correlation of preexposure antibody titers with protection against classic and nonclassic measles (Chen 1990). An explosive measles outbreak in a high school where a single index case apparently exhausted all susceptibles in the school during two days provided insight on the role of superspreaders and airborne modes in measles transmission (Chen 1989). Reevaluation of serologic data collected among placebo recipients in a measles vaccine trial in Senegal provided further insight on subclinical measles (Bennett 1999).

Whenever studying outbreaks, however, it is important to place them in the proper context. Most of the factors associated with vaccination failure are not uniformly or randomly distributed in a population. Outbreaks, therefore, usually represent exceptions rather than the rule. Modeling shows that investigation of outbreaks will tend to underestimate the true vaccine efficacy in the population. The extent of underestimation is dependent on epidemic size, vaccination coverage, clustering of vaccination failures, community size, and contact rate (Fine 1994).

The high visibility of outbreaks may detract from the larger overall accomplishment of the immunization program in decreasing disease incidence. A large measles outbreak in Burundi in 1988 (Chen 1994c) raised doubts about the effectiveness of the measles vaccination program begun in 1982. Further analysis suggests that this was most likely a "posthoneymoon period" outbreak predicted by mathematical models of partially immunized population (McLean 1988). Such periods are caused by the rapid impact of early vaccination substantially de-creasing susceptibility and limiting disease transmission (the "honeymoon"). In the absence of disease, susceptibles accumulate both because of failure to vaccinate and vaccine failure. Over time, these susceptibles may be sufficient to fuel a mega-outbreak. However, even though this outbreak may be large, it is more than compensated for by the long period of low disease incidence. In Burundi, measles immunization had, in fact, successfully reduced measles morbidity and mortality by 50% and increased the interepidemic period (Chen 1994c). An understanding of the dynamic interactions between susceptible and immune persons in a population and the oscillations introduced by immunization programs are critical to immunization program managers and policy-makers (Anderson 1991).

VACCINE EFFICACY AND VACCINE EFFECTIVENESS STUDIES

No current vaccine is perfectly effective. The "intrinsic," *nonpreventable*, primary vaccine failure rates generally range from 2% to 50% for licensed vaccines even under the ideal circumstances of clinical trials. The genetic basis for such failures is beginning to be understood (Poland 1999). Paradoxically, as the vaccine coverage in a population increases, an increasing proportion of susceptibles and, hence, cases will have a history of prior vaccination due to the intrinsic vaccine failure rate (Table 17–2). While the size of outbreaks should decrease with increasing vaccine coverage, the proportion of cases with a vaccine history will increase. In the practical world of immunization programs, vaccine failures may also occur due to *preventable* causes such as problems in manufacturing (Hlady 1992), refrigeration (Hayden 1997), or administration techniques (Wassilak 1985).

An epidemic in a highly vaccinated population along with the presence of cases in many persons who had been vaccinated previously inevitably leads to public concerns about vaccine efficacy. Postlicensure epidemiologic studies to assess vaccine effectiveness may be needed to distinguish preventable from nonpreventable causes of vaccine

Table 17–2 Relation Between Vaccine Coverage and Proportion of Cases Vaccinated for a Vaccine with < 100% Vaccine Efficacy

Total population (number)	100	100	100	100
Vaccine efficacy (%)	90	90	90	90
% Population vaccinated	20	60	90	100
No. vaccinated (total population × % population vaccinated)	20	60	90	100
No. unvaccinated, i.e., susceptible (total population − no. vaccinated)	80	40	10	0
No. protected by vaccine (no. vaccinated × vaccine efficacy)	18	54	81	90
No. vaccinated but still susceptible (no. vaccinated − no. protected by vaccine)	2	6	9	10
Total no. susceptible (no. unvaccinated + no. vaccinated but still susceptible)	82	46	19	10
% Susceptibles vaccinated (no. vaccinated but still susceptible/total no. susceptible).	2.4	13	47	100

failure and allay such concerns (Orenstein 1988). As discussed earlier, such studies may also be needed because routine use of the vaccine after licensure may be in populations or schedules that differ from prelicensure trials. The range of efficacy with the *Haemophilus influenzae* b polysaccharide vaccine depending on the population (Ward 1994) and of influenza vaccine depending on the age group (Kilbourne 1994) are some of the best examples.

Once a vaccine has been licensed, however, it would be unethical to deliberately withhold an efficacious vaccine from a needy population. Therefore, observational epidemiologic studies (with their greater attendant design challenges) are used, instead of experimental study designs, to assess vaccine efficacy postlicensure. Such studies are generally preferred to serologic surveys for logistical reasons, and also that for some vaccines, there is no accurate serologic correlate of protection.

Definitions

Immunization usually has the *direct* effect of inducing protective immunity in the *individual* vaccinee. Occasionally, a vaccinated person may not develop immunity because of primary faiure. The immunity may have the goal of preventing *infection* and/or various degrees of *disease*. For most vaccine preventable diseases, immunization also has *indirect* effects of producing herd immunity for the *population* (Fine 1993). Generally, the term *vaccine efficacy* has been applied to estimates of efficacy derived from clinical

trials where (1) vaccination occurs under optimal conditions and (2) the limited sample size usually means that only direct protection is measurable. The term *vaccine effectiveness* has been applied to observational epidemiologic studies of efficacy, reflecting measurement of both direct and indirect effects of immunization in a population under possibly suboptimal field conditions of vaccine storage, handling, and administration (Halloran 1999). In practice, this distinction between vaccine efficacy and effectiveness is frequently ignored; the term "vaccine efficacy" tends to be used universally with some resultant confusion (Comstock 1994).

Both vaccine efficacy and effectiveness (VE) can be calculated using the classic formula of Greenwood and Yule (1915); (equation 1), where the Relative Risk is of developing disease. By convention, VE results are multiplied by 100 and expressed as a percent. Several different measures of the relative success of a vaccine in protecting the recipient against disease are used in calculating VE. Classically, when the data collected are in the form of total number of cases, the VE calculation has been based on a comparison of the attack rates (or more accurately, cumulative incidence or risk) among vaccinated and unvaccinated persons (equation 2) (Greenwood 1915, Francis 1955). Alternatively, when the data available are in the form of number of cases during a certain period of observation, person-time measures like incidence rates, hazard, or force of infection are more appropriate (equation 3) (Francis 1982, Smith 1984). Other measures used for VE calculation include relative transmission probabilities (Haber 1991) and hazard ratio (Brunet 1993). These various ways of measuring VE have recently been reviewed, depending on whether data on exposure to infection are available (rarely) or not (Halloran 1999).

Smith and colleagues (1984) have noted how vaccines that confer effective protection may differ depending on a vaccine's mode of action. For example, a vaccine with 95% VE may (1) reduce the probability of infection by 95%, given equal exposure to infection in all vaccinees, or (2) completely prevent infection in 95% of vaccinees and confer no protection in the other 5%. Halloran and associates (1999) have further elaborated the theoretical implications of the various models of vaccine action on both vaccine efficacy and failure.

SCREENING FOR VACCINE EFFECTIVENESS

Before a formal epidemiologic study of vaccine effectiveness is undertaken, it is useful to review whether the surveillance data permit a rapid "screening" analysis. If the surveillance system routinely collects information on the proportion of population vaccinated (PPV) and proportion of cases vaccinated (PCV) in *the same population*, and there is good confidence in the accuracy of these data, then VE can be calculated via the following equation (4) derived algebraically (by Orenstein et al. 1985) from the classic VE equation of Greenwood and Yule (1915).

$$VE = 1 - \text{Relative Risk} \tag{1}$$

$$= 1 - \frac{\text{Attack Rate}_{vaccinated}}{\text{Attack Rate}_{unvaccinated}} \tag{2}$$

$$= 1 - \frac{\text{Incidence Rate}_{vaccinated}}{\text{Incidence Rate}_{unvaccinated}} \tag{3}$$

$$= 1 - \frac{(\text{Proportion of cases}_{vaccinated}}{(1 - \text{proportion of cases}_{vaccinated}}$$

$$\times \frac{1 - \text{Proportion of population}_{vacinated})}{\text{Proportion of population}_{vaccinated})} \tag{4}$$

Figure 17–2 depicts the relation between the two variables in equation 4 for VEs ranging from 40% to 100%. This VE "nomogram" permits field health workers to rapidly "screen" to see if the VE is within the expected range given the data on PPV and PCV, which would suggest that the vaccine failures are nonpreventable. A special epidemiologic study for validation and identification of risk factors would be indicated only if the screening suggests the VE is low. In the United Kingdom, linkage of cases, their vaccination histories, and district vaccination coverages have permitted routine use of this screening method for VE (Farrington 1993).

In using the screening method, several cautions should be noted. First, the method requires a dichotomous population of unvaccinated and fully vaccinated. Hence, partially vaccinated persons need to be excluded from calculations of both PCV and PPV. Second, the method is most vulnerable to error under conditions of very low or very high PPV and PCV. In these conditions, the VE curves tend to converge and small changes in PCV or PPV can lead to major differences in VE.

Study Design Considerations

Several epidemiologic study designs to evaluate VE are possible (Orenstein 1988, Halloran 1999). A cohort design is most appropriate when a discrete population at risk can be defined, usually retrospectively (e.g., outbreaks in institutions and schools). If, however, the outbreak is of longer duration or if vaccination status changes substantially during the outbreak because of control efforts, then person-time or life table analysis is needed (Francis 1982, Smith 1984). Case-control (Comstock 1994, Rodrigues 1999) studies may be more efficient and perhaps the only practical design for VE studies of diseases with lower case-to-infection ratio such as diphtheria (Chen 2000), polio (Deming 1992), and tuberculosis (Smith 1982). When the case attack rate is high, the "rare" disease assumption for a cumulative incidence case-control study is no longer valid. The case-cohort design (Prentice 1986), essentially an incidence density case-control

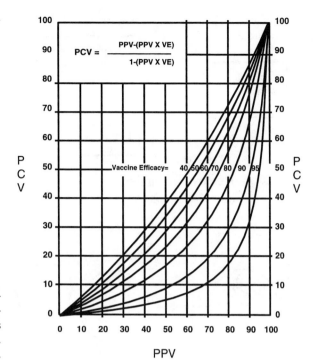

$$PCV = \frac{PPV-(PPV \times VE)}{1-(PPV \times VE)}$$

Vaccine Efficacy= 40 50 60 70 80 90 95

Figure 17–2. Percentage of cases vaccinated (PCV) per percentage of population vaccinated (PPV) for seven values of vaccine efficacy (VE). *Source*: Orenstein 1988.

study (Hogue 1983), can be used instead. A sample of the population giving rise to cases is taken irrespective of whether the sample includes some cases (Cutts 1990).

The household secondary attack rate method aims to minimize bias introduced by potential differences in risk of exposure among vaccinees and nonvaccinees. Data on attack rates among vaccinated and unvaccinated secondary contacts in many households are aggregated into a cohort. VE for measles vaccine using this method is similar to that from clinical trials (King 1991). On the other hand, household secondary attack rate studies may underestimate pertussis vaccine efficacy (Mortimer 1990, Onorato 1992), because of intense exposure, selection of households with high likelihood of vaccine failure, and retrospective case finding (Fine 1988).

Irrespective of the study design selected, an accurate VE calculation requires (1) the accurate ascertainment of susceptibility, vaccination, and disease status among the study population, and (2) similarity in other characteristics of the vaccinees and nonvaccinees. While these criteria are relatively easily met in a prospective clinical trial, they are not in an observational nonexperimental study (Fig. 17–3), especially in regard to comparability of vaccinees and nonvaccinees. The direction and the magnitude of distortion from the true VE introduced because of errors in each of these variables in study design have been extensively reviewed (Orenstein 1988, 1985, Fine 1987, Rodrigues 1999). The major errors to avoid follow.

1. Assuming persons without a vaccination record are unvaccinated. Such persons may have been vaccinated and lost their records or be truly unvaccinated. If the former, this would falsely decrease the attack rate$_{unvaccinated}$ (ARU) and lead to falsely low VE. Table 17–3 shows that the calculated VE in a study in Burundi was only 51%, using this assumption (Chen 1994c). Some studies attempt to ascertain history of vaccination among persons without records

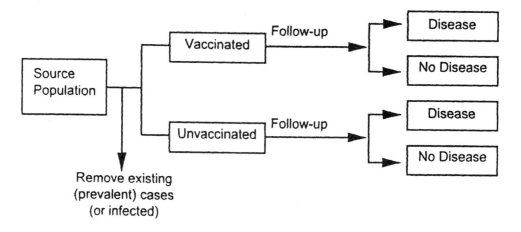

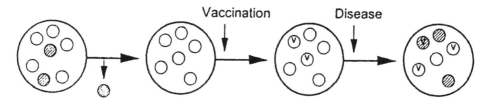

Figure 17–3. Flow diagram of vaccine efficacy study. Prospective clinical trial flows from left to right, while observational nonexperimental study during an outbreak generally seeks to reconstruct the flow retrospectively going from right to left.
Source: Chen 1996.

by interview. Such recall tends to be unreliable, however, given the large number of injections and vaccinations administered. The best strategy generally is to exclude the unknowns and restrict the analysis to persons with record-documented vaccination and nonvaccination status (Orenstein 1988). The VE in Burundi increased to 59% when this was done (Table 17–4).

2. Using a nonspecific case definition is

Table 17–3 Measles Vaccine Efficacy, Muyinga Sector, Burundi, 1988: All Children in Census (measles cases as reported by mother; children without vaccination card counted as unvaccinated)

	Measles	No Measles	Total
Vaccinated	115	893	1008
Unvaccinated	207	685	892
Total	322	1578	1900

Attack rate$_{\text{Unvaccinated}}$ = 207/892 = 23%.

Attack rate$_{\text{Vaccinated}}$ = 115/1008 = 11%.

Vaccine efficacy = (23%–11%)/23% = 1 – (11%/23%) = 51%.

an example of the "bias toward the null" in epidemiologic studies (Rothman 1998). As one would not expect a vaccine to protect against a disease other than its target disease, specificity of diagnosis is more critical to the accuracy of the vaccine efficacy estimate than sensitivity (Orenstein 1988). The endpoint "case definition" may be a laboratory result, a clinical finding, or a combination of both (Blackwelder 1991). For diseases with classic symptoms like measles, clinical diagnosis by parent and/or doctor may be adequate in some studies (MVC 1966), but not all (Chen 1994c). In Burundi, the VE further increased to 67% when a more specific case definition was used (Table 17–5). Assuming 100% sensitivity, the magnitude of the error introduced by different levels of false positive case definitions is estimated by:

$$Ve_{\text{observed}} \sim VE_{\text{true}}(x/(x + y)) \qquad (5)$$

where x is the true incidence rate of the vaccine preventable disease in the population

Table 17–4 Measles Vaccine Efficacy, Muyinga Sector, Burundi, 1988: Unvaccinated Children Restricted to Those with Vaccination Cards (on which there is no record of measles vaccination)

	Measles	No Measles	Total
Vaccinated	115	893	1008
Unvaccinated	122	316	438
Total	237	1209	1446

*Attack rate$_{Unvaccinated}$ = 122/438 = 28%.

Attack rate$_{Vaccinated}$ = 115/1008 = 11%.

Vaccine efficacy = (28%–11%)/28% = 1 – (11%/28%) = 59%.

Table 17–5 Measles Vaccine Efficacy, Muyinga Sector, Burundi, 1988: Criteria in Table 17–4 Plus Measles Patients Restricted to Those with Symptoms Meeting the Case Definition of Fever, Rash, and Cough, or Runny Nose, or Red Eyes

	Measles	No Measles	Total
Vaccinated	50	893	943
Unvaccinated	60	316	376
Total	110	1209	1319

*Attack rate$_{Unvaccinated}$ = 60/376 = 16%.

Attack rate$_{Vaccinated}$ = 50/943 = 5%.

Vaccine efficacy = (16%–5%)/16% = 1 – (5%/16%) = 67%.

and y is the incidence of the condition misdiagnosed as the vaccine preventable disease (Fine 1987).

3. Assuming vaccinees and nonvaccinees are otherwise similar, especially in terms of susceptibility and risk of exposure to disease. In nonexperimental settings, nonvaccinees generally differ from vaccinees in many ways, ranging from having contraindications to vaccination, to personal choice, to others unknown to the investigator. If the differences are related to both the exposure and outcome of interest, the VE estimate may be biased by confounding. Potential confounding factors include, but are not limited to, age, sex, race, socioeconomic status, attendance at school or institution, and place of residence. Studies should collect data on, or match on, suspected confounding variables to maximize comparability of vaccinees and nonvaccinees (Orenstein 1988). Attempting to adjust for age further increased the VE estimate in Burundi to 73% (Table 17–6).

Table 17–6 Measles Vaccine Efficacy, Muyinga Sector, Burundi, 1988: Criteria in Table 17–4 Plus Table 17–5 Plus Analysis Restricted to Children ≥9 Months of Age

	Measles	No Measles	Total
Vaccinated	41	701	742
Unvaccinated	31	118	149
Total	72	819	891

*Attack rate$_{Unvaccinated}$ = 31/149 = 21%.

Attack rate$_{Vaccinated}$ = 41/742 = 6%.

Vaccine efficacy = (21%–6%)/21% = 1 – (6%/21%) = 73%.

SURVEILLANCE OF VACCINE SAFETY

Vaccines are widely recommended or mandated, generally to otherwise healthy persons. Because no vaccine is perfectly safe, immunization programs have an obligation to carefully monitor the safety of vaccines as well as their efficacy (Chen 1999a). As the incidence of vaccine preventable diseases is reduced by increasing coverage with an efficacious vaccine, vaccine adverse events, both causal and coincidental, become increasingly prominent (Fig. 17–1) (Chen 1994b). Close monitoring and timely assessment of suspected vaccine adverse events are critical to prevent loss of confidence, decreased vaccine coverage, and return of epidemic disease. Epidemics of pertussis occurred in several countries during the 1970s when concerns with the safety of pertussis vaccine were widely publicized (Gangarosa 1998).

Recommendations for use of vaccines represent a dynamic balancing of benefits and risks. Vaccine safety monitoring is necessary to accurately weigh this balance. When diseases are close to eradication, data on complications due to vaccine relative to that of disease may lead to discontinuation of routine use of the vaccine, as was done with smallpox vaccine (CDC 1971) and oral polio vaccine in the United States (CDC 1999). Few vaccine preventable diseases are likely to be eradicated in the near future, however. Most immunizations are, therefore, likely to be needed indefinitely, with their attendant adverse events and potential for loss of public confidence.

Common adverse reactions caused by vaccine can usually be detected in prelicensure randomized, double-blind, placebo-controlled trials. However, limits in sample size, duration, and heterogeneity of prelicensure trials also mean that rare, delayed, or group-specific vaccine reactions are detectable only with wider use postlicensure. The term "adverse events" temporally related to vaccine is generally used postlicensure rather than "adverse reactions," since the word reaction implies causation by the vaccine and causality is difficult to demonstrate in the postlicensure setting.

Most commonly, postmarketing surveillance is done via passive reports. Examples include the Vaccine Adverse Event Reporting System (VAERS) (Chen 1994b) in the United States and similar systems in other countries (Duclos 1993). Such passive adverse events monitoring systems are most useful for identifying hypotheses for more detailed investigation in special studies. Such hypotheses may consist of either previously unreported vaccine adverse events (e.g., Guillain-Barré syndrome after "swine flu" vaccine (Schonberger 1979), intussusception after rotavirus vaccine (CDC-MMWR 1999) or unusual increases in known events (e.g., cluster of sterile abscesses associated with one manufacturer's product) (Bernier 1981). Passive systems are also used to monitor trends in reporting and can be used to evaluate some hypotheses. For example, the predecessor system to VAERS requested information on personal and family histories of seizures. Analysis showed that persons with such histories were significantly more likely to have seizures following DTP than persons without such histories, leading to development of precautions for vaccinating such individuals (Stetler 1985).

Interpretation of passive systems is difficult owing to (1) underreporting of events, and (2) biased reporting in favor of events occurring in closer temporal proximity to vaccination. The greatest deficiency of passive surveillance, however, relates to its general inability to determine whether a given reported event was actually caused by the vaccination or simply coincidental to it. This is because most adverse events reported do not have specific clinical (e.g., vaccine-associated polio) (Henderson 1964) or laboratory characteristics (e.g., mumps vaccine meningitis) (Forsey 1990) to differentiate them from events that occur in the absence of vaccination. In such settings, epidemiologic studies are necessary.

Passive reports like VAERS, however, generally contain only a biased fourth of the information in a 2 × 2 table of vaccination exposure and adverse event outcome needed for an epidemiologic assessment (i.e., they represent cell "a" only: those vaccinated with adverse event) . They lack built-in control groups to allow measurement of the incidence of the event in the absence of vaccination. An increase in VAERS reports may be due to (1) increase in number of doses administered, (2) increase in background rate, (3) increased reporting efficiency (e.g., due to publicity), and (4) increase in vaccine risk (Lasky 1998). Therefore, true determination of causation usually requires special studies to gather information for all four cells of a 2 × 2 table. The special studies can either be ad hoc (Bernier 1981) or, increasingly, preorganized large-linked databases. Such databases take advantage of the increasing automation of vaccination and medical records within medical care settings like health maintenance organizations (Chen 1997) and national health services (Farrington 1995) to provide more scientifically rigorous estimates of vaccine risks.

To determine vaccine causation epidemiologically requires the demonstration that either vaccinees are more likely to suffer the event than nonvaccinees (cohort design) or persons with the event are more likely to have a history of recent vaccination than persons without the event (case-control design) (Rodrigues 1999). In highly vaccinated populations, those persons remaining unvaccinated may confound studies of vaccine adverse events (Fine 1992). Person-time "risk interval" and/or "case-series" analysis is then preferred (Chen 1994a, and Farrington 1995). A risk interval for the adverse event is defined a priori based on biologic plausibility, the incidence rates of the adverse event within and without the risk interval are then compared. Adverse events with delayed or insidious onset cannot be assessed via this method, however. The substantial controversy that surrounds most vaccine safety studies highlights the import of methodologic rigor in the design of such studies (Chen 1999a).

Recent reviews have identified major "gaps and limitations" in both knowledge and research capacity on vaccine safety (Howson 1991, Stratton 1994), suggesting this as one area requiring additional attention in maturing immunization programs (Chen 1999b).

FUTURE ISSUES

Recent explosive advances in biotechnology and biomedical knowledge offer promises of development of candidate vaccines against many other infectious diseases. Epidemiology will continue to play a critical role in their evaluation. Many other difficult economic, ethical, and social issues need to be solved, however, before trials for vaccines against HIV/AIDS can begin, let alone used routinely (Rousseau 1999). Similarly, vaccines with a target population that is either limited in size or poor may never be developed (Lang 1999).

The addition of new vaccines to the routine immunization schedule suggests that combined vaccines requiring fewer injections and fewer visits are needed to maintain continued high population immunity with minimal discomfort and highest compliance. Special challenges, logistically and scientifically, exist in evaluating the safety and efficacy of such combined vaccines (Williams 1995, Guess 1999). Given the high cost of new vaccines and limited budget of many national programs, the imperative to choose rationally among existing licensed vaccines based on "best value" will require more economic and epidemiologic studies (Weniger 1998). On the other hand, new donors and changes in health care organization, especially its increasing centralization and automation

(Strom 1990), offer promising opportunities for epidemiologists to organize the studies necessary to continue the miraculous conquering of diseases by immunizations.

REFERENCES

Acres SE, and Varughese PV. Impact of vaccination on selected diseases in Canada. Can. Med. Assoc. J. 132:635–639, 1985.

Adams WG, Deaver KA, Cochi SL, et al. Decline of childhood *Haemophilus influenzae* type b (Hib) disease in the Hib vaccine era. JAMA. 269:221–226, 1993.

Advisory Committee on Epidemiology. Canadian Communicable Disease Surveillance System. Can. Dis. Wkly. Rep. 17S3, 1991.

Agocs MM, Markowitz LE, Straub I, et al. The 1988–1989 measles epidemic in Hungary: assessment of vaccine failure. Int. J. Epidemiol. 21:1007–1013, 1992.

Alter MJ, Mares A, Hadler SC, and Maynard JE. The effect of underreporting on the apparent incidence and epidemiology of acute viral hepatitis. Am. J. Epidemiol. 125:133–139, 1987.

Anderson RM, and May RM. Infectious Diseases of Humans: Dynamics and Control. Oxford: Oxford University Press, 1991:107.

Babad HR, Nokes DJ, Gay NJ, et al. Predicting the impact of measles vaccination in England and Wales: model validation and analysis of policy options. Epidemiol. Infect. 114(2): 319–344, 1995.

Barre-Sinoussi F, Chermann JC, Rey F, et al. Isolation of a t lymphotropic retrovirus from a patient at risk for acquired immunodeficiency syndrome (AIDS). Science. 220:868–871, 1983.

Bart KJ, Orenstein WA, Preblud SR, and Hinman AR. Universal immunization to interrupt rubella. Rev. Infect. Dis. 7:S177–184, 1985.

Begg NT, Gill ON, and White JM. COVER (cover of vaccination evaluated rapidly): description of the England and Wales scheme. Public Health. 103:81–89, 1989.

Begg N, and Miller E. Role of epidemiology in vaccine policy. Vaccine. 8:180–189, 1990.

Bennett J, Whittle H, Samb B, et al. Seroconversions in unvaccinated infants: further evidence for subclinical measles from vaccine trials in Niakhar, Senegal. Int. J. Epidemiol. 28:147–151, 1999.

Bernier RH, Frank JA Jr, and Nolan TF Jr. Abscesses complicating DTP vaccination. Am. J. Dis. Child. 135:826–828, 1981.

Blackwelder WC, Storsaeter J, Olin P, and Hallander HQ. Acellular pertussis vaccines: efficacy and evaluation of clinical case definition. Am. J. Dis. Child. 145:1285–1289, 1991.

Bloch AB, Orenstein WA, Stetler HC, et al. Health impact of measles vaccination in the United States. Pediatrics 76:524–532, 1985.

Bottiger M, Gustavsson O, and Svensson A. Immunity to tetanus, diphtheria and poliomyelitis in the adult population of Sweden in 1991. Int. J. Epidemiol. 27(5):916–925, 1998.

Brogan D, Flagg EW, Deming M, and Waldman R. Increasing the accuracy of the Expanded Programme on Immunization's cluster survey design. Ann. Epidemiol. 4:302–311, 1994.

Brunet RC, Struchiner CM, and Halloran ME. On the distribution of vaccine protection under heterogeneous response. Math. Biosci. 116:111–125, 1993.

CDSC. Sentinel surveillance shows small decline in MMR coverage. Commun. Dis. Rep. CDR Wkly. 8:317–320, 1998.

Centers for Disease Control. Public Health Service recommendations on smallpox vaccination. MMWR. 20:339–345, 1971.

Centers for Disease Control. Classification of measles cases and categorization of measles elimination programs. MMWR. 31:707–711, 1982.

Centers for Disease Control: Measles Surveillance Report No. 11 1977–1981. Issued September 1982.

Centers for Disease Control. Classification of measles cases and categorization of measles elimination programs. MMWR. 31:707–711, 1983.

Centers for Disease Control. Changing patterns of groups at high risk for hepatitis B in the United States. MMWR. 39: 429–432, 437, 1988.

Centers for Disease Control. Rubella vaccination during pregnancy, United States, 1971–1988. MMWR. 38:289–293, 1989.

Centers for Disease Control. Recommendations of the Immunization Practices Advisory Committee (ACIP). Measles Prevention. MMWR. 38:No. S-9:1–18, 1989.

Centers for Disease Control. Case definitions for public health surveillance. MMWR. 39 (No. RR-13):[1–43], 1990.

Centers for Disease Control. International Task Force for Disease Eradication. MMWR. 39: 209–217, 1990.

Centers for Disease Control. Biologics Surveillance Report No. 93 (1987 to 1990). Atlanta, GA: Centers for Disease Control, 1991.

Centers for Disease Control and Prevention. Retrospective assessment of vaccination coverage among school-aged children—selected US cities, 1991. MMWR. 41:103–107, 1992.

Centers for Disease Control and Prevention. Recommendations for use of *Haemophilus* b conjugate vaccines and a combined, diphtheria, tetanus, pertussis, and *Haemophilus* b vaccine. Recommendations of the Advisory Committee on Immunization Practices (ACIP). MMWR, 42:6–8, 1993.

Centers for Disease Control and Prevention. Vaccination coverage of 2-year-old children—United States, 1992–1993. MMWR. 43: 282–283, 1994.

Centers for Disease Control and Prevention. Vaccination coverage levels among children aged 19–35 months—United States, April–June 1994. MMWR. 44:396–398, 1995.

Centers for Disease Control and Prevention. The state and national vaccination coverage levels among children aged 19–35 months—United States, April–December 1994. MMWR. 44:613, 619–623, 1995.

Centers for Disease Control and Prevention. Pertussis—United States, January 1992–June 1995. MMWR. 44:525–529, 1995.

Centers for Disease Control and Prevention. Prevention of varicella: recommendations of the Advisory Committee on Immunization Practices. 45:(No. RR-11), 1996.

Centers for Disease Control and Prevention. Recommendations of the Advisory Committee on Immunization Practices: programmatic strategies to increase vaccination rates—assessment and feedback of provider-based vaccination coverage information. MMWR. 45:219–220, 1996.

Centers for Disease Control and Prevention. Evaluation of varicella reporting to the National Notifiable Disease Surveillance System—United States, 1972–1997. MMWR. 48:55–58, 1999.

Centers for Disease Control and Prevention. Intussusception among recipients of rotavirus vaccine—United States, 1998–1999. MMWR. 48:577–581, 1999.

Centers for Disease Control and Prevention. Recommendations of the Advisory Committee on Immunization Practices: revised recommendations for routine poliomyelitis vaccination. 48:590, 1999.

Centers for Disease Control and Prevention. National Vaccination Coverage levels among children aged 19–35 months—United States, 1998. MMWR 48: 829, 1999.

Centers for Disease Control and Prevention. Recommended childhood immunization schedule—United States, 2000. MMWR 49: 35, 2000.

Chauvin P, and Valleron AJ. Participation of French general practitioners in public health surveillance: a multidisciplinary approach. J. Epidemiol. Community Health. 52 Suppl 1:2S–8S, 1998.

Chen RT, Broome CV, Weinstein RA, et al. Diphtheria in the US, 1971–81. Am. J. Public Health. 75:1393–1397, 1985.

Chen RT, Goldbaum GM, Wassilak SGF, Markowitz LE, and Orenstein WA. An explosive point-source measles outbreak in a highly immunized population: modes of transmission and risk factors for disease. Am. J. Epidemiol. 129:173–182, 1989.

Chen RT, Markowitz LE, Albrecht P, et al. Measles antibody: reevaluation of protective titers. J. Infect. Dis. 162:1036–1042, 1990.

Chen RT. Special methodological issues in pharmacoepidemiology studies of vaccine safety. In: Strom BL, ed. Pharmacoepidemiology. Sussex: John Wiley, 1994a:581–594.

Chen RT, Rastogi SC, Mullen JR, et al. The Vaccine Adverse Event Reporting System (VAERS). Vaccine. 12:542–550, 1994b.

Chen RT, Weierbach R, Bisoffi Z, et al. A 'Post-Honeymoon Period' measles outbreak in Muyinga Sector, Burundi. Int. J. Epidemiol. 23:185–193, 1994c.

Chen RT, Orenstein WA. Epidemiologic methods in immunization programs. Epidemiol. Rev. 18:99–117, 1996.

Chen RT, Glasser J, Rhodes P, et al. The Vaccine Safety Datalink Project: A new tool for improving vaccine safety monitoring in the United States. Pediatrics. 765–773, 1997.

Chen RT. Safety of vaccines. In: Plotkin SA, Orenstein WA, eds. Vaccines. Philadelphia: WB Saunders, 1999a:1144–1163.

Chen RT. Vaccine risks: real, perceived, and unknown. Vaccine 17:S41–46, 1999b.

Chen RT, Hardy IRB, Rhodes PH, et al. Ukraine 1992: vaccine effectiveness and other preludes to understanding the recent resurgence of diphtheria in the former Soviet Union. J. Infect. Dis. 181(S1):2000. S178–83.

Cherry JD, Gornbein J, Heininger U, and Stehr K. A search for serologic correlates of immunity to Bordetella pertussis cough illnesses. Vaccine. 16:1901–1906, 1998.

Choi K, and Thacker SB. An evaluation of influenza mortality surveillance, 1962–1979. I. Time series forecasts of expected pneumonia and influenza deaths. Am. J. Epidemiol. 113:215–226, 1981.

Christenson B, and Bottiger M. Long-term follow-up study of rubella antibodies in naturally immune and vaccinated young adults. Vaccine. 12:41–45, 1994.

Clarkson JA, and Fine PEM. The efficiency of measles and pertussis notification in England and Wales. Int. J. Epidemiol. 14:153–168, 1985.

Clemens J, Brenner R, Rao M, et al. Evaluating new vaccines for developing countries. Efficacy or effectiveness? JAMA. 275:390–397, 1996.

Cochi SL, Edmonds LE, Dyer K, et al. Congenital rubella syndrome in the United States, 1970–1985—on the verge of elimination. Am. J. Epidemiol. 129:349–361, 1989.

Cochi SC, Preblud SR, and Orenstein WA. Perspectives on the relative resurgence of mumps in the United States. Am. J. Dis. Child. 142:499–507, 1988.

Cochi SL, Broome CV, and Hightower AW. Immunization of US children with Haemophilus influenzae type b polysaccharide vaccine. A cost-effectiveness model of strategy assessment. JAMA. 253:521–529, 1985.

Comstock GW. Evaluating vaccination effectiveness and vaccine efficacy by means of case-control studies. Epidemiol. Rev. 16:77–89, 1994.

Cutts FT. The use of the WHO cluster survey for evaluating the imapct of the expanded programme on immunization on target disease incidence. J. Trop. Med. Hyg. 91:231–239, 1988.

Cutts FT, Smith PG, Colombo S, et al. Field evaluation of measles vaccine efficacy in Mozambique. Am. J. Epidemiol. 131:349–355, 1990.

Cutts FT, Waldman RJ, and Zoffman HM. Surveillance for the Expanded Programme on Immunization. Bull. World Health Organ. 71:633–639, 1993.

Cutts FT, and Olive JM. Vaccination programs in developing countries. In: Plotkin SA, Orenstein WA, eds. Vaccines. Philadelphia: WB Saunders, 1999:1047–1073.

Deming MS, Jaiteh KO, Otten MW, et al. Epidemic poliomyelitis in the Gambia following the control of poliomyelitis as an endemic disease. II. Clinical efficacy of trivalent oral polio vaccine. Am. J. Epidemiol. 135:393–408, 1992.

Desve G. Les outils informatiques utilises dans le PEV. Sante 4(3):143–144, 1994.

Duclos P, Pless R, Koch J, et al. Adverse events temporally associated with immunizing agents. Can. Fam. Physician. 39:1907–1913, 1993.

Dudgeon JA. Selective immunization: protection of the individual. Rev. Infect. Dis. 7:S185–190, 1985.

Eddins DL. Present systems that provide indicators of immunization status of preschool children. In: Proceedings of the 18th National Immunization Conference. Atlanta, Georgia, May 16–19, 1983. Atlanta, GA: US Department of Health and Human Services, Public Health Service, Centers for Disease Control and Prevention, 83–84, 1993.

Eddins DL. Indicators of immunization status. 17th Immunization Conference Proceedings, Atlanta, Georgia, May 18–19, 1982, P47–55.

Eskola J, Peltola H, Takala A, et al. Efficacy of Haemophilus influenzae type b polysaccharide-diphtheria toxoid conjugate vaccine in infancy. N. Engl. J. Med. 317:717–222, 1987.

Evans AS. The need for serologic evaluation of immunization programs. Am. J. Epidemiol. 122:725–731, 1980.

Farrington P, Pugh S, Colville A, et al. A new method for active surveillance of adverse events from diphtheria/tetanus/pertussis and measles/mumps/rubella vaccines. Lancet. 345:567–569, 1995.

Farrington CP. Estimation of vaccine effectiveness using the screening method. Int. J. Epidemiol. 22:742–746, 1993.

Feery B. Impact of immunization on disease pattern in Australia. Med. J. Aust. 2:172–176, 1981.

Fenner F, Henderson DA, Arita I, Jezek Z, and Ladnyi ID. Smallpox and its eradication. Geneva: World Health Organization, 1988.

Ferrinho P, Valli A, Groeneveld T, et al. The effects of cluster sampling in an African urban setting. Cent. Afr. J. Med. 38:324–330, 1992.

Fine PEM, and Clarkson JA. The recurrence of whooping cough: possible implications for assessment of vaccine efficacy. Lancet. 1:666–669, 1982.

Fine PEM, and Clarkson JA. Reflections on the efficacy of pertussis vaccines. Rev. Infect. Dis. 9:866–883, 1987.

Fine PEM, Clarkson JA, and Miller E. The efficacy of pertussis vaccines under condition of household exposure. Int. J. Epidemiol. 17:635–642, 1988.

Fine PEM, and Chen RT. Confounding in studies of adverse reactions to vaccines. Am. J. Epidemiol. 136:121–135, 1992.

Fine PEM. Herd immunity: history, theory, practice. Epidemiol. Rev. 15:265–302, 1993.

Fine PEM, and Zell ER. Outbreaks in highly vaccinated populations: implications for studies of vaccine performance. Am. J. Epidemiol. 139:77–90, 1994.

Fine PEM. Implications of different study designs for the evaluation of acellular pertussis vaccine. Dev. Biol. Stand. 89:123–133, 1997.

Foege WH, Millar JD, and Lane JM. Selective epidemiologic control in smallpox eradication. Am. J. Epidemiol. 94:311–315, 1971.

Forsey T, Mawn JA, Yates PJ, Bently ML, and Minor PD. Differentiation of vaccine and wild mumps viruses using the polymerase chain reaction and dideoxinucleotide. J. Gen. Virol. 71:987–990, 1990.

Francis T, Korns RF, Voights RB, et al. An evaluation fo the 1954 poliomyelitis vaccine trials. Am. J. Public Health. 45:1–63, 1955.

Francis DP, Hadler SC, Thompson SE, et al. The prevention of hepatitis B with vaccine: Report of the Centers for Disease Control multicenter efficacy trial among homosexual men. Ann. Intern. Med. 97:362–366, 1982.

Freeman VA, and Freed GL. Parental knowledge, attitudes, and demand regarding a vaccine to prevent varicella. Am. J. Prev. Med. 17:153–155, 1999.

Fritzell B, and Plotkin S. Efficacy and safety of a Haemophilus influenzae type b capsular polysaccharide-tetanus protein conjugate vaccine. J. Pediatr. 121:355–362, 1992.

Gangarosa EJ, Galazka AM, Wolfe CR, et al. Impact of the anti- vaccine movements on pertussis control: the untold story. Lancet. 351:356–361, 1998.

Gindler JS, Atkinson WL, and Markowitz LE. Update—the U.S. measles epidemic, 1989–1990. Epidemiol. Rev. 14:270–276, 1992.

Gold MS, Martin L, Nayda CL, and Kempe AE. Electronic temperature monitoring and feedback to correct adverse vaccine storage in general practice. Med. J. Aust. 171:83–84, 1999.

Goldstein KP, Kviz FJ, and Daum RS. Accuracy of immunization histories provided by adults accompanying preschool children to a pediatric emergency room. JAMA. 270:2190–2194, 1993.

Greenwood M, and Yule GU. The statistics of anti-typhoid and anti-cholera inoculations. Proc. R. Soc. Med. 8(part 2):113–194, 1915.

Greten TF, and Jaffee EM. Cancer vaccines. J. Clin. Oncol. 17:1047–1060, 1999.

Gudnadottir M. Cost effectiveness of different strategies for prevention of congenital rubella infection: a practical example from Iceland. Rev. Infect. Dis. 7:S200–209, 1985.

Guess HA. Combination vaccines: issues in evaluation of effectiveness and safety. Epidemiol. Rev. 21(1):89–95, 1999.

Guris D, Strebel PM, Bardenheier B, et al. Changing epidemiology of pertussis in the United States: increasing reported incidence among adolescents and adults, 1990–1996. Clin. Infect. Dis. 28:1230–1237, 1999.

Haber M, Longini IM, and Halloran ME. Measures of the effects of vaccination in a randomly mixing population. Int. J. Epidemiol. 20:300–310, 1991.

Halloran ME, Haber M, Longini IM, and Struchiner CJ. Design and interpretation of vaccine field studies. Epidemiol. Rev. 21(1):73–88, 1999.

Hardy IR, Dittman S, and Sutter RW. Current situation and control strategies for resurgence of diphtheria in newly independent states of the former Soviet Union. Lancet. 347:1739–1744, 1996.

Hayden GF. Measles vaccine failure: a survey of causes and means of prevention. Clin. Pediatr. 18:155–167, 1979.

Henderson RH, Davis H, Eddins DL, and Foege WH. Assessment of vaccination coverage, vaccination scar rates, and smallpox scarring in five areas of West Africa. Bull. WHO. 48:183–194, 1973.

Henderson RH, and Sundaresan T. Cluster sampling to assess immunization coverage: a review of experience with simplified sampling method. Bull. WHO. 60:253–260, 1982.

Henderson DA, Witte JJ, Morris L, and Langmuir AD. Paralytic disease associated with oral polio vaccines. JAMA. 190:153–160, 1964.

Hennessey KA, Ion-Nedelcu N, Craciun MD, et al. Measles epidemic in Romania, 1996–1998: assessment of vaccine effectiveness by case-control and cohort studies. Am. J. Epidemiol. 150(11):1250–1257, 1999.

Hersh BS, Markowitz LE, Maes EF, et al. The geographic distribution of measles in the US, 1980–1980. JAMA. 2667:1936–1941, 1992.

Hinman AR, Orenstein WA, and Mortimer EA. When, where, and how do immunizations fail? Ann. Epidemiol. 2:805–812, 1992.

Hlady WG, Bennet JV, Samadi AR, et al. Neonatal tetanus in rural Bangladesh: risk factors and toxoid efficacy. Am. J. Public Health. 82:1365–1369, 1992.

Hogue CJR, Gaylor DW, and Schulz KF. Estimators of relative risk for case-control studies. Am. J. Epidemiol. 118:396–407, 1983.

Howson CP, Howe CJ, Fineberg HV, eds. Adverse Effects of Pertussis and Rubella Vaccines. Washington DC: National Academy Press, 1991.

Hull HF, Ward NA, Hull BP, Milstein JB, and de Quadros C. Paralytic poliomyelitis: seasoned strategies, disappearing disease. Lancet. 343: 1331–1337, 1994.

Hutcheson RH, and Barid SJ. An inexpensive methodology for immunization surveys. Public Health Rep. 89:315–319, 1974.

Hutin YJ, Harpaz R, Drobeniuc J, et al. Injections given in healthcare settings as a major source of acute hepatitis B in Moldova. Int. J. Epidemiol. 28:782–786, 1999.

Illich I. Medical Nemesis—The Expropriation of Health. New York: Pantheon Books, 1976.

Jafari HS, Adams WG, Robinson KA, et al. Efficacy of Haemophilus influenzae type b conjugate vaccines and persistence of disease in disadvantaged populations. Am. J. Public Health. 89:364–368, 1999.

Johnson RPE. Live attenuated AIDS vaccines: hazards and hopes. Nat. Med. 5:154–155, 1999.

Kelley PW, Petruccelli BP, Stehr-Green P, et al. The susceptibility of young adult Americans to vaccine-preventable infections: a national serosurvey of US Army Recruits. JAMA. 266:2724–2729, 1991.

Kilbourne EA. Inactivated influenza vaccines. In: Plotkin SA, Mortimer EA, eds. Vaccines. Philadelphia: WB Saunders, 1994:565–582.

King GE, Markowitz LE, Patriarca PA, et al. Clinical efficacy of measles vaccine during the 1990 measles epidemic. Pediatr. Infect. Dis. J. 10:883–887, 1991.

King GE, and Hadler SC. Simultaneous administration of childhood vaccines: an important public health policy that is safe and efficacious. Pediatr. Infect. Dis. J. 13:394–407, 1994.

Klaucke DN. Evaluating public health surveillance. In: Teutsch SM, Churchill RE, eds. Principles and Practices of Public Health Surveillance. Oxford: Oxford University Press, 1994:158–174.

Lang J, and Wood SC. Development of orphan vaccines: an industry perspective. Emerg. Infect. Dis. 5:749–756, 1999.

Langmuir AD. Medical importance of measles. Am. J. Dis. Child. 103:54–56, 1962.

Lasky T, Terracciano GJ, Magder L, et al. Association of the Guillain-Barré syndrome with the 1992–93 and 1993–94 influenza vaccines. N. Engl. J. Med. 339:1797–1802, 1998.

Lee A. Animal models and vaccine development. Baillieres Clin. Gastroenterol. 9:615–632, 1995.

Lemeshow S, Tserkovnyi AL, Tulloch JL, et al. A computer simulation of the EPI survey strategy. Int. J. Epidemiol. 14:473–481, 1985.

Levine MM, and Lagos R. Vaccines and vaccination in the historical perspective. In: Levine MM, Woodrow GC, Kaper JB, Cobon GS, eds. New Generation Vaccines. New York: Marcel Dekker, 1997:1–11.

Lieu TA, Cochi SL, Black SB, et al. Cost-effectiveness of a routine varicella vaccination program for U.S. children. JAMA. 271:375–381, 1994.

Mahoney RT, and Maynard JE. The introduction of new vaccines into developing countries. Vaccine 17:646–652, 1999.

Margolis HS, Coleman PJ, Brown RE, et al. Prevention of hepatitis B virus transmission by immunization: an economic analysis of current recommendations. JAMA. 274:1201–1208, 1995.

Markowitz LE, Preblud SR, Orenstein WA, et al. Patterns of transmission in measles outbreaks in the United States 1985–1986. N. Engl. J. Med. 320:75–81, 1989.

Markowitz LE, Albrecht P, Rhodes P, et al. Changing levels of measles antibody titers in women and children in the United States: impact on response to vaccination. Pediatrics 97(1):53–58, 1996.

McDonald JC, Moore DL, and Quennec P. Clinical and epidemiologic features of mumps meningoencephalitis and possible vaccine-related disease. Pediatr. Infect. Dis. J. 8:751–755, 1989.

McLean AR, and Anderson RM. Measles in developing countries. Part II. The predicted impact of mass vaccination. Infect. Immun. 100: 419–442, 1988.

McQuillan GM, Gunter WE, and Lannom L. Field issues for the plan and operation of the laboratory components of the Third National Health and Nutrition Examination Survey. J. Nutr. 120S11:1446–1450, 1990.

Measles Vaccination Committee. Vaccination against measles: a clnical trial of live measles vaccine given alone and live vaccine preceded by killed vaccine. Br. Med. J. 1:441–446, 1966.

Miller E. Rubella in the United Kingdom. Epidemiol. Infect. 107:3142, 1991.

Modlin JF, Jabbour JT, Witte JJ, and Halsey NA. Epidemiologic studies of measles, measles vaccine, and subacute sclerosing panencephalitis. Pediatrics. 59:505–512, 1977.

Monto AS. Francis field trial of inactivated poliomyelitis vaccine: background and lessons for today. Epidemiol. Rev. 21(1):7–23, 1999.

Mortimer EA, Kimura M, Cherry JD, et al. Protective efficacy of the Takeda acellular pertussis vaccine combined with diphtheria and tetanus toxoids following household exposure of Japanese children. Am. J. Dis. Child. 144:899–904, 1990.

Nathanson N, and Langmuir AD. The Cutter incident. Am. J. Hyg. 78:16–81, 1963.

National Immunization Program. Clinic Assessment Software Application (CASA). Atlanta, GA: CDC, 1994.

National Vaccine Advisory Committee. The measles epidemic: the problems, barriers, and recommendations. JAMA. 266:1547–1552, 1991.

Onarato IM, Wassilak SG, and Meade B. Efficacy of whole-cell pertussis vaccine in preschool children in the United States. JAMA. 267: 2745, 1992.

Orenstein WA, Markowitz L, Preblud SR, et al. Appropriate age for measles vaccination in the United States. Dev. Biol. Stand. 65:13–21, 1986.

Orenstein WA, Halsey NA, Hayden GF, et al. Current status of measles in the United States 1973–1977. J. Infect. Dis. 137:847–853, 1978.

Orenstein WA, Bernier RH, Dondero TJ, et al. Field evaluation of vaccine efficacy. Bull. WHO. 63:1055–1068, 1985.

Orenstein WA, Bernier RH, and Hinman AR. Assessing vaccine efficacy in the field. Further observations. Epidemiol. Rev. 10:212–241, 1988.

Orenstein WA. DTP vaccine litigation, 1988. Am. J. Dis. Child. 144:517, 1990.

Orenstein WA, Hinman AR, and Rodewald L. Public health considerations—U.S. In: Plotkin SA, Orenstein WA, eds. Vaccines. Philadelphia: WB Saunders, 1999:1006–1032.

Osborne K, Weinberg J, and Miller E. The European Sero-Epidemiology Network. European Communicable Disease Bulletin 2:29–31, 1997.

Panagiotopoulos T, Antoniadou I, and Valassi-Adam E. Increase in congenital rubella occurrence after immunisation in Greece: retrospective survey and systematic review. BMJ. 319:1462–1467, 1999.

Patriarca PA, Laender F, Palmeira G, et al. Randomized trial of an alternative formulation of polio vaccine in Brazil. Lancet 1:429–433, 1988a.

Patriarca PA, Biellik RJ, Sanders G, et al. Sensitivity and specificity of clinical case definitions for pertussis. Am. J. Public Health 78:833–836, 1988b.

Payne T, Kanvik S, Seward R, et al. Development and validation of an immunization tracking system in a large health maintenance organization. Am. J. Prev. Med. 9:96–100, 1993.

Poland GA. Immunogenetic mechanisms of antibody response to measles vaccine: the role of the HLA genes. Vaccine. 17(13–14):1719–1725, 1999.

Prentice RL. A case-cohort design for epidemiologic cohort studies and disease prevention trials. Biometrika. 73:1–12, 1986.

Prevots DR, Sutter RW, Strebel PM, Weibel RE, and Cochi SL. Completeness of reporting for paralytic poliomyelitis, U.S., 1980–1991. Arch. Pediatr. Adolesc. Med. 148:479–485, 1994.

Recommended childhood immunization schedule-United States, January–June 1996. MMWR. 44:940–943, 1996.

Reichler MR, Darwish A, Stroh G, et al. Cluster survey evaluation of coverage and risk factors for failure to be immunized during the 1995 National Immunization Days in Egypt. Int. J. Epidemiol. 27:1083–1089, 1998.

Rico-Hesse R, Pallansch MA, Nottay BK, and Kew OM. Geographic distribution of wild poliovirus type 1 genotypes. Virology. 160 (2):311–322, 1987.

Robbins RB, Brandling Bennett AD, and Hinman AR. Low measles incidence: association with enforcement of school immunization laws. Am. J. Public Health. 91:270–274, 1981.

Rodrigues LC, and Smith PG. Use of the case-control approach in vaccine evaluation: efficacy and adverse effects. Epidemiol. Rev. 21 (1):56–72, 1999.

Rohani P, Earn DJ, and Grenfell BT. Opposite patterns of synchrony in sympatric disease metapopulations. Science. 286:968–971, 1999.

Rosenthal S, and Chen RT. Reporting sensitivities of two passive surveillance systems for vaccine adverse events. Am. J. Public Health. 85:1706–1709, 1995.

Rosenthal S, Chen R, and Hadler SC. The safety of acellular pertussis vaccine versus whole cell pertussis vaccine: a post-marketing assessment. Arch. Pediatr. Adolesc. Med. 150:457–460, 1996.

Rothman KJ, and Greenland S. Modern Epidemiology. Philadelphia: Lippincott Williams & Wilkins, 1998.

Roush S, Birkhead G, Koo D, Cobb A, and Fleming D. Mandatory reporting of diseases and conditions by health care professionals and laboratories. JAMA. 282(2):164–170, 1999.

Rousseau MC, Moreau J, and Delmont J. Vaccination and HIV: a review of the literature. Vaccine. 18(9–10):825–831, 1999.

Royal College of General Practitioners. Effect of a low pertussis vaccination uptake on a large community. Br. Med. J. 282:23–26, 1981.

Salisbury DM, and Dittman S. Immunization in Europe. In: Plotkin SA, Orenstein WA, eds. Vaccines. Phialdelphia: WB Saunders, 1999: 1033–1046.

Salmon DA, Haber M, Gangarosa EJ, et al. Health consequences of religious and philosophical exemptions from immunization laws: individual and societal risk of measles. J. Am. Med. Assoc. 282:47–53, 1999.

Santoli JM, Szilagyi PG, and Rodewald LE. Barriers to immunization and missed opportunities. Pediatr. Ann. 27:366–374, 1998.

Santoli JM, Rodewald LE, Maes EF, et al. Vaccines for Children program, United States, 1997. Pediatrics. 104:e15, 1999.

Satcher D. From the Surgeon General. Polio eradication by the year 2000. JAMA. 281:221, 1999.

Schlenker TL, Bin C, Baughman AL, and Hadler SC. Measles herd immunity: the association of attack rates with immunization rates in preschool children. JAMA. 267:823–826, 1992.

Schonberger LB, Bregman DJ, Sullivan-Bolyai JZ, et al. Guillain-Barré syndrome following vaccination in the national influenza immunization program, United States, 1976–1977. Am. J. Epidemiol. 110:105–123, 1979.

Schwartz JG, Weniger BG, and Chen RT. Vaccine Identification Standards Initiative. Poster presentation at the 32nd National Immunization Conference, Atlanta, GA, July 21–24, 1998.

Scuffham PA, Lowin AV, and Burgess MA. The cost-effectiveness of varicella vaccine programs for Australia. Vaccine. 18(5–6):407–415, 1999.

Shefer A, Briss P, Rodewald L, et al. Improving immunization coverage rates: an evidence-based review of the literature. Epidemiol. Rev. 21(1):96–142, 1999.

Siber GR. Methods for estimating serological correlates of protection. Dev. Biol. Stand. 89: 283–296, 1997.

Smith PG, Rodrigues LC, and Fine PEM. Assessment of the protective efficacy of vaccines among common diseases using case-control and cohort studies. Int. J. Epidemiol. 13:87–93, 1984.

Smith PG, Retrospective assessment of the effectiveness of BCG vaccination against tuberculosis using the case-contorl method. Tubercle. 62:23–35, 1982.

Steere AC, Sikand VK, Meurice F, et al. Vaccination against Lyme disease with recombinant Borrelia burgdorferi outer-surface lipoprotein A with adjuvant. N. Engl. J. Med. 339: 209–215, 1998.

Stetler HC, Orenstein WA, Bart KJ, et al. History of convulsions and use of pertussis vaccine. J. Pediatr. 107:175–179, 1985.

Stratton KR, Howe CJ, Johnston RB, eds. Adverse Events Associated with Childhood Vaccines. Washington DC: National Academy Press, 1994.

Strebel PM, Sutter RW, Cochi SL, et al. Epidemiology of poliomyelitis in the U.S. one decade after last reported case of indigenous wild virus-associated disease. Clin. Infect. Dis. 14: 568–579, 1992.

Strebel PM, Cochi SL, Farizo KM, et al. Pertussis in Missouri: evaluation of nasopharyngeal culture, DFA testing, and clinical case definition in the diagnosis of pertussis. Clin. Infect. Dis. 16:276–285, 1993.

Strom BL, and Canson JL. Use of automated databases for pharmacoepidemiology research. Epidemiol. Rev. 12:87–107, 1990.

Sutter RW, and Cochi SL. Pertussis hospitalization and mortality in the U.S., 1985–1988: evaluation of the completeness of national reporting. JAMA. 267:386–391, 1992.

Sutter RW, Cochi SL, Brink EW, and Sirotkin BI. Assessment of vital statistics and surveillance data for monitoring tetanus mortality, United States, 1979–1984. Am. J. Epidemiol. 131: 132–142, 1990.

Szilagyi PG, and Rodewald LE. Missed opportunities for immunizations: a review of the evidence. J. Public Health Management Practice. 2:1825, 1996.

Tackett CO, Mattheis MJ, and Rennels MB. Initial clinical evaluation of new vaccine candidates. In: Levine MM, Woodrow GC, Kaper JB, Cobon GS, eds. New Generation Vaccines. New York: Marcel Dekker, 1997:35–45.

Takala AK, Koskenniemi E, Joensuu J, et al. Economic evaluation of rotavirus vaccinations in Finland: randomized, double-blind, placebo-controlled trial of tetravalent rhesus rotavirus vaccinel Clin. Infect. Dis. 27:272–282, 1998.

Taylor CE, Cutts F, and Taylor ME. Ethical dilemmas in current planning for polio eradication. Am. J. Public Health. 87:922–925, 1997.

Teutsch SM, Churchill RE, eds. Principles and Practice of Public Health Surveillance. Oxford: Oxford University Press, 1994.

Thacker SB, and Berkelman RL. Public health surveillance in the United States. Epidemiol. Rev. 10:164–190, 1988.

Tucker AW, Haddix AC, and Bresee JS. Cost-effectiveness analysis of a rotavirus immunization program for the United States. JAMA. 279:1371–1376, 1998.

Turner AG, Magnani RJ, and Shuaib M. A not quite as quick but much cleaner alternative to the Expanded Programme on Immunization (EPI) cluster survey design. Int. J. Epidemiol. 25:198–203, 1996.

Verstraeten TM, Baughman AL, Haber P. Enhancing the Vaccine Adverse Event Reporting System (VAERS) to assess risk: a capture-recapture analysis of intussusception after rotavirus vaccination (abstract). Pharmacoepidemiol. Drug Safety 9:S27, 2000.

Ward J, Lieberman JM, and Cochi S. *Haemophilus influenzae* vaccines. In: Plotkin SA, Mortimer EA, eds. Vaccines. Philadelphia: WB Saunders, 1994: 337:386.

Wassilak SGF, Orenstein WA, Strickland PL, et al. Continuing measles transmission in students despite a school-based outbreak control program. Am. J. Epidemiol. 122:208–217, 1985.

Wenger JD, DiFabio J, Landaverde JM, Levine OS, and Gaafar T. Introduction of Hib conjugate vaccines in the non-industrialized world: experience in four 'newly adopting' countries. Vaccine. 18(7–8):736–742, 1999.

Weniger BG, Chen RT, Jacobson SH, et al. Addressing the challenges to immunization practice with an economic algorithm for vaccine selection. Vaccine. 16(19):1885–1897, 1998.

Williams JC, Goldenthal KL, Burns D, et al., eds. Combined Vaccines and Simultaneous Administration: Current Issues and Perspective. New York: New York Academy of Sciences, 1995.

Witte JJ, Karchner AW, Case G, et al. Epidemiology of rubella. Am. J. Dis. Child. 118:107–111, 1969.

Wood D, Saarlas KN, Inkelas M, and Matyas BT. Immunization registries in the United States: implications for the practice of public health in a changing health care system. Annu. Rev. Public Health. 20:231–255, 1999.

Woodrow GC. An overview of biotechnology as applied to vaccine development. In: Levine MM, Woodrow GC, Kaper JB, Cobon GS, eds. New Generation Vaccines. New York: Marcel Dekker, 1997:25–34.

World Bank. World Development Report 1993: Investing in Health. New York: Oxford University Press, 1993:72–107.

World Health Organization. Department of Vaccines and Other Biologicals Annual Report 1998. Geneva, World Health Organization (WHO/V&B/99.01), 1999.

Part V

RESEARCH IN
SPECIAL POPULATIONS
OR SETTINGS

18

Research in Out-of-Home Child Care

RALPH L. CORDELL, LARRY K. PICKERING,
and M. LOUISE LAWSON

The increase in both the number and proportion of children in out-of-home child care over the last 30 years (Hofferth et al. 1991, Thacker et al. 1992, Casper 1997) has had both economic and public health consequences. The economic impact results from indirect costs, including parental absence from work because of child care–associated illness (Haskins 1989, Hofferth et al. 1991), and from direct medical costs associated with the illness (Avendano et al. 1993, Hardy 1994, Carabin et al. 1999b). The public health impact results from the child care contribution to the emergence of a number of infectious diseases (Holmes 1996) and from the widespread use of antimicrobial agents and resultant increase in antimicrobial resistance among a number of pathogens (Reves 1990).

The study of the epidemiology of infectious diseases in out-of-home child care has paralleled the increasing use of child care. Only a few investigators addressed the problem of illness in child care facilities prior to the 1940s (Anderson 1926, Conrad 1932, Anderson 1934). At the end of World

War II, a number of British researchers reported on conditions and problems in day nurseries and facilities caring for children removed from areas targeted by the Blitz (Ormiston 1942, Landon 1943, McKay 1945, Menzies 1946, Brown 1947, Forsyth 1947, McLaughlin 1947). Diehl's report (1949) comparing the prevalence of colds among children in nursery schools with that among children cared for at home was one of the first to compare the risk of illness among children in different types of child care settings. The reports of increased risk of children in child care for invasive *Haemophilus influenzae* type b infections (Redmond 1984, Istre et al. 1985, Cochi et al. 1986) and diarrheal illness (Pickering et al. 1981, 1982, 1984, Ekanem et al. 1983, Keswick et al. 1983a,b, Kim 1983, Lemp et al. 1984, Bartlett et al. 1985) and the role of child care facilities in community outbreaks of hepatitis A (Hadler et al. 1980), shigellosis (Rosenberg et al. 1976), and cytomegalovirus (CMV) infections (Strangert et al. 1976, Strom 1979, Pass et al. 1982, 1984, CDC 1985) during the late 1970s and early

1980s heralded the emergence of child care epidemiology as an area of study. This led to the Symposium on Infectious Diseases in Child Care, which was held in Minneapolis in 1984 (Osterholm et al. 1986). Child care epidemiology in the 1990s was highlighted by publication of the *National Performance Standards* (currently being revised) by the American Public Health Association and American Academy of Pediatrics (1992) and the *ABC's of Safe and Healthy Child Care* by the U.S. Centers for Disease Control and Prevention (CDC) (Hale 1996), the 1992 International Conference on Child Day Care Health in Atlanta, and development of an action plan for health and safety in out-of-home child care (CDC 1994). Much of the interest during the latter half of the 1990s centered around the role of child care facilities in the emergence of infectious diseases and the development of antimicrobial resistance. Although it is difficult to predict the course the field will take as we enter the next decade, child care epidemiologists likely will be called on to address issues of quality child care, the cost-effectiveness of interventions, and the provision of care for mildly ill children. Emerging infections and antimicrobial resistance will continue to play a role in our investigations.

This chapter describes (1) the general epidemiology of child care–associated illnesses and risk factors for transmission of infections in child care facilities, (2) the different types of epidemiologic studies used in child care settings, and (3) the methodologic challenges encountered in conducting studies in this area.

GENERAL EPIDEMIOLOGY OF CHILD CARE–ASSOCIATED ILLNESS

Child care–associated illnesses may be defined as those infections resulting from transmission within an out-of-home child care setting. Intrafacility transmission of infections in child care amplifies the prevalence of infections already circulating in the community. Since strains of pathogens circulating in child care facilities are often identical to those found in the community, it is generally difficult to attribute a given illness episode to child care exposure except in the case of well-defined, focal outbreaks. For this reason, the risk associated with exposure to child care generally is expressed in the context of comparison with a control group of similarly aged persons, in the same community, not exposed to child care.

Four patterns of illness occurrence have been characterized based on groups most likely to experience clinical illness (Table 18–1) (Goodman et al. 1984, Pickering 1987). One significance of these patterns is that they represent groups that need to be monitored or interviewed for indications of outbreaks in child care facilities. They also reflect levels of immunity and the natural history of various infections that occur in child care facilities. Once introduced by an ill child, infections are transmitted to other children and staff by fomites, direct contact, aerosols, and food. This spread is facilitated by infectious prodromes and inapparent infections, a high proportion of susceptible individuals, conducive behaviors such as mouthing and incontinence, and the need for hands-on care. Unless effective interventions are applied, multiple transmission cycles may occur and pathogens may be transmitted into homes and the general community.

A number of models have been developed to describe disease transmission in child care facilities. One of the first described transmission patterns for hepatitis A virus (Hadler et al. 1982). Factors influencing the occurrence of hepatitis A virus were divided into those influencing the risk of introducing pathogens into a facility and those influencing transmission once a pathogen has been introduced. The former group included total enrollment, enrollment of young children, number of hours open per day, and operation for profit. Spread of infection once introduced was correlated only with minimum age. Ekanem and coworkers (1983) developed a model depicting spread of enteric bacteria within child care centers. This model demonstrated how, once introduced into a facility, pathogens can be spread to other children, staff, and fomites, including toys, classroom floors, and diaper-changing

Table 18-1 Patterns of Occurrence of Child Care–Associated Infections Among Children and Contacts

Occurrence Pattern	Example
Illnesses affecting children, child care staff, and adult contacts	Gastrointestinal and respiratory tract infections, skin infections, and infestnations
Symptomatic illness predominately among children.	Varicella, *Haemophilus influenzae* type b disease, otitis media
Symptomatic illness predominately among adults with mild or asymptomatic infections among children.	Hepatitis A, some enterovirus infections
Mild or asymptomatic infections common among both children and adults with severe infections among fetuses of infected women or persons with immune deficiencies.	Cytomegalovirus, parvovirus B-19

Source: Modified from Pickering 1987.

areas. This model was expanded to include foodborne transmission and the role of hand-washing, frequency of contact, host susceptibility, and agent survival (Laborde et al. 1993). Studies demonstrating contamination of hands, surfaces, and fomites in child care centers and using DNA markers to track spread of organisms have supported these models (Wilde et al. 1992, Jiang et al. 1998). While these models were all developed for enteric pathogens, they probably are applicable with minor modifications to other modes of transmission. Although these models describe the classroom as the primary focus of interest, the reality is more complex, and infection may spread between classrooms through siblings. The practices of combining groups of children before and after normal operating hours, "graduating" individual children from younger to older classes, and interactions among groups of children in play and other common areas may also promote spread among classes or groups of children.

TYPES OF EPIDEMIOLOGIC STUDIES APPLIED TO CHILD CARE SETTINGS

A number of designs have been used in studies of infectious diseases in child care settings. The appropriateness of each design depends on questions to be addressed, resources available, and local circumstances. In some instances, for example, large sur-

veys, child care is only one of many variables studied, while in others, exposure to child care defines the study population. Reports often involve a combination of study designs and it is not unusual for a report on a cohort study to start by describing the prevalence or to report frequency distributions of pathogens identified through surveillance of a cohort of children. Many issues, such as parental notification, informed consent, and valid data collection, cut across study designs. Investigators accustomed to working in clinical or research settings probably will be dismayed at the incompleteness and inaccuracy of information in the records for children and child care providers in most child care settings. Perhaps the best advice we can give those planning research projects in child care facilities is to carefully read the methods sections of reports based on similar study designs. As the field is developing, there are few conventions. The following section highlights the few conventions as well as the many pitfalls and areas for improvision.

Surveillance Activities

Infectious disease surveillance in child care settings in the United States is primarily linked to the notifiable disease reporting system. Not all states require reporting from child care providers, however, and there is no nationwide surveillance for child care-associated illness. Although data from the notifiable disease reporting system have the potential to demonstrate trends and patterns, they are subject to variability and dependent on the goodwill, motivation, and interests of the multitude of child and health care providers, public health officials, and investigators who make up this system (Sherman 1952). Providers are often unaware of reporting requirements (Addiss et al. 1994) that are based on specific diagnoses (frequently unknown to the provider) or poorly defined terms such as "outbreaks" or "unusual occurrence." Symptom-based reporting has been suggested as a means to overcome these problems. However, participation in symptom-based surveillance systems in San Diego and Seattle child care facilities was low and the situation with respect to surveillance in child care settings is not likely to change until child care providers view disease monitoring and reporting as an important part of quality child care and until they receive appropriate training in that area (MacDonald et al. 1997, Cordell et al. 1999). That is not to say that surveillance in child care is not worthwhile. Targeted surveillance for specific conditions in motivated sentinel child care facilities could serve as an indication of illness in the community at large and provide useful information on the effectiveness of prevention and control programs as demonstrated in active surveillance systems in physicians' offices, hospitals, and the CDC's Food Net program to identify new foodborne pathogens.

Outbreak Investigations

The primary purpose of outbreak investigations is to identify the cause, interrupt spread, and develop recommendations for future prevention efforts (Polder 1996). However, outbreak investigations have provided information about both the epidemiologic and clinical characteristics of child care–associated illness and contributed to recognition of pathogens previously not associated with illness (Davis 1994). Although outbreaks in child care settings are seldom predictable, planning and preparation are certainly possible and will contribute to both the effectiveness of public health responses

and the ability to draw broader conclusions from results of investigations. Most outbreak investigations will be conducted in collaboration with local public health authorities. If this is not the case, local health officials should be notified of the investigation, since outbreaks are reportable conditions in most states.

Whenever possible, protocols should be developed for investigating outbreaks of illness associated with child care facilities. Protocols may be extensive and include the development and piloting of standardized data collection instruments and criteria for obtaining clinical and environmental samples (Davis 1994). If research is a prime focus and results are generalizable to other groups, consideration should be given to obtaining review by an Institutional Review Board. This is especially true if the work has been funded or results are to be published. Polder and Mohle-Boetani (1996) have addressed some of the practical aspects of outbreak investigations and identified several steps involved in investigating outbreaks in child care facilities. These include (1) determining the existence of an outbreak, (2) confirming the diagnosis and establishing the causative agent, (3) defining a case, developing a questionnaire, and counting cases, (4) orienting data according to time, place, and person, (5) determining who is at risk, (6) developing and testing hypotheses, (7) planning more systematic studies, (8) preparing a written report, and (9) executing prevention and control measures. The relative significance of each step will depend on circumstances. For example, in some instances, more systematic studies may not be feasible or necessary, whereas they may be vital in others. However, even the most cursory investigations can benefit by reference to these steps.

All protocols should include a communications path listing individuals and organizations that need to be contacted. Procedures for notifying licensing and public health agencies should be detailed. Criteria for arranging field activities, the purpose of such activities, staff involved, and their respective roles and responsibilities should all be determined. Individuals with expertise in epidemiology, sanitation, and child care should all take part in field activities and follow up. A method for communicating written information on follow-up activities, actions, and recommendations to child care providers should be developed.

Screening of exposed children and staff is a common component of outbreak investigations. However, screening in itself is not a disease control activity. Before the first specimen is collected, the reason for screening should be determined, the target population should be carefully identified, and plans for managing persons found to be infected should be in place and understood by all. Other considerations include specimen collection, storage and transport of specimens to the laboratory, and communication of results to parents, providers, and, possibly, public health officials. Although it is relatively easy for providers to collect stool specimens while changing diapers, older diapered children may not have a bowel movement at the facility or children (especially ill children) may be absent from the facility and parents may need to collect specimens at home. Specimen collection systems or instructions for collecting stools need to be provided for staff and parents of toilet-trained children. Confidentiality concerns need to be addressed in making decisions regarding disclosure of results. Although informed consent may not be required in some instances, parents should always be notified of testing. Parents who prefer to have their child screened by their pediatrician or health care provider should be allowed to do so provided assurance can be given that methods are comparable to those used for testing the remainder of the group.

Letters to parents are often an important part of follow-up activities. These letters provide information to parents and are often given to health care providers by parents seeking further advice or follow-up treatment. In order to be optimally useful, a letter should include background information on the specific exposure, the illness, directions for follow up, and a person or office to contact for further information. Background information should not identify the index case or provide information on his or her present condition or prognosis but should include the last date of attendance and the classroom or group. Specific information on the illness and causative agent should be included and the symptoms and mode of transmission described in terms understandable to a lay audience. Instructions for follow up should be given. These instructions may range from "contact your pediatrician or family physician if your child develops any of the above symptoms" to "contact your pediatrician or family physician as soon as possible concerning treating your child with _____." Include the telephone number of a contact person or agency able to answer questions. A number of sources contain information that may be useful in drafting these letters (Benenson 1990, Donowitz 1993, Hale 1996, American Academy of Pediatrics 1997).

Most states have laws and regulations governing reporting outbreaks and isolation of individuals with various communicable diseases. Investigators from academic or health care institutions who find themselves facing an outbreak in a child care setting should notify local public health officials as soon as possible in order to avoid problems and obtain assistance.

Case-Control Studies

Case-control studies involving child care–associated illness generally have been conducted in the context of a health care setting, such as a hospital (Anderson et al. 1988) or physician's office (Reves et al. 1993), or involved persons reported as being ill (Cochi et al. 1986, Arnold 1993, Chute 1987, Istre et al. 1985). Wenger and coworkers (1990) provided an interesting twist on this study design in their study of facility characteristics and invasive *H. influenzae* disease. They used the facility as the unit of analysis: case facilities had an ill child and control facilities did not have an ill child. This approach has promise and could be used more often to identify facility characteristics associated with illness.

One advantage to the case-control design is that cases and controls have been evaluated by a health care provider and are likely to be appropriately classified with respect to illness. It is also advantageous in dealing with relatively rare events such as hospitalization or in evaluating the association between illness and multiple risk factors. A disadvantage to case-control studies is that cases are often not representative of the entire spectrum of illness. Differences in exclusion and readmission policies may result in bias toward those facilities most likely to refer children to health care providers as a condition for readmission. Representativeness may be a problem when using facilities as the unit of analysis in case-control studies in that there may be a link between diligence in reporting and levels of hygiene. Another concern is to develop case definitions that are both sensitive and specific so as to minimize misclassification bias. This may be difficult when dealing only with information from child care providers. Conversely, when cases are selected through medical records or other reports, collecting information on facility characteristics and conditions may be difficult.

Analysis of case-control studies in the child care setting is similar to the analysis of data from other settings, with the odds ratio being the effect measure and logistic regression being the multivariate tool. Because many case-control studies in child care settings use some form of matching, it is important to consider the matching scheme in the analysis. Matching has the potential to introduce bias if the crude analysis is not stratified by the matching variable or the regression analysis is not conditional on the matching factor.

Prevalence Studies

Prevalence data from national interview surveys have provided most of our national data on child care–associated illness (Johansen 1988, Alexander et al. 1990, Hurwitz 1995) and conditions in child care (Addiss et al. 1994, Cain 1994). Cain (1994) reviews the methodologic issues surrounding these large population-based sample surveys. Data quality is perhaps the greatest concern in these studies, especially when interviewing par-

ents. Devising a question that will differentiate between or include the many different types of child care and their various regional and local appellations is difficult. Defining mild illness or other outcomes, such as absence due to illness, also may be difficult and the larger the number of respondents, the greater the variation in responses. Problems with recall and recall bias are also a serious concern (Cordell et al. 1997a, 1999). Population-based studies based on parental interviews may be best confined to more serious outcomes involving hospitalization, emergency medical attention, or outpatient procedures, because these are less likely to be subject to problems with definitions and recall.

Issues to confront in conducting population-based facility surveys generally involve sample frames. In most instances, these will be lists of licensed facilities obtained from state agencies and referral systems. Multistate surveys will likely encounter problems with differences in which types of facilities are required to be licensed. Complete and current lists also can be an issue, especially in the case of child care homes. Studies in San Diego and Seattle found that significant proportions of child care homes on lists from licensing agencies could not be contacted (MacDonald et al. 1997, Cordell et al. 1999). Surveys of Milwaukee child care facilities did not experience these difficulties (Cordell et al. 1997b). Lags between starting operations and adding new facilities onto licensure rolls may mean that newer facilities are underrepresented on these lists. Another consideration is the information source, that is, there may be differences in responses and quality of information obtained from directors or administrators of child care facilities and teachers or persons who actually are providing care. In a nationwide survey of child care providers, incidence data from directors were found to correlate with that from teachers (Ikeda 1994).

More focal, prevalence studies based on laboratory screening of children in child care have provided useful data on the prevalence of various pathogens during nonoutbreak conditions. Although these studies often collect information from a control group (e.g., children not in child care), they are not case-control studies in the strict sense of the term. Sometimes these studies take the form of sequential screening or prevalence measures. Although data may be collected over time, these technically are not prospective or cohort studies unless results can be expressed in terms of incidence rates. The major obstacles in these studies are gaining cooperation of facilities, obtaining informed consent, obtaining demographic data, and arranging specimen collection and transport.

If the focus of a prevalence study is to describe the prevalence of disease in a particular population, then prevalence rates with exact confidence intervals can be reported. If the purpose of a cross-sectional study is to describe predictors of disease, then the decision about the type of analysis becomes more complex. In general, if the population can be considered to be in a steady state and the investigator is interested in assessing the cause of incident cases, the prevalence odds ratio is the best estimator (Miettinen 1976). In this case, standard procedures for calculating the odds ratio using logistic regression should be used. For situations in which the steady state cannot be assumed (which is the case in most infectious disease outbreaks) or the investigator is interested in estimating the predictors of disease prevalence, then the prevalence rate ratio is the best estimator (Zocchetti 1976).

Cohort Studies

While some cohort studies have focused on children (Wald et al. 1988, 1991), a more frequent approach is to focus on facilities. This latter approach is especially suitable if variables of interest include facility characteristics. Many of the issues encountered in conducting cohort or prospective studies in child care settings are common to other study designs. Issues such as definition of illness, bias in data sources, representativeness of sampling frames, and participating facilities have been discussed in other sections and are equally applicable to this study design.

Dropout and failure to retain children, child care staff, and child care facilities can be a significant problem in conducting cohort studies in child care facilities. From 20% to 40% of facilities participating in studies in Seattle and San Diego withdrew before participating for one year (MacDonald et al. 1997, Cordell et al. 1999). The additional time and effort of participation was a major cause of dropout of child care centers in those studies. Every effort should be made to reduce or eliminate data collection burden on regular child care staff. Dropout may be reduced by routine contact (especially by trained personnel who can address providers' concerns about health issues) and tokens of appreciation. Although paying facilities to participate has been discussed, it is seldom done and may be prohibited in some instances. Field staff should be knowledgeable, personable, and willing to assist in child care activities, including changing diapers if the occasion arises. Staff turnover in excess of 50% per year is not unusual in child care facilities and can cause serious problems in studies involving child care homes. Discontinuation of providing child care was one of the major reasons for child care homes to cease participation in prospective studies. This may be minimized, but not eliminated, by limiting participation to those facilities that plan on maintaining operations for at least the duration of the study.

Collecting environmental information can be especially difficult in child care homes, and one must temper the need for rigorous data collection with the need for goodwill from providers. Differences in perception of data collection may occur in day care centers and child care homes. Overexuberance in data collection may contribute to dropout in either type of facility.

Depending on the duration and nature of the study, investigators may need to be concerned about the possibility of a Hawthorne-type effect in that participation in studies may result in an increased awareness of hygiene and infection control. Several investigators have noticed decreased illness levels after participation for a year or longer (Sullivan et al. 1984, Cordell et al. 1999).

Other issues unique to cohort studies include case counting and definitions. It is not unusual to have an illness begin as a mild respiratory tract infection with rhinitis then develop otitis media or a lower respiratory tract infection manifested by a cough along with otitis and end with gastrointestinal tract symptoms including vomiting and diarrhea. The purpose of the study will determine how such an episode is to be counted. Episode definition will also influence data entry, and investigators should decide how they want to categorize illness episodes before data entry or if this is to be included as part of computer programming. The former is somewhat easier in terms of data entry and analysis, while the latter allows for flexibility and consistency in the application of definitions.

Consideration also needs to be given to calculating denominators and adjusting for weekends, holidays, and times children are not in attendance in measuring duration of illness and attendance. At present, there are no conventions although most investigators use child-week in the denominator for incidence density rates and count any week or portion of a week for which information is received about a child as a child-week. We have used a life table approach in dealing with weekends and holidays. For example, if a child was sick on Friday but well the following Monday, we would count the child as being ill on Saturday and well on Sunday unless we had information to the contrary. Another approach would be to not count these days when doing calculations.

Cohort studies also need to deal with the issue of how long a child must be symptom-free before an illness can be considered a new episode. There is no consensus on this issue and consideration should be given to the illness being studied as well as methods of detection and definitions used in previously published reports. Researchers should be aware that symptoms of some illnesses such as cryptosporidiosis may be intermittent. If available, laboratory support can be valuable in clarifying these issues.

In analyzing cohort studies, all available data should be used despite the challenge of finding appropriate statistical tools. For standard cohort studies in which the expo-sure occurs at the beginning of the study and the outcome is development of a chronic illness or death, simple Poisson regression and survival analysis have been the tools of choice for multivariate analysis. Proportional hazards models allow for time-varying covariates, so repeated measures of predictor variables have been modeled using this technique. In child care studies, it is common to have more than one measurement of both predictors and disease, resulting in the need for some sort of repeated measures analysis. Generalized estimating equations (GEE) have gained popularity as repeated measures marginal models. GEE treats the correlations between observations on an individual or facility as nuisance parameters and calculates an averaged effect measure. In some instances, this is not the desired tool because the effect of the facility might be of interest. In this case, generalized linear models are useful to model specific effects of the facility on disease outcome (Zeger 1988). Methods that allow for correlation between multiple factors are under development (Shults 1998).

Intervention Studies

Intervention studies may be considered a population counterpart of clinical trials and subject to the same difficulties and issues. In addition, the move to the population level adds problems unique to intervention trials. A typical intervention trial in a child care setting consists of recruiting a number of child care facilities that are randomized to receive the intervention to be tested or to serve as controls. The unit of analysis should ideally be the facility, although data also can be analyzed at the level of the child. One of the first issues to be addressed is whether the control facilities should receive some intervention unrelated to the intervention to be tested. The reason for considering an intervention in the control group is that simply being exposed to any intervention may cause a change in behavior. Also, it has been shown that the Hawthorne effect results in increased handwashing in child care workers (Bartlett et al. 1988) and monitoring alone can result in disease reduction (Sullivan et al. 1984, Carabin et al. 1999a). The Hawthorne effect in an intervention trial is similar to the placebo effect in a clinical trial. Thus having the control group receive an intervention unrelated to the one being tested results in a more valid trial. Investigators must be careful, however, to choose a topic for intervention that would not be expected to have any effect on the behavior being targeted for study. If possible, it is best to use a comparison intervention that would be appropriate for subsequent monitoring (e.g., use an intervention on injury prevention as the control for an intervention in handwashing).

Another issue to be considered in intervention trials is that cultural norms can change during the period of the study. The change in norms may occur at a different rate in facilities that serve different populations or different geographic areas. Also, because the intermediate target of interventions is usually behavior, the measurement of outcomes can be challenging. If the goal of the intervention is to change behavior that leads to infection or injury, measurement of the ultimate target (disease or injury) should be considered. However, these outcomes depend not only on the behavior of those at risk but also on the background risk, which changes over time and place. Therefore, the investigator must consider how the risk has changed in the facility during the study period, how the background risk differed between facilities, and how the intervention has modified the risk. Investigators have often used instruments like the Harms and Clifford Early Childhood Environmental Rating Scale to make a somewhat objective measure of the physical environment of child care centers. Documenting background knowledge and practices of staff (pre- and posttests), demographic and cultural characteristics of facility staff and clients, and changes in facility practices also can help to reduce bias in intervention studies.

Finally, unlike clinical trials, which often test the efficacy of a drug to change the clinical outcome of disease in individuals under almost experimental conditions, intervention trials test the effectiveness of a program in changing the behavior of a population under real world conditions. Because of this, interpreting data from intervention trials can be challenging. The analysis used is similar to that of a cohort trial, with the relative risk being the effect measure of choice, and Poisson regression being used for multivariate analysis. It generally is not necessary to conduct repeated measures regression in analyzing data if the unit of analysis is the center, although special cluster techniques must be used if the unit of analysis is the individual. Cluster analysis techniques that control for both the repeated measures in the individual and the effect of the center are under development (Shults 1998). When analyzing data from an intervention trial it is important to distinguish, if possible, between an effective technique and an effective program. For example, increased handwashing by child care workers results in decreased diarrhea, so handwashing has been shown to be an effective prevention technique (Bartlett et al. 1988). Programs to increase handwashing, however, have met with limited long-term success in decreasing illness (Kotch et al. 1994, Carabin et al. 1999a), because such programs do not result in long-term increases in handwashing. Thus the failure is in the program, not in the technique. Investigators must also pay close attention to whether the intervention under study is passive (decreasing risk of scalds by lowering temperature of water heaters) or active (decreasing risk of scalds by training workers to test water before bathing children). In the latter case, success or failure of the intervention should be reported in terms of both intervention/nonintervention rates of injury and whether the behavior was adopted. This is a change from the classic advice to analyze clinical trials only from an intent-to-treat basis. For intervention studies, the nature of the success or failure is important in designing future interventions and should be reported in detail.

Environmental Studies

Environmental studies generally are classified into one of the above categories but are unique in that they involve data on pathogens or indicator organisms in the environment. They may take the form of prevalence-type studies, where microbes are most likely to be found, or intervention studies, where particular interventions result in a decrease in the frequency of microbes in the child care environment.

Molecular Studies

The powerful techniques of molecular biology are being used in child care settings with promising results. These techniques may be used in conjunction with standard epidemiologic study designs or in modifications. There are several advantages to using molecular techniques in epidemiologic studies of infection in the child care setting. A major advantage of molecular techniques is that they allow investigators to determine if viral pathogens are present in an outbreak. This has been especially useful in the study of gastroenteritis, because major outbreaks in child care centers are often caused by rotaviruses, enteric adenoviruses, astroviruses and caliciviruses, which can not be cultured easily. In addition, molecular techniques can be used to demonstrate past infection and the development of immunity by showing the presence of antibodies to specific pathogens and viral types (O'Ryan et al. 1990). The seroepidemiology of rotavirus proved instrumental in developing a vaccine, as multiple types of rotavirus are present in nature. Thus the ability of molecular techniques to distinguish between subtypes of pathogens can be extremely important in the understanding and prevention of disease outbreaks. In addition, immunoassays are often less expensive and labor intensive than standard culture techniques, and allow easier collection and processing of samples.

Thus the use of molecular techniques is becoming common in child care studies. Molecular techniques have been used to show that CMV infection occurs in children in child care settings by demonstrating common strains among children in a large child care center compared to the multiple strains found among children not attending child care (Adler 1985). These techniques have also been used to show mucosal immunity

to *Giardia lamblia* (Hashkes et al. 1994), to isolate the source of an *Escherichia coli* outbreak in Wisconsin (Gouveia et al. 1998), to illustrate two distinct campylobacter outbreaks occurring simultaneously in Brussels child care centers (Goossens et al. 1995), to determine the risk of CMV seroconversion in child care workers (Murph et al. 1991), to document hepatitis B transmission in an elementary school (Williams et al. 1977), and to detect rotavirus in the environment (Wilde et al. 1992). A novel use of molecular techniques is the use of a DNA marker from a cauliflower mosaic virus to model the spread of disease pathogens with a child care center (Jiang et al. 1998). The advantage of such a technique is that the marker can be used without risk of disease, so researchers can study transmission without waiting for an outbreak of illness.

METHODOLOGIC AND DESIGN CHALLENGES OF CONDUCTING RESEARCH IN OUT-OF-HOME CHILD CARE SETTINGS

Child care facilities are a constantly changing kaleidoscope of children, providers, and environmental conditions that appears to defy the standardization and structure that is so important to scientific research. We have discussed some of the challenges and issues unique to various study designs in the preceding section. Here we discuss issues common to multiple study designs. In some instances, topics may be the same but the perspectives differ.

Definitions and Generalizability

The variability in form and organization of child care facilities makes it difficult to compare results from one study to those from another. The American Academy of Pediatrics (AAP) has defined three basic types of out-of-home child care: small family child care homes, large family child care homes, and child care centers (1997). In addition to these three types, there are preschools, nursery schools, and facilities associated with a variety of establishments ranging from gambling casinos to religious institutions. The majority of published literature has focused on child care centers. There also are significant differences in structure and management of child care facilities within the United States and across international boundaries. The three family systems in Scandinavian countries are considerably different from the family child care homes in the United States. Investigators should clearly describe their study settings, using standard categories such as those developed by the AAP.

Illness definitions are another area for consideration. Although studies should obtain illness information from health care providers and base definitions of disease on rigorous clinical or laboratory data, many studies obtain illness information from parents or child care providers without using well-structured definitions. Studies of diarrheal illness generally have used definitions based on providers' opinions of what was unusual with respect to form or frequency of stooling for a particular child. One advantage with this approach is that care providers are in a position to have observed the child's stool pattern before and after the diarrheal illness.

Definitions of respiratory illness are variable. Some investigators have combined otitis, pharyngitis, rhinitis, and cough into respiratory illness, while others report them separately or in various combinations. A given illness episode may involve a combination of the above symptoms and may change over time.

Size

Although group size has been frequently cited as a risk factor for illness, this concept has been used in several different contexts and there are different measures of group size. The concept underlying the use of size as a risk factor is that it reflects the likelihood of introducing a pathogen into a facility and the likelihood of exposure to an infected child. Some investigators have evaluated facility size while others have evaluated primary group (classroom) size. Primary group size may be more important than facility size in determining risk of otitis

(Marx 1995). If one considers child care facilities to be analogous to pot luck suppers and each child brings the pathogens circulating in his or her household to the mix, the situation becomes even more complex, as one generally finds groups of siblings as well as singletons in child care facilities. The exposure dynamics between eight children in a child care home (primary group) may be considerably different than those between eight children in a child care center class. The eight children in the child care home generally represent groups of siblings of different ages, perhaps representing three or four different households, who will continue to have contact outside the facility. The eight children in the child care centers are of similar age, generally represent eight households and will cease to have contact once they leave the facility.

Measures of group size include licensed capacity, average daily attendance, total enrollment, and mixing of different age groups. Licensed capacity usually is found in licensing records and can be used to compare participating and nonparticipating facilities. Licensed capacity generally refers to the maximum number of children that may be cared for at any point in time. The actual attendance may be less or greater than the licensed capacity. Average daily attendance may give a good measure of the level of crowding and number of exposures in a given time period. Children are often placed in drop-off groups before and after normal operating hours, and a child in a class with an average daily attendance of 10 may have exposure to many more children during a day. Total enrollment may be the best measure of the number of different persons a child is likely to encounter during a longer time period.

Age Groups

Most child care centers group children by age groups dictated by licensing regulations. However, these are generally broad and there is a great deal of variation. Where classroom is used as a unit of analysis, combining data across different facilities may not be appropriate because of differences in grouping by age. The age structure of a toddler class in one facility may be quite different from that in another. This may be one reason why many investigators use child as the unit of analysis. Facilities also differ in their practices with respect to moving children up to the next age group. Some move the entire group forward (much like elementary schools) while others move one child at a time depending on birth date or level of development. Although age is an important risk factor for illness, the issue may be circumvented somewhat by using the presence of a non-toilet-trained child in the classroom as a surrogate for age. In child care homes, the ages of enrolled children have a wider range and may include infants to preschool aged children.

Sources of Data

The three major sources of information about illness among children in child care are parents (or other adult household members), health care providers, and child care providers. All three may be potential sources of bias. With respect to provider reporting, children in child care might be more likely to be taken to emergency rooms for minor illness than children in home care (Mackenzie 1994). In addition, providers may be more likely to remember and report major illness and injury than relatively minor events. These problems may be overcome by using daily illness/injury logs and collecting data prospectively. The major problems with provider-reported illness, however, are that providers are likely to miss illness that is minor or subclinical, providers can not provide information about the pathogen causing illness, and providers can supply little information about illness resulting in the child being kept at home. Interest and motivation may have a positive influence on reporting as well as in maintaining healthy conditions in child care settings. Facilities with the highest scores (most hygienic conditions) on environmental surveys may have the highest incidence of provider-reported illness. These problems are more difficult to solve and illustrate why many investigators prefer to collect data from children and parents di-

rectly, in spite of the added expense and difficulty of such studies. Parental information generally has been obtained through telephone surveys, usually asking about illness in the last two weeks, although in some instances the period of inquiry has included the past year. Parents may be more likely to remember conditions involving time off from work or those requiring medical attention than those not involving a major change in routine. Because child care centers are more likely to exclude mildly ill children than are child care homes, parents of children in child care homes may be more likely to underreport illness than are those of children in center care. Health care providers have been important sources of information for conducting case-control studies. However, a potential for bias exists, in that factors influencing parents' decision to seek health care for an ill child include severity of illness and exclusion from child care. Capture-recapture methods have recently been proposed as a possible solution to this dilemma and as a means to adjust for ascertainment bias (Cordell et al. 1999). Illness information prospectively collected from child care providers could be combined with that from cross-sectional telephone surveys of randomly selected parents with interviews covering a period no longer than one week prior to the call. This method should provide more complete information than either method alone. For outcomes such as illness or injury requiring medical attention or antibiotic use, parents are probably the best source of information. In most instances, mothers or female heads of household are the best sources of information on health status.

Unit of Analysis

The determination as to whether the primary unit of analysis will be the child, the classroom, or the facility is important to the study design and analysis and interpretation of results. The majority of studies have used the child as the unit of analysis. This approach generally provides the greatest power though there is a problem with a lack of independence between observations. This may be resolved somewhat during the analysis phase by using software that allows one to specify the sampling method and control for a lack of independence in observations.

The unit of analysis also depends on the study design. Case-control studies generally use the child as the unit of analysis although there is at least one example where the facility was the unit of analysis (Wenger et al. 1990). Outbreak and environmental studies often focus on classrooms. Cohort studies may focus on the individual (Cordell et al. 1999) or the classroom (Kotch et al. 1994). The facility has been used as the unit of analysis in national surveys (Addiss et al. 1994), case control studies (Wenger et al. 1990), and prevalence studies (Hadler et al. 1980). Some studies have used multiple units of analysis (Van et al. 1992).

Outcome Measures

A number of different outcome measures have been used in child care studies. The choice of outcome is critical to the interpretation of study results and must be balanced among various issues including cost, convenience, privacy, reliability, sensitivity, and reproducibility. Types of outcomes that have been collected about children can be divided into several broad categories. Studies tend to focus on infectious disease transmission and prevention, injury severity, and causes and costs and benefit of child care and vaccines. Some pathogens (e.g., hepatitis A, parvovirus B-19, and CMV) may cause insignificant illness in immunocompetent children and more dangerous infections in adults and immunocompromised hosts. In the case of hepatitis A virus infection, disease in the child is an exposure variable, and the outcome is illness in adults. Sources of data include reports from the facility director and staff, hospital admission records and public health surveillance systems. As always, the gold standard of data collection methods is a prospective cohort study with data collected directly from children, staff, and parents.

Common measures collected at facilities include rates of gastroenteritis, respiratory tract illness, or injury as reported by child care workers (Chang 1989, Sacks et al. 1989, Briss et al. 1994, Jorm 1994, Kotch

et al. 1994, Cordell et al. 1997a, 1999). Causes of gastroenteritis in children include bacteria (*Campylobacter jejuni, Shigella* sp., *Clostridium difficile, Escherichia coli,* and *Salmonella* sp.), viruses (rotavirus, calicivirus, astrovirus, enteric adenovirus), and parasites (*Cryptosporidium* and *Giardia)* (American Academy of Pediatrics 1997, Pickering 1997). Child level studies of gastroenteritis have used numerous definitions of outcome, including incidence of loose or watery stools (Collet et al. 1994, Kotch et al. 1994), presence of pathogens in stools (Goossens et al. 1995, Gouveia et al. 1998), fecal contamination of the environment (Van et al. 1991, Laborde et al. 1993, Holaday et al. 1995), and antibody in the blood (O'Ryan et al. 1994, Goossens et al. 1995) and saliva (Hashkes et al. 1994). An important issue to consider in selecting an outcome for a study of gastroenteritis is the sensitivity and specificity of the measure. Detecting pathogens in stool is very specific, but some bacteria and many viruses are difficult to isolate in culture systems. Using molecular tools (for stool or body fluids) increases sensitivity but can lead to false positive results, detection of subclinical infections, and detection of previous infections. Finding a pathogen during a clinical illness does not always mean the pathogen is responsible for disease. For example, a nested case-control study of diarrhea and astrovirus infection in child care centers found that cases and controls were equally likely to have astrovirus (Lew et al. 1991). Thus it is important that control data be gathered in most research protocols.

Respiratory tract infections in child care centers are usually caused by viral pathogens (e.g., rhinovirus, adenovirus, parainfluenza virus, influenza virus, and respiratory syncytial virus), but they can also be the result of nonviral pathogens (e.g., *Streptococcus pneumoniae, Neisseria meningitidis, Bordetella pertussis, Mycobacterium tuberculosis)* (American Academy of Pediatrics 1997). Outcomes related to respiratory tract illness are varied and often difficult to define. Respiratory tract infection is the most common illness reported in child care facilities but the symptoms vary. Characteristics defining upper respiratory tract infection (URI) from two cohort studies included coughing, runny nose, wheezing or rattling in the chest, sore throat, earache, otitis media (as diagnosed by a physician), or laryngitis (Collet et al. 1993, Kotch et al. 1994). URI is often initially caused by a viral agent but secondary infections due to bacteria may occur. Thus assigning a particular illness to a particular cause can be problematic. In addition, classic interventions have had little effect on the frequency of URI (Collet et al. 1993, Kotch et al. 1994, Carabin et al. 1999a), presumably because URI is usually infectious prior to being symptomatic and the infectious agent is airborne. Future research should focus on novel approaches to preventing URI in the child care setting. For example, there is some indication that the risk of otitis media can be reduced with the influenza A vaccine (Clements et al. 1995) and smaller classroom groups (Marx 1995). A clinical trial of a drug designed to stimulate nonspecific immunity also showed some promise (Collet et al. 1993). Interventions based on other such novel approaches might have more success than those based on improved hygiene and isolation.

Injury studies have historically used data from hospital records (Mackenzie 1994), registries (Chang 1989, Kopjar 1996), or surveillance systems (Sacks et al. 1989, Briss et al. 1995). A major issue with injury outcomes is how injury is defined and rated. The most comparable injury outcome across studies is "injury requiring hospitalization." Beyond that investigators have tended to rate injuries either by type (e.g., laceration, bruise, broken bones) or severity (e.g., requiring no treatment, requiring minimal treatment). Injury report forms to be filled out prospectively by care providers have included type of injury, body part, location of injury, activity, and contributing factors (Alkon et al. 1994). Another important issue in reporting injury in child care settings is the collection of data from a comparison group, since there is evidence that injury may be more likely in the home setting (Rivara et al.

1989, Kopjar 1996). Reporting injury rates for child care centers without comparison groups could be unnecessarily alarming to parents and regulatory agencies.

Studies focusing on the costs of illness are relatively rare in child care research. The 1990 National Child Care Survey included information on time lost from work due to illness (Hofferth et al. 1991). Other studies have been conducted on subsets of a cohort study (Nurmi 1991) or cross-sectional surveys to estimate costs combined with cohort data on illness (Bell et al. 1989, Hardy 1994). A model for conducting cost-focused research has been published along with results from a representative cohort study (Carabin et al. 1999b). The authors suggest a breakdown of costs into direct costs (medication and physician visits) and indirect costs (missed work, cost of alternative care). This suggestion mirrors previous approaches, but this recent study collected data on actual costs as recorded prospectively on calendars and enhanced via telephone interview surveys every two weeks. This prospective data collection is an improvement in cost accounting and reflects growing interest among public health researchers and policymakers in documenting costs, benefits, and economic efficiency.

There are several useful tools to be recommended for improving the overall validity of research in child care facilities. Scales for ranking the physical environment of a child care center, such as the Harms and Clifford Early Childhood Environmental Rating Scale (Harms 1980) are available commercially. Checklists can be created from the APHA/AAP National Health and Safety Performance Standards (American Public Health Association 1992, Hawks et al. 1994, Lie et al. 1994) and can be used to document background risk and to measure confounders. Compliance with the standards has also been the target of research (Addiss et al. 1994). Lastly, data from government sources (e.g., *Morbidity Mortality Weekly Reports*) and previously published reports should be used to calculate seasonal and age-specific incidence rates for illness

(Morrow 1991). These data can also be used as a starting place for power calculations in determining necessary sample sizes.

Comparability and Representativeness

Investigators frequently are called to demonstrate that one group of facilities is comparable to another. An example would be to compare participating facilities with the remainder of those in the area. Commonly used criteria include whether or not the facility accepts children who are toilet trained, for-profit/not-for-profit status, licensed capacity, and management structure (sole facility or part of a local or nationwide chain). The advantage to these variables is that they usually are available from licensing records. However, except for the first, one can question the relevance of these variables in demonstrating meaningful comparability. As previously discussed, the risk of illness in child care facilities is due to a number of factors, only some of which are under the control of a facility. Although each of the criteria has, at one time or another, been associated with an increased risk of illness, they can hardly be considered valid indicators of comparability.

It is extremely difficult to conduct studies in a truly random sample of child care facilities. Although the initial sample may be random, dropout, especially of facilities, most often leaves the investigator with facilities that are willing to participate. Surveillance studies in both child care centers and homes in Seattle suggest that participation may be determined by factors other than the amount of work involved, as the proportion of facilities that provided data in an active surveillance system involving daily recording and weekly reporting of data was comparable to the proportion that provided data in a more passive system (MacDonald et al. 1997).

Informed Consent

Obtaining informed consent from parents can be even more difficult and labor intensive than recruiting a truly representative group of child care facilities. Contact with

parents is often limited in terms of time, that is, they are usually in a hurry to get to work and seldom in a position to engage in lengthy discussions as to the relative risks and benefits of participation. An effective process requires wholehearted support of the facility director and staff. Whenever possible, project staff should present study objectives and methods at parent meetings (simultaneous with obtaining consent). Ideally, project staff should be on site to recruit parents and answer questions during periods when parents drop children off and pick them up. However, this is often not possible and recruitment is frequently left to facility staff who are generally less enthusiastic and knowledgeable about the project than are project staff. Consent forms should include places for parents to indicate unwillingness as well as willingness to participate. Reasons for unwillingness to participate and demographic information of families who refuse participation should be recorded whenever possible. This will allow an estimation of the intensity of recruitment efforts, indicate concerns or problems parents may have with allowing their children to take part in research projects, and characterize those who refuse to participate. Sending consent forms home with children is generally ineffective and does not give parents an opportunity to ask questions that are an integral part of the informed consent process.

SUMMARY

Research in child care facilities is a methodologically challenging undertaking because of the tremendous amount of variation encountered over both place and time and among facilities. The multiple levels of possible analytic units (e.g., child, classroom or facility) add yet another dimension. Combining these analytic challenges with high levels of staff and child turnover and facility dropout results in a situation that almost defies the standardization that is so comforting to investigators in other settings. For these reasons, the caution needed to extrapolate results from studies conducted in the past, in other areas, or in small groups of facilities ensures that there will be a continuing and increasing need for work in this area.

REFERENCES

Addiss DG, Sacks JJ, Kresnow MJ, et al. The compliance of licensed US child care centers with National Health and Safety Performance Standards. Am. J. Public Health. 84 (7):1161–1164, 1994.

Adler SP. The molecular epidemiology of cytomegalovirus transmission among children attending a day care center. J. Infect. Dis. 152 (4):760–768, 1985.

Alexander CS, Zinzeleta EM, MacKenzie EJ, et al. Acute gastrointestinal illness and child care arrangements. Am. J. Epidemiol. 131(1): 124–131, 1990.

Alkon A, Genevro JL, Kaiser PJ, et al. Injuries in child-care centers: rates, severity, and etiology. Pediatrics. 94(6, Pt 2):1043–1046, 1994.

American Academy of Pediatrics. 1997 Red Book, Report of the Committee on Infectious Diseases. Elk Grove Village, IL, American Academy of Pediatrics, 1997.

American Public Health Association, American Academy of Pediatrics. Caring for Our Children National Health and Safety Performance Standards: Guidelines for Out-of-Home Child Care Programs. Washington: American Public Health Association, 1992.

Anderson HH. The attendance of nursery school children. Child Dev. 5:81–88, 1934.

Anderson JE. Attendance of nursery school children. School Soc. 24:182–184, 1926.

Anderson LJ, Parker RA, Strikas RA, et al. Day-care center attendance and hospitalization for lower respiratory tract illness. Pediatrics. 82 (3):300–308, 1988.

Arnold C, Makintube S, and Istre GR. Day care attendance and other risk factors for invasive *Haemophilus influenzae* disease. Am J. Epidemiol. 138(5):333–340, 1993.

Avendano P, Matson DO, Long J, et al. Costs associated with office visits for diarrhea in infants and toddlers. Pediatr. Infect. Dis. J. 12 (11):897–902, 1993.

Bartlett AV, Jarvis BA, Ross V, et al. Diarrheal illness among infants and toddlers in day care centers: effects of active surveillance and staff training without subsequent monitoring. Am. J. Epidemiol. 127(4):808–817, 1988.

Bartlett AV, Moore M, Gary GW, et al. Diarrheal illness among infants and toddlers in day care centers. II. Comparison with day care homes and households. J. Pediatr. 107(4):503–509, 1985.

Bell DM, Gleiber DW, Mercer AA, et al. Illness associated with child day care: a study of incidence and cost. Am. J. Public Health. 79(4): 479–484, 1989.

Benenson AS, ed. Control of Communicable Diseases in Man. Washington, DC: American Public Health Association, 1990.

Briss PA, Sacks JJ, Addiss DA, et al. A nationwide study of the risk of injury associated with day care center attendance. Pediatrics. 93(3): 364–368, 1994.

Briss PA, Sacks JJ, Addiss DA, et al. Injuries from falls on playgrounds. Effects of day care center regulation and enforcement. Arch. Pediatr. Adolesc. Med. 149(8):906–911, 1995.

Brown EH. *Giardia lamblia*: The incidence and results of infestation of children in residential nurseries. Arch. Dis. Child. 23:119–128, 1947.

Cain VS. Child care and child health: use of population surveys. Pediatrics. 94(6 Pt 2):1096–1098, 1994.

Carabin H, Gyorkos TW, Soto JC, et al. (1999a). Effectiveness of a training program in reducing infections in toddlers attending day care centers. Epidemiology. 10(3):808–817, 1999a.

Carabin H, Gyorkos TW, Soto JC, et al. Estimation of direct and indirect costs because of common infections in toddlers attending day care centers. Pediatrics. 103(3):556–564, 1999b.

Casper L. PPL-81, Who's Minding Our Preschoolers? Fall 1994 (Update), US Bureau of the Census, 1997.

Centers for Disease Control. Prevalence of cytomegalovirus excretion from children in five day-care centers—Alabama. MMWR 34(4): 49–52, 1985.

Centers for Disease Control and Prevention. CDC action plan for child care health and safety. Atlanta, GA. 1994.

Chang A, Lugg MM, and Nebedeum A. Injuries among preschool children enrolled in day-care centers. Pediatrics. 83(2):272–277, 1989.

Chute CG, Smith RP, and Baron JA. Risk factors for endemic giardiasis. Am. J. Public Health. 77(5):585–587, 1987.

Clements DA, Langdon L, Bland C, et al. Influenza A vaccine decreases the incidence of otitis media in 6- to 30-month-old chidren in day care. Arch. Pediatr. Adolesc. Med. 149(10): 1113–1117, 1995.

Cochi SL, Fleming DW, Hightower AW, et al. Primary invasive *Haemophilus influenzae* type b disease: a population-based assessment of risk factors. J. Pediatr. 108(6):887–896, 1986.

Collet JP, Ducruet T, Kramer MS, et al. Stimulation of nonspecific immunity to reduce the risk of recurrent infections in children attending day care centers. Pediatr. Infect. Dis. J. 12(8):648–652, 1993.

Collet JP, Burtin P, Kramer MS, et al. Type of day-care setting and risk of repeated infections. Pediatrics 94(6 Pt 2):997–999, 1994.

Conrad HS, and Jones MC. A two year record of attendance and colds in a nursery school. Child Dev. 3:43–52, 1932.

Cordell RL, MacDonald JK, Solomon SL, et al. Illnesses and absence due to illness among children attending child care facilities in Seattle-King County, Washington. Pediatrics. 100(5):850–855, 1997a.

Cordell RL, Thor PM, Addiss DG, et al. Impact of a massive waterborne cryptosporidiosis outbreak on child care facilities in metropolitan Milwaukee, Wisconsin. Pediatr. Infect. Dis. J. 16(7):639–644, 1997b.

Cordell RL, Waterman SL, Chang A, et al. Provider-reported illness and absence due to illness among children attending child care homes and child care centers in San Diego, California. Arch. Pediatr. Adolesc. Med. 153 (3):275–280, 1999.

Davis JP, MacKenzie WR, and Addiss DG. Recognition, investigation, and control of communicable-disease outbreaks in child day-care settings. Pediatrics. 94(6 Pt 2): 1004–1006, 1994.

Diehl I. The prevalence of colds in nursery school children and non-nursery school children. J. Pediatr. 34:52–61, 1949.

Donowitz LG, ed. Infection Control in the Child Care Center and Preschool. Baltimore: Williams & Wilkins, 1993.

Ekanem EE, DuPont HL, Pickering LK, et al. Transmission dynamics of enteric bacteria in day-care centers. Am. J. Epidemiol. 118(4): 562–572, 1983.

Forsyth FMJ. Work at a day nursery Br. Med. J. i:147, 1947.

Goodman RA, Osterholm MT, Granoff DM, et al. Infectious diseases and child day care. Pediatrics. 74(1):134–139, 1984.

Goossens H, Giesendorf BA, Vandamme P, et al. Investigation of an outbreak of Campylobacter upsaliensis in day care centers in Brussels: analysis of relationships among isolates by phenotypic and genotypic typing methods. J. Infect. Dis. 172(5):1298–1305, 1995.

Gouveia S, Proctor ME, Lee MS, et al. Genomic comparisons and shiga toxin production among Escherichia coli O157:H7 isolates from a day care center outbreak and sporadic cases in southeastern Wisconsin. J. Clin. Microbiol. 36(3):727–733, 1998.

Hadler SC, Erben JJ, Francis DP, et al. Risk factors for hepatitis A in day-care centers. J. Infect. Dis. 145(2):255–261, 1982.

Hadler SC, Webster HM, Erben JJ, et al. Hepatitis A in day-care centers. A community-wide assessment. N. Engl. J. Med. 302(22):1222–1227, 1980.

Hale C, and Polder J. ABC's of Safe and Healthy Child Care. Atlanta: Centers for Disease Control and Prevention, 1996.

Hardy AM, Lairson DR, and Morrow AL. Costs associated with gastrointestinal-tract illness among children attending day-care centers in Houston, Texas. Pediatrics 94(6 Pt 2):1091–1093, 1994.

Harms T, and Clifford RM. Early Childhood Rating Scale. New York: Teachers College Press, 1980.

Hashkes PJ, Spira DT, Deckelbaum RJ, et al. Salivary IgA antibodies to Giardia lamblia in day care center children. Pediatr. Infect. Dis. J. 13(11):953–958, 1994.

Haskins R. Acute illness in day care: how much does it cost? Bull. NY Acad. Med. 65(3):319–343, 1989.

Hawks D, Ascheim J, Giebienk GS, et al. American Public Health Association/American Academy of Pediatrics National Health and Safety Guidelines for Child-Care programs: featured standards and implementation. Pediatrics. 94(6 Pt 2):1110–1112, 1994.

Hofferth SL, Brayfield A, Deich S, et al. National Child Care Survey, 1990. The Urban Institute, 1991. Washington, D.C.

Holaday B, Waugh G, Moukaddem VE, et al. Fecal contamination in child day care centers: cloth vs paper diapers. Am. J. Public Health. 85(1):30–33, 1995.

Holmes SJ, Morrow AL, and Pickering LK. Child-care practices: effects of social change on the epidemiology of infectious diseases and antibiotic resistance. Epidemiol. Rev. 18 (1):10–28, 1996.

Hurwitz E, and Cordell R. Infectious diseases and out-of-home child care. Curr. Issues Public Health. 1:263–266, 1995.

Ikeda RM, Sacks JJ, and Briss PA. Assessment of telephone survey data. Pediatrics. 94(3):405–406, 1994.

Istre GR, Conner JS, Broome CV, et al. Risk factors for primary invasive Haemophilus influenzae disease: increased risk from day care attendance and school-aged household members. J. Pediatr. 106(2):190–195, 1985.

Jiang X, Dai X, Goldblatt S, et al. Pathogen transmission in child care settings studied using a cauliflower virus DNA as a surrogate marker. J. Infect. Dis. 177(4):881–888, 1998.

Johansen AS, Leibowitz A, and Waite LJ. Child care and children's illness. Am. J. Public Health. 78(9):1175–1177, 1988.

Jorm LR, and Capon AG. Communicable diseases in long day care centres in western Sydney: occurrence and risk factors. J. Paediatr. Child Health. 30(2):151–154, 1994.

Keswick BH, Pickering LK, DuPont HI, et al. Prevalence of rotavirus in children in day care centers. J. Pediatr. 103(1):85–86, 1983a.

Keswick BH, Pickering LK, DuPont HI, et al. Survival and detection of rotaviruses on environmental surfaces in day care centers. Appl. Environ. Microbiol. 46(4):813–816, 1983b.

Kim K, DuPont HL, and Pickering LK. Outbreaks of diarrhea associated with *Clostridium difficile* and its toxin in day-care centers: evidence of person-to-person spread. J. Pediatr. 102(3):376–382, 1983.

Kopjar B, and Wickzier T. How safe are day care centers? Day care versus home injuries among children in Norway. Pediatrics. 97(1):43–47, 1996.

Kotch JB, Weigle KA, Weber DJ, et al. Evaluation of an hygienic intervention in child day-care centers. Pediatrics. 94(6 Pt 2):991–994, 1994.

Laborde DJ, Weigle KA, Weber DJ, et al. Effect of fecal contamination on diarrheal illness in day-care centers. Am. J. Epidemiol. 138(4):243–255, 1993.

Landon JF, and Thompson H. Preschool day care. Arch. Paediatr. 60:537–566, 596–621, 665–693, 1943.

Lemp GF, Woodward WE, Pickering LK, et al. The relationship of staff to the incidence of diarrhea in day-care centers. Am. J. Epidemiol. 120(5):750–758, 1984.

Lew JF, Moe CL, Monroe SS, et al. Astrovirus and adenovirus associated with diarrhea in children in day care settings. J. Infect. Dis. 164(4):673–678, 1991.

Lie L, Runyan CW, Petridou E, et al. American Public Health Association/American Academy of Pediatrics Injury Prevention Standards. Pediatrics. 94(6 Pt 2):1046–1048, 1994.

MacDonald JK, Boase J, Stewart LK, et al. Evaluation of active and passive surveillance for communicable diseases in child care facilities: Seattle-King County, Washington State. Am. J. Public Health. 87(12):1951–1955, 1997.

Mackenzie SG, and Sherman GJ. Day-care injuries in the data base of the Canadian hospitals injury reporting and prevention program. Pediatrics. 94(6 Pt 2):1041–1043, 1994.

Marx J, Osguthorpe JD, and Parsons G. Day care and the incidence of otitis media in young children. Otolaryngol. Head Neck Surg. 112(6):695–699, 1995.

McKay HMM, and Dobbs RH. The effect of national bread, of iron medicated bread, and of iron cooking utensils on the haemoglobin level of children in wartime day nurseries. Arch. Dis. Child. 20:56–63, 1945.

McLaughlin ME. The physical health of children attending day nurseries. A report to the Day Nurseries Committee of the Medical Women's Federation. Br. Med. J. i:591–594, 631–634, 1947.

Menzies HF. Children in day nurseries. With special reference to the child under two tears old. Lancet. ii:499–501, 1946.

Miettinen O. Estimability and estimation in case-referent studies. Am. J. Epidemiol. 103:226–234, 1976.

Morrow AL, Townsend IT, and Pickering LK. Risk of enteric infection associated with child day care. Pediatr. Ann. 20(8):427–433, 1991.

Murph JR, Baron JC, Brown CK, et al. The occupational risk of cytomegalovirus infection among day-care providers JAMA. 265(5):603–608, 1991.

Nurmi T, Salminen E, and Ponka A. Infections and other illnesses of children in day-care centers in Helsinki. II. The economic losses. Infection. 19(5):331–335, 1991.

Ormiston G, Taylor J, and Wilson GS. Enteritis in a nursery home associated with *Giardia lamblia*. Br. Med. J. 2:151–154, 1942.

O'Ryan ML, Matson DO, Estes MK, et al. Molecular epidemiology of rotavirus in children attending day care centers in Houston. J. Infect. Dis. 162(4):810–816, 1990.

O'Ryan ML, Matson DO, Estes MK, et al. Acquisition of serum isotype-specific and G type-specific antirotavirus antibodies among children in day care centers. Pediatr. Infect. Dis. J. 13(10):890–895, 1994.

Osterholm MT, Klein JO, Aronson SS, et al. Infectious diseases in child day care: management and prevention. Introduction. Rev. Infect. Dis. 8(4):513, 1986.

Pass RF, August AM, Dworsky M, et al. Cytomegalovirus infection in a day-care center. N. Engl. J. Med. 307(8):477–479, 1982.

Pass RF, Hutto SC, Reynolds DW, et al. Increased frequency of cytomegalovirus infection in children in group day care. Pediatrics. 74(1):121–126, 1984.

Pickering LK. Infections in day care. Pediatr. Infect. Dis. J. 6(6):614–617, 1987.

Pickering LK, Evans DG, DuPont HL, et al. Diarrhea caused by Shigella, rotavirus, and Giardia in day-care centers. Prospective study. J. Pediatr. 99(1):51–56, 1981.

Pickering LK, and Woodward WE. Diarrhea in day care centers. Pediatr. Infect. Dis. 1(1):47–52, 1982.

Pickering LK, Woodward WE, DuPont HL, et al. Occurrence of *Giardia lamblia* in children in day care centers. J. Pediatr. 104(4):522–526, 1984.

Pickering LK, and Osterholm M. Infectious diseases associated with out-of-home child care. In: Long SS, Pickering LK, Prober CG, eds. Principles and Practice of Pediatric Infectious Diseases. New York: Churchill-Livingstone, 1997:31–39.

Polder JA, and Mohle-Boetani J. Investigations in child care facilities. In: Gregg MB, Dicker RC, Goodman RA, eds. Field Epidemiology. New York: Oxford University Press 1996:227–238.

Redmond SR, and Pichichero ME. *Hemophilus influenzae* type b disease. An epidemiologic study with special reference to day-care centers. JAMA. 252(18):2581–2584, 1984.

Reves RR, and Jones JA. Antibiotic use and resistance patterns in day care centers. In: Pickering LK, ed. Seminars in Pediatric Infectious Diseases. Philadelphia: WB Saunders, 1990: 212–221.

Reves RR, Morrow AL, Bartlett AV, et al. Child day care increases the risk of clinic visits for acute diarrhea and diarrhea due to rotavirus. Am. J. Epidemiol. 137(1):97–107, 1993.

Rivara FP, DiGuiseppi C, Thompson RS, et al. Risk of injury to children less than 5 years of age in day care versus home care settings. Pediatrics. 84(6):1011–1016, 1989.

Rosenberg ML, Weissman JB, Gangarosa EJ, et al. Shigellosis in the United States: ten-year review of nationwide surveillance, 1964–1973. Am. J. Epidemiol. 104(5):543–551, 1976.

Sacks JJ, Smith D, Kaplan KM, et al. The epidemiology of injuries in Atlanta day-care centers. JAMA. 262(12):1641–1645, 1989.

Sherman IL, and Langmuir AD. Usefulness of communicable disease reports. Public Health Rep. 67(12):1249–1257, 1952.

Shults J, and Chaganty NR. Analysis of serially correlated data using quasi-least squares. Biometrics. 54:1622–1630, 1998.

Strangert K, Carlstrom G, Jeansson S, et al. Infections in preschool children in group day care. Acta Paediatr. Scand. 65(4):455–463, 1976.

Strom J. A study of infections and illnesses in a day nursery based on inclusion-bearing cells in the urine and infectious agent in faeces, urine and nasal secretions. Scand. J. Infect. Dis. 11(4):265–269, 1979.

Sullivan P, Woodward WE, Pickering LK, et al. Longitudinal study of occurrence of diarrheal disease in day care centers. Am. J. Public Health. 74(9):987–991, 1984.

Thacker SB, Addiss DG, Goodman RA, et al. Infectious diseases and injuries in child day care: opportunities for healthier children. JAMA. 268(13):1720–1726, 1992.

Van R, Wun CC, Morrow AL, et al. The effect of diaper type and overclothing on fecal contamination in day-care centers. JAMA. 265 (14):1840–1844, 1991.

Van R, Wun CC, O'Ryan M, et al. Outbreaks of human enteric adenovirus types 40 and 41 in Houston day care centers. J. Pediatr. 120(4 Pt. 1):516–521, 1992.

Wald ER, Dashefsky B, Byers C, et al. Frequency and severity of infections in day care. J. Pediatr. 112(4):540–546, 1988.

Wald ER, Guerra N, and Byers C. Frequency and severity of infections in day care: three-year follow-up. J. Pediatr. 118(4, Part 1):509–514, 1991.

Wenger JD, Harrison LH, Hightower A, et al. Day care characteristics associated with *Haemophilus influenzae* disease. Am. J. Public Health. 80(12):1455–1458, 1990.

Wilde J, Van R, Pickering L, et al. Detection of rotavirus in the day care environment by reverse transcriptase polymerase chain reaction. J. Infect. Dis. 166(3):507–511, 1992.

Williams I, Smith MG, Sinha D, et al. Hepatitis B virus transmission in an elementary school setting. JAMA. 278(24):2167–2169, 1977.

Zeger SL, Liang KY, and Albert PS. Models for longitudinal data: a generalized estimating equation approach. Biometrics. 44(4):1049–1060, 1988.

Zocchetti C, Consonni R, and Bertazzi P. Relationship between prevalence rate ratios and odds ratios in cross-sectional studies. Int. J. Epidemiol. 26(1):220–223, 1976.

19

Infections Among the Elderly

LAURA C. HANSON

The proportion of the U.S. population that is aged 65 and older is growing faster than any younger age group. Elderly citizens made up 12% of the U.S. population in the 1980s, but will be 22% of the population by the year 2030. Improvements in nutrition, sanitation, and the management of some common chronic diseases have combined to permit more people to live into their seventies, eighties, and nineties. Among the elderly, the numbers of the oldest old, people aged 85 and older, are growing at the fastest rate. This demographic trend will change the epidemiology of many diseases, including infections.

As the population ages, the public health impact of infections that are more frequent or more severe among the elderly will increase. More research focused on the specific manifestations of infectious diseases in elderly patients will be needed. In addition, the design and interpretation of epidemiologic research will be affected by the inclusion of more elderly subjects. Physiologic changes and chronic illnesses associated with aging will add to the heterogeneity of study populations and mandate different approaches in study design and analysis. Finally, there are unique social characteristics of older persons that affect their willingness and ability to participate in research. Consideration of all these factors will lead to more useful and successful research about infections in elderly patients, and more appropriate interventions to reduce related morbidity and mortality.

POPULATION DISTRIBUTION OF INFECTIONS

Diseases of Increasing Frequency or Severity

Many infectious diseases disproportionately affect older persons.(Table 19–1) The incidence of bacterial pneumonia, endocarditis, cholecystitis, and diverticulitis increases with advancing age. Only a few infections are less common among the elderly, such as appendicitis and influenza. Sixty-four percent of nosocomial infections occur in people aged 60 and older, although they account for 23% of the hospitalized population.

Table 19-1   Infections Disproportionately Affecting Elderly Patients

Increased Incidence	Increased Severity
Bacterial pneumonia	Urinary tract infection
Endocarditis	Bacterial pneumonia
Cholecystitis	Tuberculosis
Diverticulitis	Influenza
Herpes zoster	Appendicitis

Rates of nosocomial urinary tract infections and wound infections are most strongly age-linked (Gross 1983, Saviteer 1988). Twenty-eight percent of new TB cases nationally, and even higher proportions in some states, are in people over 65 (Yoshikawa 1992, Weber 1989). Herpes zoster, the cutaneous recurrence of Varicella virus, occurs far more often in elderly than young adults, and the elderly account for almost all cases of prolonged neuralgia(Straus 1988).

Some diagnoses present in elderly and young patients, but the causative pathogens differ by age. In infections of the central nervous system, *Listeria monocytogenes* and enteric gram-negative rods emerge as important pathogens only in older patients (Behrman 1989). Although *Streptococcus pneumoniae* is the most common cause of community-acquired pneumonia at all ages, Mycoplasma becomes very rare and enteric gram-negative rods more frequent with advancing age. Pathogens causing endocarditis in later years include *Streptococcus bovis* and enterococci (Terpenning 1987).

Many common bacterial infections are also more severe for elderly persons. Urinary tract infections are more likely to be complicated by sepsis (Gleckman 1982). Bacterial pneumonia, meningitis, and pneumococcal bacteremia have higher mortality rates among older patients (Durand 1993, Fedullo 1985, Plouffe 1996). Some diseases that rarely kill younger adults have exceptionally higher mortality among the elderly, so that almost all deaths occur in this age group. Less than 10% of cases of appendicitis occur in older adults, but they account for nearly 100% of deaths (Lewis 1975, Peltokallio 1970). Tuberculosis demonstrates a tenfold increase in mortality from age 25 to age 65, so that 60% of deaths are in the elderly (Yoshikawa 1992). Similarly, 95% of influenza deaths occur in 45+ year-olds, although they experience less than 12% of infections (Couch 1986). These increases in severity of infections have variously been attributed to aging changes in host defenses, delay in diagnosis, and comorbid diseases.

EFFECTS OF AGING ON CLINICAL PRESENTATION OF INFECTIONS

Altered Host Defenses

With advanced age, basic changes occur in the ability of the human body to defend against infectious pathogens. These changes may explain some differences in incidence or severity of disease with advancing age. In nearly all older people some aspects of host defenses decline because of the aging process. For certain subpopulations, the effects of chronic diseases, medications, and medical procedures are superimposed on normative aging changes. Knowledge of these factors is essential to understand the relationship of the variable "age" to the frequency, severity, and outcomes of infections. Although data on *chronologic age* are easily collected and analyzed, it must be distinguished from *physiologic age*, defined as the combined effect of aging and chronic illness on an individual's physiologic functioning. The functional heterogeneity of the aged population is greater than that of younger persons, and researchers must exercise caution in interpretation of chronologic age.

Infectious diseases occur when a pathogenic organism interacts with a susceptible host. The older host is made vulnerable to infections by changes in barrier defenses and in immune function. Aging causes predictable changes in most elderly persons. Other failures of host defenses are attributable to specific disease states or medical procedures, and affect only a subset of those who are old. For a given infectious disease, alterations in host defenses might account for increased incidence, or severity, or different causal pathogens in the older host.

Barrier defenses are anatomic defenses that separate host tissues from the environment. They include the skin, mucosal surfaces, and organ-specific structural barriers. As skin ages, it becomes thinner, less hydrated, less elastic, and the subcutaneous tissues atrophy. Aged skin is more easily punctured or torn, and penetrating wounds close more slowly. Protein malnutrition, circulatory disease, or immobility will exacerbate these aging changes. Among chronically ill or medically frail older patients skin wounds are common, and healing is slowed. The barrier defenses protecting the lungs are somewhat less effective in healthy elderly, and various disease states compound aging changes. Changes in lung defenses permit *colonization* of the upper airway. A tissue is considered to be colonized when a potentially pathogenic organism becomes dominant and can be cultured in large quantities, yet does not cause clinical signs of infection. The presence of colonization is often the first step in pathogenesis of infection (Muder 1991) and increases the risk that the host will become infected. Pathogenic bacteria more readily colonize the upper airway. While only 3% of healthy young hospital employees have evidence of colonization on cultures of oral flora, 6% of healthy elderly subjects demonstrate this change. The rate of colonization dramatically increases if the older person is in a long-term care or acute care institution (Valenti 1978). The swallow and gag mechanisms that prevent aspiration of oral contents remain intact in healthy elderly but may be impaired by stroke, parkinsonism, or other central nervous system diseases (Huxley 1978). Mucociliary streaming, lung elastic recoil, the cough reflex, and respiratory muscle strength all decrease somewhat, even in the healthy older person (Weiss 1982). These changes are more severe in the elderly smoker. Differences in barrier lung defenses between older and younger individuals may be an important cause of the differences in the frequency and severity of pneumonia.

Barrier defenses for the urinary tract also change with age. For women, withdrawal of estrogen with menopause will raise the pH of the vaginal mucosa and permit colonization by enteric bacteria (Raz 1993). Atrophy of urethral mucosa and prolapse of pelvic organs may decrease sphincter barriers. As men age, enlarging prostate tissue may partially or completely obstruct the urethra, resulting in retained urine that is easily colonized. Asymptomatic colonization of urine is more common in healthy older than middle-aged men (0.1% to 10%), and is very common in older women (5% to 20%). Rates of colonization are 20%-50% above age 80 (Boscia 1987). The subset of elderly who have chronic cognitive impairment or impaired mobility often have poor perineal hygiene. Urinary or fecal incontinence may also result in frequent contamination and colonization of the urethral mucosa. Finally, the use of chronic indwelling urinary catheters is more common among the elderly, particularly in institutions. These catheters often result in chronic colonization of urine, and high rates of clinical infection.

The clinical epidemiology of urinary tract colonization highlights the importance of correct interpretation of associations found using epidemiologic methods. Early studies of urinary tract colonization found an association with increased mortality (Dontas 1981). Later randomized controlled trials of treatment showed no improvements in health outcomes, confirming confounding by other health status variables in earlier studies (Abrutyn 1994). Colonization should be understood as a marker of risk rather than a disease causing poor outcomes.

If barrier defenses are overcome, then immune defenses still may prevent infection. Immune senescence is the age-related decline in the efficacy of cellular and serologic host defenses once a pathogenic organism invades host tissues. A functional decrement in cellular immunity occurs with advancing age. Although T cells remain normal in number, the distribution of T cell subsets may change (Saltzman 1987). T cell function in response to stimuli is reduced (Murasko 1986, Phair 1978), and this is clinically evident in the diminished response of elderly patients to immunization and their susceptibility to infection by viruses or *Mycobacterium*.

Other changes include a variable increase in total antibody production, a decrease in antibody response to T-cell-dependent antigens, and less effective polymorphonuclear response to major bacterial infections (Saltzman 1987). Cellular immune function may be further impaired in elderly persons with hematologic malignancy or those taking immunosuppressive drugs. Immune senescence is clinically important in specific infections that depend on the cellular immune system response, such as herpes viral infections or mycobacterium infections (Miller 1980). Diseases normally associated with severely impaired cellular immunity have rarely been reported to occur in frail elderly persons (Jacobs 1991, Prince 1989).

Two other characteristics of aging may affect the severity of infections. The combined impact of aging and chronic disease on organ systems may diminish compensatory functional reserves in multiple organ systems. Reserve function permits other organs to compensate when one organ is affected by acute illness. For example, if pneumonia compromises oxygen exchange, the elderly person with underlying coronary artery disease may suffer an acute myocardial infarction as well, increasing the risk of pneumonia-related death. A 35–year-old patient is more likely than an 85–year-old to have renal function adequate to correct metabolic imbalances and dehydration from viral gastroenteritis. A skin wound that heals quickly without superinfection in a younger person may become infected, increase in size, and cause sepsis in an elderly patient who is incontinent and poorly mobile. Studies of infectious diseases must include data on comorbid diseases and baseline organ system function, to distinguish the impact of infection from the impact of chronic organ system failure on clinical outcomes.

Malnutrition, while not a part of normal aging, is common with advancing age. Inadequate protein intake occurs in about 10% of community living elderly (Bianchetti 1990), and rates of malnutrition range from 17% to 65% among institutionalized elderly (Morley 1988, Abbasi 1993). Protein-calorie malnutrition increases the incidence and severity of many infections (Martin 1987). Markers of protein-calorie malnutrition, such as serum albumin level, have been shown to predict death among institutionalized elderly, most of whom die of infectious diseases (Constans 1992, Klonoff-Cohen 1992). Tracheobronchial colonization, the first step in the pathogenesis of pneumonia, is increased among nutritionally deficient patients (Niederman 1984, 1989). Low serum albumin level is also a risk factor for hospital-acquired pneumonia in the elderly (Hanson 1992). A few intervention studies demonstrate that correction of nutritional deficiencies can improve outcomes. Dietary protein supplements have been shown to speed healing of bedsores (Breslow 1993) and prevent infectious complications of surgery (Mullen 1980). Other intervention studies with vitamin or mineral supplements have also demonstrated significant improvements in cellular immune function and rates of infection (Chandra 1992, Talbott 1987, Meydani 1990). Nutritional variables may play an important role in the association between age and infection. Since nutritional deficiencies are common among older patients, but reversible, further study of this relationship may favorably affect disease incidence or severity.

The decline in barrier defenses is due to a combination of normal aging and disease states that are relatively common among the elderly. Defects in immunity due to cancer, immunosuppressive drugs, diabetes, or malnutrition become more common with advancing age. Host responses to infectious diseases will be impaired in most older patients but will be more severely impaired when chronic diseases are also present. Design and interpretation of epidemiologic studies must be informed by these differences between older and younger study subjects. When possible, studies should distinguish between age-related susceptibility to infection and the effects of comorbid diseases or malnutrition.

Altered Presentation of Infections

These differences in older patients' host defenses may also affect disease presentation, and therefore change case definitions used in infectious disease epidemiology. In the design of epidemiologic research that includes elderly subjects, knowledge of age-specific differences in presentation is essential to avoid selection and misclassification bias.

Older subjects who have infections are usually accurately diagnosed, but atypical signs and symptoms are more common than for younger study populations. The case definition of major bacterial infection may be contingent on localizing symptoms and signs, such as auscultatory changes in pneumonia, abdominal pain in appendicitis, and dysuria in cystitis. While the majority of persons aged 65 and older will present with classic features of these infections, a sizable minority will not. In these cases, nonspecific systemic features predominate, such as malaise, anorexia, frequent falls, mental status changes or a syndrome of "failure to thrive." Many examples of this presentation have been described for major infectious diseases. In acute cholecystitis, patients aged 65 and older more often present with mental status changes and less frequently demonstrate abdominal tenderness (Morrow 1978). Delirium occurs earlier in Rocky Mountain spotted fever, but onset of the characteristic rash is delayed or may not occur in elderly patients (Morrison 1991). Endocarditis presents with more confusion and less fever in elderly patients (Terpenning 1987).

Fever is considered the hallmark of infection and yet is sometimes absent in elderly persons with major infection. Tuberculosis commonly presents without fever in older patients (Alvarez 1987). While 91% of 29–49 year-olds have high fevers with pneumococcal bacteremia, similar temperatures occur in only 71% of 65+ year-olds (Finkelstein 1983). The converse is also true; when fever does occur in elderly individuals, it usually signals more serious infections (Keating 1984). Fever elevations may occur but be of a lesser magnitude in elderly subjects. A study of nursing home residents found that many older individuals had baseline body temperatures below 98.6°F, and that a 2.4° rise from baseline temperature was a better indicator of serious infection than a fever of 101°F (Castle 1991).

Finally, essential test results are occasionally altered with advanced age. Three such tests are the tuberculin skin test, the chest X-ray, and the white blood cell count. Immunocompetent T cells in the skin are reduced, and T-cell function also declines, leaving a significant minority of elderly persons anergic in response to tuberculin skin testing with purified protein derivative (PPD) (Creditor 1988, Slutkin 1986, Gordin 1988). When clinical tuberculosis is suspected, diagnostic PPD testing must be done with control antigens to distinguish true negative skin tests from anergy. Two-step testing, placing a second PPD 2–4 weeks after the first, may also be needed to detect tuberculosis immunity that has waned over time. Chest X-ray evidence of infiltrates is often required in study definitions of pneumonia or tuberculosis. In older subjects, tuberculosis infiltrates are less often apical, and early bacterial pneumonias may present without any distinct infiltrate. Finally, a small fraction of elderly persons with serious bacterial infections will fail to demonstrate an elevated white blood cell count, again affecting the selection of cases if this is used as a criterion.

Case definitions for major infections in the elderly should be carefully planned, yet flexible, so as not to exclude elderly persons with the infection of interest. Requiring fever, or localizing abdominal pain, or an elevated cell count will result in selection bias by excluding the most frail and acutely ill elderly subjects. Initial literature review can help to identify the frequency and type of atypical presentations seen in a specific condition. When literature is lacking, interviews with experienced geriatricians may assist in the development of an appropriate case definition.

ANALYSIS ISSUES

Confounding Bias and Competing Causes
Epidemiologic bias arises from the greater frequency of comorbid diseases among elderly study subjects. When multiple diseases are present along with an infection, they become competing causes of morbidity and mortality. When an older person suffers ill-

ness or death concurrent with evidence of infection, the outcome may be fully or partially attributable to the infection, or may be unrelated. For example, an older person with an acute myocardial infarction and a urinary tract infection may die from cardiac causes after the infection is successfully treated. Similarly, a study of aminoglycoside nephrotoxicity must exclude other causes of renal disease and examine appropriateness of dosing practices to conclude that chronologic age is a true risk factor. Comorbid diseases may also cause abnormal test results or symptoms. An older person who develops pneumonia and congestive heart failure (CHF) together may have the symptoms and chest X-ray findings obscured by the CHF. To describe the true relationship between age and infection, it is important to collect adequate data on comorbid diseases and concurrent medical therapies that might affect measures of exposure or outcomes. An alternative method is to exclude older patients with chronic diseases from the study, although this practice creates problems with generalizability.

Use of Age in Analysis

In analysis of epidemiologic data, age is often included as a main effect or source of confounding. The way in which age, a continuous variable, is handled in analysis may create or obscure important conclusions about elderly subjects. Adjusting results for age may be a convenient way to account for aging changes and age-related comorbid diseases that are not of interest in the study. However, if age is to be examined as a risk factor or predictor of outcome, then it merits closer examination. As a continuous variable, it may have a linear relationship to the incidence of disease or with an outcome such as mortality. If so, then it may be simply analyzed and reported as a continuous variable. Convenient cut-points are often used that give a reasonable reflection of the linear relationship, such as 10–year intervals. Although comparisons of "less than 65 years old" and "65 and older" are often made, this presentation suggests that within these two large ranges the effect of age is uniform, and obscures a linear, exponential, or other type of relationship.

Continuous variables do not always meet the assumption of linearity. Some diseases, such as tuberculosis, increase in incidence only for the oldest age groups. Careful examination of the raw data will then suggest appropriate cut-points to describe the relationship. If risk is fairly constant before age 50, and then increases linearly, age might be described as a dichotomous variable around this cut-point. An exponential variable should be modeled if incidence or mortality increase in a J-shaped manner relative to age. Spline functions (Streitberg 1990) offer an alternative, statistically sophisticated method by which appropriate cut-points may be determined for a continuous variable.

Although many epidemiologic studies cover the entire adult age range, pooling elderly and younger adults may obscure important differences in causal pathways or outcomes of infections. Risk factors that are common for young patients, such as a history of intravenous drug use related to endocarditis, might be so rare as to be irrelevant for the same disease in elderly patients. Studies of nosocomial pneumonia in only elderly patients have found that different risk factors are important in this age group, suggesting that the mechanism of disease, and thus preventive interventions, might differ by age (Harkness 1990, Hanson 1992). Studies that include only older subjects have essentially controlled for age by stratification. Little can be concluded in such studies about age as a predictor, but this design may reveal important differences in the pathophysiology of infection in older persons.

RECOMMENDATIONS FOR EPIDEMIOLOGIC RESEARCH

When planning or interpreting research involving elderly subjects, several study design characteristics are important (Table 19–2). First, as life expectancy shortens, outcomes of function, satisfaction, and quality of life may become as important as survival. In addition to mortality, intervention studies should be designed to report quality of life

Table 19–2   Research Strategies for Older Populations

Study Design Issue	Research Strategy
Heterogeneity of older populations	Define target population and selection criteria carefully
Recruitment	Avoid prolonged interviews, involve family, provide supportive telephone follow up, provide transportation
Sample size	Anticipate high dropout, competing morbidity, mortality
Choice of outcome	Measure multiple outcomes, such as function, quality of life
Confounding bias	Measure comorbid illness, interventions
Proxy respondents for persons with cognitive impairment	Pilot interview items with proxies and respondents to estimate bias

or patient satisfaction measures, functional status, or cost-effectiveness. These measurements are more costly and complex than recording deaths, and studies should use reliable and valid instruments.

Second, the "elderly" are arguably more heterogeneous than other age groups, and the target population should be carefully defined. Is the study designed to address vigorous elders, persons with a specific chronic illness, or medically frail elders such as nursing home residents or equally dependent elders in the community? Researchers must consider the trade-off of studying a homogeneous but poorly generalizable group, or a diverse group of elderly with more potential for confounding bias (Williams 1984).

Third, sample size calculations must anticipate rates of important comorbid conditions that are exclusion criteria or confounding variables. Elderly subjects may also have higher morbidity and mortality rates during follow up, leading to higher dropout or crossover effects (Ouslander 1993). One large, very well designed study of community elderly reported a 40% dropout rate (Applegate 1990). Studies that do not anticipate these differences may fail to demonstrate important relationships or obscure randomization because of excessive crossover.

Although clinical research should involve elderly subjects, they demand a careful approach to recruitment and retention of study participants. Older subjects are more difficult to recruit, but once involved are more reliably retained during follow up (Applegate 1990). Researchers seeking to study older individuals, especially those who are

chronically ill or functionally dependent, must become familiar with techniques that make participation feasible and enjoyable for these individuals. Higher rates of visual and hearing impairment may make data collection more difficult, unless techniques of communication are modified. Transportation problems may make frequent clinic visits difficult for older participants. Prolonged data collection sessions may need to be fragmented if older persons become fatigued. Rates of significant cognitive impairment are high among the oldest old, with a prevalence of 3% in 65–74 year-olds, but rising to over 40% among those aged 85 and older (Evans 1989). To obtain meaningful informed consent, researchers may need a screening procedure for decisional capacity. If surrogate interviews are used they should be analyzed for systematic differences, since surrogates have been shown to overestimate older persons' disabilities (Magaziner 1988). Data collection procedures should be flexible and sensitive, to minimize disruptive or painful experiences for cognitively impaired individuals (Ouslander 1993).

A final obstacle to valid research involving elderly subjects is determined by systematic differences in medical treatment for old and young patients. Because of atypical presentations or lack of physician expertise, diagnoses such as endocarditis, myocardial infarction, alcoholism, and Alzheimer's disease are often missed or delayed in elderly persons. Advanced age is associated with nontreatment or undertreatment of cancer (Greenfield 1987), and with increasing use of decisions to limit life-sustaining treatment (Holtzman 1996). Dissecting the importance of these treatment differences in studies of the outcomes of infection may be very difficult.

Long-term care has established different standards for diagnostic testing, treatment, and record keeping than acute care medicine. Although infections are the primary cause of death and hospitalization for nursing home residents (Irvine 1984), testing and treatment are often withheld (Warren 1991). Constraints on care are due to a poorly defined mix of ethical decision making, different practice standards, and neglect (Fabiszewski 1990, Brown 1979, Magaziner 1991). Researchers accustomed to nursing and physician records from acute care hospitals may be frustrated by missing data and less skilled or overworked nursing staff. Anticipating these differences will allow researchers to coordinate their data collection efforts with nursing home staff and residents, so that research is mutually beneficial (Ouslander 1993).

REFERENCES

Abbasi AA, and Rudman D. Observations on the prevalence of protein-calorie undernutrition in VA nursing homes. J. Am. Geriatr. Soc. 41: 117–121, 1993.

Abrutyn E, Mossey J, Berlin JA, et al. Does asymptomatic bacteriuria predict mortality and does antimicrobial treatment reduce mortality in elderly ambulatory women? Ann. Intern. Med. 120:827–833, 1994.

Alvarez S, Shel C, and Berk SL. Pulmonary tuberculosis in elderly men. Am. J. Med. 82: 602–606, 1987.

Applegate WB, and Curb JD. Designing and executing randomized clinical trials involving elderly persons. J. Am. Geriatr. Soc. 38:943–950, 1990.

Behrman RE, Meyers BR, Mendelson MH, Sacks HS, and Hirschman SZ. Central nervous system infections in the elderly. Arch. Intern. Med. 149:1596–1599, 1989.

Bianchetti A, Rozzini R, Carabellese C, Zanetti O, and Trabucchi M. Nutritional intake, socioeconomic conditions, and health status in a large elderly population. J. Am. Geriatr. Soc. 38:521–526, 1990.

Boscia JA, Kobasa WD, Knight RA, et al. Therapy vs no therapy for bacteriuria in elderly ambulatory nonhospitalized women. JAMA. 257:1067–1071, 1987.

Breslow RA, Hallfrisch J, Guy DG, Crawley B, and Goldberg AP. The importance of dietary protein in healing pressure ulcers. J. Am. Geriatr. Soc. 41:357–362, 1993.

Brown NK, and Thompson DJ. Nontreatment of fever in extended-care facilities. N. Engl. J. Med. 300(22):1246–1250, 1979.

Castle SC, Norman DC, Yeh M, Miller D, and Yoshikawa TT. Fever response in elderly nursing home residents: are the older truly colder? J. Am. Geriatr. Soc. 39:853–857, 1991.

Chandra RK. Effect of vitamin and trace-element supplementation on immune responses and infection in elderly subjects. Lancet. 340: 1124–1127, 1992.

Constans T, Bacq Y, Brechot JF, et al. Protein-energy malnutrition in elderly medical patients. J. Am. Geriatr. Soc. 40:263–268, 1992.

Couch RB, Kasel JA, Glezen WP, et al. Influenza: its control in persons and populations. J. Infect. Dis. 153:431–440, 1986.

Creditor MC, Smith EC, Gallai JB, Baumann M, and Nelson KE. Tuberculosis, tuberculin reactivity, and delayed cutaneous hypersensitivity in nursing home residents. J. Gerontol. 43:M97–100, 1988.

Dontas AS, Kasviki-Charvati P, Papanayiotou PC, and Mareketos SG. Bacteriuria and survival in old age. N. Engl. J. Med. 304:939–943, 1981.

Durand ML, Calderwood SB, Weber DJ, et al. Acute bacterial meningitis in adults: a review of 493 episodes. N. Engl. J. Med. 328:21–28, 1993.

Evans DA, Funkenstein H, Albert MS, et al. Prevalence of Alzheimer's disease in a community population of older persons: higher than previously reported. JAMA. 262:2551–2556, 1989.

Fabiszewski KJ, Volicer B, and Volicer L. Effect of antibiotic treatment on outcome of fevers in institutionalized Alzheimer patients. JAMA. 263:3168–3172, 1990.

Fedullo AJ, and Swinburne AJ. Relationship of patient age to clinical features and outcome for in-hospital treatment of pneumonia. J. Gerontol. 40:29–33, 1985.

Finkelstein MS, Petkun WM, Freedman ML, and Antopol SC. Pneumococcal bacteremia in adults: age-dependent differences in presentation and in outcome. J. Am. Geriatr. Soc. 31: 19–27, 1983.

Gleckman R, Blagg N, Hibert D, et al. Acute pyelonephritis in the elderly. South. Med. J. 75: 551–554, 1982.

Gordin RM, Perez-Stable EJ, Flaherty D, et al. Evaluation of a third sequential tuberculin skin test in a chronic care population. Am. Rev. Respir. Dis. 137:153–157, 1988.

Greenfield S, Blanco DM, Elashoff RM, and Ganz PA. Patterns of care related to age of breast cancer patients. JAMA. 257:2766–2770, 1987.

Gross PA, Rapuano C, Adrignolo A, and Shaw B. Nosocomial infections: decade-specific risk. Infect. Control. 4:145–147, 1983.

Hanson LC, Weber DJ, Rutala WA, and Samsa GP. Risk factors for nosocomial pneumonia in the elderly. Am. J. Med. 92:161–166, 1992.

Harkness GA, Bentley DW, and Roghmann KJ. Risk factors for nosocomial pneumonia in the elderly. Am. J. Med. 89:457–463, 1990.

Holtzman J. and Lurie N. Causes of increasing mortality in a nursing home population. J. Am. Geriatr. Soc. 44:258–264, 1996.

Huxley EJ, Viroslav J, Gray WR, and Pierce AK. Pharyngeal aspiration in normal adults and patients with depressed consciousness. Am. J. Med. 64:564–568, 1978.

Irvine PW, van Buren N, and Crossley K. Causes for hospitalization of nursing home residents: the role of infections. J. Am. Geriatr. Soc. 32:103–107, 1984.

Jacobs JL, Libby DM, Winters RA, et al. A cluster of Pneumocystis carinii pneumonia in adults without predisposing ilnesses. N. Engl. J. Med. 324:246–250, 1991.

Keating HJ, Klimek JJ, Levine DS, and Kiernan FJ. Effect of aging on the clinical significance of fever in ambulatory adult patients. J. Am. Geriatr. Soc. 32:282–287, 1984.

Klonoff-Cohen H, Barrett-Connor EL, and Edelstein SL. Albumin levels as a predictor of mortality in the healthy elderly. J. Clin. Epidemiol. 45:207–212, 1992.

Lewis RF, Holcroft JW, Boey J, and Dunphy JE. Appendicitis: a critical review of diagnosis and treatment in 1,000 cases. Arch. Surg. 110:677–682, 1975.

Magaziner J, Simonsick RM, DaSheur JM, and Hebel JR. Patient-proxy response comparability on measures of patient health and function status. J. Clin. Epidemiol. 41:1065, 1988.

Magaziner J, Tenney JH, DeForge B, et al. Prevalence and characteristics of nursing home-acquired infections in the aged. J. Am. Geriatr. Soc. 39:1071–1078, 1991.

Martin TR. The relationship between malnutrition and lung infection. Clin. Chest Med. 8:359–372, 1987.

Meydani SN, Barklund MP, Liu S, et al. Vitamin E supplementation enhances cell-medicated immunity in healthy elderly subjects. Am. J. Clin. Nutr. 52:557–563, 1990.

Miller AE. Selective decline in cellular immune response to varicella-zoster in the elderly. Neurology. 30:582–587, 1980.

Morley JE,. Mooradian AD, Silver AJ, Heber D, Alfin-Slater RB. Nutrition in the elderly. Ann. Intern. Med. 109:890–904, 1988.

Morrison RE, Lancaster L, Lancaster DJ, and Land MA. Rocky Mountain spotted fever in the elderly. J. Am. Geriatr. Soc. 39:205–208, 1991.

Morrow DJ, Thompson J, and Wilson SE. Acute cholecystitis in the elderly: a surgical emergency. Arch. Surg. 113:1149, 1978.

Muder RR, Brennen C, Wagener MM, et al. Methicillin-resistant staphylococcal colonization and infection in a long-term care facility. Ann. Intern. Med. 114:107–112, 1991.

Mullen JL, Buzby GP, Matthews DC, Smale BF, and Rosato EF. Reduction of operative morbidity and mortality by combined preoperative and postoperative nutritional support. Ann. Surg. 192:604–613, 1980.

Murasko DM, Nelson BJ, Silver R, Matour D, and Kaye D. Immunologic response in an elderly population with a mean age of 85. Am. J. Med. 81:612–618, 1986.

Niederman MS, Mantovani R, Schoch P, Papas J, and Fein AM. Patterns and routes of tracheobronchial colonization in mechanically ventilated patients: the role of nutritional status in colonization of the lower airway by Pseudomonas species. Chest. 95:155–161, 1989.

Niederman MS, Merrill WW, Ferranti RD, et al. Nutritional status and bacterial binding in the lower respiratory tract in patients with chronic tracheostomy. Ann. Intern. Med. 100:795–800, 1984.

Ouslander JG, and Schnelle JF. Research in nursing homes: practical aspects. J. Am. Geriatr. Soc. 41:182–187, 1993.

Peltokallio P, and Jauhiainen K. Acute appendicitis in the aged patient: study of 300 cases after the age of 60. Arch. Surg. 100:140–143, 1970.

Phair JP, Kauffman CA, Bjorson A, et al. Host defenses in the aged: evaluation of components of the inflammatory and immune responses. J. Infect. Dis. 138:67–73, 1978.

Plouffe JF, Breiman RF, and Facklam RR, for the Franklin County Pneumonia Study Group. Bacteremia with Streptococcus pneumoniae: implications for therapy and prevention. JAMA. 275:194–198, 1996.

Prince DS, Peterson DD, Steiner RM, et al. Infection with Mycobacterium avium complex in patients without predisposing conditions. N. Engl. J. Med. 321:863–868, 1989.

Raz R, and Stamm WE. A controlled trial of intravaginal estriol in postmenopausal women with recurrent urinary tract infections. N. Engl. J. Med. 329:753–756, 1993.

Saltzman RL, and Peterson PK. Immunodeficiency of the elderly. Rev. Infect. Dis. 9:1127–1139, 1987.

Saviteer SM, Samsa GP, and Rutala WA. Nosocomial infections in the elderly: increased risk per hospital day. Am. J. Med. 84:661–666, 1988.

Slutkin G, Perez-Stable EJ, and Hopewell PC. Time course and boosting of tuberculin reactions in nursing home residents. Am. Rev. Respir. Dis. 134:1048–1051, 1986.

Straus SE, Ostrove JM, Inchauspe G, et al. Varicella-zoster virus infections: biology, natural history, treatment, and prevention. Ann. Intern. Med. 108:221–237, 1988.

Streitberg B, and Meyer-Sabellek W. Smoothing twenty-four hour ambulatory blood pressure profiles: a comparison of alternative methods. J. Hypertens. Suppl. 8:S21–27, 1990.

Talbott MC, Miller LT, and Kerkvliet NI. Pyridoxine supplementation: effect on lymphocyte responses in elderly persons. Am. J. Clin. Nutr. 46:659–664, 1987.

Terpenning MS, Buggy BP, and Kauffman CA. Infective endocarditis: clinical features in young and elderly patients. Am. J. Med. 83:626–707, 1987.

Valenti WM, Trudell RG, and Bentley DW. Factors predisposing to oropharyngeal coloniza-tion with gram-negative bacilli in the aged. N. Engl. J. Med. 298:1108–1111, 1978.

Warren JW, Palumbo FB, Fitterman L, and Speedie SM. Incidence and characteristics of antibiotic use in aged nursing home residents. J. Am. Geriatr. Soc. 39:963–972, 1991.

Weber DJ, Rutala WA, Samsa GP, Sarubbi FA, and King LC. Epidemiology of tuberculosis in North Carolina, 1966 to 1986: analysis of demographic features, geographic variation, AIDS, migrant workers, and site of infection. South. Med. J. 82:1204–1214, 1989.

Weiss ST. Pulmonary system. In: Rowe JW, Besdine RW, eds. Health and Disease in Old Age. Boston: Little, Brown, 1982:369–379.

Williams ME, and Retchin SM. Clinical geriatric research: still in adolescence. J. Am. Geriatr. Soc. 32:851–857, 1984.

Yoshikawa TT. Tuberculosis in aging adults. J. Am. Geriatr. Soc. 40:178–187, 1992.

20

HIV/AIDS Research

STEN H. VERMUND, HOWARD WIENER, M. LOUISE LAWSON,
and MADHAV P. BHATTA

Methodologic challenges of human immunodeficiency virus (HIV) epidemiology are
distinct in key ways from those that previously faced infectious disease or chronic disease researchers. HIV is an infection communicable in three ways (blood-borne, sexual,
mother-to-child), manifesting clinical disease
after many years or even decades, and resulting in lifelong infection (Peterman and Allen
1989, Royce et al. 1997, IOM 1998, Vermund et al. 1999). Its incidence is affected by
community prevalence, behavior, cofactors
in transmission, and treatment adherence,
quite different from nonvenereal infectious
agents that have been the focus of intense
public health activity such as most of the
vaccine preventable diseases. Acute infectious diseases are affected by the dynamics
of population crowding and mixing patterns,
the number of susceptible individuals, the
number of immune persons, and the infectiousness of the given agent. Behavioral factors, short of vaccination adherence, have
little to do with risk of measles, pertussis, rubella, diphtheria, or a host of other infectious agents. Furthermore, with exceptions

such as hepatitis C, dengue, and protozoal
parasites, most infections either kill their
host within the acute infectious event or result in an immunologically protected state
such that risk of future disease is diminished
or eliminated. Acute infectious diseases that
result in chronic infection and later recrud-
escence such as poliomyelitis, tuberculosis,
leprosy, or syphilis present research challenges that resemble in certain ways the
methodologic issues faced in HIV research.
Yet even these infections are quite distinct in
key aspects. Polio, for example, has a clear
correlate of protective immunity, namely,
antibody titers to all three polio types. Tuberculosis, while affected by immunosuppression, does not cause immune deficiency
as part of its major pathogenic pathway.
Leprosy infects many more persons than
those who suffer serious disease. Syphilis is
easily curable with antibiotics. HIV, unique
among the infectious diseases, causes a primary immunosuppression, a chronic illness,
is usually lethal if not treated, and is heavily
influenced by behavioral factors in both acquisition and response to therapy. Since HIV

epidemiology has complex elements that remind us of both classical and modern chronic disease epidemiology, one must incorporate modern epidemiologic methods in its study. HIV disease is both an infectious disease and, at the same time, a chronic disease that, like hepatitis B and C, is not generally transmissible through casual, respiratory or gastrointestinal exposure.

Many challenges in HIV epidemiology are faced by researchers. This chapter, although it does not address these challenges comprehensively, seeks to introduce a few of the key issues in HIV of relevance to both students and practitioners of infectious disease epidemiology (Table 20–1).

EARLY HISTORY OF HIV EPIDEMIOLOGY

The earliest case series of HIV were reports of a new syndrome from Los Angeles and New York City (Gottlieb et al. 1981, Masur et al. 1981). The clusters of *Pneumocystis carinii* pneumonia with immunosuppression among young homosexual men reporting many sexual partners was a complete mystery with no precedent in the medical literature (CDC 1981a,b). Speculation regarding the etiology abounded with most observers suspecting a viral infection such as CMV or HTLV-I, though neither disease resembled the new syndrome (Sonnabend et al. 1983). However, drug use and abuse, autoimmune, and other theories abounded as to the etiology; even after discovery of LAV/HTLV-III, later named HIV, alternative speculation as to etiology persisted (Weiss 1990).

The earliest cases shared much in common. Large city residence, white race, male gender, male-to-male sexual contact preference, history of sexual adventurism, frequent nitrite drug use, prior sexually transmitted infections but otherwise good general prior health, and seemingly rapid disease progression were noted in the earliest case series. No women, children, or heterosexuals were yet recognized. To their credit, key public health and medical research agency employees in Europe, the Americas, and, soon, in Africa responded promptly. They sought to characterize more fully the epidemic, discover an etiology, promulgate prevention messages based on apparent risk factors, and try therapies that might work.

Within months, the syndrome was identified in a host of other population groups: Haitians (CDC 1982a, Pape et al. 1983, Vieira et al. 1983), infants and children (Oleske et al. 1983, Rubinstein et al. 1983), women (Masur et al. 1982), heterosexuals (Harris et al. 1983), persons with hemophilia (CDC 1982b), blood transfusion recipients (CDC 1982c, Ammann et al. 1983), injection drug users (CDC 1982d, Moll et al. 1982), Europeans (Brunet et al. 1983, Bygberg 1983), Africans (Clumeck 1983, Clumeck et al. 1984, Obel et al. 1984, Piot et al. 1984, Van De Perre et al. 1984), Latin Americans (Amato et al. 1983, Estevez 1983), Asians (Miyoshi et al. 1983), child abuse and rape victims (Gutman et al. 1991, Irwin et al. 1995), health care workers after needle sticks (Anonymous 1984, McCray 1986, Oksenhendler et al. 1986, Stricof and Morse 1986), and sexual partners of afflicted persons (Masur et al. 1982, CDC 1983a, Harris et al. 1983). Given the evident similarities, hepatitis B was invoked as an analogous agent from its transmission patterns, even though the natural history of the disease was quite distinct (Francis et al. 1983). In this way, prevention messages were promulgated even in the first year of the recognition of AIDS (1981), preceding the discovery of HIV in 1983 (CDC 1982e, 1983b) and serologic test licensure in 1985.

Shortly after the initial case series, CDC established a surveillance case definition, and cases outside of Los Angeles and New York were reported to CDC within weeks (CDC 1982d). Many studies of HIV in the United States were conducted by the CDC in collaboration with local medical centers and health departments. Behavioral research was illuminating from the very beginning, as in the case of the sexual linkage studies of Darrow and colleagues that confirmed that dozens of the very first AIDS reports had reported sexual relations with a single homosexual man whose airline career brought him to major cities throughout North Amer-

Table 20–1 Challenges in HIV Epidemiology Presented by the Virus, the Host, the Nature of Investigation, and the Environment/Society

Virus

- The chronic, incurable nature of the infection
- The unknown timing and origin of the seroconversion event in most individuals,
- The deep tissue reservoirs of virus (e.g., lymph nodes)
- The variable incubation distribution for one time from infection to serious disease (or AIDS)
- The relatively low infectiousness of the virus in most transmission settings
- The rapid mutational rates of HIV
- The inherent complexities of a "Trojan horse" infection that lives within the very human T cells that are designed to recognize and destroy foreign infectious agents through antigenic recognition

Host

- The complexity of host immunogenetic factors that affect the risk of acquisition of infection and/or progression of disease
- The lack of a correlate(s) of protective immunity, yet the obvious impact of a partially effective immune response
- The unknown role of both humoral and cellular immunity
- The unknown role of mucosal immunity

Investigational

- The complexity of field research studies with high risk populations
- The methodologic difficulties in measuring infection in mucosal sites
- The urgency to approve promising new chemotherapeutic agents or regimens even before definitive clinical trial findings are available
- The opportunities and challenges to develop and use mathematical models of transmission, disease progression, and prevention
- The stigmatization and discrimination associated with HIV infection and the consequent reluctance of society or the public health professional community to embrace classic approaches to disease surveillance and control
- The challenges of clinical measurement in biologic and behavioral areas
- The difficulties of bias and precision in HIV-related measurements
- The features that confront community-based prevention clinical trials including randomization at the community level, ethical concerns in trial design, cost of large field trials, and the complexity of securing definitive, HIV-related trial outcomes

Environment/Society

- The impact of behavior on acquisition origin of most HIV infections and progression
- The complex, facilitative role of other infections, both genital (e.g., gonorrhea) and systemic (e.g., tuberculosis), for HIV transmission
- The suggested, but not well confirmed role of other infections in accelerated HIV disease progression
- The stigma attached to AIDS and HIV infection that inhibits effective prevention and control
- The advent of potent antiretroviral combinations requiring sustained, lifelong adherence to complex chemotherapeutic regimens for their success
- The prospects for HIV control through diverse interventions, both biologic and behavioral

ica in the late 1970s and early 1980s (Auerbach et al. 1984).

As important as these early studies were, there were substantial limitations of inference due to biased ascertainment, surveillance limitations, poor recognition of the syndrome, lack of a screening test, and poor research funding support prior to 1985. Furthermore, there were inherent problems with the ecologic observations of AIDS in the United States given the differences in AIDS presentations elsewhere, such as in sub-Saharan Africa (Piot et al. 1984, Quinn et al 1986). It would take years before investigators appreciated that the African epidemic was older and much more advanced than that in the United States (Gao et al. 1999). From 1980 to 1989, there were 3533 references with the United States as a keyword in the bibliographic database, AIDSLINE, while there were only 783 references with Africa as a keyword (4.5:1). From 1990 to 1998 the ratio was 3:1.

CASE-CONTROL STUDIES

Studies with more substantial value for discovering the behavioral and biologic antecedents of AIDS were initiated in the early 1980s. The first to be complete were case-control studies. CDC sponsored the first to be published, implicating strongly an infectious agent that was sexually transmitted, though not ruling out amyl nitrite use as a contributor (Jaffe et al. 1983, Rogers et al. 1983). Case-control studies emerged from a variety of populations with various risk behaviors or exposures implicated in transmission: injection drug users (needle sharing) (Friedland et al. 1985, Vanichseni et al. 1989, van Ameijden et al. 1992), children (parent with AIDS or at risk) (Hersh et al. 1993), blood recipients (number of transfusions or receipt of concentrated blood products) (Donegan et al. 1990, Busch et al. 1996), persons with hemophilia (number of factor VIII infusions received) (Remis et al. 1990), heterosexuals (promiscuity or at-risk partner) (Ellerbrock et al. 1992), Africans and Haitians (no special risk, though risk highest among promiscuous persons) (Bonneux et al. 1988, Halsey 1992, Harrison et al. 1991), and health care workers (deep needlestick from AIDS patient) (CDC 1994, Cardo et al. 1997).

HIV-related research relying on case-control study methods has the same design hazards as case-control studies on other topics. For example, selection of controls may not be straightforward. In a matched nested case-control study of whether or not HIV vaccine recipients in an uncontrolled Phase II study of recombinant gp-120 subunit vaccines had experienced any modification of their clinical course (determined by plasma viral load), despite having "broken through"

by becoming infected, controls selected were from those who had seroconverted but had not received the vaccine. Matching on risk exposure category and year of seroconversion, gender, age within five years, and geographic location (when possible) was attempted after considerable debate within the investigator group. Importantly, control subjects had to be identified within an ongoing cohort study of persons at high risk, since this is how vaccinees had been selected and followed. Some investigators argued that they already had studied persons who had seroconverted but who had not received vaccine. These persons, already identified, should be the controls for the case-control study of vaccine outcome. Since such individuals were much more likely to come to the attention of laboratory investigators if they were symptomatic, and since symptomatic seroconverters tend to have higher viral loads than asymptomatic seroconverters, inclusion of persons who seroconverted but had not been identified in a fashion similar to how the infected vaccinees had been identified would introduce bias into the study. If more symptomatic seroconverters were included in the control group owing to biased ascertainment based on recognition of seroconversion symptoms, then viral load at defined times postseroconversion would be expected to be higher in control subjects, suggesting that vaccine had a salutary benefit (lower postinfection virus loads) compared to no vaccine, even if the vaccine had had no such effect. In choosing the more laborious route of identifying matched controls from defined epidemiologic cohorts in which at-risk persons were under periodic surveillance, this methodologic hazard was avoided and unbiased control subjects were recruited. No impact of vaccination on postinfection virus load could be ascertained in the study (Connor et al. 1998, Graham et al. 1998). This example is but one of many in the HIV literature that illustrate a key principle in case-control methodology: the subjects in the control group would show up in the study as a case if they were to experience the outcome of interest (assuming all cases were enrolled).

Limitations of case-control methods are the same in the HIV field as they are in any other epidemiologic context. Uncertain cause versus effect, presence of confounding or interacting factors, and noncomparability of cases and controls are among the many potential issues. However, case-control studies continue to provide rapid, valuable, and usually valid information to inform AIDS research as long as investigators are sensitized to the methodologic challenges and hazards facing them.

COHORT STUDIES

Extraordinary insights have emerged from HIV/AIDS-motivated cohort studies. Given the pandemic, explosive, and lethal nature of the condition, studies all over the world have sought to illuminate the transmission, acute infection, natural history, terminal events, and prevention of HIV (Table 20–2).

Some cohorts have been followed predating the HIV epidemic itself because of prior studies of hepatitis B vaccine among gay men (Hessol et al. 1989, Rutherford et al. 1990). While heart disease and cancer have had greater scientific research investments over time, HIV is surely the most studied infectious disease in modern scientific history. For example, in the 1990s, HIV-related research represented about 10% of the National Institutes of Health budget in the United States, averaging about $1.5 billion per year. While only a fraction of this has been in support of cohort studies, such studies do tend to be costly given their long-term timetables, their large sample sizes, and their extensive scope.

The cohort study permits the estimation of incidence rates. Unlike surveillance studies in which data are collected at the time of diagnosis or reporting, the cohort can be followed even after an initial event (such as the AIDS-defining condition) to characterize the total population burden of disease. Cohorts can follow at-risk subjects from the time they are uninfected to assess risk factors for acute infection, while infected persons are asymptomatic to examine risk

for disease progression, and among symptomatic persons to study risk for specific opportunistic infections, malignancies, or death. The natural history of HIV was studied thoroughly before the treatment era began with the advent of zidovudine and *P. carinii* primary prophylaxis in 1987. However, the proper cryopreservation of well-characterized and processed samples has permitted ongoing exploitation of these cohort samples, using modern molecular techniques, as was the case with the MACS and viral load as a predictor of clinical course (Mellors et al. 1996). This illustrates a key feature of the cohort study, namely, the opportunity for nested case-control studies in which the cases and controls have been followed in unbiased fashion prior to the onset of the disease condition. It is precisely this study design that demands excellence in specimen acquisition and cryopreservation. Unfortunately, major cohorts may lose research support and tens of thousands of specimens then go underexploited because of the lack of sustained linkages between basic science laboratories and epidemiologists or because of improper processing or storage of materials.

In the pretreatment era, the major focus of research was in the etiology of AIDS and in the transmission and natural history of HIV. The rapid laboratory discovery of HIV in 1983, just two years after recognition of AIDS (Barre-Sinoussi et al. 1983), and evidence of this virus as the primary etiology of AIDS published in 1984 (Popovic et al. 1984) led researchers within these incipient cohorts to concentrate more on transmission and natural history issues than on etiology per se. Some observations have proven to be key in prevention and disease control. The association of sexually transmitted infections and HIV acquisition has led to STD control as a tool in HIV prevention (Laga 1995). The observation that multiple sexual partners increase HIV acquisition risk led to key health behavior messages (Ostrow 1989). The utility of CD4+ cell counts and quantitative viral loads has been well characterized, enabling clinical monitoring (Coffin 1995, Cook et al. 1999). The association of

Table 20–2   Major HIV/AIDS Cohorts from Around the World

Cohort	Reference
Multicenter AIDS Cohort Study (MACS)	Kaslow et al. 1987
San Francisco City Clinic Cohort	Jaffe et al. 1985
San Francisco Men's Health Study	Winkelstein et al. 1987
DC Gay Men's Study	Goedert et al. 1985
Fenway Clinic Cohort	McCusker et al. 1989
ALIVE Cohort of Injection Drug Users	Vlahov et al. 1991
Montefiore Methadone Maintenance Cohort	Selwyn et al. 1992
Amsterdam Cohorts	Keet et al. 1993
Hemophilia Growth and Development Study	Loveland et al. 1994
Mother and Infants Transmission Study	Parekh et al. 1991
Women and Infants Transmission Study	Diaz et al. 1998
Women's Interagency HIV Study	Barkan et al. 1998
HIV Epidemiological Research Study (women)	Smith DK et al. 1997
REACH Cohort (adolescents)	Rogers AS et al. 1998
Vancouver Cohort	Boyko et al. 1986
Montreal Cohort	Bruneau et al. 1998
Canadian Women's HIV Study	Hankins et al. 1998
Sydney Cohort	Burcham et al. 1989
European Heterosexual Transmission Study	de Vincenzi et al. 1994
HIV Italian Seroconversion Study	Pezzotti et al. 1996
Projet SIDA (in Zaire)	Laga et al. 1993
Rwandan and Zambian Discordant Couples Studies	Allen et al. 1992a
Heterosexual AIDS Transmission Study	Skurnick et al. 1998
European Perinatal Cohort	European Collaborative Study 1988
Thai Cohort	Beyrer et al. 1996
Côte d'Ivoire Cohort	Adjorlolo-Johnson et al. 1994
Kenyan Cohort	Martin et al. 1994

viral resistance patterns with drug administration and adherence has enabled more rational therapeutic regimens. Less definitive is the 20-year search for infectious cofactors for HIV disease progression. Many infectious agents have been implicated, but few have been compelling cofactors in HIV progression. These coinfections include HTLV-I, CMV, EBV, *Mycoplasma fermentans*, HSV-II, HHV-6, tuberculosis, malaria, and others (Diaz-Mitoma et al. 1990, Kucera et al. 1990, Margalith et al. 1990, Levy et al. 1991, Hawkins et al. 1992, Montagnier and Blanchard 1993, Schechter et al. 1994, Carrigan et al. 1996, Chandramohan and Greenwood 1998, Del Amo et al. 1999, Dorrucci et al. 1999, Kovacs et al. 1999, Sinicco et al. 1997). Vaccinations have been implicated in HIV viral load increases, implying that disease progression may increase (Stanley et al. 1996). Data for increased rapidity of disease progression exist and may prove to have significance in local settings. However, no coinfection emerges to compete with HIV itself as the single most compelling predictor of disease progression. The more likely frontier is host immune response reflected in host immunogenetic profiles (Dean et al. 1996, Smith et al. 1997, Saah et al. 1998, Winkler et al. 1998, Carrington et al. 1999, Keet et al. 1999, Martin et al. 1998, Tang et al. 1999).

An example of a recurring challenge in HIV research that can arise in both case-control and cohort studies is the issue of death of infected persons with short incubation periods between infection and disease. Selective deletion of such persons from participation in research will occur, since they may have died prior to potentially being recruited. Hence, an underrepresentation of persons with rapid disease progression in the case group may ensue, unbeknownst to the epidemiologist or clinical investigator. In an effort to assess the impact of zidovudine on mortality in a real world setting, this possibility was not appreciated by authors, reviewers, or editors (Graham et al. 1992a). Upon presentation of this argument in a letter to the editor, reanalysis of the observational cohort data had to be performed with more conservative assumptions in an effort to correct for the possibility that persons with rapid disease progression had died before 1987 when zidovudine became widely available in the cohort (Gail and Mark 1992, Graham et al. 1992b). If "rapid progressors" (Schrager et al. 1994) were systematically excluded from a study of treatment effect due to their death prior to drug availability (about 1987 in this case) (Rosenberg et al. 1991), but such individuals provided data to the control or comparison group, then the treatment group would be inherently healthier than the untreated control group, biasing an analysis in favor of the treatment group seeming healthier.

Many limitations exist in cohort studies that must been considered. A few of these are obvious, while others are not. That nearly all cohort data from the 1980s were among men inhibited their generalizability to women. The existence of an "unseen cohort" of persons who will have died before being able to be enrolled into a given study can cause mischief in inference, since these "rapid progressors" are different from the longer-term survivors overrepresented in the eligible study pool (Hoover et al. 1991). Persons surviving longer are also living long enough to be able to take advantage of novel chemotherapeutic and prophylactic agents, at least in industrialized countries. Selection bias due to recruitment strategies, selective dropout particularly among drug users, participant utilization of many health care providers (a particularly common challenge in U.S. studies), underrepresentation of minorities or of persons living in rural environments, and many other examples illustrate complexities in cohort research designs.

One innovation is the use of an open or "dynamic" cohort, in which the enrollment of new subjects is continued as the study is ongoing, particularly when the purpose of the research study is to identify and follow high risk seronegative persons in anticipation of prevention clinical trials (Heyward et al. 1994). Vaccine trial preparedness may depend on such cohorts in which persons are recruited for a limited number of years with new subjects recruited as replacement members. The MACS recruited its subjects in 1983–84, but owing to underrepresentation of African Americans, chose to keep open enrollment for black gay or bisexual men for an additional five years (Kaslow et al. 1987, Dudley et al. 1995).

MONITORING THE EPIDEMIC WITH SURVEILLANCE-BASED RESEARCH

AIDS Surveillance

Continuously from 1981, the surveillance infrastructure has been developed and case definitions refined. Case ascertainment improved, though the revolution of HIV testing in 1985 was not immediately exploited for surveillance purposes in most public health venues because of civil liberties concerns about reporting infected persons by name. Early characterizations of AIDS included such terms as gay-related immune deficiency. The original surveillance case definition of AIDS included a list of conditions thought to be found overwhelmingly among persons with AIDS. The case definition was revised in 1985 and 1987 to include HIV seropositivity and a few more opportunistic infections (OIs) and malignancies. In 1993, after a bitter public debate about women's issues, the new case definition added three more conditions, tuberculosis, recurrent pneumonias, and cervical carcinoma. More significant in its impact was the inclusion of CD4+ cell count under 200/µl. Thus, in 1993, a huge bolus of individuals were reported in the United States who met only this new criterion, distorting the comparisons with surveillance data from past years. This change acknowledged that in the treatment era, an individual could die from HIV disease without ever being eligible for a surveillance case definition of AIDS, since drugs coud stave off OIs and malignancies. However, the Europeans continued to use the earlier case definitions for AIDS, believing that the value of a consistent case definition for projection modeling overcame the theoretical benefits of more complete reporting of severe HIV disease, which is how AIDS is now considered clinically. In those states and countries in which testing is widely available and is widely exploited in many screening settings and where HIV infection is reportable, HIV surveillance is proving to be a better indicator of epidemic evolution than AIDS surveillance.

Other AIDS case definitions have been offered. The Walter Reed classification system used delayed-type hypersensitivity responses from skin test antigen responses to help characterize HIV infection and AIDS. The World Health Organization (WHO) noted that HIV testing in developing countries was often unavailable. The WHO and other groups have proposed a number of AIDS and HIV classification schemes that attempt to characterize AIDS with maximum validity at minimal cost. The WHO classification scheme uses lymphocyte count in lieu of HIV testing or CD4+ cell count when the latter are not available. The Kigali, Uganda, Thai, and other definitions have been validated against clinical outcome with some success, suggesting that it is possible to use "appropriate technology" surveillance, including HIV testing when possible, but identifying AIDS cases even when HIV testing is not available.

AIDS surveillance has been developed in many forms. North America, Western Europe, and Australia have striven for complete case ascertainment using a variety of mechanisms. Hospital- and physician-based reporting, assistance from laboratories that perform CD4+ cell counts and HIV tests, and substantial outreach infrastructures to study records and investigate reports have contributed to over 85% complete reporting according to estimates (Buehler et al. 1992, Rosenblum et al. 1992, Schwarcz et al. 1999). In developing nations with limited resources, there are alternative approaches. Some countries with minimal surveillance infrastructures largely report persons who have been prescreened in richer countries, as with returning Pakistani workers who have tested positive in routine HIV screening in the rich Gulf states. There is no distinction between HIV and AIDS testing in such circumstances (Shah et al. 1999). In Thailand, in contrast, one of the world's best AIDS surveillance systems has been established with nationwide testing availability and good educational level for clinical AIDS presentation among health care providers. However, not all practioners appreciate the need for HIV testing in persons who are not symptomatic (Stringer et al. 1999).

HIV Surveillance

HIV testing and surveillance are prevalent in parts of Europe and in selected states but have not been adopted universally. At the time of the development of the HIV test (licensed first in the United States in 1985), there was a strong bias among many community and professional groups that HIV testing had little to offer in therapeutic intervention but much to risk in terms of stigmatization and prejudice. The advent of therapy in 1987 did surprisingly little to alter these antitesting views. A few states such as Colorado took a classic public health approach to HIV as an STD with mandatory named HIV reporting and even contact tracing to inform exposed persons of their need to be tested and to protect themselves from future exposure. Other states continue to report only AIDS, not HIV, including high prevalence states such as California and

New York. Still other states have hybrid approaches requiring reporting of pediatric but not adult HIV cases (e.g., Connecticut) or have mandatory testing of newborns but no such approaches (including no HIV reporting) in adults (e.g., New York).

In an effort to encourage testing but enable this to be done without social harm, anonymous counseling and testing centers have been established in many locales. It is not known whether these counseling and testing centers have been a public health success in bringing persons at high risk into care or whether they have largely served the low risk "worried well" or persons who would otherwise have been served in a standard health environment without difficulty.

HIV surveillance has a number of benefits and limitations. In the treatment era, time to AIDS is commonly lengthened. AIDS surveillance alone would therefore be expected to reflect poorly recent trends and changing epidemic dynamics. HIV seropositivity is an objective marker of infection, while AIDS depends on a surveillance case definition occasionally open to interpretation, for example, is this pneumonia a recurrence, is this chest X-ray confirming *P. carinii*, or is this pathologic sample definitive for Kaposi's sarcoma? However, HIV testing coverage may be capricious, positives may not be reported to health officials, and inconsistencies in HIV test policies from locale to locale may not permit cross-venue comparisons. Given that biased ascertainment may persist in a given geographic location, however, trends over time may be assessed with some accuracy.

Case ascertainment bias is the principal problem in HIV surveillance. Early detection can occur with early testing. Late detection, even as late as post-AIDS diagnosis, occurs when testing is anonymous or not done or available. This typically differs by subgroup even within the same community. Early in the epidemic, health care providers typically overlooked HIV in persons who did not fit a stereotypical risk profile, including women (Schoenbaum and Webber 1993). Testing was often not performed in many resource-poor settings or when physi-

cians or families wanted to hide the truth for fear of disclosure. In a recent paradox, the imperative to protect infants born to HIV-infected mothers has led to widespread screening of women of child-bearing age. Thus from underrepresented in HIV testing to well represented, women are now more likely to receive an HIV test than men in many settings.

Whether HIV testing and named reporting is good public health and clinical practice or whether it is an open door to unnecessary discrimination and a civil liberties assault on confidentiality ("AIDS exceptionalism") continues to be debated. However, the drastic changes in treatment options have moved the debate strongly toward testing and reporting. Since HIV disease resembles diabetes as a chronic, manageable disease, more and more practitioners and community representatives are urging testing as a first step to education and therapy. The 1998 Institute of Medicine report on perinatal transmission prevention states, "the United States should adopt a national policy of universal HIV testing, with patient notification, as a routine component of prenatal care" (IOM 1998). Despite this new paradigm in the era of highly active antiretroviral therapy (HAART), only 32 U.S. states mandate HIV reporting to state authorities, suggesting continued popular ambivalence regarding the public health value of such surveillance when weighed against civil liberties fears.

Sentinel surveys of defined populations are a valuable adjunct to surveillance, particularly with known HIV underreporting. Such studies have been done worldwide in a multitude of populations, sometimes combining some element of knowledge, attitudes, and behaviors assessment with anonymous HIV testing. The largest data base cataloguing HIV seroprevalence studies, whether formally published or not, is maintained by the U.S. Census Bureau (http://www.census. gov/ipc/www/hivaidsd.html). Caution in interpretation of such surveys is needed, since studies differ as to the exact sampling strategies, the timing of the survey, the nature of the study population, the testing methods used, and the generalizability of the results.

Sometimes surveillance statistics have been merged with other surveillance, hospital, or clinical data to indicate possible associations. One such study suggested that high pneumonia hospital discharge rates correlated with AIDS surveillance data at the zip (postal) code level (Drucker et al. 1989). While potentially suffering from the risk of an ecologic fallacy (poor people in the Bronx, New York, have more pneumonia and have more AIDS, but they are not necessarily linked at individual level), the clinical evidence was mounting simultaneously with the surveillance-hospital discharge data that, together convinced the CDC to include recurrent pneumonias as an AIDS-defining clinical condition in the 1993 surveillance case definition revision (CDC 1988, Selwyn et al. 1988, Drucker et al. 1989). A similar paradigm was noted for tuberculosis, with clinical observations, surveillance data, linkage studies, and cohort studies all pointing toward a common conclusion, that pulmonary tuberculosis and HIV were closely linked, resulting in inclusion of pulmonary tuberculosis as an AIDS-defining condition (CDC 1987, Selwyn et al. 1992, Stoneburner et al. 1992).

MITIGATING THE EPIDEMIC

Clinical Care Approaches

A discussion of issues in HIV-related human experiments is a huge topic beyond the scope of this chapter. The urgency and lethality of AIDS, the organization of activist groups, the substantial investments in drug discovery and development, and the rapidity of progress in developing hitherto unknown classes of chemotherapeutic agents have all introduced innovations and shortcuts in the licensure and research evaluation process (Arno and Feiden 1992). The Food and Drug Administration has modified its review processes for urgent circumstances, the threshold of evidence has been lowered for more lethal diseases, and the review process has been accelerated for drugs in general. Enrollment must now include women, children, and minorities unless a justification

for their exclusion can be given. This is in response to the absence of generalizable results from studies conducted largely among white, gay men. Loss to follow up is a recurrent problem in clinical trials; community-based infrastructures like the Community Program for Clinical Resaerch on AIDS were begun by the NIH in order to maximize accrual and retention of hard-to-access populations. Notably, community representatives were included at nearly every level of research planning, review, and even licensure at a scale unique for the NIH, the CDC, and the FDA.

As a direct consequence of the sense of urgency, new commitment to the study of true surrogate markers was made. A surrogate marker varies in response to a therapeutic intervention in direct predictive proportion to the eventual therapeutic impact on the disease outcome. Thus trials with excellent surrogate markers can be terminated based on the treatment effect on the marker rather than waiting for the definitive clinical outcomes. CD4+ cell counts were the best available surrogates at one time. However, the early termination of AIDS clinical Trial Groups (ACTG) 019 trial based on zidovudine impact on CD4+ cell counts suggested that zidovudine given early (>200 CD4+ cells/μl) was advisable (Fischl et al. 1987). Yet the European Concorde study suggested that early versus late zidovudine made no difference and argued that early termination of the ACTG 019 study had been misleading owing to the inadequacy of CD4+ cell counts as a true surrogate for clinical outcome, that is, time to AIDS or death (Aboulker and Swart 1993). The advent of quantitative HIV viral load (Piatak et al. 1993, Mellors et al. 1996) and its strong long-term prognostic value for disease progression velocity have revolutionized AIDS clinical research. Its use as a true surrogate marker enables much improved clinical trial rapidity, particularly since clinical outcomes are increasingly rare in the HAART era. Other surrogates of viral activity such as soluble markers like β-microglobulinemia or neopterin have proven helpful in refining risk of progression (Fahey et al. 1998), but are indirect assessments of viral activity and are now less helpful in the face of the direct viral load assessment.

Another key policy change of the AIDS era was the impact of compassionate use availability on clinical trial design. Many persons in trials did not trust randomization to provide them the personal maximum benefit. They preferred to take the experimental therapies even before they were proven to work. Hence, after unmasking themselves by testing their clinical trial assigned drugs or through inference based on CD4+ cell count changes, they would secure drugs from companies that were making them available to persons not on clinical trials. This behavior may have slowed the time of completion of clinical trials because of self-reassignment of persons in "standard care" groups who chose to take the experimental drugs secured outside of the clinical trial paradigm. Thus intent-to-treat analyses would have compromised statistical power, owing to the increased bias toward the null hypothesis from patient-initiated reallocation of treatment groups. The ethical implications of slowing down clinical trials are interesting to ponder; the individual good in such an instance may inhibit wider community benefits such that persons desiring specific allocation to a given treatment may do well not to enroll in clinical trials that randomize them into an unknown treatment group.

Key methodologic issues in HIV-related clinical trials are reviewed in many other chapters and reviews (Anonymous 1990, Pizzo 1990, Vermund 1994, Katzenstein 1995, Dabis et al. 1995, Lange 1995, Schaper et al. 1995, Schooley 1995, Fleming et al. 1997, Mildvan et al. 1997, Zackin 1998, Boily et al. 1999). Readers are referred to these references to study experimental trials techniques in the AIDS era further.

Prevention Techniques

The cost of treating HIV is extremely high, with current highly active antiretroviral therapy (HAART) accessible to only a small portion of those infected with HIV worldwide.

Thus preventing the spread of HIV in populations is widely considered to be of utmost importance. Relatively little effort has been expended in developing and testing biomedical interventions for the prevention of HIV, in part because of the difficulty of evaluating prevention intervention effectiveness. Prevention strategies can be active medical interventions (i.e., vaccines or administration of zidovudine during childbirth) that require little or no effort on the part of the individual targeted for the intervention. In such instances, use of the standard clinical trial approach to evaluating the effectiveness of the prevention strategy (see previous section) is appropriate and provides easily interpretable results.

The vast majority of prevention strategies, however, require a change in behavior from the person being targeted for the intervention (i.e., use of condoms during every act of intercourse). In addition, many prevention strategies do not lend themselves to a classic clinical trial approach because of the lack of an appropriate placebo and ethical issues. For example, a clinical trial of the effectiveness of condoms in preventing HIV would require one group at high risk of HIV infection to use condoms for each act of intercourse, and one group not to use condoms. Given that condoms prevent transmission of body fluids that are known to contain HIV, it would be unethical to require one group to abstain from using condoms. In addition, the requirement that the only treatment group actively use condoms at each act of intercourse introduces a behavioral bias that makes the clinical trial extremely difficult to interpret using the classic "intent-to-treat" analysis.

An example of this is provided by a study of the female condom, in which 126 women treated for trichomoniasis were randomized either to use the female condom or not to do anything to prevent reinfection. There was no difference in reinfection rates between the two groups. Unfortunately, only 20 of the 104 women who completed a 45-day follow-up period used the condom for every act of intercourse. No reinfection occurred among 20 women (0%) who used the female condom all the time, 7 reinfections occurred among 50 women (14%) who did not use the device, and 5 reinfections occurred among 34 women (15%) who used it inconsistently (Soper et al. 1993). Interpretation of these data is difficult, because the women who were randomized to use the female condom and used it every time were different from the women who were randomized to use the female condom and did not use it every time. Their behavior in following the study protocol was different, and this could have been because of differences in background risk, differences in willingness to engage in risky behavior, ability to follow instructions, ability to negotiate condom use, or multiple other factors that could be related to trichomonas reinfection. In addition, the women who were in the nontreatment group (not asked to use the female condom) may have behaved differently from the women who were asked to use the female condom (i.e., been more or less willing to have sex with a casual partner).

Because of such ethical and design issues observational studies are more commonly performed than clinical trials in HIV prevention research. Follow-up studies are different in prevention research from the classic design described in the prior section. In a follow-up study of condom use as a risk reduction technique, for example, individuals are observed for some period of time for both condom use and development of HIV. Typically, all couples enrolled in such a study would be encouraged to use condoms. At the end of the study, rates of HIV are compared between those who used condoms and those who did not. In a case-control study of condom use, the use history of an HIV-positive group (cases) and an HIV-negative group (controls) is used to estimate the odds of the diseased having used condoms when compared to the nondiseased (or vice versa).

Of course, both follow-up studies and case-control studies of this type have an inherent bias, because the study subjects self-select into use groups. These self-selected groups probably have different levels of risk. Investigators usually try to measure background risk and deal with the potential bias by restricting subjects (e.g., recruiting only prostitutes) or "adjusting" for the risk differences in the analysis of the study. In addition, it is difficult to determine how use should be defined. If a couple uses condoms the majority of the times they have sex, should they be classified as condom users? Observational studies provide valuable information about the real world efficacy of a prevention technique, however, because in the real world the choices individuals make about whether or not to use a technique will ultimately have a substantial effect on the overall impact of the intervention.

Measurement issues in the evaluation of prevention techniques
In addition to the issues of bias and reliability, evaluation of prevention techniques presents special challenges in measuring both predictors and outcomes. Measuring risk behaviors is a science fraught with special challenges. Self-report of behavior is sometimes inaccurate, especially with regard to sexual activity and drug use. In some instances, the behavior in question can be confirmed with a biologic marker. For example, it is possible to use a semen marker (such as prostate specific antigen) to confirm reports of no sexual activity in the last day. In addition, some studies of condom use have required the participants to return the used condom for examination (Richters et al. 1988, Rugpao et al. 1993). For treatment studies, the state-of-the-art includes pill dosage containers that can actually record when pills are removed and direct observation of medication adherence.

Measurement of outcomes is also difficult because of the large number of surrogate outcomes (such as behavior change or STD development) and the intricacies of the laboratory assays involved. If disease is the outcome of a prevention study, then the definition of disease must be determined in advance. In studies of STD prevention (which are often used as surrogates for HIV and as predictors of HIV risk), the choice of laboratory assay is of paramount importance.

(See Table 13–3 for the sensitivity and specificity of various laboratory tests for sexually transmitted diseases.) Wet preps for trichomonas can be sensitive when done properly, but proper training is time consuming and often overlooked. In developing countries, STD diagnosis is often done with gram-stains, which are vastly inferior to culture and molecular assays such as polymerase chain reaction (PCR) and ligase chain reaction (LCR). Even among the best assays, PCR is superior to culture, and LCR is usually superior to PCR in terms of sensitivity. The opposite is often true for specificity. Comparing outcomes across studies when different laboratory techniques are used is often impossible.

When and how samples are taken can also be important. To continue the STD example, samples for both gonococcal and chlamydia should be taken from the cervix. Sensitivity of the assays will be significantly affected if the samples are taken only in the vagina, as is sometimes done. In addition, chlamydia resides in the basal layers of the cervix, so taking the sample for chlamydia last is the best way to insure a good test. If HIV is the outcome and an antibody test is used, the timing of the test is extremely important. For example, infants retain maternal antibodies for up to 18 months. Thus studies of vertical transmission that rely on antibody testing in the first few months of life may have a significant number of false positives. The opposite is true of prevention studies in adults, when taking antibody tests too early in infection can lead to false negative results.

In summary, designing a good prevention study requires attention to both ethical and study design issues. In addition, it is important to learn all of the details of laboratory assays and give attention to detail in measuring risk behavior, predictors of disease (such as STD), or actual disease. It is also wise to remember that in any study population, there will be a background risk of infection that may vary across self-selecting study groups. Any measurement of background risk that can be included in the study design will strengthen the interpretability of

the results. In spite of the methodologic problems in evaluating prevention techniques, it is important that such studies be conducted and the results made available to policymakers and the public.

Decision making

Decisions about what techniques to use in preventing and treating HIV should be made based on the *efficacy* of a particular technique. Efficacy refers to the ability of a technique or protocol to produce the desired result (e.g., fewer opportunistic infections). A protocol is first evaluated for its efficacy in the laboratory setting, then under perfect conditions of use, and finally during typical use in the real world. Sometimes the term efficacy is used to describe how well a technique works under perfect conditions, while the term effectiveness is used to describe how well the technique works in the real world. For the purposes of this discussion, efficacy will be used as a general term, and three specific types of efficacy will be described. In Chapter 16, a distinction is made between efficacy as measured in individual-level and community-level interventions. We use the term here in the context of individual-level interventions.

Theoretical efficacy refers to the effectiveness of a technique in the laboratory setting. For example, male latex condoms have been tested in the laboratory and found to be very effective barriers to HIV under controlled conditions (Van de Perre et al. 1987). Thus the theoretical efficacy of condoms as an HIV prevention technique is good. If a protocol has good theoretical efficacy, it may be explored further to determine how well it works outside of the laboratory setting. In general, decisions about whether to introduce a new technique in the general population should not be made based on theoretical efficacy alone.

Method efficacy indicates how well a technique works under strictly controlled conditions in human trials. Method efficacy is often measured in clinical trials with strictly limited study populations, and represents the efficacy during perfect and consistent use by individuals. Method efficacy is an important concept, as it provides pertinent information for individual decision making and potential public health benefits. Many individuals want to know how well a technique works if they use it exactly as prescribed, and method efficacy is useful in this context. Sometimes method efficacy mimics theoretical efficacy (e.g., use of condoms to prevent HIV in discordant couples) and sometimes method efficacy is very different from theoretical efficacy (e.g., Nonoxynol-9 as a microbicide works extremely well in the lab and less well in human trials).

Use efficacy (or effectiveness) is the term used to describe how well a technique works in the real world. If a protocol has high method efficacy and low use efficacy, the protocol may be difficult or inconvenient to use correctly, or it may be unacceptable to some segment of the population. Low use efficacy due to incorrect or inconsistent use can potentially be improved by interventions to encourage correct and consistent use (Ngugi et al. 1988, Allen et al. 1992b). An example of the discrepancy in method and use efficacy is seen in users of HAART, who often have difficulty being compliant with the protocol because of side effects and the need for strict timing in taking multiple medications. Use efficacy should be used by policymakers in deciding when, how, and where to invest money for population-based interventions.

Sometimes, decisions are less straightforward than simply determining efficacy. Often, treatment protocols involve multiple decisions over time based on the clinical picture. In addition, clinicians and policymakers often have more than one option available at any given time and must find a way to make a choice. *Decision analysis* is a technique used to quantify what is known about a particular protocol and make decisions based on probabilities. In decision analysis, protocols are broken into decision trees, with each branch of the tree representing probabilities of given outcomes. At each fork in the tree, a decision is made based on the answer to a particular question (e.g., Is the patient's CD4 cell count above 500?). The decision could be initiating therapy for patients with a low CD4 count based on the fact that patients with a low CD4 count have a higher probability of improved outcome. Decision analysis can also be used to examine hypothetical situations, as was done with the use of zidovudine for the prevention of vertical transmission of HIV infection (Rouse et al. 1995). The decision analysis approach was used to show that all HIV-positive women should be treated with zidovudine to prevent transmission of the virus during delivery. This analysis was able to answer concerns that zidovudine might lead to adverse outcomes in uninfected children.

Application of mathematical modeling to HIV

Mathematical modeling is a tool that is coming to be depended on often by public health planners. The term *mathematical model* can be used in a variety of ways, but it simply means a set of equations that predict some observed phenomenon. This is a very general concept, which includes a formidable number of techniques. In particular, we are interested here in dynamic models: models that predict the behavior of some phenomenon over time. The phenomenon of interest to us here is the progression of HIV infection in a population.

Reasons why a public health planner might try to build a model include: projecting the number of individuals who will need medical services; comparing different assumptions about the dynamics of disease propagation (Aylward et al. 1995, Lipsitch and Nowak 1995, Gregson et al. 1997, West and Thompson 1997); estimating parameters pertinent to the disease (Renton et al. 1995, West and Thompson 1997); evaluating possible interventions (Anderson et al. 1995, Garnett et al. 1995, Kault 1995, Nagelkerke et al. 1995, Atkinson 1996, Wein et al. 1997); deciding on the disposition of public health resources. Basically, we can say that dynamic models can be used to try to answer questions that fall into these categories: what is happening, what did happen, and what may happen.

In order to discuss how to design a dynamic model, let us consider an infectious disease with a much more acute presentation than HIV disease. Measles, rubella, or any other highly contagious disease could fit into this discussion. Models of diseases of this type have been very useful in the area of vaccinology. For example, modeling predicts the paradox observed in vaccinology that a vaccine program, if not implemented correctly, can actually make matters worse relative to the disease the program is designed to prevent. Later in this section, reasons why HIV models must differ from these models will be discussed. The information that we want the model to supply is the number of individuals in a population with and without the disease. We classify each member of the population as being in one of several groups or compartments, for example, those susceptible to infection and those already infected (Boily and Masse 1997). The type of model often used for a disease like measles is called an SIR model because it contains three compartments: susceptible, infectious, and recovered (understood to mean recovered with lasting immunity) (Anderson and May 1995).

Once the compartments are decided on, the investigator must specify how individuals are able to move from compartment to compartment. These relationships, which give the dynamics of the disease within the population, are then formally written as equations that express the change in the number of individuals in the compartments over time. We will see later that models can be either discrete or continuous, depending on how the time change is described.

A common way that the relationships between compartments are portrayed is as a flowchart (Anderson and May 1995). Such a chart shows which transitions are possible, that is, which compartments individuals can move to from a given compartment, and shows the names of the parameters that govern the rates of these transitions. Consider the SIR model. Susceptible individuals can become infected, so a transition from the susceptible to the infectious compartment is possible. An infectious individual can recover from the infection with lasting immunity (infectious to recovered). A sus-

ceptible individual can also be successfully vaccinated (susceptible to recovered). There is no reason to keep those who are immune due to vaccination and those who are immune due to recovery from the disease in separate compartments; they have the same relevance in the model. If an individual is immune, that individual is unable to contract the disease from an infectious individual, and is unable to infect a susceptible individual. As the proportion of the population that is immune (for whatever reason) increases, the probability that an encounter between two individuals is an encounter between a susceptible individual and an infectious individual decreases. When this probability is very low (not necessarily zero!), it is possible for the disease to stop being propagated in the population because the disease entity never gets to a susceptible individual in which it can reproduce. This is known as herd immunity and is the typical objective of a vaccination program (Anderson and May 1995).

Transitions can be expressed in terms of rates or proportions, depending on the way that the model expresses change. If the modeler decides on a basic time interval and expresses all of the changes relative to that interval (e.g., how do the number of individuals in each compartment change from week 1 to week 2; week 2 to week 3; etc.), the parameters are typically proportions. Thus, for example, we may say that in a typical week, 10% of the infectious individuals recover with immunity. Such a model is called a discrete model because the only times that appear in the final result are defined by the time interval. For this example, the result from the model might be expressed as a table that shows the total number of individuals in each compartment at week 1, then the number at week 2, then at week 3, etc. This type of model is very well suited to presentation as a spreadsheet. If the modeler did not feel that a particular time interval was appropriate, change over time would be expressed as a derivative, which is interpreted as an instantaneous rate of change (West and Thompson 1997). In this case, the parameters would not be proportions, but rates. A model of this type is called a continuous model. Either way, a term that expresses a change will be written as a parameter times the number in a compartment. For example, if we say that 10% of the infectious individuals recover in one time interval in a discrete model, and we use Y to denote the number of infectious individuals, then $(0.1)Y$ represents the amount that Y will decrease due to recovery. This is true of every term except those terms that involve individuals actually becoming infected.

An infection is due to the infectious agent being passed from an infectious individual to a susceptible individual. This passage can only occur if there is a meeting between an infectious individual and a susceptible individual. Thus the total number of infections that occur must depend in some way on the total number of such meetings that can occur. Let's say that we have M infectious individuals and N susceptible. The first infectious individual could possibly meet any one of the susceptible individuals, for a total of N possible meetings. The same is true of the second infectious individual, and the third, etc. Following this reasoning through, we see that the total number of possible meetings between susceptible and infectious individuals is $N + N + \ldots = MN$, the product of the total number of infectious individuals and the total number of susceptible individuals. If we are dealing with a discrete model, we can reason that in one time interval some proportion of the total possible meetings will happen, and some proportion of the meetings will result in the infectious agent actually being passed successfully to the susceptible individual. The number of new infections in one interval will thus be expressed as some parameter times the product of the number in the two compartments (Boily and Masse 1997). The corresponding term in a continuous model can be much more complicated but will typically be a term involving the number of infectious individuals times the number of susceptible individuals. For example, a constant times the proportion of the population that is infectious (i.e., the prevalence of infection) times the number of susceptibles

is used (Boily and Masse 1997, West and Thompson 1997).

When the equations are developed to describe the following model, a general notation will be used for change over time. If X represents the number of individuals in a particular compartment, the change in the number of individuals in that compartment will be expressed as DX whether the change is discrete or continuous. In a discrete model, the values at particular times would be denoted X_t (e.g., X_0, X_1, X_2, etc.), and DX indicates a difference of the form $X_{t+1} - X_t$. For a continuous model, the value at a particular time is denoted $X(t)$ where time is not constrained to be an integer. In this case, DX could denote the time derivative dX/dt, or when the model is dependent on age as well as time $\partial X/\partial t + \partial X/\partial a$. The choice will affect the particular values of the parameters, and will have a profound effect on how the equations are solved, but the technique for expressing the model is the same. Before proceeding, it is best to decide on what variables will be used to denote which compartments. Following the notation of Anderson and May, we will use X for the number of susceptible individuals, Y for the number of infectious individuals, and Z for the number of immune (recovered or vaccinated) individuals. We are now ready to describe the possible transitions between the compartments.

Table 20–3 summarizes exactly which transitions are possible. Note that a transition between two compartments will involve two terms in the final equations: one positive and one negative. For example, when a susceptible individual is infected, that individual is lost to the number of susceptibles (a negative term for the change in X) and is added to the number of infectious (a positive term for the change in Y). There are no compartments for birth or death in this table. Birth is considered an infinite source, death an infinite sink; more people can always be born, and more can always die. A hyphen is the character used to indicate these sources and sinks. Note that although individuals in any of the compartments can die, individuals can only be born into the susceptible

Table 20–3 Summary of Transitions Between Compartments

From	to	Process
—	X	Birth
X	—	Death
X	Y	Infection
X	Z	Immunization
Y	—	Death
Y	Z	Recovery
Z	—	Death

category. This model does not admit the possibility of vertical transmission.

This same information can be expressed as a flowchart, which also gives the values of the rates of transition (Anderson and May 1995, Boily and Masse 1997). There is no specifically agreed-upon format for such a flowchart, but many authors present their models in this way (Fig. 20–1). This chart indicates, for example, that if the model were a discrete model, at the next time interval, the number of infectious individuals that die will be μY, and the number that recover will be σY. The birth term will be slightly more complicated, because individuals in any of the compartments can have children. Thus the number of individuals that will be born in the next interval will be $\beta(X+Y+Z)$. As mentioned before, the infection term (which has the coefficient r) involves both X and Y, and is necessarily more complicated than the other terms. In a discrete model, the infection term would take the form rXY. If the model does not depend on age, the term will be similar for a continuous model. When we assemble all of the terms, we have these three equations:

$$DX = \beta(X + Y + Z) - \mu X - rXY - \xi X$$

$$DY = rXY - \mu Y - \sigma Y$$

$$DZ = \sigma Y + \xi X - \mu Z$$

Note that every term, except birth and death terms, is balanced; that is to say, each term that is added in one equation is subtracted in another. If the population is assumed to be in steady state, that is, that the number of in-

dividuals in the population remains constant over time, the mathematical assumption made is that $b = \mu$, and all terms will then be balanced.

This model is quite adequate for investigating a large variety of questions. Anderson and May use this model and others derived from it to investigate some of the problems of vaccine program planning. It is not adequate for investigating the dynamics of HIV disease for a variety of reasons. One reason is the third compartment: those who are immune to the disease. Despite the very small number of long-term nonprogressors found, there is no lasting immunity to this disease. This compartment must be done away with entirely for an HIV model. Another problem was alluded to earlier. This model does not admit the possibility of vertical transmission. This is less of a problem because models are often used to investigate the dynamics of the disease in adult populations. However, it would be necessary to include this consideration in a model of the disease in a large population over a long time period.

Some other reasons that this model is inadequate for describing the dynamics of HIV disease arise from the fact that one major mode of transmission of HIV is as an STD. A compartment that was not discussed earlier that is pertinent to STDs is the group of latent individuals. These are the individuals who have been infected (so they are no longer susceptible) but are not yet infectious to others (so they do not participate in the rXY term). For a disease such as measles, this is not a major consideration. The latent period is relatively short, and everyone in the population breathes the same air, so latency will not significantly affect the dynamics of that disease. The situation is quite different with an STD for one very important reason: if a susceptible individual is having sex with a latent individual, it is pretty safe to rule out the possibility that the same person is simultaneously having sex with an infectious individual. An interaction with one person precluding interaction with another is a characteristic of STDs that is not true of aerosol spread diseases, and so

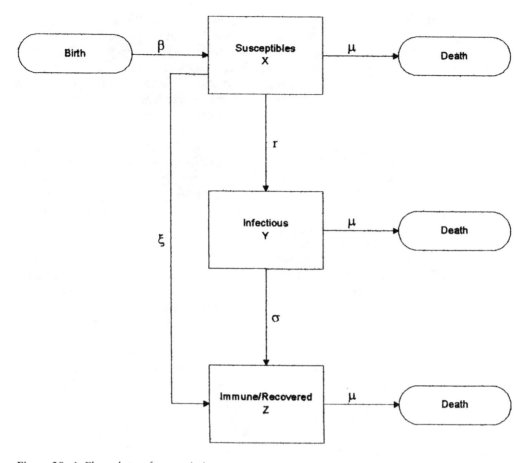

Figure 20–1. Flow chart of transmission compartments.

latency must be considered in the modeling of STDs. The concept of a core group—a subgroup within the population that engages in more active disease transmission behavior—is also vitally important in the modeling of an STD (Anderson et al. 1995, Renton et al. 1995, Stigum et al. 1997). Specific to HIV is the further consideration of varying infectivity (Kault 1995, Iannelli et al. 1997). It is now accepted that there is a peak infectivity early in the infection, relatively low infectivity during the asymptomatic period of the disease, and higher infectivity when symptoms begin to appear (the development of frank AIDS). This is a complication that can be handled in a variety of ways. The period during which a person has the disease can be split into several compartments (e.g., early, middle, and late each with its own infectivity), or the infec-

tivity can be expressed as a function of the amount of time that the person has been infected. Both approaches have been used by modelers (Boily and Masse 1997).

Still another complication of HIV disease is the fact that it has three distinct transmission modes, each with its own dynamics. Two were mentioned before: vertical transmission and sexual transmission. The third, parenteral transmission, can be the most important in certain settings. The transmission of HIV among intravenous drug users (IVDU) has been the sole subject of many studies (Atkinson 1996). When studied by itself, HIV transmission among IVDU individuals can be modeled in essentially the same way as the sexual transmission of HIV. The concept of a core group is important in both models because there is a strong behavioral component to both processes. The picture becomes much more complicated if a model tries to take into account both modes of transmission. In particular, there would be two separate core groups to consider.

There are other facets of the dynamics of STD transmission that must also be considered by a modeler concerning heterogeneity within the population. One such heterogeneity is gender. There is typically a higher probability of transmitting an STD from male to female than from female to male (Garnett and Anderson 1995, Renton et al. 1995). There are different transmission probabilities between vaginal and anal sex. As important as this biologic heterogeneity is, even more important to the dynamics of the disease is behavioral heterogeneity. As mentioned before, the concept of a core group—a subgroup with higher sexual activity—is important to consider in such a model (Garnett and Anderson 1995, Renton et al. 1995, Boily and Masse 1997, Thomas and Tucker 1995). If we treat the entire population of interest as being composed of groups with different levels of sexual activity, the model must not only accommodate the susceptible and infective individuals in these groups as separate compartments but must include infection terms for each possible interaction (e.g., a low-activity susceptible individual may be infected by a low-activity infective individual, or a high activity infective individual), and must allow for differential mixing between the groups (i.e., individuals in a particular group may preferentially choose partners within their own group). The coefficient that indicates how often a person in one group chooses a partner in the other group must be included in the model (Boily and Masse 1997). Transitions among these new compartments must be included in the model as well. For example, a person who has been in the high activity group may decide to change to a lower level of sexual activity if he or she becomes infected.

These are not the only characteristics of HIV that make it unique and a challenge to modeling. Most characteristics are shared by all STDs (with the possible exception of the differential infectivity over the course of

the disease). But HIV is unique in that HIV disease, though infectious, is a chronic disease. In part, this means that the only transition out of the infectious state is death. There may be a transition to a compartment with a different level of activity or a different infectiousness, but the infectiousness will never be zero. Another aspect of this characteristic of the disease is that, although it is not curable (at this time), it is treatable. A modeler must take into account the fact that the infectiousness of the disease depends on the treatment that the individual is undergoing.

It is easy to see that a complete model takes into account a great many mathematical relationships, each with a characteristic coefficient. The problem is that in order to completely specify the model, the values of all of these coefficients must be specified. Finding the value of a single coefficient may be, in of itself, the subject of an entire study. The potential complexity of a model is always sacrificed in favor of forming a model that is tractable. When a model is specified, it can be used for a variety of purposes, as mentioned previously. However, models can also be used in a way completely opposite to the manner discussed here.

Suppose that a modeler has good information about some, but not all, of the coefficients used in a model. The model itself can be used to estimate these unknown coefficients. The problem is this: we have a collection of observed data, and a theoretical model for the behavior of that data. We wish to estimate the particular constants that will complete the specification of that theoretical model. This is the same type of problem as the problem of linear regression. In a linear regression problem, we have a collection of data (y-values), the corresponding independent variable values (x-values), and the form of an assumed theoretical model ($y = \xi_0 + \xi_1 x$). We wish to estimate the coefficients (ξ_0, and ξ_1) that complete the specification of the model. We do this by setting up a formula for the total difference between the observed data and the theoretical data, and find the values of the coefficients that minimize this total difference. The observed values are given the notation y_i, and the corresponding theoretical values from the model are given by $\beta_0 + \beta_1 x_i$. The total difference is thus given as

$$\sum_{i=1}^{n}(y_i - \beta_0 - \beta_1 x_i)^2$$

The values of the coefficients that minimize this sum of squares gives the so-called least squares regression line. The same thing can be done with the dynamic model for the disease process (Iannelli et al. 1997). We have observed numbers of susceptible and infectious individuals, and compare those with the number of susceptible and infectious individuals predicted by the model at each time for which data are available. We need to form a total difference between these sets of numbers, and then a best estimate of the unknown coefficients can be estimated. One choice for the total difference is the sum of the squares of the differences, but it is not the only one. A technique of this type can be used to estimate unknown constants of disease dynamics or compare different assumptions about the disease.

There is an additional challenge when dealing with HIV disease and AIDS that must be taken into account. Very often, the numbers predicted by the model are not observable. Asymptomatic HIV disease will "count" in the model but may remain undetected. It is thus necessary to link the actual numbers measured to the theoretical numbers. A technique that makes this link is called backcalculation (Rosenberg 1994, Iannelli et al. 1997).

It is important to realize that the results of a calculation that infers population parameters from observed data are dependent on the assumed model. In other words, the results are precisely the best estimate(s) of the given coefficent(s) *assuming that the model in question is appropriate for the data*.

Mathematical models can occasionally be quite influential in public policy. Two good examples are from the fields of HIV and malaria prevention. In the absence of definitive clinical trials of needle exchange to protect injection drug users from HIV, mathematical models of HIV PCR positivity from exchanged needles have demonstrated dramatic reduction in HIV transmission risk, presumably due to the wider circulation of clean needles and the removal of the community of dirty needles (Kaplan and Heimer 1992, Heimer et al. 1993). These models have led directly to liberalized needle exchange programs in the United States (IOM 1995).

A second example is the use of models by MacDonald in the 1960s to demonstrate the relative inefficiency of mass chemotherapy as a sole tool for malaria transmission reduction (MacDonald et al. 1968). When the Nicaraguan government, evidently ignorant of MacDonald's work, launched the largest mass chemotherapy campaign for malaria in the world history (1.9 million persons in 1982) the impact of malaria was almost precisely as predicted by the MacDonald model, that is, incidence rate of malaria returned to the baseline level within seven months (Garfield and Vermund 1983).

CONCLUSION

In the new millennium, HIV will be seen increasingly as a chronic infectious disease that has much in common with hepatitis B, hepatitis C, selected herpes viruses, and other agents that infect and may not be cleared by host defense mechanisms. "Natural experiments" among both immune competent and suppressed individuals have enabled us to recognize the infectious nature of other chronic diseases such as peptic ulcers and Kaposi's sarcoma. Future research may identify infectious contributors to such chronic disease scourges as diabetes mellitus, multiple sclerosis, and atherosclerosis. In important ways, techniques developed for HIV research have assisted in this broader search for infectious etiologies of chronic diseases, and, we hope, their ultimate control.

REFERENCES

Aboulker JP, and Swart AM. Preliminary analysis of the Concorde trial. Concorde Coordinating Committee. Lancet. 341(8849):889–90, 1993.

Adjorlolo-Johnson G, de Cock KM, Ekpini E, et al. Prospective comparison of mother-to-child transmission of HIV-1 and HIV-2 in Abidjan, Ivory Coast. JAMA. 272(6):462–466, 1994.

Allen S, Serufilira A, Bogaerts J, et al. Confidential HIV testing and condom promotion in Africa. Impact on HIV and gonorrhea rates. JAMA. 268(23):3338–3343, 1992a.

Allen S, Tice J, Van De Perre P, et al. Effect of serotesting with counseling on condom use and seroconversion among HIV discordant couples in Africa. BMJ. 304:1605–1609, 1992b.

Allen S, Serufilira A, Gruber V, et al. Pregnancy and contraception use among urban Rwandan women after HIV testing and counseling. Am. J. Public Health. 83(5):705–710, 1993.

Amato NV, Uip DE, Boulos M, et al. Acquired immunodeficiency syndrome (AIDS): report of the 1st autochthonous case in Brazil and immunological study. Rev. Paul. Med. 101 (4):165–168, 1983.

Ammann AJ, Cowan MJ, Wara DW, et al. Acquired immunodeficiency in an infant: possible transmission by means of blood products. Lancet. 1:956–958, 1983.

Anderson RM, and May RM. Infectious Diseases of Humans. Oxford: Oxford Science Publications, 1995.

Anderson RM, Swinton J, and Garnett GP. Potential impact of low efficacy HIV-1 vaccines in populations with high rates of infection. Proc. R. Soc. Lond. B. Biol. Sci. 261(1361): 147–151, 1995.

Anonymous. Needlestick transmission of HTLV-III from a patient infected in Africa. Lancet. 2:1376–1377, 1984.

Anonymous. Methodological issues in AIDS clinical trials. A symposium sponsored by the National Institute of Allergy and Infectious Diseases and Food and Drug Administration. Bethesda, Maryland, November 20–21, 1989. Proceedings. J. Acquir. Immune Defic. Syndr. 3 Suppl 2:S1–147, 1990.

Arno PS, and Feiden KL. Against the Odds: the Story of AIDS Drug Development, Politics, and Profits. New York: Harper Collins, 1992.

Atkinson J. A simulation model of the dynamics of HIV transmission in intravenous drug users. Comput. Biomed. Res. 29(4):338–349, 1996.

Auerbach DM, Darrow WW, Jaffe HW, and Curran JW. Cluster of cases of the acquired immune deficiency syndrome. Patients linked by sexual contact. Am. J. Med. 76(3):487–492, 1984.

Aylward B, Kane M, McNair-Scott R, Hu DJ, and Hu DH. Model-based estimates of the risk of human immunodeficiency virus and hepatitis B virus transmission through unsafe injections. Int. J. Epidemiol. 24(2):446–452, 1995.

Barkan SE, Melnick SL, Preston-Martin S, et al. The Women's Interagency HIV Study. WIHS Collaborative Study Group. Epidemiology. 9(2):117–125, 1995.

Barré-Sinoussi F, Chermann JC, Rey F, et al. Isolation of a T-lymphotropic retrovirus from a patient at risk for acquired immune deficiency syndrome (AIDS). Science. 220(4599): 868–871, 1983.

Beyrer C, Brookmeyer R, Natpratan C, et al. Measuring HIV-1 incidence in northern Thailand: prospective cohort results and estimates based on early diagnostic tests. J. Acquir. Immune. Defic. Syndr. 12(5):495–499, 1996.

Boily MC, and Masse B. Mathematical models of disease transmission: a precious tool for the study of sexually transmitted diseases. Can. J. Public Health. 88(4):255–265, 1997.

Boily MC, Masse BR, Desai K, Alary M, and Anderson RM. Some important issues in the planning of phase III HIV vaccine efficacy trials. Vaccine. 17(7–8):989–1004, 1999.

Bonneux L, Van der SP, Taelman H, et al. Risk factors for infection with human immunodeficiency virus among European expatriates in Africa. BMJ. 297(6648):581–584, 1988.

Boyko WJ, Schechter MT, Craib KJ, et al. The Vancouver Lymphadenopathy-AIDS Study: 5. Antecedent behavioural, clinical and laboratory findings in patients with AIDS and HIV- seropositive controls. Can. Med. Assoc. J. 135(8):881–887, 1986.

Bruneau J, Lamothe F, Franco E, et al. High rates of HIV infection among injection drug users participating in needle exchange programs in Montreal: results of a cohort study. Am. J. Epidemiol. 146(12):994–1002, 1997.

Brunet JB, Bouvet E, Leibowitch J, et al. Acquired immunodeficiency syndrome in France. Lancet. 1(8326:Pt 1):t–1, 1983.

Buehler JW, Berkelman RL, and Stehr-Green JK. The completeness of AIDS surveillance. J. Acquir. Immune. Defic. Syndr. 5:257–264, 1992.

Burcham JL, Tindall B, Marmor M, et al. Incidence and risk factors for human immunodeficiency virus seroconversion in a cohort of Sydney homosexual men. Med. J. Aust. 150: 634–639, 1989.

Busch MP, Operskalski EA, Mosley JW, et al. Factors influencing human immunodeficiency virus type 1 transmission by blood transfusion. Transfusion Safety Study Group. J. Infect. Dis. 174(1):26–33, 1996.

Bygbjerg IC. AIDS in a Danish surgeon (Zaire, 1976). Lancet. 1:925, 1983.

Cardo DM, Culver DH, Ciesielski CA, et al. A case-control study of HIV seroconversion in health care workers after percutaneous exposure. N. Engl. J. Med. 337(21):1485–1490, 1997.

Carrigan DR, Harrington D, and Knox KK. Variant A human herpesvirus six as a cofactor in the pathogenesis of AIDS. J. Acquir. Immune. Defic. Syndr. 13(1):97–98, 1996.

Carrington M, Nelson GW, Martin MP, et al. HLA and HIV-1: heterozygote advantage and B*35–Cw*04 disadvantage. Science. 283 (5408):1748–1752, 1999.

CDC. *Pneumocystis* pneumonia—Los Angeles. MMWR. 30:250–252, 1981a.

CDC. Kaposi's sarcoma and *Pneumocystis* pneumonia among homosexual men—New York City and California. MMWR. 30:305–308, 1981b.

CDC. Opportunistic infections and Kaposi's sarcoma among Haitians in the U.S. MMWR. 31:353-354, 360–361, 1982a.

CDC. *Pneumocystis carinii* pneumonia among persons with hemophilia A. MMWR. 31: 365–367, 1982b.

CDC. Possible transfusion-associated acquired immune deficiency syndrome (AIDS)—California. MMWR. 31:652–664, 1982c.

CDC. Update on acquired immune deficiency syndrome (AIDS)—United States. MMWR. 31:507–514, 1982d.

CDC. Acquired immunodeficiency syndrome (AIDS): precautions for clinical and laboratory staff. MMWR. 32(577):580, 1982e.

CDC. Immunodeficiency among female sexual partners of males with acquired immune deficiency syndrome (AIDS)—New York. MMWR. 31:697–698, 1983a.

CDC. Prevention of acquired immune deficiency syndrome (AIDS): report of inter-agency recommendations. MMWR. 32:101–103, 1983b.

CDC. Tuberculosis and acquired immunodeficiency syndrome—New York City. MMWR. 36:785–790, 795, 1987.

CDC. Increase in pneumonia mortality among young adults and the HIV epidemic—New York City, United States. MMWR. 37(38): 593–596, 1988.

CDC. Case-control study of HIV seroconversion in health-care workers after percutaneous exposure to HIV-infected blood—France, United Kingdom, and United States, January 1988–August 1994. MMWR. 44(50):929–933, 1995.

Chandramohan D, and Greenwood BM. Is there an interaction between human immunodeficiency virus and Plasmodium falciparum? Int. J. Epidemiol. 27(2):296–301, 1998.

Clumeck N. Acquired immuno-deficiency syndrome: a fatal but preventable disease. Acta Clin. Belg. 38:145–147, 1983.

Clumeck N, Sonnet J, Taelman H, et al. Acquired immunodeficiency syndrome in African patients. N. Engl. J. Med. 310(8):492–497, 1984.

Coffin JM. HIV population dynamics in vivo: implications for genetic variation, pathogenesis, and therapy. Science. 267(5197):483–489, 1995.

Connor RI, Korber BT, Graham BS, et al. Immunological and virological analyses of persons infected by human immunodeficiency virus type 1 while participating in trials of recombinant gp120 subunit vaccines. J. Virol. 72(2):1552–1576, 1998.

Cook J, Dasbach E, Coplan P, et al. Modeling the long-term outcomes and costs of HIV antiretroviral therapy using HIV RNA levels: application to a clinical trial. AIDS Res. Hum. Retroviruses. 15(6):499–508, 1999.

Dabis F, Msellati P, Newell ML, et al. Methodology of intervention trials to reduce mother to child transmission of HIV with special reference to developing countries. International Working Group on Mother to Child Transmission of HIV. AIDS. 9(Supp):l–74, 1995.

Dean M, Carrington M, Winkler C, et al. Genetic restriction of HIV-1 infection and progression to AIDS by a deletion allele of the CKR5 structural gene. Science. 273(5283):1856–1862, 1996.

Del Amo J, Malin AS, Pozniak A, and de Cock KM. Does tuberculosis accelerate the progression of HIV disease? Evidence from basic science and epidemiology. AIDS 13(10): 1151–1158, 1999.

de Vincenzi I. A longitudinal study of human immunodeficiency virus transmission by heterosexual partners. European Study Group on Heterosexual Transmission of HIV. N. Engl. J. Med. 331(6):341–346, 1994.

Diaz-Mitoma F, Ruiz A, Flowerdew G, et al. High levels of Epstein-Barr virus in the oropharynx: a predictor of disease progression in human immunodeficiency virus infection. J. Med. Virol. 31(2):69–75, 1990.

Diaz C, Hanson C, Cooper ER, et al. Disease progression in a cohort of infants with vertically acquired HIV infection observed from birth: the Women and Infants Transmission Study (WITS). J. Acquir. Immune Defic. Syndr. Hum. Retrovirol. 18(3):221–228, 1998.

Donegan E, Stuart M, Niland JC, et al. Infection with human immunodeficiency virus type 1 (HIV-1) among recipients of antibody-positive blood donations. Ann. Intern. Med. 113 (10):733–739, 1990.

Dorrucci M, Rezza G, Andreoni M, et al. Serum IgG antibodies to human herpesvirus-6 (HHV-6) do not predict the progression of HIV disease to AIDS. Eur. J. Epidemiol. 15 (4):317–322, 1999.

Drucker E, Webber MP, McMaster P, and Vermund SH. Increasing rate of pneumonia hospitalizations in the Bronx: a sentinel indicator for human immunodeficiency virus. Int. J. Epidemiol. 18:926–933, 1989.

Dudley J, Jin S, Hoover D, et al. The Multicenter AIDS Cohort Study: retention after 9 1/2 years. Am. J. Epidemiol. 142(3):323–330, 1995.

Ellerbrock TV, Leib S, Harrington PE, et al. Heterosexually transmitted human immunodeficiency virus infection among pregnant women in a rural Florida community. N. Engl. J. Med. 327:1704–1709, 1992.

Estevez ME, Bruno S, Sen L, et al. Acquired immunodeficiency syndrome (AIDS) with Kaposi's sarcoma in homosexuals in Argentina. Medicina. 43(4):477, 1983.

European Collaborative Study Group. Mother-to-child transmission of HIV infection. Lancet. 2(8619):1039–1043, 1988.

Fahey JL, Taylor JM, Manna B, et al. Prognostic significance of plasma markers of immune activation, HIV viral load and CD4 T-cell measurements. AIDS. 12(13):1581–1590, 1998.

Fischl MA, Richman DD, Grieco MH, et al. The efficacy of azidothymidine (AZT) in the treatment of patients with AIDS and AIDS-related complex. A double-blind, placebo-controlled trial. N. Engl. J. Med. 317:185–191, 1987.

Fleming TR, DeGruttola V, and DeMets DL. Surrogate endpoints. AIDS Clin. Rev. 129–143, 1997.

Francis DP, Curran JW, and Essex M. Epidemic acquired immune deficiency syndrome: epidemiologic evidence for a transmissible agent. J. Natl. Cancer Inst. 71:1–4, 1983.

Friedland GH, Harris C, Butkus-Small C, et al. Intravenous drug abusers and the acquired immunodeficiency syndrome (AIDS). Demographic, drug use, and needle-sharing patterns. Arch. Intern. Med. 145(8):1413–1417, 1985.

Gail MH, and Mark SD. Early zidovudine and survival in HIV infection. N. Engl. J. Med. 327(11):815–816, 1992.

Gao F, Bailes E, Robertson DL, et al. Origin of HIV-1 in the chimpanzee Pan troglodytes troglodytes. Nature. 397(6718):436–441, 1999.

Garfield RM, and Vermund SH. Changes in malaria incidence after mass drug administration in Nicaragua. Lancet. 2(8348):500–503, 1983.

Garnett GP, and Anderson RM. Strategies for limiting the spread of HIV in developing countries: conclusions based on studies of the transmission dynamics of the virus. J. Acquir. Immune Defic. Syndr. Hum. Retrovirol. 9(5):500–513, 1995.

Goedert JJ, Biggar RJ, Winn DM, et al. Decreased helper T lymphocytes in homosexual men. I. Sexual contact in high-incidence areas for the acquired immunodeficiency syndrome. Am. J. Epidemiol. 121(5):629–636, 1985.

Gottlieb MS, Schroff R, Schanker HM, et al. Pneumocystis carinii pneumonia and mucosal candidiasis in previously healthy homosexual men. N. Engl. J. Med. 305:1425–1431, 1981.

Graham BS, McElrath MJ, Connor RI, et al. Analysis of intercurrent human immunodeficiency virus type 1 infections in phase I and II trials of candidate AIDS vaccines. J. Infect. Dis. 177(2):310–319, 1998.

Graham NMH, Zeger SL, Park LP, et al. The effects on survival of early treatment of human immunodeficiency virus infection. N. Engl. J. Med. 326:1037–1042, 1992a.

Graham NMH, Zeger SL, and Park LP. Early zidovudine and survival in HIV infection. N. Engl. J. Med. 327(11):815–816, 1992b.

Gregson S, Anderson RM, Ndlovu J, Zhuwau T, and Chandiwana SK. Recent upturn in mortality in rural Zimbabwe: evidence for an early demographic impact of HIV-1 infection? AIDS. 11(10):1269–1280, 1997.

Gutman LT, Saint-Claire KK, Weedy C, et al. Human immunodeficiency virus transmission by child sexual abuse. Am. J. Dis. Child. 145:137–141, 1991.

Halsey NA, Coberly JS, Holt E, et al. Sexual behavior, smoking, and HIV-1 infection in Haitian women. JAMA. 267(15):2062–2066, 1992.

Hankins C, Tran T, and Lapointe N. Sexual behavior and pregnancy outcome in HIV-infected women. Canadian Women's HIV Study Group. J. Acquir. Immune Defic. Syndr. Hum. Retrovirol. 18(5):479–487, 1998.

Harris C, Small CB, Klein RS, et al. Immunodeficiency in female sexual partners of men with the acquired immunodeficiency syndrome. N. Engl. J. Med. 308:1181–1184, 1983.

Harrison LH, Da Silva AP, Gayle HD, et al. Risk factors for HIV-2 infection in Guinea-Bissau. J. Acquir. Immune Defic. Syndr. 4(11):1155–1160, 1991.

Hawkins RE, Rickman LS, Vermund SH, and Carl M. Association of mycoplasma and human immunodeficiency virus infection: detection of amplified Mycoplasma fermentans DNA in blood. J. Infect. Dis. 165:581–585, 1992.

Heimer R, Kaplan EH, Khoshnood K, Jariwala B, and Cadman EC. Needle exchange decreases the prevalence of HIV-1 proviral DNA in returned syringes in New Haven, Connecticut. Am. J. Med. 95:214–220, 1993.

Hersh BS, Popovici F, Jezek Z, et al. Risk factors for HIV infection among abandoned Romanian children. AIDS. 7(12):1617–1624, 1993.

Hessol NA, Lifson AR, O'Malley PM, et al. Prevalence, incidence, and progression of human immunodeficiency virus infection in homosexual and bisexual men in hepatitis B vaccine trials, 1978–1988. Am. J. Epidemiol. 130(6):1167–1175, 1989.

Heyward WL, Osmanov S, Saba J, et al. Preparation for phase III HIV vaccine efficacy trials: methods for the determination of HIV incidence. AIDS. 8(9):1285–1291, 1994.

Hoover DR, Munoz A, Carey V, et al. The unseen sample in cohort studies: Estimation of its size and effect. Stat. Med. 10(12):1993–2003, 1991.

Iannelli M, Milner FA, Pugliese A, and Gonzo M. The HIV/AIDS epidemics among drug injectors: a study of contact structure through a mathematical model. Math. Biosci. 139(1): 25–58, 1997.

IOM. Preventing HIV Transmission: The Role of Sterile Needles and Bleach. National Academy Press, 1995.

IOM. Reducing the Odds Preventing Perinatal Transmission of HIV in the United States. Washington, DC: National Academy Press, 1998.

Irwin KL, Edlin BR, Wong L, et al. Urban rape survivors: characteristics and prevalence of human immunodeficiency virus and other sexually transmitted infections. Multicenter Crack Cocaine and HIV Infection Study Team. Obstet. Gynecol. 85(3):330–336, 1995.

Jaffe HW, Choi K, Thomas PA, et al. National case-control study of Kaposi's sarcoma and Pneumocystis carinii pneumonia in homosexual men. Part 1. Epidemiologic results. Ann. Intern. Med. 99:145–151, 1983.

Jaffe HW, Darrow WW, Echenberg DF, et al. The acquired immunodeficiency syndrome in a cohort of homosexual men. A six-year follow-up study. Ann. Intern. Med. 103(2):210–214, 1985.

Kaplan EH, and Heimer R. A model-based estimate of HIV infectivity via needle sharing. J. Acquir. Immune Defic. Syndr. 5:1116–1118, 1992.

Kaslow RA, Ostrow DG, Detels R, et al. The Multicenter AIDS Cohort Study: rationale, organization, and selected characteristics of the participants. Am. J. Epidemiol. 126:310–318, 1987.

Katzenstein DA. Viral phenotype and genotype as markers in clinical trials. J. Acquir. Immune Defic. Syndr. 10:Suppl-34, 1995.

Kault DA. Modelling AIDS reduction strategies. Int. J. Epidemiol. 24(1):188–197, 1995.

Keet IP, Krijnen P, Koot M, et al. Predictors of rapid progression to AIDS in HIV-1 seroconverters. AIDS. 7(1):51–57, 1993.

Keet IP, Tang J, Klein MR, et al. Consistent associations of HLA class I and II and transporter gene products with progression of human immunodeficiency virus type 1 infection in ho-

mosexual men. J. Infect. Dis. 180(2):299–309, 1999.

Kovacs A, Schluchter M, Easley K, et al. Cytomegalovirus infection and HIV-1 disease progression in infants born to HIV-1–infected women. N. Engl. J. Med. 341(2):77–84, 1999.

Kucera LS, Leake E, Iyer N, Raben D, and Myrvik QN. Human immunodeficiency virus type 1 (HIV-1) and herpes simplex virus type 2 (HSV-2) can coinfect and simultaneously replicate in the same human CD4+ cell: effect of coinfection on infectious HSV-2 and HIV-1 replication. AIDS Res. Hum. Retroviruses. 6(5):641–647, 1990.

Laga M. STD control for HIV prevention—it works. Lancet. 346(8974):518–519, 1995.

Laga M, Alary M, Nzila N, et al. Condom promotion, sexually transmitted diseases treatment, and declining incidence of HIV-1 infection in female sex workers. Lancet. 344:246–248, 1994.

Laga M, Manoka A, Kivuvu M, et al. Non-ulcerative sexually transmitted diseases as risk factors for HIV-1 transmission in women: results from a cohort study. AIDS. 7(1):95–102, 1993.

Lange JM. Current HIV clinical trial design issues. J. Acquir. Immune Defic. Syndr. 10 (Supp):1–51, 1995.

Levy E, Margalith M, Sarov B, et al. Cytomegalovirus IgG and IgA serum antibodies in a study of HIV infection and HIV related diseases in homosexual men. J. Med. Virol. 35:174–179, 1991.

Lipsitch M, and Nowak MA. The evolution of virulence in sexually transmitted HIV/AIDS. J. Theor. Biol. 174(4):427–440, 1995.

Loveland KA, Stehbens J, Contant C, et al. Hemophilia growth and development study: baseline neurodevelopmental findings. J. Pediatr. Psychol. 19(2):223–239, 1994.

Macdonald G, Cuellar CB, and Foll CV. The dynamics of malaria. Bull. World Health Organ. 38(5):743–755, 1968.

Margalith M, Sarov B, Sarov I, et al. Serum IgG and IgA antibodies specific to Epstein-Barr virus capsid antigen in a longitudinal study of human immunodeficiency virus infection and disease progression in homosexual men. AIDS Res. Hum. Retroviruses. 6(5):607–616, 1990.

Martin HL Jr, Jackson DJ, Mandaliya K, et al. Preparation for AIDS vaccine evaluation in Mombasa, Kenya: establishment of seronegative cohorts of commercial sex workers and trucking company employees. AIDS Res. Hum. Retroviruses. 10(Suppl 2):S235–237, 1994.

Martin MP, Dean M, Smith MW, et al. Genetic acceleration of AIDS progression by a promoter variant of CCR5. Science. 282(5395): 1907–1911, 1998.

Masur H, Michelis MA, Greene JB, et al. An outbreak of community-acquired *Pneumocystis
carinii* pneumonia: initial manifestation of
cellular immune dysfunction. N. Engl. J.
Med. 305:1431–1438, 1981.

Masur H, Michelis MA, Wormser GP, et al. Opportunistic infection in previously healthy
women. Initial manifestations of a community-acquired cellular immunodeficiency. Ann.
Intern. Med. 97:533–539, 1982.

McCray E. Occupational risk of the acquired immunodeficiency syndrome among health care
workers. N. Engl. J. Med. 314:1127–1132,
1986.

McCusker J, Stoddard AM, Zapka JG, Zorn M,
and Mayer KH. Predictors of AIDS-preven-
tive behavior among homosexually active
men: a longitudinal study. AIDS. 3(7):443–
448, 1989.

Mellors JW, Rinaldo CR Jr, Gupta P, et al. Prognosis in HIV-1 infection predicted by the
quantity of virus in plasma. Science. 272
(5265):1167–1170, 1996.

Mildvan D, Landay A, De Gruttola V, Machado
SG, and Kagan J. An approach to the valida-
tion of markers for use in AIDS clinical trials.
Clin. Infect. Dis. 24(5):764–774, 1997.

Miyoshi I, Kobayashi M, Yoshimoto S, et al.
ATLV in Japanese patient with AIDS. Lancet.
2(8344):275, 1983.

Moll B, Emeson EE, Small CB, et al. Inverted
ratio of inducer to suppressor T-lymphocyte
subsets in drug abusers with opportunistic infections. Clin. Immunol. Immunopathol. 25:
417–423, 1982.

Montagnier L, and Blanchard A. Mycoplasmas
as cofactors in infection due to the human immunodeficiency virus. Clin. Infect. Dis. 17:
Suppl-15, 1993.

Nagelkerke NJ, Moses S, Embree JE, Jenniskens
F, and Plummer FA. The duration of breastfeeding by HIV-1–infected mothers in developing countries: balancing benefits and risks.
J. Acquir. Immune Defic. Syndr. Hum. Retrovirol. 8(2):176–181, 1995.

Ngugi EN, Plummer FA, Simonsen JN, et al. Prevention of transmission of human immunodeficiency virus in Africa: effectiveness of condom promotion and health education among
prostitutes. Lancet. 2:887–890, 1988.

Obel AO, Sharif SK, McLigeyo SO, et al. Acquired immunodeficiency syndrome in an African. E. Afr. Med. J. 61(9):724–726, 1984.

Oksenhendler E, Harzic M, Le Roux JM, Rabian
C, and Clauvel JP. HIV infection with seroconversion after a superficial needlestick injury to the finger. N. Engl. J. Med. 315:582,
1986.

Oleske J, Minnefor A, Cooper R, Jr., et al. Immune deficiency syndrome in children.
JAMA. 249:23452349, 1983.

Ostrow DG. Risk reduction for transmission of
human immunodeficiency virus in high-risk
communities. Psychiatr. Med. 7:79–96, 1989.

Pape JW, Liautaud B, Thomas F, et al. Characteristics of the acquired immunodeficiency
syndrome (AIDS) in Haiti. N. Engl. J. Med.
309(16):945–950, 1983.

Parekh BS, Shaffer N, Pau CP, et al. Lack of correlation between maternal antibodies to V3
loop peptides of gp120 and perinatal HIV-1
transmission. AIDS. 5(10):1179–1184, 1991.

Peterman T, and Allen J. Recipients of blood and
blood products. In: Kaslow RA, Francis DP,
eds. *The Epidemiology of AIDS.* New York:
Oxford University Press, 1989: 179–193.

Pezzotti P, Phillips AN, Dorrucci M, et al. Category of exposure to HIV and age in the progression to AIDS: longitudinal study of 1199
people with known dates of seroconversion.
BMJ. 313(7057):583–586, 1996.

Piatak M Jr, Saag MS, Yang LC, et al. High levels of HIV-1 in plasma during all stages of infection determined by competitive PCR. Science. 259:1749–1754, 1993.

Piot P, Quinn TC, Taelman H, et al. Acquired
immunodeficiency syndrome in a heterosexual population in Zaire. Lancet. 2(8394):65–
69, 1984.

Pizzo PA. Considerations for the evaluation of
antiretroviral agents in infants and children
infected with human immunodeficiency virus: a perspective from the National Cancer
Institute. Rev. Infect. Dis. 12:Sl–9, 1990.

Popovic M, Flomenberg N, Volkman DJ, et al.
Alteration of T-cell functions by infection
with HTLV-I or HTLV-II. Science. 226(4673):
459–462, 1984.

Quinn TC, Mann JM, Curran JW, and Piot P.
AIDS in Africa: an epidemiologic paradigm.
Science. 234(4779):955–963, 1986.

Remis RS, O'Shaughnessy MV, Tsoukas C, et al.
HIV transmission to patients with hemophilia by heat-treated, donor-screened factor concentrate. Can. Med. Assoc. J. 142(11):1247–
1254, 1990.

Renton A, Whitaker L, Ison C, Wadsworth J, and
Harris JR. Estimating the sexual mixing patterns in the general population from those in
people acquiring gonorrhoea infection: theoretical foundation and empirical findings. J.
Epidemiol. Comm. Health. 49(2):205–213,
1995.

Richters J, Donovan B, Gerofi J, and Watson L.
Low condom breakage rate in commercial
sex. Lancet. 2(8626-8627):1487–1488, 1988.

Rogers AS, Futterman DK, Moscicki AB, et al.
The REACH Project of the Adolescent Medicine HIV/AIDS Research Network: design,
methods, and selected characteristics of participants. J. Adolesc. Health. 22(4):300–311,
1998.

Rogers MF, Morens DM, Stewart JA, et al. National case-control study of Kaposi's sarcoma and *Pneumocystis carinii* pneumonia in homosexual men. Part 2. Laboratory results. Ann. Intern. Med. 99(2):151–158, 1983.

Rosenberg PS. Backcalculation models of age-specific HIV incidence rates. Stat Med. 13(19-20):1975–1990, 1994.

Rosenberg PS, Gail MH, Schrager LK, et al. National AIDS incidence trends and the extent of zidovudine therapy in selected demographic and transmission groups. J. Acquir. Immune Defic. Syndr. 4(4):392–401, 1991.

Rosenblum L, Buehler JW, Morgan MW, et al. The completeness of AIDS case reporting, 1988: a multisite collaborative surveillance project. Am. J. Public Health. 82:1495–1499, 1992.

Rouse DJ, Owen J, Goldenberg RL, and Vermund SH. Zidovudine for the prevention of vertical HIV transmission: a decision analytic approach. J. Acquir. Immune Defic. Syndr. 9:401–407, 1995.

Royce RA, Sena A, Cates W Jr, and Cohen MS. Sexual transmission of HIV. N. Engl. J. Med. 336(15):1072–1078, 1997.

Rubinstein A, Sicklick M, Gupta A, et al. Acquired immunodeficiency with reversed T4/T8 ratios in infants born to promiscuous and drug-addicted mothers. JAMA. 249:2350–2356, 1983.

Rugpao S, Pruithithada N, Yutabootr Y, Prasertwitayakij W,and Tovanabutra S. Condom breakage during commercial sex in Chiang Mai, Thailand. Contraception. 48(6):537–547, 1993.

Rutherford GW, Lifson AR, Hessol NA, et al. Course of HIV-I infection in a cohort of homosexual and bisexual men: an 11 year follow up study. BMJ. 301(6762):1183–1188, 1990.

Saah AJ, Hoover DR, Weng S, et al. Association of HLA profiles with early plasma viral load, CD4+ cell count and rate of progression to AIDS following acute HIV-1 infection. AIDS. 12(16):2107–2113, 1998.

Schaper C, Fleming TR, Self SG, and Rida WN. Statistical issues in the design of HIV vaccine trials. Annu. Rev. Public Health. 16:1–22, 1995.

Schechter M, Harrison LH, Halsey NA, et al. Coinfection with human T-cell lymphotropic virus type I and HIV in Brazil. Impact on markers of HIV disease progression. JAMA. 271(5):353–357, 1994.

Schoenbaum EE, and Webber MP. The under-recognition of HIV infection in women in an inner-city emergency room. Am. J. Public Health. 83:363–368, 1993.

Schooley RT. Correlation between viral load measurements and outcome in clinical trials of antiviral drugs. AIDS. 9:Suppl-S19, 1995.

Schrager LK, Fowler MG, Young JY, Mathieson BJ, and Vermund SH. Long-term survivors of HIV infection: Definitions and research challenges. AIDS. 8(suppl 1):S95–S108, 1994.

Schwarcz SK, Hsu LC, Parisi MK, and Katz MH. The impact of the 1993 AIDS case definition on the completeness and timeliness of AIDS surveillance. AIDS. 13(9):1109–1114, 1999.

Selwyn PA, Alcabes P, Hartel D, et al. Clinical manifestations and predictors of disease progression in drug users with human immunodeficiency virus infection. N. Engl. J. Med. 327:1697–1703, 1992.

Selwyn PA, Feingold AR, Hartel D, et al. Increased risk of bacterial pneumonia in HIV-infected intravenous drug users without AIDS. AIDS. 2(4):267–272, 1988.

Selwyn PA, Sckell BM, Alcabes P,et al. High risk of active tuberculosis in HIV-infected drug users with cutaneous anergy. JAMA. 268(4):504–509, 1992.

Shah SA, Khan OA, Kristensen S, and Vermund SH. HIV-infected workers deported from the gulf states:impact on Southern Pakistan. Int. J. STD AIDS. 10:812–814, 1999.

Sinicco A, Raiteri R, Sciandra M, et al. The influence of cytomegalovirus on the natural history of HIV infection: evidence of rapid course of HIV infection in HIV-positive patients infected with cytomegalovirus. Scand. J. Infect. Dis. 29(6):543–549, 1997.

Skurnick JH, Kennedy CA, Perez G, et al. Behavioral and demographic risk factors for transmission of human immunodeficiency virus type 1 in heterosexual couples: report from the Heterosexual HIV Transmission Study. Clin. Infect. Dis. 26(4):855–864, 1998.

Smith DK, Warren DL, Vlahov D, et al. Design and baseline participant characteristics of the Human Immunodeficiency Virus Epidemiology Research (HER) Study: a prospective cohort study of human immunodeficiency virus infection in US women. Am. J. Epidemiol. 146(6):459–469, 1997.

Smith MW, Dean M, Carrington M, et al. Contrasting genetic influence of CCR2 and CCR5 variants on HIV-1 infection and disease progression. Science. 277(5328):959–965, 1997.

Sonnabend J, Witkin SS, and Purtilo DT. Acquired immunodeficiency syndrome, opportunistic infections, and malignancies in male homosexuals. A hypothesis of etiologic factors in pathogenesis. JAMA. 249(17):2370–2374, 1983.

Soper DE, Shoupe D, Shangold GA, et al. Prevention of vaginal trichomoniasis by compliant use of the female condom. Sex. Transm. Dis. 20(3):137–139, 1993.

Stanley S, Ostrowski MA, Justement JS, et al. Effect of immunization with a common recall antigen on viral expression in patients infected with human immunodeficiency virus type 1. N. Engl. J. Med. 334(19):1222–1230, 1996.

Stigum H, Magnus P, and Bakketeig LS. Effect of changing partnership formation rates on the spread of sexually transmitted diseases and human immunodeficiency virus. Am. J. Epidemiol. 145(7):644–652, 1997.

Stoneburner R, Laroche E, Prevots R, et al. Survival in a cohort of human immunodeficiency virus-infected tuberculosis patients in New York City. Implications for the expansion of the AIDS case definition. Arch. Intern. Med. 152:2033–2037, 1992.

Stricof RL, and Morse DL. HTLV-III/LAV seroconversion following a deep intramuscular needlestick injury. N. Engl. J. Med. 314:1115, 1986.

Stringer JS, Stringer EM, Phanuphak P, et al. Prevention of mother-to-child transmission of HIV in Thailand: physicians' attitudes on zidovudine use, pregnancy termination, and willingness to provide care. J. Acquir. Immune Defic. Syndr. 21(3):217–222, 1999.

Tang J, Costello C, Keet IP, et al. HLA class I homozygosity accelerates disease progression in human immunodeficiency virus type 1 infection. AIDS Res. Hum. Retroviruses. 15(4):317–324, 1999.

Thomas JC, and Tucker M. The development and use of the concept of a sexually transmitted disease core. J. Infect. Dis. 174(Suppl 2):S134–143, 1995.

van Ameijden EJ, van den Hoek JA, van Haastrecht HJ, and Coutinho RA. The harm reduction approach and risk factors for human immunodeficiency virus (HIV) seroconversion in injecting drug users, Amsterdam. Am. J. Epidemiol. 136(2):236–243, 1992.

Van De Perre P, Lepage P, Kestelyn P, et al. Acquired immunodeficiency syndrome in Rwanda. Lancet. 2:62–65, 1984.

Van de Perre P, Jacobs D, and Sprecher-Goldberger S. The latex condom, an efficient barrier against sexual transmission of AIDS-related viruses. AIDS. 1(1):49–52, 1987.

Vanichseni S, Wright N, Akarasewi P, et al. Case control study of HIV positivity among male

intravenous drug addicts (IVDA) in Bangkok. Int. Conf. AIDS. 1989; 5(abstract no. W.G.P.19).

Vermund S, Tabereaux PB, and Kaslow RA. Epidemiology of HIV Infection. In: Merigan T, Bolognesi D, Bartlett J, eds. Textbook of AIDS Medicine. Baltimore: Williams & Wilkins, 1999: 101–109.

Vermund SH. The efficacy of HIV vaccines: methodological issues in preparing for clinical trials. In: Nicolosi A, ed. HIV Epidemiology: Models and Methods. New York: Raven Press, 1994: 187–209.

Vieira J, Frank E, Spira TJ, and Landesman SH. Acquired immune deficiency in Haitians: opportunistic infections in previously healthy Haitian immigrants. N. Engl. J. Med. 308(3):125–129, 1983.

Vlahov D, Anthony JC, Munoz A, et al. The ALIVE study, a longitudinal study of HIV-1 infection in intravenous drug users: description of methods and characteristics of participants. NIDA Res. Monogr. 109:75–100, 1991.

Wein LM, Zenios SA, and Nowak MA. Dynamic multidrug therapies for HIV: a control theoretic approach. J. Theor. Biol. 185(1):15–29, 1997.

Weiss RA, and Jaffe HW. Duesberg, HIV and AIDS. Nature. 345(6277):659–660, 1990.

West RW, and Thompson JR. Modeling the impact of HIV on the spread of tuberculosis in the United States. Math. Biosci. 143(1):35–60, 1997.

Winkelstein W Jr, Samuel MC, Padian NS, et al. The San Francisco Men's Health Study. III. Reduction in human immunodeficiency virus transmission among homosexual/bisexual men, 1982–86. Am. J. Public Health. 77:685–689, 1987.

Winkler C, Modi W, Smith MW, et al. Genetic restriction of AIDS pathogenesis by an SDF-1 chemokine gene variant. Science. 279(5349):389–393, 1998.

Zackin R, Marschner I, Andersen J, et al. Perspective: human immunodeficiency virus type 1 (HIV-1) RNA end points in HIV clinical trials: issues in interim monitoring and early stopping. J. Infect. Dis. 177(3):761–765, 1998.

21

Research Collaborations in Developing Countries

MARIA J. WAWER

There are compelling reasons to conduct infectious disease epidemiologic research in developing countries. Many conditions (such as malaria or leprosy) affect populations primarily or almost exclusively in such settings. The epidemiology of some infections differs substantially between developing and developed countries (for example, in sub-Saharan Africa, a far higher proportion of HIV transmission occurs through heterosexual contact than is the case in North America or Europe), and control measures need to be tested in the appropriate context. Conversely, lessons learned in developing regions can have substantial relevance to developed countries; for example, in the design and evaluation of outreach strategies to underserved segments of the population, or by spearheading the testing of interventions such as human immunodeficiency virus (HIV) vaccines or short course chemotherapy to prevent maternal-child HIV transmission. Growing cadres of highly trained clinicians, epidemiologists, and other public health specialists residing in developing countries are actively pursuing research agendas and seeking collaborations.

This chapter is written from the perspective of a researcher in a developed country seeking to collaborate on epidemiologic research in a developing country with researchers from that country. The chapter addresses steps and issues that need to be considered in undertaking an international research collaboration, with the goal of providing a summary of key areas essential to project development. Points considered include contact between research groups and host country policymakers, research design and implementation, infrastructure development, ethics, and funding.

In this chapter, the term *host country researcher* is used for nationals or permanent residents of the developing country, whereas investigators from the Western country are referred to as *guest researchers*. Although the terminology may seem whimsical, its intent is serious. The foreign scientists are indeed guests in the developing country, regardless of the duration and extent of the collaboration. Their long-term involvement is entirely dependent on the goodwill and collaboration of the in-country government and research community. Ways of enhancing good collaboration are discussed throughout the chapter.

DEFINING THE RESEARCH ISSUE

A critical first step in any research program is the development of a clear statement regarding the significance of the health problem, why it is of importance in the host country, and why research on this issue should be supported by the scientific community (both in-country and internationally) and by potential donors. An explicit definition of the problem helps to justify research goals (e.g., the reason schistosomiasis was selected for study, rather than malaria), preempt misunderstanding between collaborators regarding the project's purpose, and provide a solid foundation for funding proposals. Moreover, scientific questions should be formulated as testable hypotheses whenever possible.

IDENTIFYING RESEARCH COUNTERPARTS

Genuine collaboration is the cornerstone for productive, satisfying, and long-term international research. Participants bring different but crucial strengths to the collective effort. The contributions of the host country researchers include cultural and linguistic knowledge, insights into the epidemiology and clinical manifestations of the target condition, and information on how to get things done in a given country, including clearing the inevitable logistic and bureaucratic hurdles. The guest researchers bring specialized technical resources, such as access to novel laboratory assays, and may have greater access to funding through a variety of grant mechanisms. Both groups need to combine their specialized technical skills acquired through prior training and experience. A good research collaboration avoids exploitation; for example, where one group predominates in acquiring findings and publications, or where data are not applied to improve the health of the host country population. All collaborations go through diffi-

cult periods. For example, in the early days of AIDS research in Uganda, there was substantial suspicion in some quarters that foreign groups were spreading the infection or trying to impose condoms for immoral reasons. International collaborative studies were saved by host country researchers who undertook major efforts to address the concerns of the press and the community. These efforts were greatly facilitated by intensive communications, trust, and clear and explicit goals established between host scientists, key policymakers, and the guest researchers.

The first and most crucial step in developing a research collaboration is thus to identify study counterparts. Whether the research idea originates with the host country researcher or the international investigator, the process is much the same, and is as delicate and important as the first steps in any marriage. The "index" researcher needs to sound out potential investigators in the host country (or conversely, the developed country) and identify an investigator(s) with congruent interests and a desire to conduct collaborative research. Key research personnel on both sides must be committed to the work and be able to devote the required time—with the caveat that international collaborations inevitably require substantial time commitment, including extensive travel. At the very least, the lead investigators on both sides need to identify full-time, energetic, organized, and, if at all possible, experienced personnel to whom they can delegate day-to-day study management. The roles and responsibilities of each member of the collaboration must be realistic, clearly specified, and agreed upon in advance. If a member of the research group experiences difficulties in meeting commitments, the problem needs to be discussed in a frank but supportive manner, in order to identify solutions.

Career incentives taken for granted by guest investigators (publications, promotions, salary support) may be far less available or valued in other countries. Developing country researchers and faculty in government institutions are often paid low salaries and may be forced to moonlight. In some countries, promotions may be less dependent on research productivity than on clinical activity. Research grants need to budget for adequate support for local counterparts. If government regulations limit salary compensation for host country investigators, other forms of recompense (e.g., travel to conferences, educational opportunities, consulting opportunities) need to be explored. Enabling host country counterparts to build a strong and visible research career (through presentations at domestic and international conferences and first-authored publications) enables them to acquire future grants and to establish a career path that brings rewards independently of local constraints.

CONTACT WITH KEY DECISION MAKERS AND ACQUISITION OF NECESSARY PERMISSIONS

Early in the process of establishing the collaboration, it is important to meet with key in-country policymakers and health professionals to discuss research goals. The list includes officials in the ministry of health, medical school faculty, investigators in existing research collaborations, and the representatives of relevant international health agencies (e.g., the in-country representative of the World Health Organization). This step ensures full understanding by all interested parties, minimizes real or perceived duplication of effort or competition for scarce resources, and greatly facilitates the acquisition of all necessary permits, accreditations, and memoranda of understanding.

The needed permits include approval of the study proposal by a host country scientific board; host country ethical review (more details follow); export permits (for biologic specimens taken out of the country for specialized laboratory testing or quality control); resident visas, work permits, and investigators' licenses for expatriate personnel; and import licenses and/or memoranda facilitating import of supplies, medications, and equipment and establishing import tax status. The host country researcher plays a key role in establishing contacts and carrying out negotiations for these permits. Additional documents for the study should include an agreement on use of data and publications, and a memorandum of understanding with the counterpart institution that spells out roles and responsibilities of key members of the collaboration.

The researchers must also ensure that the proposed research has all necessary clearances from the developed country side of the collaboration. Studies must be cleared by institutional human subjects committees. In addition, American government research monies (e.g., funds from the National Institutes of Health) cannot be expended outside the United States without State Department clearance and agreement by the American embassy in the host country. The requirements for these arrangements differ by country and donor agency.

DEVELOPING THE RESEARCH PLAN

The process of developing the study goals, research design, and time lines must involve key personnel from all cooperating institutions. Broadly, epidemiologic research entails observation or intervention. Conducting these types of research in developing countries generates the following issues.

Observational studies encompass assessment of the prevalence, incidence, and risk factors for infection (morbidity or mortality) and their respective distributions. Observational studies can be carried out in selected subpopulations (e.g., clinic attendees, industrial or agricultural employees, commercial sex workers, and the like) or in the general population. The latter approach is logistically challenging but offers the great advantage of defining the prevalence and distribution of an infectious disease in the general, non-self-selected population. As in developed countries, clinic users in developing countries may not be representative of the general population and are likely to provide a biased assessment of the factors associated with infection. Population-based surveys are often less expensive and thus more feasible in developing countries than in the settings of Western, developed countries.

Political and local community leaders are frequently open to such designs, community cohesion (such as that found in rural villages) facilitates participation, and the extensive personpower required for a community survey is far less expensive than in industrialized countries. Many population-based household surveys that incorporate interview and sample collection have been described in the literature, and a number of these have developed into long-term population-based cohort studies that follow entire villages for many years, providing valuable epidemiologic and demographic data and acting as an ideal setting to test community-based interventions (Becker and Weng 1998, Kengeya-Kayondo et al. 1996, Todd et al. 1997, Wawer et al. 1999).

Simplified survey methodologies have been developed to increase the feasibility of population-based data collection. Among the best known is the cluster survey technique of the World Health Organization Expanded Program on Immunization (Henderson and Sundaresan 1982, Boerma and Van Ginneken 1992). The survey sample consists of 30 clusters randomly selected with probability proportional to population size. (For example, if each village represents one cluster, larger villages have a higher probability of being chosen.) In each cluster, an initial household is randomly selected, and, in order to simplify logistics and reduce costs, all subsequent households are selected in a predetermined pattern (such as concentric circles) from among neighboring houses. Depending on the goals of the survey, either a fixed number of households is included in each cluster, or households are added until a fixed quota of target persons has been interviewed. Childhood immunization surveys in which at least seven children are included per cluster can estimate coverage with a precision of approximately 10% (Lemeshow et al. 1985). Cluster sampling techniques have been adapted to specific geographic situations (Kok 1986).

Regardless of the setting, intervention studies and trials need to follow rigorous design and quality control procedures. Particular challenges toward this end in many developing country settings include the identification, training, and retention of personnel; ensuring the safety of study personnel; provision of an adequate infrastructure to ensure quality clinical assessment and care; maintenance of required diagnostic and laboratory equipment in settings that may experience fluctuating power, extremes of temperature, and unsure water supply; and establishment of a data center, including the capacity to transfer between collaborators and the data safety and monitoring center. Key aspects are described in more detail later in this chapter.

Community-based intervention studies and trials are generally as feasible, or even more feasible, in developing countries than in developed countries, particularly trials conducted in rural areas. A community trial design is ideal for testing interventions where population coverage is required to maximize treatment effects. Examples include control of malaria and trachoma (Misra et al. 1999, Whitty et al. 1999) and control of sexually transmitted diseases to limit transmission of HIV (Grosskurth et al. 1995, Wawer et al. 1999, Hayes et al. 1997). Political will, community cohesion, and relatively inexpensive personnel costs enhance the conduct of such trials in many developing countries. In addition, the relative lack of extensive public media or transport, as is the case in many developing country settings, reduces the likelihood of contamination between intervention and control groups but, as discussed later, it also creates some challenges. This topic is addressed more fully in Chapter 16, Community Intervention Studies.

SELECTION OF STUDY POPULATIONS; ACQUISITION OF BASIC DATA

Selection of the study population is based on the goals of the proposed research. Basic data on disease prevalence and on population stability are needed to calculate sample sizes, to develop the sampling and randomization plans (if needed), and to plan strategies to maximize coverage and follow up. Such data may be acquired from clinical records and previous studies in the host country. However, clinic-based data do not always accurately reflect prevalence, incidence, or rates of follow up. If reliable data are unavailable or if the quality of existing data is suspect, it may be necessary to conduct small scale prestudy behavioral and prevalence surveys. Such surveys can provide rough estimates of disease prevalence and of risk factors, and can serve to evaluate the quality of the available service statistics to determine whether the latter can be relied upon. By determining population mobility, including how long people have lived in the community and how much they travel, such surveys can also provide data on potential loss to follow up in order to adjust sample size estimates.

RESEARCH IMPLEMENTATION

The following section briefly describes key steps in research implementation.

1. Plan of action, division of responsibilities, job descriptions, and time line. Based on the research goals and study design, the principal investigators should develop a written list of steps required for project implementation and of additional personnel required for implementation; job descriptions; and clear deadlines for each project step (i.e., a project time line).

2. Personnel, and their training, supervision, and retention. Finding and keeping good personnel represents a crucial step in implementing the research. Well-trained personnel may be hard to find, particularly in developing countries where the opportunities for training are limited, placing trained people in high demand. Community-based surveys and intervention studies generally have the most intensive needs, given that they include many of the same personnel required in a clinic-based study, with the addition of field cadres. The following list delineates the types of personnel required for a community-based infectious disease project:

• Research staff, including epidemiologists, clinicians, social scientists, laboratory scientists, and statisticians. Their roles include development of study instruments; laboratory, clinical, and field protocols;

analysis plans; and the preparation of reports and publications. A multidisciplinary team strengthens infectious disease research and enhances funding prospects: a grant that considers biologic and clinical aspects of disease within the behavioral and social contexts that influence risk and clinical course appeals to a broad range of grant reviewers. Appropriate personnel, both in terms of numbers and qualifications, must also be identified for the translation and transcription of study materials and of qualitative or open-ended interview data. Research staff overlap with many of the other personnel categories listed below, and include the principal investigators from the host and guest institutions.

• Medical personnel include doctors, nurses, midwives, and health technicians, who provide diagnostics and health care as needed.

• Field personnel: field director, field supervisors, census takers (to develop lists of participants, collect pertinent household information, and track subjects over time), survey teams, and field editors. Survey personnel can be trained to administer fairly complex interview instruments and to collect a broad range of samples under field conditions.

• Laboratory technicians, who may include technicians who travel with the survey teams to collect and handle specimens.

• Data personnel, for the development of data entry programs and screens; for data input, cleaning, and analyses; and for liaison with data staff in collaborating institutions.

• Motivators or health educators to explain the study goals, provide appropriate health education, and encourage participation among target individuals, whether in the clinic, the community as a whole, or in relevant subgroups.

• Drivers and mechanics are essential personnel in community-based studies in settings where there is no or only limited public transport.

• Administrative personnel, to oversee all personnel and budgetary issues, ensure all permits and clearances are up to date, order supplies and supervise shipments.

• Support staff, including secretarial staff, cleaners, and security personnel.
• Translators where more than one language or dialect is spoken.

In many situations, staff can be shared with existing facilities and programs. However, it is imperative to ensure that adequate time is allotted to the research project, which in turn implies both a serious commitment on part of the host institution and, generally, the availability of funding to fully cover the percentage time required by the project. As a general rule, key staff (field directors, essential laboratory and data personnel) should be employed by the project full-time.

Training needs will vary with the complexity of the project and the experience of available staff. In the Rakai community-based STD Control for AIDS Prevention Trial (Wawer et al. 1998, 1999), field survey staff were chosen from among cadres having at least two years of postsecondary education, including nurses, midwives, and non-medical personnel, such as school teachers. Approximately 2.5 weeks of full-time, intensive training were required to teach personnel to administer a detailed behavioral and health questionnaire, and to collect a number of biologic samples, including venous blood, in the home. A week of formal retraining was conducted every 10 months.

Retraining and ongoing supervision are key to project success and to ongoing quality control and need to be formally scheduled at regular intervals. Staff in any research project, regardless of where it is conducted, have a tendency to drift from the official protocol. The impact of seemingly inconsequential alterations or omissions (slight changes in wording of interview questions, tiny modifications in clinical recording) accrues over time. Unless staff receive continuous supervision and support, by the end of the study the data collected can be quite different from what was planned. Protocol drift is particularly common in field-based studies, where unexpected contingencies arise every day and require rapid resolution. Field staff must be encouraged to make decisions to keep field work rolling, but must

be regularly supervised to ensure decisions are clearly documented and do not adversely alter the research plan. During the Rakai STD Control for AIDS Prevention trial, which included an STD mass treatment intervention, the Muslim holy season of Ramadan began just as the field treatment team was conducting the annual survey in a community with a high proportion of Muslims. Devout Muslims who were fasting declined to take the directly observed treatment during daylight hours. The team decided to alter the schedule of field visits, and delay treatment in this community until the end of the holy season. Careful supervision ensured that the decision was fully documented, that the change in schedule was factored into data analyses, and that subsequent schedules were appropriately adjusted.

Staff retention becomes a growing problem as project personnel acquire new expertise and start to be avidly courted by other programs competing for scarce personpower. Annual turnover rates of 25%–30% are not uncommon and can badly interfere with project activities. A good work environment, a sense of participation in decision making and ownership of the research, adequate monetary compensation, commendations and other recognition, and opportunities for additional training (including those made available by foundations and agencies such as Fogarty International of the US National Institutes of Health), are all key to successful retention. Salaries should be set in consultation with in-country principal investigators, taking into account levels paid by similar in-country research collaborations. In some countries, national policies dictate low levels of compensation for international collaborative project staff, in order to keep such collaborations from placing undue pressures on governmental and in-country employers. Although commendable in principle, such an approach frequently results in limited commitment by staff, who are forced to maintain multiple jobs in the public and private sectors to meet their financial needs. Appropriate strategies to stay within national policy while encouraging the needed level of personnel commitment must be discussed frankly with the in-country principal investigators.

3. Data and specimen collection. There is growing experience with the collection of complex interview data coupled to biologic samples, in clinic and community-based studies. Population-based projects (such as the aforementioned Rakai Project in Uganda; the Medical Research Council (UK) project in Masaka, Uganda; and the Mwanza Project in Tanzania) have each collected sociodemographic, behavioral, sexual practice, and health data, and a broad series of biologic samples, from over 10,000 participants in their homes or in small rural areas (Hayes et al. 1997).

Identifying and Tracking the Study Population

Establishing mechanisms to identify and track the study population represents something of a challenge in communities without street addresses, house numbers, mailboxes, or telephones. Migrant communities undergo rapid alterations in the layout of buildings and roads. Portions of *favelas* (low income communities) in Rio de Janeiro literally float on anchored rafts along the bay. Census data are often nonexistent or desperately out of date. These problems offer particular challenges for community-based studies, but clinic-based research also needs to develop adequate strategies to follow up participants who fail to return for appointments.

A number of strategies assist to define the catchment population and identify the target group for the study. A door-to-door census conducted prior to the study delineates the size of the study population, identifies the head of the household, and defines family relationships. The latter step greatly facilitates the design of studies that include, for example, both members of a couple, or that plan to enroll minors and thus require parental permission.

Maps of the study area greatly facilitate follow up in places with no formal streets or house numbers. Maps can be hand drawn or developed from aerial photographs or global positioning satellite (GPS) coordinates (Hightower et al. 1998, Croner et al. 1996). GPS and geographic information systems (GIS) technologies are rapidly improving and are, in general, affordable, offering detailed locational referencing useful in tracking disease distribution and spread. The utility of maps can be further enhanced if participants permit the researchers to paint or otherwise attach visible numbers to houses.

Methods of enhancing follow up have been briefly discussed. Return for clinic visits can be enhanced if the project provides transportation, either by paying for use of public transport (where it exists) or by sending a project vehicle. Since use of the latter may be stigmatizing, participants should be given a choice of travel modalities.

A key relative, who can subsequently help to track the whereabouts of participants who migrate out of the study area or who are temporarily away, can also be identified, provided that the participant consents to such tracking. The Rakai project identified household "scouts" who traveled to the project headquarters and informed research staff of deliveries occurring in the home to women enrolled in a maternal-infant study.

Developing Study Instruments

As a general rule, infectious disease research is substantially strengthened if it combines biologic, clinical, sociodemographic, and behavioral data. Furthermore, qualitative data, collected through in-depth interviews, focus groups, and related methodologies, often provide valuable insights into the phenomena being studied (Powell and Single 1996, Daly 1996, Steckler et al. 1991, Morgan 1998).

Study instruments include tracking forms (to determine follow up), census forms (to identify and track household members in community-based studies), structured questionnaires, clinical recording forms, focus group guides, and in-depth interview guides. Although such instruments can be based in part on preexisting materials (e.g., WHO survey modules or instruments from other similar research projects), they have to incorporate data of relevance to local conditions. All instruments need to be translated into the host country language(s), back-translated by an independent translator into the language of the collaborating team (that is, retranslated into English, as a check on whether the original intent of the question has been retained), corrected and modified in the host country language, and pretested. Focus groups (Powell and Single 1996) and in-depth interviews can provide valuable information prior to the development of structured questionnaires, by exploring local beliefs and behaviors, and by providing information on terminology that is comprehensible to study subjects. It is often helpful to conduct periodic focus group interviews during the course of an observational study, since inevitably the standardized questionnaire data will point to new behavioral and attitudinal issues that should be explored.

Many steps required for data quality are inherent to research and are not unique to developing country settings. Questionnaires and biologic specimens must be meticulously labeled to ensure they are linked to the correct participants: preprinted labels, with unique computer-generated alphanumeric identification numbers are very useful in this regard. In some cultures, however, individuals have multiple names (official, traditional, religious, family, clan). This can cause a problem in studies that follow an individual over time. Photo identification cards have been successfully used to reduce the chance of misidentification (Wawer et al. 1998). Field- or clinic-based project personnel have the essential role of reviewing all questionnaires (ideally on the day of collection), tracking samples, and ensuring all materials are correctly labeled and handled confidentially.

Biological Specimen Collection

High compliance has been achieved with home-based or field station collection of diverse specimens, including venous and finger stick blood samples, urine, self-administered vaginal swabs, genital ulcer swabs, and placentas (Cushman et al. 1998, Grosskurth et al. 1995, Wabwire-Mangen 1999, Wawer et al. 1995, 1998). Biologic sampling requires careful planning of collection methods, short- and long-term storage, transport to testing facilities, temperature control, and assurance of biosafety for project workers. The complexity of sample collection varies from the simple (for example, urine or finger stick blood collection) to the fairly complex (for example, placentas). Combined interview and biologic data are often invaluable in interpreting epidemiologic findings and in monitoring trial outcomes. Ultimately, the complexity of data and sample collection will depend on local resources: types and numbers of personnel, and the feasibility of transporting samples, as well as on the funding available for collection and testing.

4. Piloting the study. Prior to full-scale implementation of data and sample collection, researchers are strongly advised to conduct a pilot exercise in which study components are tried first on a similar population outside of the study sample or on a small proportion of the final projected sample. The pilot provides a dry run for all key members of the staff and helps ensure that mechanisms for data management and sample collection, handling, processing, and shipping are in place and well integrated. Initial laboratory quality control can also be established at this time.

When a study is piloted on future study participants, the effects of the pilot on the study findings can be attenuated by including only a small proportion of the target population; using participation in prestudy activities as one of the randomization criteria if the study is a randomized trial; and by using participation in the pilot in data analyses.

5. Laboratory testing. The last decade of the twentieth century witnessed a revolution in the development of laboratory techniques that permit biologic assessment of large populations surveyed in nonclinical settings. To give some examples from the reproductive health field, urine (which is readily collected in the home or the workplace) can be tested for HIV (Meehan et al. 1999), gonorrhea and chlamydia (Buimer et al. 1996, Gaydos and Quinn 1995); and early pregnancy (Gray et al. 1998b). Self-administered vaginal swabs, which have been successfully collected by women in populations as diverse as rural Uganda and Manhattan, New York (Cushman et al. 1998, Wawer et al. 1998), can be tested for gonorrhea, chlamydia, human papilloma virus, trichomonas, and bacterial vaginosis (Ching et al. 1995, Gray et al. 1998a, Serwadda et al. 1999, Sewankambo et al. 1997, Wawer et al. 1995, 1998). Some of the tests (such as InPouch TV culture for trichomonas and gram stain for bacterial vaginosis (Borchardt et al. 1991, Hillier 1993) are relatively inexpensive and "low tech" and can thus, with appropriate training, be implemented in a small field laboratory. Others based on amplification or hybrid capture technologies (Buimer et al. 1996, Lorincz 1996) are more expensive and require shipment to specialized laboratories. Even these drawbacks, however, pale in comparison to the advantages of acquiring detailed information on infections of interest. The coming decades will see further improvements in rapid and lower cost diagnostics in many areas of infectious disease.

Whether a project sets up its own laboratory or develops a relationship with an existing in-country facility will depend on local resources and the tests required. If the study proposes to rely heavily on laboratory data, it must provide adequate salary support, supplies, and personpower resources to the collaborating facility. Clear guidelines for laboratory turnaround time must be established. Realistic expectations are essential: in a clinical laboratory, patient management generally gets priority over research, and delays should be expected. Mechanisms for ordering and shipping supplies, test kits, and reagents must be specified, with a clear definition of staff roles and responsibilities in this regard.

Meticulous staff training and supervision are essential for the implementation of laboratory testing. Quality control measures should include testing a subsample of specimens in an independent reference laboratory. Researchers can also submit positive and negative controls to the study's laboratory for masked testing.

Archival storage of samples should be built into the project. In general, samples will need to be stored at least for the life of the project to allow retesting for quality control. Many studies will opt to retain samples for longer periods of time. Adequate freezer space must be made available: a prudent project does not count on long-term storage in freezers belonging to another program, since freezer space is generally at a premium and it is difficult to ensure quality control in shared equipment. Although many samples can be stored for long periods at $-20°C$, a temperature of $-70°C$ is generally recommended for long-term storage of serologic specimens. All laboratory equipment must be provided with peripherals appropriate to local conditions, including universal power sources, surge suppressors, and voltage regulators. Projects may need to install their own generators. If steady water supply represents a problem, water tanks and water purification equipment will be required.

6. Data management. The study infrastructure is of no utility if the data collected cannot be processed and used in a timely manner.

Research projects require an identified data manager, who takes ultimate responsibility to ensure information is entered and cleaned, and that data sets (census, interview, laboratory) are correctly linked. Range and consistency checks, and double data entry, minimize errors.

Appropriate computer programs and software packages must be selected to permit complex linkages. Data analysis responsibilities need to be clearly delineated between the collaborating institutions. Data should be available to all study researchers and can be readily exchanged electronically via file transfer protocol (FTP). Multisite trials may use DataFax for rapid transmission of clinical information to a central data monitoring institution. It should be noted, however, that electronic data transfer will require some patience and luck, given the rudimentary connectivity available in many developing countries.

Desktop and laptop computers each have their liabilities and assets. Laptop computers maximize project flexibility, but they are generally more expensive and fragile than desktop models with similar capabilities. They also present a greater security risk due to theft or damage. Therefore, different computers may be needed to suit particular project tasks.

7. Transportation and communication. The need to ensure reliable transport of personnel, equipment, data, and (sometimes) study participants cannot be overemphasized. Where the local transportation infrastructure is poor, clinical and field studies alike will need to purchase motorized vehicles, or bicycles, as appropriate. New research collaborations are encouraged to seek advice from established programs regarding the selection, purchase, and registration of vehicles. Budgeting must take into account high international fuel and maintenance costs, as well as insurance rates. Driver safety training may be required and a reliable mechanic identified.

Researchers from the collaborating countries should establish frequent communication via e-mail, telephone, and travel. In countries with poor land lines, cellular and mobile phones are needed for key staff. Visits to the field site are crucial and provide the only means of fully understanding constraints and problems. Particularly in the early phases of the project, senior investigators should plan to meet at least three to five times per year.

8. Office equipment and electrical power. In many developing countries it is generally prudent not to assume that any services will be readily and steadily available, and it is best to have contingency plans to cover emergencies, including the installation of generators and water tanks. Similarly, the project may need to purchase its own basic office support (copying facilities, printers).

In some rural regions of Africa, electric power can fluctuate from 90 to 300 volts in a single day. Electronic equipment must be protected with power stabilizers, surge suppressors, universal power sources, and transformers. Wiring and plugs must fit local specifications. Spare adaptors, surge suppressors, and transformers should be kept on hand at all times: visitors on short-term missions to the project frequently forget to bring such equipment and will be eternally grateful for assistance.

9. Shipping. Laboratory supplies, therapeutics and equipment will need to be shipped to the host country. Conversely, specimens may need to be sent out for quality control purposes or for analyses in specialized laboratories. Shipping of samples (whether dry or frozen on wet ice or dry ice) presents special challenges. Prior to shipping, all host country permissions must be acquired. Entry into the United States requires a permit from the Centers for Disease Control and Prevention. If the samples are shipped via intermediary countries, additional clearances may be needed for those countries. Samples must be appropriately packed in International Aviation and Transport Agency (IATA)-approved containers and labeled with biohazard stickers as needed. Airlines differ in their requirements, which must be clarified prior to shipment. Regulations also change (sometimes in a seemingly arbitrary fashion). Researchers need to identify a reliable international shipping company, and they are advised not to be penny wise and pound foolish in their selection: experience shows that if something can go wrong, it will, and the more qualified a shipping company, the greater its capacity to avoid or correct problems. Discussions with personnel in other collaborative studies in the host or neighboring countries can often provide valuable information on shipping to and from the region.

10. Liaison with host and donor country institutions. Ongoing contact and sharing of publications and reports should be maintained with host country ministries, agencies, other research collaborations, and the appropriate embassies (particularly those representing the main donor agencies). A surprised or discomfited ministry or embassy may be less helpful in times of crisis.

11. Community liaison and participant motivation. Community liaison represents a crucial and ongoing activity in any research activity. Whether the "community" represents the entire population of a village, a subgroup such as commercial sex workers, or the clientele of an infectious disease clinic, it is important that relevant and influential local authorities (civil, religious, traditional) be informed about the study. Good word of mouth from such persons is invaluable. Conversely, suspicion and rumors can rapidly sink a project. A research collaboration that envisages long-term involvement with a specific population can undertake additional community projects (assistance with rebuilding a health clinic or primary school, support for a local youth sports team) to indicate its interest in the community and encourage rapport.

The project should train community liaison personnel who contact potential subjects to explain the study and encourage participation. Such contact can occur at the village level, through scheduled community meetings; within clinics, via presentations to groups of potential participants waiting for service; and/or at the individual level. Liaison personnel can also act as health educators, disseminating broader health messages while informing individuals of the planned research and of its goals. The health education provided represents a benefit offered by the project.

A frequently raised issue concerns payment or other incentives provided to study participants. Host country policies differ in this regard. Frequently, access to health care provided by the project is sufficient to encourage participation. Reimbursement for time lost may also be offered. Where financial incentives are offered, their scale should be carefully established to avoid unethical coercion and to ensure that future studies are not priced out of the market.

12. Data dissemination. Members of the collaboration need to share in the analyses, publication, and dissemination of data. Study results should be made available to key host country policymakers prior to international dissemination. Learning the results of research conducted in one's own country through the international press or at an international conference is annoying, but more important, gives the message that the host country is a secondary player on the research team. Furthermore, in-country policymakers and health professionals must be prepared to respond to queries that may arise and cannot do so if they have not been briefed.

If possible, key results should be provided through an open in-country meeting or conference. Such a setting provides the information to a broad range of local, interested parties, and allows investigators to discuss study ramifications. If such a meeting cannot occur prior to publication of results, one should be organized as soon as possible afterward. Research collaborations may also develop a system of "national conferences" every few years, to bring key health personnel, policymakers, and interested local and international agencies up to date on project progress and findings.

ETHICS AND PARTICIPANT SAFETY

Research-related ethical issues are complex, and the reader is referred to a broad literature and to guidelines such as those produced by the Council of International Organizations of Medical Sciences (CIOMS) (Faden and Kass 1998, Weed 1994, Sleep 1991, CIOMS 1991). A number of key points are summarized here, with special reference to studies conducted in developing countries.

Research studies must be reviewed and approved by human subjects committees in the host country institution and, if required, by a ministerial or national review board. (In Uganda, for example, the AIDS Research Subcommittee of the Uganda National Council for Science and Technology fulfills this function for all HIV-related research at the national level.) Studies must also be approved by the human subjects board at the institution housing the developed country investigator. Funding agencies such as the United States National Institutes of Health have an additional review board that must approve a study prior to enrollment of subjects. An independent data safety and monitoring board (DSMB) may be convened to oversee the long-term ethical implementation of a study and to ensure participant safety (such a board is virtually mandatory for clinical trials). The DSMB is given the authority to terminate a study if there is evidence to suggest harm to participants.

Voluntary and informed consent represents a cornerstone of ethical research. Participants must be informed of potential risks and benefits, potential advantages, subject selection, randomization strategies and use of placebos (where applicable in randomized trials), and their right to refuse participation in the study without loss of benefits. These concepts may be difficult to explain, especially in cultures where patients are used to unquestioning acceptance of doctors' recommendations, or where they cannot envisage that a doctor may potentially provide a placebo. Qualitative research and extensive pretesting of informed consent instruments are required to optimize comprehension. If participants are not literate, the presence of a literate witness is highly desirable and "written" informed consent can consist of a thumb print. In community and household surveys, a multitiered approach to consent may be required: consent of community leaders to enroll the village; consent from the head of the household to contact family members; and finally, confidential individual consent. Assent should be obtained from child study participants, often in conjunction with consent from their parents. Researchers must ensure that the individual freely consents, without undue pressure from his or her community or family. To maximize individual consent, the final consent procedures are carried out in private.

Safeguarding individual confidentiality is a second crucial element in any study. Great care must be taken to ensure interview and laboratory data are stored separately and securely from individual identifiers. Access to linkage codes and files should be restricted to key project staff. Questionnaires and other data must be stored in securely locked cabinets. The study team should not discuss individual participation or results with other family or community members (the one exception being the parents or legal guardian of a minor).

Questions repeatedly arise regarding the ethics of clinical and community-based trials in developing countries. Should developed country agencies fund or participate in trials of drugs or strategies that do not reflect Western standards of care? Such trials may give the appearance of testing substandard technologies. Conversely, research limited to Western standards, which may test treatment or prevention modalities that are unsustainable and unreplicable in a developing country, is unlikely to benefit the host country. The issue becomes particularly thorny when deciding on the minimum standard of care that should be provided to those not receiving the intervention. A recent example of this controversy centered on the use of a placebo in trials to prevent mother-to-child HIV transmission (Angell 1997, Lurie and Wolfe 1997, Merson 1997, Varmus and Satcher 1997). The question is whether it is ethical to withhold a preventive measure of known efficacy from the control group, even if the measure is unfeasible in the host developing country and its use in the control group may prevent adequate evaluation of more affordable and replicable interventions. This particular controversy has been partially alleviated with the advent of less cumbersome and less expensive regimens to prevent mother-to-child transmission of HIV (which themselves required trials and raised questions), but the basic issues are likely to arise in many future trials, and a perfect resolution to the dilemma is unlikely. Research collaborators need to be aware of such concerns, discuss them openly with the host country and developed country ethical review boards, try to arrive at approaches that safeguard subject safety and maximize benefits to the population, and clearly document the basis for the decisions adopted. At a minimum, subjects should be offered the prevailing standard of care.

All participants should receive some benefits from participation. Services can include additional health care, or health education and preventive services, such as condoms. Participants in infectious disease studies should have access to their results and to appropriate counseling. The latter points are of particular relevance in HIV studies. Research programs that cannot themselves provide counseling should set up referral to and collaboration with agencies that do offer such services. HIV research teams should become familiar with host country policies regarding testing and counseling. Specific policy issues include mandatory versus voluntary counseling. (In the United States, HIV prevention trial participants must be informed of their serologic results. In many developing countries, participants are not obliged to receive their results, but may voluntarily elect to do so, and the researchers provide the participants with the opportunity to receive confidential counseling.)

CULTURAL CLASHES: WHEN YES MEANS NO, AND OTHER SURPRISES

Integrating diverse cultural approaches represents one of the pleasures of international research—and one of the frustrations. Both the host and the guest country researchers come to a collaboration with cultural norms and preconceptions that influence styles of negotiation and discussion, perceptions of illness and care giving, and which may also affect the roles played in the project.

Western investigators can be perceived as somewhat domineering, partly because Western culture values competition, and partly because of the way funding of projects from the West is structured. If the Western researcher is the principal investigator on the project grant, he or she feels direct pressure to meet contractual obligations (in part to ensure future funding success) and may feel impatient with the process of building consensus and other inevitable "delays" and compromises. In groups, there is a tendency among Western-trained scientists to talk to one other, without adequate effort to draw host country counterparts into the discussion. This problem is particularly acute if the meeting is conducted in English (or French, etc . . .) and this is not the first language in the host country. Efforts to increase self-awareness, soliciting feedback from one's colleagues (" . . . did you have a chance to say what was on your mind?"), and accepting constructive critique of one's communication style help to alleviate the problem. Wherever possible, adequate preparatory time should be built into the research grant to facilitate the process of consensus building.

In many (although certainly not all) cultures, there is a reluctance to directly contradict colleagues or those perceived as being in charge. Visiting researchers need to be very sensitive to the dynamics of agreement. Agreement (or silence) can mean "yes, we really can and want to do this" or "this really is not a good or feasible idea, but we will agree in order to avoid confrontation or disappointing you." The problem can be minimized by picking up on subtle reluctance and constructively bringing it into the open ("I sense that some of you may be a little worried about this. Is some of what is being proposed going to be difficult?"), encouraging discussion and having repeat sessions to go over key issues. Ultimately, actions speak louder than words. If agreed-upon courses of action are not followed up on, the research group needs to examine whether the cause is logistic (lack of personnel or resources) or an unarticulated lack of consensus.

Many other cultural factors influence collaboration. Some societies live by the clock, others have a less rigid sense of time, and still others juggle too many simultaneous activities and are always running behind. Some are very direct, others require time for social contact prior to getting down to work. In some cultures, the exact use of contractual language can take on a seemingly overwhelming importance, resulting in days spent discussing what the Western researcher feels are unimportant nuances; in other settings, contracts and agreements are merely seen as a tool to secure funding and get on with the work. Relationships between men and women differ according to sociocultural setting. Given the plethora of attitudes on both sides of a collaboration, it is not possible to write a definitive primer on how to achieve mutual goals. However, frequent and frank discussion of accomplishments, problems, and concerns; development of transparent goals; and sharing of data and project financial information, all assist in building the collaboration.

FUNDING

The best intentions and research ideas in the world are of limited usefulness without hard cash. Funding issues are of paramount importance at the onset of the collaboration and remain germane throughout. Several agencies and foundations fund international research. While the proposed research is still a gleam in the researchers' eyes, contact should be established with representatives of the World Health Organization, the World Bank, the US National Institutes of Health, the UK Wellcome Trust, or other relevant institutions. Discussions should include a frank appraisal of whether the proposed topic is of relevance to the agency's research agenda, and of proposal requirements, formats, deadlines, and monetary limits on awards. Suggestions regarding other potential donors should be sought. It is paradoxic that research grant submissions are generally more successful if the research is already underway, both as a proof of feasibility and as a means of tantalizing donors with partial data. It is worthwhile to identify a source of seed money to undertake part of the proposed research agenda, prior to developing a large grant proposal.

In general, projects should try to secure multiple funding sources. Having several donors with different grant periods provides security and greatly maximizes project flexibility, particularly if the funding portfolio includes governmental and nongovernmental sources. Canny investigators are continually looking for studies (and thus funding) that can be piggybacked onto existing research: care must be taken, however, to ensure research goals are compatible and that the existing resources are not overwhelmed. Multiple sources of funding are also very

useful in dealing with the idiosyncrasies of different donors. For example, funds from US government sources, including the US National Institutes of Health, can cover overhead ("indirect") costs in US-based universities and institutions but generally cannot be used to cover overhead costs in developing country institutions—as if the latter did not have the same or even greater needs than their US-based counterparts. Such costs (e.g., water, electricity, security, space rental) must be covered either with nongovernmental or "direct" funds.

Some research costs in developing countries are lower than in the developed countries: this is particularly true of staff salaries. However, other costs (transportation, fuel, shipping, communications) are much more expensive. Researchers should not count on overseas studies as a cost-cutting strategy.

Early in the collaboration, the study team needs to establish in-country bank accounts, develop and test mechanisms for transfer of funds, and develop local accounting and check writing procedures. Researchers should become well versed in national banking and money exchange policies. In countries with unstable currencies or high rates of inflation, it is prudent to set up a system of relatively small but frequent money transfers. The ideal schedule will depend in part on the ease and efficiency of such transfers. Many host country institutions do not have the resources to continue a study for some weeks or months if there is a break in funding procedures (e.g., if the in-country bank reports that the latest transfer never arrived, weeks of detective work will be required to prove that the money was indeed transferred). Contingency planning for finances is thus crucial.

HUMAN RESOURCE AND INFRASTRUCTURE DEVELOPMENT

An international research collaboration offers excellent opportunities for infrastructure development in all participating institutions. The collaboration is likely to bring physical improvements, including equipment and new technologies, to the host institution. The Western counterpart institution has the opportunity to provide field experience to its junior faculty and students, including data collection for thesis purposes. Faculty and student exchanges need to be clearly delineated and approved by researchers in all participating institutions, and resulting publications should include the junior faculty member or student, as well as agreed upon host country collaborators. Authorship order and responsibilities should be mutually defined early in the process and recorded in writing to enhance career development for all concerned.

In-country and external training for host country staff greatly strengthens the collaboration. Support for long-term professional development, including scholarships for masters and doctoral studies, is available through private foundations, the World Health Organization, the Fogarty International program at the US National Institutes of Health, and other agencies. Such development is most valuable if the professionals return to a position that allows immediate and direct application of newly acquired skills. The great advantage of long-term research collaborations is that they provide an ideal arena for this process: a staff member can acquire hands-on experience in the project, enter a postgraduate program, and use project data for thesis purposes, then return to the project in a position to take on greater responsibilities, including leadership of new studies nested in the overall collaboration. In cases where the research collaboration is associated with a host country university, a joint faculty position can complement ongoing project work.

Human resource development can also take less formal forms. Including smart, motivated midlevel personnel in project decision making, organization, and development of study instruments and protocols instills a sense of ownership and provides direct experience with research planning and implementation. Although such involvement increases the length of deliberations, the ultimate payoff in nurturing an "A-team" is invaluable. These individuals represent the up-and-coming research cadres for the project and the host country and also have direct and practical insights into improvement of day-to-day project activities.

SUMMARY

International research offers the opportunity to address unique and important health problems and to implement innovative research designs. Developing a collaboration is a complex undertaking, requiring substantial inputs from researchers in all participating countries and institutions. Attention to a myriad of details is essential, particularly early in the process. The long-term benefits of such collaborations, to the researchers, their institutions, and the population, often make the challenges eminently worthwhile.

REFERENCES

Angell M. The ethics of clinical research in the Third World. N. Engl. J. Med. 337:847–849, 1997.

Becker S, and Weng S. Seasonal patterns of deaths in Matlab, Bangladesh. Int. J. Epidemiol. 27:814–823, 1998.

Boerma JT, and Van Ginneken JK. Comparison of substantive results from demographic and epidemiological survey methods. In: Measurement of Maternal and Child Mortality, Morbidity and Health Care, International Union for the Scientific Study of Population (IUSSP), Derouaux-Ordina Editions, Lieges, 1992:27–60.

Borchardt KA, and Smith RF. An evaluation of an InPouch™ TV culture method for diagnosing *Trichomonas vaginalis* infection. Genitourin. Med. 67:149–152, 1991.

Buimer M, van Doornum GJ, Ching S, et al. Detection of *Chlamydia trachomatis* and *Neisseria gonorrhoeae* by ligase chain reaction-based assays with clinical specimens from various sites: implications for diagnostic testing and screening. J. Clin. Microbiol. 34:2395–2400, 1996.

Ching S, Lee H, Hook, EW, et al. Ligase chain reaction for detection of *Neisseria gonorrhoeae*. J. Clin. Microbiol. 33:3111–3114, 1995.

CIOMS. Ethics and epidemiology. XXVth CIOMS Conference. Wkly. Epidemiol. Rec. 66:17–19, 1991.

Croner CM, Sperling J, and Broome FR. Geographic information systems (GIS): new perspectives in understanding human health and environmental relationships. Stat. Med. 15: 1961–1977, 1996.

Cushman L, Kalmuss D, and Wawer M. Home-based STD screening of women in Washington Heights: a feasibility study. Abstr B7, 1998 National STD Prevention Conference, Dallas, Texas, Dec 6–9, 1998.

Daly J. Qualitative research methods. J. Health Serv. Res. Policy. 1:165–166, 1996.

Faden R, and Kass N. HIV research, ethics and the developing world. Am. J. Public Health. 88:548–550, 1998.

Gaydos CA, and Quinn TC. DNA amplification assays: a new standard for diagnosis of *Chlamydia Trachomatis* infections. Venerology. 8: 234–239, 1995.

Gray RH, Wawer MJ, Girdner J, et al. Self-collected vaginal swabs for detection of *C. Trachomatis*. STD. (8):450, 1998a.

Gray RH, Wawer MJ, Sewankambo NK, et al. Population-based study of fertility in women with HIV-1 infection in Uganda. Lancet. 351: 98–103, 1998b.

Grosskurth H, Mosha F, Todd J, et al. Impact of improved treatment of sexually transmitted diseases on HIV infection in rural Tanzania: randomised controlled trial. Lancet. 346: 530–536, 1995.

Hayes R, Wawer M, Gray R, et al. Randomized trials of STD treatment for prevention: report of an international workshop. HIV/STD Trials Workshop Group. Genitourin. Med. 73: 432–443, 1997.

Henderson RH, and Sundaresan T. Cluster sampling to assess immunization coverage: a review of experience with a simplified sampling method. Bull. World Health Organ. 60:253–260, 1982.

Hightower AW, Ombok M, Otieno R, et al. A geographic information system applied to a malaria field study in western Kenya. Am. J. Trop. Med. Hyg. 58:266–272, 1998.

Hillier S. Diagnostic microbiology of bacterial vaginosis. Am. J. Obstet. Gynecol. 169:455–459, 1993.

Kengeya-Kayondo JF, Kamali A, Nunn AJ, et al. Incidence of HIV-1 infection in adults and socio-demographic characteristics of seroconverters in a rural population in Uganda: 1990–1994. Int. J. Epidemiol. 25:1077–1078, 1996.

Kok PW. Cluster sampling for immunization coverage. Soc. Sci. Med. 22:781–783, 1986.

Lemeshow S, Tserkovnyi AG, Tulloch JL, et al. A computer simulation of the EPI survey strategy. Int. J. Epidemiol. 14:473–481, 1985.

Lorincz A. Hybrid Capture™ method for detection of human papillomavirus DNA in clinical specimens. Papillomavirus Rep. 7:1–6, 1996.

Lurie P, and Wolfe SM. Unethical trials of interventions to reduce perinatal transmission of the human immunodeficiency virus in developing countries. N. Engl. J. Med. 337:853–856, 1997.

Meehan MP, Sewankambo N, Wawer M, et al. Sensitivity and specificity of HIV-1 testing of urine compared with serum specimens: Rakai, Uganda. STD. 13:37–39, 1999.

Merson MH. Ethics of placebo-controlled trials of zidovudine to prevent the perinatal transmission of HIV in the Third World. N. Engl. J. Med. 338:840–841, 1998.

Misra SP, Webber R, Lines J, Jaffar S, and Bradley DJ. Malaria control: bednets or spraying? Spray versus treated nets using deltamethrin—a community randomized trial in India. Trans. R. Soc. Trop. Med. Hyg. 93:456–457, 1999.

Morgan DL. Practical strategies for combining qualitative and quantitative methods: applications to health research. Qual. Health Res. 8:362–376, 1998.

Powell RA, and Single HM. Focus groups. Int. J. Qual. Health Care. 8:499–504, 1996.

Serwadda D, Wawer MJ, Shah K, et al. Use of a hybrid capture assay of self-collected vaginal swabs in Uganda for detection of HPV. JID. 180:1316–1319, 1999.

Sewankambo NK, Gray RH, Wawer MJ, et al. Human immunodeficiency virus type-1 infection associated with abnormal vaginal flora morphology and bacterial vaginosis. Lancet. 350:546–550, 1997.

Sleep J. Development of international ethical guidelines for epidemiological research and practice. Report of the proceedings of the 25th Council for the International Organization of Medical Sciences (CIOMS) conference, WHO headquarters, Geneva, Switzerland, 7–9 November, 1990. Midwifery 7:42, 1991.

Steckler A, McLeroy KR, Goodman RM, Bird ST, and McCormick L. Toward integrating qualitative and quantitative methods: an introduction. Health Educ. Q. 19(1):1–8, 1992.

Todd J, Balira R, Grosskurth H, et al. HIV-associated adult mortality in a rural Tanzanian population. AIDS. 11:801–807, 1997.

Varums H, and Satcher D. Ethical complexities of conducting research in developing countries. N. Engl. J. Med. 337:1003–1005, 1997.

Wabwire-Mangen R, Gray RH, Kigozi G, Serwadda D, Wawer MJ, and Sewankamo NK. Randomized trial of STD treatment during pregnancy: effects on pregnancy outcomes and maternal HIV incidence. Thirteenth Meeting of the International Society for Sexually Transmitted Disease Research, Denver, CO, July 11–14, 1999. Abstract 209, p. 128.

Wawer MJ, Sewankambo NK, Serwadda D, et al. Control of sexually transmitted diseases for AIDS prevention in Uganda: a randomized community trial. Lancet. 353:525–535, 1999.

Wawer MJ, Gray RH, Sewankambo NK, et al. A randomized, community trial of intensive STD control for AIDS prevention, Rakai, Uganda. AIDS. 12:1211–1225, 1998.

Wawer MJ, McNairn D, Wabwire-Mangen F, et al. Self administered vaginal swabs for popu-

lation-based assessment of *Trichomonas vaginalis* infection. Letter. Lancet. 345:131–132, 1995.

Weed DL. Science, ethics guidelines and advocacy in epidemiology. Ann. Epidemiol. 4:166–171, 1994.

Whitty CJ, Glasgow KW, Sadiq ST, Mabey DC, and Bailey R. Impact of community-based mass treatment for trachoma with oral azithromycin on general morbidity in Gambian children. Pediatr. Infect. Dis. J. 18:955–958, 1999.

Glossary

Antibacterial A substance that inhibits the growth of bacteria or leads to bacterial death.

Antibiotic Synonymous with antimicrobial.

Antibody See immunoglobulin.

Antigen An antigen (Ag) is a molecule capable of inducing an immune response and of being recognized by an immunogen (antibody) and/or sensitized cells manufactured as a consequence of the immune response.

Antigenicity Ability of an antigen to react with the product(s) of an immune response.

Antimicrobial A substance that inhibits the growth of a microbe or leads to microbial inactivation. Antimicrobials may demonstrate antiviral, antibacterial, antifungal or antiparasitic activity.

Antiseptic Agent used on the skin that inhibits the growth of a microbe or leads to microbial inactivation.

Asymptomatic Infection The presence of an infection in a host without discernible clinical symptoms or signs.

Biotyping Characterization of a microbial strain by its pattern of metabolic activities. It may include specific biochemical reactions, colonial morphology, and environmental tolerance.

Carrier A person or animal that harbors a specific infectious agent in the absence of clinical disease and serves as a potential source of infection.

Case Fatality Rate The proportion of persons infected with a particular organism who die of the disease caused by the organism (not a true rate). Most commonly calculated during a specific epidemic.

Colonization The presence of a microbe on a nonsterile surface of the body without causing any symptoms or signs (i.e., no infection or disease).

Communicable Disease Considered by some to be synonymous with infectious disease. Considered by others to be a subset of infectious diseases that may be transmitted via person-to-person spread.

Communicable Period The period of time during which an infectious agent may be transmitted from an infected host to another host. Some diseases (e.g., varicella) may be communicable prior to when the source develops symptoms (i.e., during the incubation period).

Concurrency A term used to describe a pattern of sexual relationships. Concurrent relationships overlap in time, in contrast to sequential relationships in which one ends before the other begins.

Contact An association between an infected host or a contaminated environment and a susceptible host that provides an opportunity to transmit the infective agent (synonymous with exposure). The term is sometimes for a person; the susceptible with whom the infective made contact.

Contact Rate The number of susceptible people with whom an infected person has contact during his or her period of infectiousness.

Contamination The presence of microorganisms on inanimate objects (e.g., clothing) or in substances (i.e., food, water).

Dependent Happening The dependence of the probability of becoming infected on the number of people already infected. Related to the likelihood of exposure.

Disinfection The killing (or inactivation) of infectious agents outside the body by direct exposure to chemical or physical agents.

Effect, Direct Benefits of an intervention resulting from receiving the intervention (e.g., less susceptibility to an infection because of being immunized).

Effect, Indirect Benefits of an intervention that accrue to a person who has not received the intervention (e.g., decreased exposure to infectious people because others have been immunized).

Effectiveness The degree to which an intervention achieves its intended purpose when applied under 'real world' conditions in a community or set of communities.

Efficacy The degree to which an intervention achieves its intended purpose under ideal (e.g., experimental) conditions.

Endemic The usual presence of disease within a geographic area or population group (see also hyperendemic).

Entomological Risk The degree of exposure a host has to vectors that are competent in transmitting infection.

Epidemic An excess over the expected occurrence of disease within a geographic area or population group.

Epizootic An excess over the expected occurrence of disease within an animal population.

Eradication The end of transmission of an agent by eliminating the infectious agent, modes of transmission, or susceptible hosts from a geographical area. The term "elimination" is sometimes used in situations where reintroduction of the agent and resumption of transmission is possible.

Exposure Synonymous with contact.

Herd Immunity The lower likelihood of an infectious agent to spread in a group because of the immunity in a high proportion of the members of the group.

Host A person or animal that provides subsistence to an infectious agent under natural conditions.

Hyperendemic A sustained high rate of disease in a geographic area or population group.

Immunogenicity Ability of an agent or material to induce an immune response.

Immunoglobulin Immunoglobulin (Ig) molecules are products of antibody-secreting cells (B cells). Igs are constructed of one or several units, each of which consists of two heavy polypeptide chains and two light polypeptide chains. Each unit possesses two combining sites for antigen.

Incubation Period The time interval between initial contact with an infectious agent and the appearance of the first sign or symptom of the disease in question.

Incubation Period, Extrinsic The period of time between infection of a vector and the point at which transmission of the agent will result in infection in a susceptible host. Analogous to the latent period, rather than the incubation period, in the host.

Index case A referent infected host who serves as the source of infection for others.

Infection The entry and multiplication of an infectious agent in the tissues of the host.

Infectious Agent An organism (virus, bacterium, fungus, protozoan, helminth) that is capable of producing infection or an infectious disease.

Infectious Disease An infection that produces clinical signs and/or symptoms in humans or animals.

Infectious Dose The dose (number) of a pathogen capable of infecting a host. The infecting dose is specific to the pathogen, host, and transmission route. The minimum infecting dose is the lowest dose required; the median infectious dose (ID_{50}) is the dose yielding infection in half of the people exposed.

Infectious Period The time interval during which an infected host can infect another host or vector.

Infective An infectious host.

Infestation The presence of a pathogenic agent on the exterior surface (i.e., skin or gastro-intestinal tract) of a host.

Isolation Precaution Refers to the precautions taken that are adequate to prevent transmission of an infectious agent from an infected host. Measures taken usually address direct contact (including droplet) transmission (e.g., gloves, mask) and airborne transmission (e.g., N-95 respirator).

Latent Period The time interval from initial infection to becoming infectious.

Morbidity Rate The proportion of all persons in a population who become clinically ill during a stated period of time (not a true rate). The population may be limited to a specific age group, sex, or those with certain characteristics. (In contrast to pathogenicity, for which the denominator is restricted to those with a particular infection).

Mortality Rate The proportion of all people dying from a particular disease in a population during a stated period of time, usually a year (not a true rate). (In contrast to the case fatality rate, for which the denominator is restricted to those with a particular infection.)

Network Study A study in which the contacts of each infected person are identified, and the contacts of the contacts, *ad libitum*. "Contacts" in such studies sometimes include those from whom an infection was acquired as well as those to whom an infection was transmitted.

Nosocomial Infection An infection that was not present or incubating at the time of admission to a medical care facility (i.e., hospital or extended care facility) and which was acquired as a result of that admission.

Nosohusial Infection An infection that was not present or incubating at the time of initiation of home medical care.

Outbreak Considered by some to be synonymous with an epidemic. Considered by others to be a type of epidemic characterized by a sharp rise and fall in incidence within a relatively short period of time.

Pandemic An epidemic that affects several countries or continents.

Parasite Burden The number of parasites the host carries. Usually used to describe infections with macroparasites such as helminths.

Partner Study A study design used most often for sexually transmitted diseases where one sexual partner is infected and the other is not (i.e., a discordant couple). The outcome of interest is the probability of transmission to the susceptible partner.

Pathogen Any microorganism that has the capacity to cause disease. However, often regarded as synonymous with an infectious agent.

Pathogenicity The capability of an infectious agent to cause disease in a susceptible host.

Polymerase Chain Reaction A method for amplification of DNA which among other things, can be used for typing microorganisms or detection of microbes (i.e., diagnosis).

Persistence The continuous presence of an infectious agent within a population or geographical area.

Phage Typing Bacteriophages are viruses that infect bacteria. Some bacterial strains may be characterized by their patterns of resistance or susceptibility to a standard set of phages.

Plasmid Analysis Typing systems of microbes based on size and electrophoretic pattern of plasmids (extrachromosomal genetic elements) present in the cytoplasm.

Prophylaxis The provision of medications (usually antimicrobials or immunoglobulins) to prevent the development of disease following exposure to an infectious agent.

Quarantine Restriction of the activities of well persons or animals who have been exposed to a case of communicable disease during its period of communicability to prevent disease transmission during the incubation period if infection should occur.

Reproductive Number (R_0) The expected number of new infectious hosts that one infectious host will produce during his or her infectious period in a large population that is completely susceptible (sometimes called the reproductive rate).

Reservoir Any person, animal, anthropod, plant, soil, or substance (or combination of these) in which an infectious agent normally lives and multiplies, on which it depends primarily for survival, and where it reproduces.

Resistance The sum total of host defenses which protect against infection. Includes nonspecific defense mechanisms (e.g., integrity of skin) and specific host defenses mechanisms (immunoglobulins and cell mediated immunity).

Secondary Attack Rate The proportion of susceptible people who become infected following contact with an infectious host (not a true rate).

Seroprevalence The proportion of people with a positive serologic test for a particular infectious agent.

Serotyping Serological typing is based on the observation that microbes of the same species can differ in antigenic determinants expressed on their cell surface.

Source The person, animal, object, or substance from which a pathogen is transmitted to a susceptible host.

Superinfection Simultaneous infection with more than one strain of a particular organism.

Surveillance The orderly collection, analysis and dissemination of information on incident disease cases.

Surveillance, Active When conducting surveillance, obtaining data from health care providers or other sources by frequent direct contact (e.g., telephone).

Surveillance, Passive When conducting surveillance, obtaining data from health care providers or other sources by reports initiated by the health care provider.

Susceptible A human or animal not possessing sufficient host resistance against a particular pathogen to prevent contracting infection or disease when sufficiently exposed to that pathogen.

Toxin A material produced by a microorganism that it "releases" to affect other microbes or cells at a distance. Exotoxins are microbial products (proteins) that are released from microbes during growth and are toxic to other microbes, target cells, or experimental animals. Endotoxins refer to the intracellular and cell-associated toxic components of microbes, especially Gram-negative bacteria.

Transmission, Direct Immediate transfer of an infectious agent from an infected host or reservoir to a susceptible host. Modes of direct transmission include physical contact and droplet spread.

Transmission, Indirect Transmission of an infectious agent to a susceptible host that occurs with the aid of a vehicle (inanimate objects), a vector (usually arthropods), or the air (distinguished from droplet spread by a longer distance).

Transmission Probability The probability that, given a contact between an infective source and a susceptible host, successful transfer of the agent will occur so that the susceptible host becomes infected. Also called transmissibility.

Transmission Probability Ratio (TPR) A measure of the relative risk of transmission to susceptibles between different two levels (including presence versus absence) of a factor among infectives.

Vector A living animal, usually an arthropod, that is capable of transmission of an infectious agent from an infected host to a susceptible host, resulting in infection. The agent may multiply in the vector (biological transmission) or be carried without multiplication (mechanical transmission).

Vehicle An inanimate object that facilitates transmission of an infectious agent (also referred to as a fomites [singular, fomes]). Can include toys, surgical instruments, food, and water.

Vertical Transmission In humans, transmission from an infected mother to her fetus. In vectors, the passage of the agent from one life stage to another or directly from parent to progeny.

Virulence The degree of pathogenicity of an infectious agent, indicated by its ability to invade and damage host tissues and/or kill the host.

Virulence Factors Factors produced by a pathogen which, while not "toxic" to target cells, possess biologic activities that interfere with normal host function to the advantage of the pathogen.

Zoonosis An infection or infectious disease transmittable under natural conditions from vertebrate animals to humans.

Acknowledgments and Credits

Figure 1-1 Reproduced with permission given by Harcourt Health Sciences to use Figure 1-1 on page 1-2 in Bowlus B, ed. APIC Infection Control and Applied Epidemiology: Principles and Practice, 1996.

Figure 1-2 Reproduced with permission given by Harcourt Health Sciences to use Figure 1-2 on page 1-3 in Bowlus B, ed. APIC Infection Control and Applied Epidemiology: Principles and Practice, 1996.

Figure 1-3 Reproduced with permission given by McGraw-Hill Companies to use Figure 3-1 on page 37 in Holmes KK, Mardh P, Sparling PF, et al., eds. Sexually Transmitted Diseases, 3rd ed., 1997.

Figure 1-4 Reproduced with permission given by Harcourt Health Sciences to use Figure 1-5 on page 1-8 in Bowlus B, ed. APIC Infection Control and Applied Epidemiology: Principles and Practice, 1996.

Figure 1-7 Reproduced with permission given by Aspen Publishers, Inc. to use Figure 11-4 on page 345 in Friis RH, Sellers TA. Epidemiology for Public Health Practice, 2nd ed., 1999.

Figure 1-8 Reproduced with permission given by Harcourt Health Sciences to use Figure 11-1 on page 265 in Mausner JS, Kramer S. Epidemiology—An Introductory Text 2nd ed., 1985.

Figure 1-9 Reproduced with permission given by Arnold Medical Publishing to use Figure 2.2 on page 15 in Johan G. Modern Infectious Disease Epidemiology, 1994.

Figure 1-10 Reproduced with permission given by Harcourt Health Sciences to use Figure 1-3 on page 13 in Mausner JS, Kramer S. Epidemiology—An Introductory Text 2nd ed., 1985.

Table 3.1 Reproduced with permission given by the author, Michel Ibrahim, to use Table 4.1 in Ibrahim M. Epidemiology and Health Policy. Rockville, MD: Aspen Systems, Corp., 1985.

Figure 4-6 Reproduced with permission given by The American Museum of Natural History.

Figure 4-9 Reproduced with permission given by Lippincott Williams & Wilkins to use Figure 27-6 in Rothman K, Greenland S, eds. Modern Epidemiology 2nd ed., 1998.

Figure 5-1 Reproduced with permission given by Oxford University Press to use Figure 2 on page 798 in Halloran ME, Struchiner C, Longini IM. Study designs for evaluating different efficacy and effectiveness aspects of vaccines. *American Journal of Epidemiology* 146(10):789–803, 1997.

Table 5.1 Reproduced with permission given by Oxford University Press to use Table 1 on page 790 in Halloran ME, Struchiner C, Longini IM. Study designs for evaluating different efficacy and effectiveness aspects of vaccines. American Journal of Epidemiology 146(10):789–803, 1997.

Figure 7-1 Reproduced with permission given by The American Public Health Association to use Figure 1 on page 1314 in Birkhead G, Chorba TL, Root S, Klaucke DN, Gibbs NJ. Timeliness of national reporting of communicable diseases: the experience of the national electronic telecommunications system for surveillance. American Journal of Public Health 81(10): 1313-1315, 1991.

Figure 7-2 Reproduced with permission given by Wiley-Liss, Inc., a subsidiary of John Wiley & Sons, Inc. to use Figure 1 on page 115 in Chorba TL, Holman RC, Strine TW, Clarke

MJ, Evatt BL. Changes in longevity and causes of death among persons with Hemophilia A. American Journal of Hematology 45(2): 112-121, 1994.

Figure 8-1a Reproduced with permission given by Harcourt Health Sciences to use Figure 1a on page 264 in Weber S, Pfaller M, Herwaldt H. Role of molecular epidemiology in infection control. Infectious Disease Clinics of North America 11(2):257–278, June 1997.

Figure 8-1b Reproduced with permission given by Harcourt Health Sciences to use Figure 1b on page 265 in Weber S, Pfaller M, and Herwaldt L. Role of molecular epidemiology in infection control. Infectious Disease Clinics of North America 11(2):257–278, June 1997.

Figure 8-2 Reproduced with permission given by Harcourt Health Sciences to use Figure 2 on page 267 in Weber S, Pfaller M, and Herwaldt L. Role of molecular epidemiology in infection control. Infectious Disease Clinics of North America 11(2):257–278, June 1997.

Table 8.1 Reproduced with permission given by Harcourt Health Sciences to use Table 1 on page 270–271 in Weber S, Pfaller M, and Herwaldt L. Role of molecular epidemiology in infection control. Infectious Disease Clinics of North America 11(2): 257-278, June 1997.

Table 8.2 Reproduced with permission given by Harcourt Health Sciences to use Table 2 on page 272 in Weber S, Pfaller M, and Herwaldt L. Role of molecular epidemiology in infection control. Infectious Disease Clinics of North America 11(2):257–278, June 1997.

Table 8.3 Reproduced with permission given by Harcourt Health Sciences to use Table 3 on page 273 in Weber S, Pfaller M, and Herwaldt L. Role of molecular epidemiology in infection control. Infectious Disease Clinics of North America 11(2):257–278, June 1997.

Figure 9-1 Reproduced with permission given by Lippincott Williams & Wilkins to use Figure 3-1 on page 44 in Fletcher RH, Fletcher SW, Wagner EH. Clinical Epidemiology: The Essentials. 3rd ed., 1996.

Figure 9-2 Reproduced with permission given by Lippincott Williams & Wilkins to use Figure 3-2 on page 47 in Fletcher RH, Fletcher SW, Wagner EH. Clinical Epidemiology: The Essentials. 3rd ed., 1996.

Figure 9-3 Reproduced with permission given by Lippincott Williams & Wilkins to use Figure 3-8 on page 57 in Fletcher RH, Fletcher SW, Wagner EH. Clinical Epidemiology: The Essentials. 3rd ed., 1996.

Figure 9-4 Reproduced with permission given by The Publishing Division of the Massachusetts Medical Society to use Figure 3 on page 466 in Stamm WE, Counts GW, Running KR, Fihn S, Turck M, and Holmes KK. Diagnosis of coliform infection in acutely ill dysuric women. New England Journal of Medicine 307(8):463–468, 1982.

Figure 9-5 Reproduced with permission given by The Publishing Division of the Massachusetts Medical Society to use Figure 2 on page 1111 in Pauker SG and Kassirer JP. The threshold approach to clinical decision-making. New England Journal of Medicine 302(20):1109–1117, 1980.

Table 9.1 Reproduced with permission given by The Publishing Division of the Massachusetts Medical Society to use Table 1 on page 1437 in Shands KN, Schmid GP, Dan BB, et al. Toxic-shock syndrome in menstruating women: association with tampon use and *Staphylococcus aureus* and clinical features in 52 cases. New England Journal of Medicine 303(25):1436–1442, 1980.

Figure 10-1 Reproduced with permission given by Elsevier Science to use Figure 2 on page 291 in Gwaltney JM, Buier RM, Rogers JL. The influence of signal variation, bias, noise, and effect size on statistical significance in treatment studies of the common cold. Antiviral Research 29(2-3):287–295, 1996.

Figure 14-1 Reproduced with permission given by SLACK Incorporated to use Figure 1 on page 650 in Sellick JA. The use of statistical process control charts in hospital epidemiology. Infection Control and Hospital Epidemiology 14(11):649–656, 1993.

Figure 14-2 Reproduced with permission given by SLACK Incorporated to use Figure 1 on page 322 in Jacquez GM, Waller LA, Grimson R and Wartenberg D. The analysis of disease clusters, Part I: State of the art. Infection Control and Hospital Epidemiology 17(5): 319–327, 1996.

Figure 14-3 Reproduced with permission given by Harcourt Health Sciences to use Figure 4-1 on page 4-4 in Bowlus B, ed. APIC Infection Control and Applied Epidemiology: Principles and Practice, 1996.

Figure 14-4 Reproduced with permission given by Harcourt Health Sciences to use Figure 4-2 on page 4-5 in Bowlus B, ed. APIC Infection Control and Applied Epidemiology: Principles and Practice, 1996.

Table 14.1 Reproduced with permission given by SLACK Incorporated to use Table 1 on page 866 in Humble C. Caveats regarding the use of control charts. Infection Control and Hospital Epidemiology 19(11):865–868, 1998.

Table 18-1 Reproduced with permission given by Lippincott Williams & Wilkins to use Table 2 on page 615 in Pickering LK. Infections in day care. The Pediatric Infectious Disease Journal 6(6):614–617, 1987.

Index

Page numbers followed by f and t indicate figures and tables, respectively.